Y0-BXD-249

MEDICAL SOCIOLOGY

MINAKO K. MAYKOVICH
California State University at Sacramento

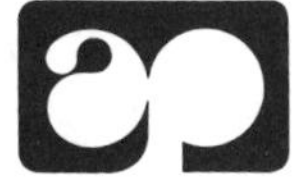

ALFRED PUBLISHING CO., INC.

15335 Morrison Street, Sherman Oaks, CA 91403

Printed and bound in the United States of America

Library of Congress Cataloging in Publication Data

Maykovich, Minako K.
Medical sociology.

Includes bibliographical references and index.
1. Social medicine. I. Title [DNLM: 1. Social medicine. 2. Sociology. WA31 M469m]
RA418.M328 362.1'042 79-24351
ISBN 0-88284-099-1

CONTENTS

Preface

By providing an integrative theoretical framework, this book is designed to be a small step forward in medical sociology as a science. More than ten years ago Mechanic (1968a) described medical sociology as a "series of threads going in many directions," rather than a "single fabric" woven together. Today, the diversity of the field still remains in its varied approaches, perspectives, and subject areas. This is partly due to the fact that medical sociology converged out of medical and social sciences that differ vastly.

Medical sociology has been inclined to a descriptive, fact-finding approach without any general conceptual scheme. Many authors of textbooks in medical sociology have compiled factual information in a rather ad hoc manner or have used a vague notion of environmental adaptation as a conceptual framework. The link between medicine and sociology was suggested, but only tentatively and hesitantly. Some textbook authors abandoned the link altogether, claiming that classical sociological jargon is irrelevant to an applied field such as medical sociology.

The multiphasic nature of the field should not preclude the development of a conceptual framework. The approach adopted in this textbook is to weave a general sociological fabric in which health and illness are seen as social behavior in the context of social structure, interaction, and processes. The book brings together major sociological theories and analyzes sociomedical data in terms of these theories. This approach is based on the belief that the growth of medical sociology requires a close collaboration between sociology and the health sciences. Otherwise, knowledge gained from the various subdisciplines is not cohesive.

This is not a text in the usual sense of discussing pertinent literature about standard topics, but rather this is a basic theoretical text for realistic students who wish to know how theories about medical sociology relate to empirical situations. The audience is sought from both the social science and health science fields. Students and researchers in sociology, political science, economics, and other social sciences can be challenged by applying sociological models to the world of medicine. Health practitioners, researchers, and students, on the other hand, can learn fundamental concepts, theories, and methodology without first taking an introductory sociology course.

The book does not require prior knowledge of either sociology or medicine. It builds from an introduction of basic concepts and theoretical frameworks to an extensive presentation and analysis of current research findings. Therefore, this book is addressed to an audience with various levels of knowledge: undergraduate students, graduate students, practitioners, professors, researchers, government officials, and the lay public who are concerned with the health care delivery system in this country.

The book is divided into three parts. Part 1 introduces the sociological theoretical framework and furnishes an overview of the relationship between health and social variables. Chapter 1 traces the history of medical sociology as it has converged from two distinct disciplines: medicine and social science. Chapter 2 presents three major sociological theories: functionalism, conflict theories, and interactionism. They serve as guidelines for the analysis of later chapters. Chapters 3 and 4 present sociological variables, such as sex, race, social class, and marital status, that have been associated with health and illness. Chapter 3 discusses the methods and conceptual frameworks by which sociological correlates of illness are examined; Chapter 4 presents current research findings.

Part 2 views medicine as a social system and examines interrelations among various components that make up the institution of medical practice. Chapter 5 questions whether or not the physician–patient relationship can be considered as an integrated social system. In Chapter 6 the medical profession is perceived as a social system that is maintained by mechanisms such as the socialization of physicians-to-be and consolidation of the professional organization. Chapter 7 analyzes structure and processes of modern, complex hospital organizations. Finally, Chapter 8 deals with healing practitioners other than physicians; each group is identified as a separate social system attempting to attain professional status.

Part 3 views medicine as a subsystem within the larger social system and discusses the interactions between medicine and other social institutions such as education, economy, and government. The analysis shifts from the micro to the macro levels, that is, community health care is discussed in Chapter 9, national health care and forms of social insurance in Chapter 10, and international modes of health service in Chapter 11. The book concludes with a discussion of medical ethics in Chapter 12, where a critical question is posed: is scientific control over nature and human beings an unmixed blessing? Here we examine the convergence not only of medicine and sociology but also of other spheres of human life, such as ethics, philosophy, and religion.

The unique feature of this textbook is that it is historical, sociological, and theoretical as well as medical. The subject matter in each chapter is examined in a historical light first. A comprehension of "what is" is frequently enhanced by the knowledge of "what used to be." Then the data under each topic is analyzed in the broader social context according to the three sociological frameworks. These theoretical models, presented in Chapter 2, constitute the core of the book, to which readers will be referred again and again.

It is a pleasure to acknowledge my debt of gratitude to many persons without whose help this book would not have been completed. I wish to express by appreciation for the reviewers, whose constructive comments have been extremely helpful: Dr. Stephen M. Shortell, Associate Professor and Director, Center for Health Services Research, University of Washington; Dr. Russell Ward, Assistant Professor of Sociology, State University of New York at Albany; and Sylvia Clavan, Associate Professor of Sociology, St. Joseph's College, Philadelphia. I am grateful to Joseph R. Ferrell for his careful reading and editorial assistance in the writing of this manuscript. Finally, to John J. Maykovich, I am indebted for his support and encouragement throughout this project.

PROLOGUE: The Current Status of Medical Sociology

Medical sociology is a vast field. It is the study of health care organizations in which doctors, administrators, nurses, and patients interact and where conflict appears and is resolved. But medical sociology examines more than sick people and the medical profession; it also looks at healthy people and their attitudes concerning, among other things, pills, jogging, and health foods. It also analyzes controversies such as those over Laetrile, national health insurance, and the Natural Death Act. Succinctly, medical sociology is an attempt to understand health and illness behavior in relation to social structure and processes.

Students are perplexed about the substance of medical sociology because it is a relatively new course offering in various departments of our universities, and it is a combination of medical and sociological disciplines. Medical sociology was officially recognized as an independent discipline by the American Sociological Association (ASA) only in 1960. The discipline is a result of the convergence of medicine and sociology, both of which had been established as separate entities during the nineteenth century. The medical sociology section within the ASA has grown now to over 1000 members and is the largest section within the Association (Hollingshead, 1973).

Medicine, Sociology, and Medical Sociology

Medicine may be defined as the science and art of maintaining health and preventing, alleviating, or curing disease. Sociology is defined as the science of society, social institutions, and social relationships, specifically, the systematic study of the development, structure, interaction, and collective behavior of organized groups of human beings.

What is common to both fields is that they are sciences. Science hopes to discover general truths and to analyze the operation of general laws by means of observation, experimentation, and the formulation and testing of hypotheses.

There are some differences in emphasis between the two sciences. Medicine earned recognition as an independent discipline when the germ theory of disease was discovered, that is, when it was recognized that disease is caused by microorganisms. Ever since, medicine has been inclined to deal with physical factors as they affect individual organisms. In contrast, sociologists seldom study a person in isolation. Sociologists are interested in persons who are in contact and communication with others. Sociology is the study of humans functioning in the social group.

The task of medical sociology, then, is to identify and to study social groups in their activities of maintaining health and preventing, alleviating, or curing disease. A social group can be viewed as a social system whose components are interdependent. Also, the social group is viewed as an ongoing process of conflict and resolution.

The social group as a unit of analysis can be identified at various levels, such as dyad, organization, social status, community, and society. At the dyadic level, the smallest unit of the social group, the relationships between doctor and patient, nurse and patient, doctor and nurse, and others are studied. The organizational level includes hospitals, the American Medical Association, weight watchers' clubs, etc. Social status refers to occupational categories such as those of the physician, nurse, and orderly and to socioeconomic status, age status, and the like. At the community level, neighborhood health centers, public health, and the accessibility of primary care can be studied. Finally, national health insurance and socialized medicine involve the entire society as a study unit.

Each of these social groups should be examined in terms of its internal structure and processes and of its relation to other social groups.

Sociology of Medicine versus Sociology in Medicine

Medical sociology, as a child of mixed blood born of the marriage between medicine and sociology, suffers from an identity dilemma. Among various dimensions that have coalesced under the title of medical sociology, a distinction has been made between sociology *of* medicine and sociology *in* medicine (Strauss, 1957).

Sociology of medicine is a basic science in which knowledge is pursued for its own sake. By studying medicine as a social institution and illness as a social behavior, sociologists of medicine attempt to gain knowledge of basic principles of social structure and human interaction. They are likely to be affiliated with a department of sociology and to have access to medical institutions where they are able to collect data for research.

Sociology in medicine is an applied science in which knowledge is pursued for use in solving practical problems. Sociology in medicine consists of collaborative research or teaching with medical practitioners, whose main concerns are the prevention and treatment of illness, the allocation of resources, and other practical problems. Sociologists in medicine try to provide medical practitioners with a broader perspective for understanding some of the social and cultural factors affecting health problems.

Initial Dominance by Medicine

During its first years, medical sociology was more inclined to medical science than to social science. In fact, medical science took the lead in building the common meeting ground for medical practitioners and sociologists. It was the American Public Health Association and its membership of physicians and social workers that formed a section on sociology as early as 1910. On the other hand, it was not until 1960 that the section on medical sociology was established as a part of the American Sociological Association (Hollingshead, 1973).

During 1955 and 1956, sociologists and physicians met informally at the conventions of the American Sociological Association (Strauss, 1957, p. 200) to establish channels of communication concerning the many developments in the new subspecialty of medical sociology. In 1956 Strauss identified 144 people known to be medical sociologists. Of these, 34 were physicians, anthropologists, psychologists, and social workers. The other 110 were sociologists. Of those, 60 were affiliated with medical organizations such as medical schools, schools of public health, schools of nursing, hospitals, governmental agencies of public health and mental health, and voluntary health organizations. Of the others, 16 were with research groups, and only 34 had a department of sociology as their primary base.

During the 1950s the primary concern of medical sociology was the contribution of sociology to medical research rather than the other way around. A number of writers (Anderson, 1952; Blackwell, 1953; Evans, 1952; Mangus, 1955; Reader & Goss, 1959; Simmons & Wolff, 1954) suggested the benefits that sociology might offer to medicine—to provide a social point of view for the medical clinician.

Partly because of the newness of this subfield of medical sociology but possibly because of the pragmatic pressure exerted by medical practitioners, medical sociology in the 1950s was characterized by factual emphasis, and it lacked conceptual structures. Data were gathered as practical necessity arose, but they were not used to develop a conceptual scheme or to provide a missing link in a theoretical construct (Reader & Goss, 1959). Reviews of published research in the 1950s (Caudill, 1953; Reader & Goss, 1959) show the selectiveness of research topics. Greater emphasis was placed on the study of the socialization process of medical students rather than the behavior of interns and residents; on the study of doctors' views of patients rather than patients' views of doctors; on the study of nurses rather than of physicians; and on the study of hospitals rather than of physicians' private offices. Such selectivity, long before the skyrocketing of malpractice insurance rates, suggests that it was the doctor who commanded the type of information to be gathered to suit his or her own needs. The idea that physicians know what is best for everyone underlay the research conducted by medical sociologists.

The Growth of Sociological Influence in the 1960s

The dominance of medical practitioners was readily perceived by the sociologists, who, by the end of the 1950s, were keenly concerned about the issue. At the medical sociology section of the American Sociological Association in 1958, they explored the desirability of various locations for a sociologist in the social structure of the medical school. There was a concensus that the medical sociologist should be fitted into the regular department structure (Freeman, Levine, & Reeder, 1972).

Since then, the notation of a behavioral science department with interdisciplinary approaches has become accepted. As a result, the social scientist has a more secure and satisfactory status and can compete more effectively for rank, salary, and curricular hours.

By 1962 there were over 700 social scientists who identified themselves as members of the medical sociology section of the American Sociological Association. Over 800 sociologists in addition to anthropologists and social psychologists were at work in major research projects in the medical field. In addition, 57 departments of sociology offered graduate courses in medical sociology in 1965 (American Sociological Association, 1965).

The sociologist's decision to go beyond mere fact-gathering was becoming apparent, particularly in the field of medical education (Huntington, 1957; Martin, 1957; Merton, Bloom, & Rogoff, 1956; Parsons, 1951). There were even some studies that tried to achieve a balance between empiricism and scientific conceptualization (Hughes, 1956; Merton, Reader, & Kendall, 1957). Reader and Goss stated in 1959 that physicians and sociologists could best contribute to medical sociology if the sociologists who do research in medicine remain sociologists first and foremost (Reader & Goss, 1959).

Sociological fact-finding began to be accompanied by a variety of conceptual emphases, such as the sociology of occupation, sociology of institution, sociology of complex formal organization, and small group theory.

Current Status and the Future

The field had grown rapidly by the 1970s. While in 1965 one third of the sociology departments with graduate programs offered medical sociology courses, by 1978 the proportion rose to nearly one half, that is, 101 out of 209 departments (American Sociological Association, 1965, 1978).

Due to the availability of federal government funds for research, the number of sociomedical research projects was expanding. In a survey of social and economic research undertaken by the Health Information Foundation in 1961, over 1,000 different projects were reported and over 2,000 research persons were involved. Though not all of these projects can be classified as sociological, a great percentage of the resources was being spent in sociomedical research. The annual reports of the Russell Sage Foundation also attest to the active role played by social scientists in the field of health (Freeman, Levine, & Reader, 1972).

Another index of growth of the field is the appearance of sociomedical journals, such as the *Journal of Health and Human Behavior* (1960), later changed to the *Journal of Health and Social Behavior* (1966), and the introduction of medical journals such as *Administration in Mental Health* (1972), the *Community Mental Health Journal* (1965), *Health Services Research* (1966), *Medical Care* (1967), and *International Journal of*

Addiction (1965). In addition, sociological articles are now seen more frequently in traditional medical journals, such as the *American Journal of Public Health,* the *Journal of the American Medical Association,* and the *Journal of Chronic Diseases.* These journals state that their publication objectives are to provide a forum and to disseminate useful theoretical and empirical research results with implication for medical sociology and other related areas. They emphasize the interaction between theory, practice, and research.

With the maturing of the field, the occupational role of medical sociologists is being differentiated. Sociologists of medicine are found in the traditional departments of sociology as well as newly developed interdisciplinary departments where they teach and do research. Medical schools have changed their curricula significantly and require that sociology courses be taught by sociologists of medicine. Some universities such as the University of California at San Francisco have begun Ph.D. programs in medical sociology and in the sociology of aging as interdisciplinary ventures. Sociologists in medicine are engaged in teaching, research, consulting, and administrative work in various medical institutions.

The Dilemma of Medical Sociologists

Sociology was born as the science of society; the history of that process will be discussed in Chapters 1 and 2. Its goal was defined as discovering laws of social phenomena by means of objective and impirical methods (Lundberg, 1939, 1963). In an effort to establish the field as a science, some sociologists stressed the importance of objectivity, that is, freedom from value judgment. This led to the dichotomization of basic science versus applied science. The early sociologists envisioned their discipline as a basic science and excluded applied work from the realm of sociology.

Medical sociology, on the other hand, could not maintain this idealistic position because it came into existence as a union of basic sociology and the applied field of medicine, which is highly value-oriented. When sociologists move out of their own departments within the academic setting of a college or university into the world of medicine, considerable friction can develop in the interaction with persons whose roles, goals, and requirements are quite different. Furthermore, the native inhabitants of the system of medicine may resent the sociological newcomer.

The medical practitioners may demand that sociologists abandon their jargon and provide immediate sociological answers for urgent problems. If sociologists play successful roles as administrators or as consultants in the medical setting, they are likely to acquire a new set of values and goals. The dilemma is that if sociologists sacrifice their identity as sociologists, they are also prone to lose the ability to make a unique contribution to medicine.

This crisis of identity is currently being expressed by critics within medical sociology. They contend that the sociologists' subordinate position to medical practitioners hampers the growth of medical sociology both as a scholarly pursuit and as a policy science. For example, Johnson (1975) laments the theoretical impoverishment of British and American medical sociology due to domination by medical values and perspectives. Pflanz (1975) calls for the liberation of German medical sociology from medical power structures. After analyzing all research articles in the *Journal of Health and Social Behavior,* the "official" journal of medical sociology, Gold (1977) reveals the presence of implicit or explicit medical value assumptions behind research processes and a tendency for medical bias in collaborative research sponsored by medical funding.

Such an identity crisis affects the field of medical sociology as a whole as well as individual sociologists. The problem is much more complex for sociology in medicine than for sociology of medicine. It should be noted, however, that the dilemma discussed here is one faced by any sociologist working in an applied setting.

Alternatives

No clear-cut solutions have been discovered, but there have been conscious efforts to alleviate this crisis. Several alternatives have been proposed, varying according to the academic and professional distance between medical sociologists and the field of medicine.

First of all, there are those who think of sociology as a basic science. They regard theoretical frameworks of great importance and regret the fact that, to date, medical sociology has been inclined to descriptive, fact-finding activities. Maturity of a well-rounded medical sociology, according to these idealists, will be reached when the full range of existing sociological theory can be brought to bear on the field of medicine. The development of general networks among interrelated concepts is needed, they feel. In order to maintain integrity as a sociologist, the idealists recommend that medical sociologists insulate themselves from contact with medical practitioners as much as possible (Freeman, Levine, & Reeder, 1972).

The second approach calls for medical sociologists to maintain their identification with sociology but to make adjustments to medical environments. Strauss (1957, p. 203) described the role of the medical sociologist as resembling the chameleon. Like chameleons, they have a basic structure and identity that are constant, but their survival depends on their ability to adapt to the environment by changing their outward appearance. After all, sociologists teaching in medical school are challenged to apply sociological concepts to the problems of medicine.

A more distinct identity than that of a chameleon is advocated by others (Badgley & Bloom, 1973; Gold, 1977). They feel that the first step toward strengthening the identity of medical sociology as sociology is to effectively negotiate working relationships within medical organizations so as to allow greater freedom and autonomy for medical sociologists. Only through collaboration based on equality and autonomy will mutually beneficial results be generated.

The third perspective is that basic and applied sciences are not vastly different, since each should develop both values and theories. Concerning this value argument, Gouldner (1962) and others offered an eloquent discussion claiming the impossibility of a social scientist being completely value-free. Drawing examples from medical sociology, Gouldner illustrated his thesis that observation could never be unaffected by the frame of the value reference of a researcher. He called value-free sociology a myth. At the same time, Gouldner stipulated theoretical requirements in applied sociology. Labeling Marx and Freud as great applied sociologists, Gouldner (1957) claimed that some kind of a conceptual framework is needed in any field as a guideline for research (Friedrichs, 1970; Lynd, 1939; Street & Weinstein, 1975).

The fourth alternative is to create a new form of sociology called applied sociology. Gouldner (1956) suggested that applied sociology should be articulated, elaborated, and refined by those sociologists who are devoted to affecting social change in their own right. Thus the sociologist in medicine can become a new action specialist rather than being a servant to the medical practitioner. While playing this active role, Gouldner claimed, the sociologist could develop a body of practical theory to supplement existing sociological knowledge.

When Gouldner introduced this new brand of sociology in the 1950s, most sociologists were dubious about it. However, the notion of applied sociology with a systematic framework and raison d'etre appeared to be a more desirable alternative than the subjugation of the sociologist to the power of the medical world.

Since the 1950s the status of applied sociology has changed drastically, partly because of the natural evolutionary process of differentiation of sociology but mainly because of the changes in socioeconomic conditions of the 1960s and 1970s. In the early 1960s there sprang up radical civil rights movements by political, racial, ethnic, sexual, and other minorities. This was the first systematic attack by the minorities against the existing social system, and the targets included the educational system and the discipline of sociology. They asserted that sociology had been developed and maintained by whites, and they criticized the lack of its relevance to other members of the society. During the 1970s, the question of "Sociology for Whom?" grew in importance and was selected as the theme for the 1976 program of the American Sociological Association convention. In choosing this theme, the president of the Association, Alfred M. Lee, stated that sociology could not remain within the ivory tower and that it needed to broaden its concerns and to sweep away elitism and scientism (American Sociological Association, 1975).

Another important phenomenon was the reduction in job opportunities in university teaching for new sociology Ph.D.'s in the 1970s, due to the decline of sociology student enrollment. Whatever the causes of this situation, sociologists were squeezed out of academia and began to examine job possibilities outside the university. As more sociologists moved into the community, the role of sociologists had to be redefined (Gelfand, 1975).

The status of applied sociology has risen, although there may still be some stigma attached. In 1978 there were 74 departments offering graduate programs in applied sociology out of 209 departments of sociology in the United States. Sociologists in medicine, as applied scientists, need no longer feel that they are second-class citizens in relation to medical practitioners or sociologists.

At this point it is difficult to predict the future direction of medical sociology. Further convergence or divergence of medicine and sociology will depend upon internal logical necessity in scientific knowledge as well as the external social environment.

In order to appreciate the current identity of medical sociology, in Chapter 1 we will trace the development of medicine, sociology, and medical sociology.

PART 1

Sociological Perspectives

CHAPTER 1
The Emergence of Medical Sociology

Sociology as a discipline is less than 150 years old. Medical sociology, an offspring of that relatively young social science, was officially acknowledged by the American Sociological Association to be a distinct field only about 20 years ago. However, the roots of medical sociology can be traced to medical and sociological thinking from the beginning of recorded history.

The emergence of any particular system of knowledge is influenced by at least two factors: the internal, logical thought processes and the external social environment. Internal logic is made up of the assumptions and objectives of intellectuals, the logical and technical methods they employ, their focuses of interest, the necessary sequences that result in discovery, and the way their ideas evolve (Barber, 1959; Butterfield, 1960). Both sociology and medicine were a part of the great evolution of thought in Western civilization that passed first from religion to philosophy and then to science (Cornford, 1957; Martindale, 1960). Physical science pioneered the evolutionary movement and thereby constructed the formula for its liberation from philosophy. Sociology followed suit and separated itself from philosophy. That process of evolution and liberation, however, was also influenced by the external social environment (Merton, 1973).

This environment consists of social values, structures, and interactions that encourage or discourage the birth of a new field. Attitudes toward health and concepts of illness are derived from the central value orientations of a particular society at a particular time. For example, social stratification determines the position of physicians with respect to others such as patients, priests, politicians, aristocrats, and the proletariat.

This chapter examines the social backgrounds and social and medical thought of pertinent historical periods in order to delineate the evolutionary thought processes that led to the emergence of medical sociology. To that end, Western civilization is divided into three major stages: the embryonic stage, the divergent stage, and the convergent stage of medical and social thought. Figure 1.1 outlines these stages and should be referred to while reading this chapter.

Figure 1.1: Emergence of Medical Sociology

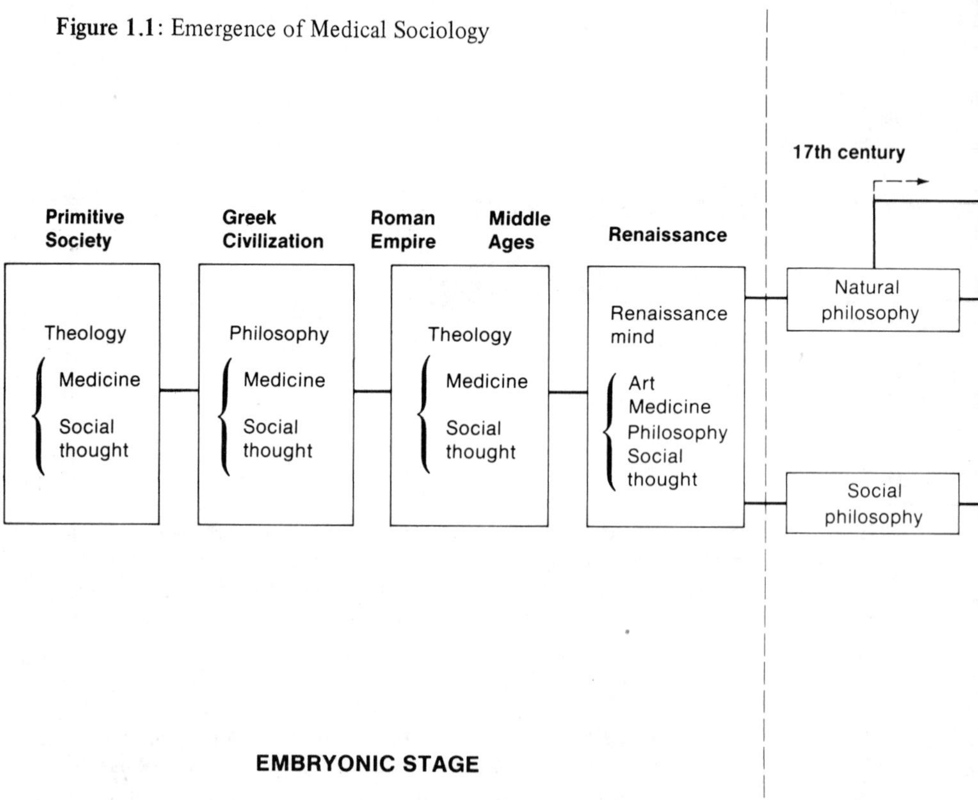

Although the emergence of medicine can also be examined in such non-Western parts of the world such as Mesopotamia, Egypt, India, and China, this chapter will focus on Western civilization.

EMBRYONIC STAGE OF SOCIAL AND MEDICAL THOUGHT

In the minds of prescientific people, medicine and sociology were undifferentiated in the domain of religion. From the beginning of recorded history it is shown that human beings have given considerable attention to their relation to the universe. They conceived their universe, whether the natural or social environment, as "peopled with the spirits" (Bogardus, 1929, p. 18). They held the belief that natural objects, natural phenomena, and the universe itself possessed souls and consciousness. God was thought to be the transcendent reality of which the material universe and human beings were only manifestations. According to this belief, both sociological issues (interpersonal relations) and medical issues (relations between the biological organism and the natural environment) were subserviant to the task of discovering the proper

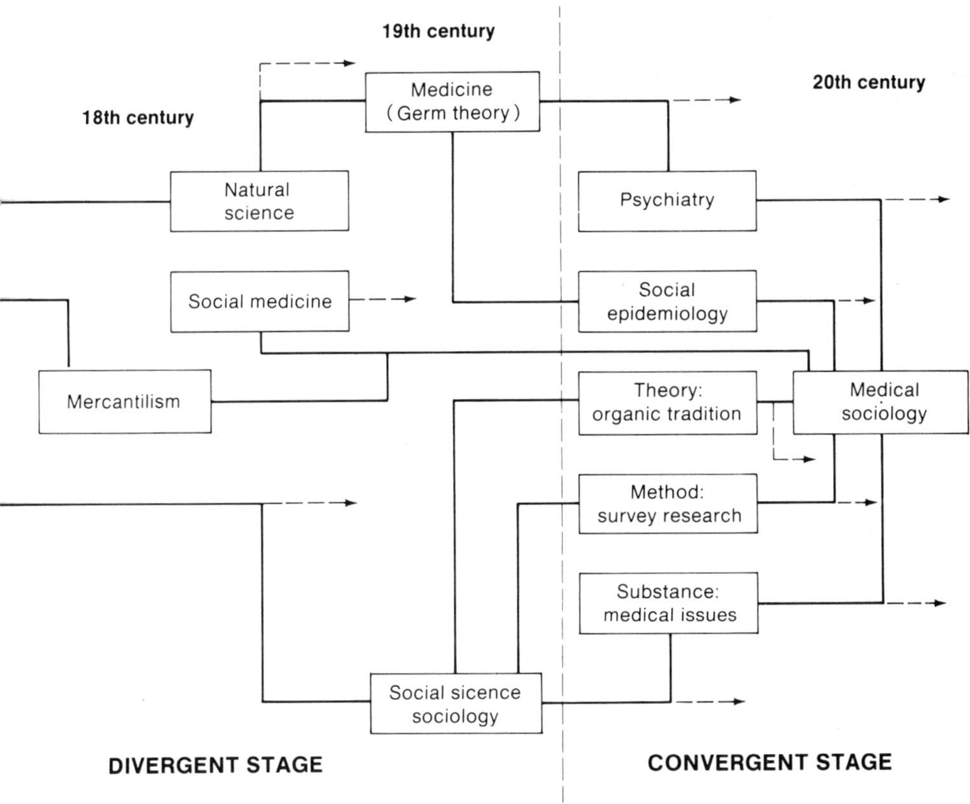

relations of human beings to a universe ruled by spirits and gods.

The universe presented two types of problems: trivial concerns of daily routine on the one hand and unusual and serious events on the other. Folk wisdom or common sense took care of the first problem. Even in the simplest of societies, people reflected on the ordinary incidents and encounters in daily life and were able to discover cures for minor illnesses and injuries. But, when they were faced with the second type of problem—the tragic, the unexpected, the frustrating, they sought for answers in religion. The magician-priests are the "world's first professional intellectuals" (Martindale, 1960, p. 5); they provided the form of abstract thought about the universe, and it included elements of sociology and medicine.

This embryonic stage of sociology and medicine in the womb of religion continued throughout the Renaissance, although it passed through various phases. During both the Greek civilization and the Renaissance, there was a slight departure of philosophy from theology. In philosophy the *rational,* investigation of the truths and principles of being is conducted without resorting to explanations by means of supernatural or divine power. But it was not until the Age of Enlightenment in the seventeenth century that theology lost its control over humanity.

The waxing and waning of the firm grip religion had on people in Western civilization will be traced through five stages: the primitive, Greek, Roman, Medieval, and Renaissance periods.

Primitive Society

To the primitive mind, magic, religion, medicine, and social thought blended into one. The belief in spirits that resided in animate and inanimate objects was used to explain the health or illness of people.

As a matter of fact, there was an interesting intrusion of social factors into the relationship between the physical and religious worlds. People believed that physical illness was caused by offending the spirits, that these spirits were provoked by humans violating social norms and taboos. The sick person in primitive society was believed to be the victim of transcendental forces that exercised social sanctions. In order to diagnose the cause of illness, the primitive healer asked for the history of the patient with emphasis on whether or not the patient remembered having broken any taboo, committed any offence to other people, or whether a member of the patient's family had committed an offence (Sigerist, 1961, vol. 1).

The healers were priests, sorcerers, and physicians all in one. They were concerned not only with the health of an individual but with the welfare of the entire group, and their authority ranged from the control of the quality of crops to that of the outcome in war. It was their function to avert evil spirits that could threaten the tribe in any form. They were often the chiefs of the tribes (Sigerist, 1961, vol. 1).

The position of the primitive healer was much more important than that of a medical doctor in contemporary society. The primitive healer had to be a sociologist who knew what principles of human interaction protected the welfare of the entire society as well as a physician with knowledge and skills in curing illness (Atkinson, 1956; Castiglioni, 1958).

This undifferentiated social, medical, and religious universe of primitive people is seen in various societies, such as the ancient civilizations of Egypt and Babylon. It is in Greek civilization that a differentiation of philosophy from magic, theology, and folk wisdom can first be seen.

Greek Civilization

Greek Social Thought

During the Greek period, the evolution of thought reached a slightly higher level in that philosophy became distinct from magic and religion. When speculation about human nature and the universe moves out of the realm of sacred institutions, ideas must be validated by their own merit. There is no established dogma against which to measure the cogency of ideas (Martndale, 1960).

In Greek civilization, a transition from theology to philosophy was made through several rational channels (Rossides, 1978). The Socratic method formulates the criteria by which truth may be determined. Aristotle (384–322 B.C.) is given credit for having laid the foundations of logic as the rational proof for a system of thought. Another criterion for establishing the acceptability of ideas was mathematics; the works of Thales (640?–546 B.C.) Phthagoras (ca. 497 B.C.), and Euclid (ca. 300 B.C.) were instrumental in defining this criterion. The analysis of empirical data, particularly comparative data as collected by the Sophists, was also a successful method of rational proof (Fletcher, 1971).

Since they were liberated from magico-religious concepts of the universe, Greek philosophers were concerned with the moral obligations of individuals to society (Conford, 1957). Plato (427?–347 B.C.) assumed that human beings live only in an organized society. According to Plato, society originated in the minds of people who perceived the advantage of mutual accommodation among themselves. He further assumed that people could mold society to their rational will for the attainment of a good life (Becker & Barnes, 1961). For example, Plato's proposal for mate selection, which was based on physical fitness, is the beginning of eugenics. According to Plutarch, a Greek biographer,

> boys and girls exercised in the presence of each other in the nude, not only to harden their bodies but also to enable the young man to select the right mate. When the time came he raped the girl and carried her into his house. Her hair was cut, and from then on she was primarily a breeding machine who might sleep with other men, if eugenic reasons made it seem desirable (Sigerist, 1961, vol. 2, p. 216).

As a philosopher-scientist, Aristotle developed a soul theory of the human body. He postulated that human beings are able to nourish themselves (a vegetable soul), and are able to enlighten themselves (a rational soul) (Jowett, 1927).

Having departed from theology, Greek philosophers used logic, mathematics, and empirical data to substantiate the validity of their ideas. Their discovery of rational proof was one of the essential steps toward science. However, the founding of social science was still quite distant because of the predominantly speculative nature of social thought during this period.

Greek Medicine

Greek medicine can be divided roughly into two categories: religious practices and scientific practices.

The beginnings of Greek medicine had religious, magical, and empirical attributes. During the first several centuries of the Christian era, the cult of Asclepius flourished. The temples of Asclepius, the Greek god of health, were built in places where the natural beauty of the surroundings was suitable for the sick. People came to the temples on foot or on donkey.

> When the patient arrived he first underwent purification rites. . . . Only the pure were admitted to the temple. But it was mainly a spiritual purity that was required. . . . The suppliant bathed and put on a white chiton. He then offered sacrifices to god, according to his means, honey, cakes, fruit, or a rooster. . . .
>
> . . . When the sun had set and night had come, the patient was brought to the *abaton,* the holiest part of the sanctuary, where he was instructed to lie down on a

> couch. There he waited for the god to come. The hours went by—and suddenly the god appeared looking like his statue in the temple, . . . He approached the patient, touched him, gave him medicine, or operated on him. . . . And when the glow of morning appeared on the hills, the blind would open their eyes. . . . The deaf would hear the singing of the birds. . . . Old pains had vanished (Sigerist, 1961, vol. 2, pp. 64–65).

The temples of Asclepius were the last resort for patients who had been given up by their physicians or for those who could not afford a physician. Religious medicine is timeless in that there have always been religious individuals who seek help from a priest rather than from a physician. And some people were really cured by such religious rituals. It may be because of the placebo effect of their belief in god or the result of the natural healing power of the human body. It could also be the consequence of therapies such as bathing, special dieting, exercising, psychotherapy, drugs, or manipulation provided at the temples (Clendening, 1960).

With Hippocrates (460?–377?B.C.) Greek medicine is said to have reached its zenith, unsurpassed for 500 years thereafter (Major, 1954, vol. 1, p. 115). Among the achievements that earned for Hippocrates the title of the father of medicine are the liberation of medicine from theology and philosophy and the establishment of an ethical code for physicians as professionals

Hippocrates expressed reverance to the gods but combated supernatural elements in medicine such as demonic possession of the soul. Furthermore, he divorced medicine from philosophic speculation. Philosophy to him signified the close study of nature combined with logical reasoning. He claimed that disease had natural causes and natural cures. In search of a logical explanation of natural phenomena, he relied on empirical experience, practical clinical observation at the bedside, and rational examination of cause and effect. In his development of a medical system, accuracy of observation and profundity of reasoning partially compensated for his faulty knowledge of anatomy, physiology, and pathology.

The doctrine underlying Hippocratic medicine is that of the four humors: blood, phlegm, yellow bile, and black bile. Health is defined as a proper mixture of the humors, while disease is the state of disequilibrium among them. When the patient becomes ill, however, there is a natural tendency to recovery. The role of a physician is to aid this process.

An improper mixture of the humors may arise from an individuals's environment, which consists of four elements—earth, air, fire, and water—characterized by four qualities—respectively, dryness, coldness, heat, and dampness. An imbalance of the qualities in the environment will cause an imbalance in the humors, namely, disease. For instance, phlegm, the coldest of all humors, increases in winter; it is then that phlegm diseases (e.g., sneezing and blowing nose) are prevalent. In the spring phlegm still is powerful but the blood increases, for blood is moist and hot, like spring (Sigerist, 1961, vol. 2, p. 322). The atmospheric changes due to the seasons were interpreted as a link between the macrocosm of the universe and the microcosm of the organism. These theories were adopted by social philosophers such as Plato and Aristotle for the enhancement of social welfare.

The Hippocratic Oath has exerted a great influence throughout the centuries.

It has served as a form of indenture for people apprenticing themselves to practitioners of the healing art. It is a pledge to the gods and goddesses to refrain from such conduct as giving fatal drugs, performing abortions, practicing surgery, engaging in sexual contacts with patients, or violating professional confidence. The Hippocratic Oath elevates patient care above priestly rites at the same time that it maintains scientific honesty by admitting to the limitations of medicine. The Oath proves the existence of a medical sect independent of the priestly caste during Hippocrate's time (Clendening, 1960; Sigerist, 1961, vol. 2).

In sum, philosophy became distinct from theology during the Greek period, and both medicine and social thought were freed from the control of religion. Philosophy became the new patron for medicine and social thought. With the development of the rules of logic and of empiricism, Greek philosophy indicated a potential for the development of science, but it did not allow at this stage for the differentiation of medicine as a natural science and sociology as a social science, both distinct from and independent of philosophy.

Roman Empire

Roman Social Thought

Roman culture may be considered an outgrowth of Greek philosophic movements. Although the Romans did not expand or extend the horizons of the Greeks, some credit is due to the Romans for receiving, reworking, maintaining, and transmitting parts of Hellenic civilization to later generations.

The Roman Empire was built by soldiers and administrators at a cost for the majority of the Roman people. However, there was a constructive aspect to the legal and administrative work of the Romans—the codification of important phases of social control. The Romans established a special kind of social science—a legal code that emphasized the rights of contract, of private property, of monetary interest, for example. This legal science, while serving to develop individualistic institutions, was nevertheless instrumental in constructing a stable framework for the Empire (Bogardus, 1929).

In general, Roman thought accentuated the military principle of authority and developed the concept of organized power. Religion was used as a means of maintaining unity and solidarity in the Empire, and it was in that environment that Christianity became firmly established as the official religion.

Roman Medicine

The first Greek doctors in Rome were slaves who were captives of war or piracy, and they were used only to treat gladiators and other slaves. Mistrust of foreign doctors by the Romans continued until the second century before Christ, when Greek influence increased. Finally, their status was firmly established when Julius Caesar, who wished to keep skilled physicians in the Roman army, granted citizenship to all physicians practicing in Rome (Castiglioni, 1958; Sigerist, 1961, vol. 2).

In the early days of the Roman army, sick soldiers were simply sent home for treatment. As the Empire expanded, however, that became impossible, and military hospitals were built at various strategic centers and eventually were founded in the Roman provincial towns; later, public hospitals for citizens were established.

The unique contribution of the Romans to medicine was the development of public health programs. The Roman Empire was concerned with the physical welfare of its people, and it had many constructive public hygienic programs—roads were built; long aqueducts were established to bring pure water into the cities; baths were constructed for the public; better sanitary conditions were created for the home; food was provided; and gymnastics was encouraged (Major, 1954; Rosen, 1958).

During this period, there seems to have been no fundamental progress in medical science. The Romans' contribution to medicine is in their codification of medical knowledge transmitted by the Greeks. Through the compilation of encyclopedias, they preserved information for posterity (Sigerist, 1961, vol. 2).

One exception to the view of the Romans as mere catalogers is found in Galen (ca. A.D. 130?–201?). Galen went beyond Hippocrates, who was a great physician but not a philosopher. Galen erected a complete system of medicine upon the foundations of philosophy and mathematics. In carrying out this grandiose scheme, Galen sometimes had to bend medical facts to fit them into his exact framework. However, he did not entirely depend upon a priori reasoning but insisted that every theoretical conclusion, though logical, be proved by experiment (Major, 1954).

A main feature of Galen's theory was the assumption that the blood passes from the right chamber to the left chamber of the heart through small openings in the interchamber wall. He missed the point that the blood circulates completely through the body. During his lifetime it was illegal to dissect human bodies, and his anatomical work was based on dissections of apes and pigs. With errors included, Galen's theories dominated medical thought for more than thirteen centuries.

During this period, sociology and medicine were embraced by the organized power of the Roman Empire. The Romans stalled any further differentiation of philosophy and science such as had been germinating in Greek culture.

The Middle Ages

Medieval Social Structure and Social Thought

The downfall of the Roman Empire left Europe devoid of structure and without a central government. An overall ruling authority was needed under whose protection some new form of social organization might eventually develop. There remained only the church as an institution sufficiently strong to maintain order. Since the powerful Roman bias for organization and administration had been built into the church, it followed that the church became the center of power after the fall of the Roman Empire (Heer, 1961).

For protection against physical attacks, however, warriors were needed.

Thus, the church and the monarchy gave power to a class of warriors by granting them lands and rights of jurisdiction. In return, the warlords supported their monarchs and protected the unarmed peasantry. Because of their common beliefs in Christianity, the contractual bonds of feudalism were strong.

The social thought of the Middle Ages not only reflected the unsettled social conditions but also the philosophy of the five centuries prior to the fall of the Roman Empire. Retrogression occurred during the Middle Ages, and the church fathers taught their followers that the authority of all governments was derived from God (Becker & Barnes, 1961; Bogardus, 1929; Fletcher, 1971).

Social reform or progress was regarded as unimportant. It was held that one should not dissipate one's energy in an attempt to improve temporary earthly conditions lest one should jeopardize one's salvation. The poor were believed to be part of the divine order in order to promote the spiritual welfare of the almsgivers. The prevalent opinion during the Middle Ages was that government existed to help the individual attain salvation (Rosen, 1958, 1974).

Medieval Medicine

For almost eight centuries, classical learning and science had managed to survive the rise and fall of the Roman Empire; that body of knowledge passed into the church's reservoir. It was fortunate that the church as a conserving force existed during the period of unrest (Walker, 1955).

However, the monks were not really interested in medical research. Their concern was primarily the practical one of how to relieve sick persons from pain when they came to the monasteries for help. Medical research was at an end. With the disappearance of science, the magico-religious treatment of medicine regained its status. Ecclesiastic medicine was a mixture of physical remedies, magic, and ritual. Under the rule of the church, the old view of the supernatural origin of diseases was revived. Illness was ascribed to demons or considered as punishment for sin. The sick were treated by such means as prayers, exorcism, the laying on of hands, and exhibition of holy relics. Some monks looked upon illness as a discipline to be endured with patience and to be mitigated by constant prayer. Hospitals were founded by the church, but they served as refuge for the destitute rather than places that would offer expert medical care (Castiglioni, 1958; Sigerist, 1961, vol. 2).

The *royal touch* was a special ritual practiced by kings in the Middle Ages. It was applied only for two types of illness: epilepsy and scrofula, or the tuberculous swelling of the glands of the neck ("King's evil"). The following is an account of the royal touch:

> A young woman had married a husband of her own age, but having no issue by union, the humours collected abundantly in her neck, she contracted a sore disorder and the glands swelled in a dreadful manner. Admonished in a dream to have the part affected washed by the King, she entered the palace, and the King himself fulfilled the labour of love by rubbing the young woman's neck with his fingers dipped in water. Joyous health followed his healing hand; the lurid skin opened so that worms flowed out with the purulent matter, and the tumor subsided (Walker, 1955, pp. 73–74).

Since the majority of patients would recover from minor illnesses without any remedies at all, the great majority of those treated by the priests or kings recovered, thereby adding to the glory of the church.

Despite its lack of scientific knowledge, the church should be credited for providing humane nursing care for the sick. For instance, nursing orders were developed and sponsored by the church and their Christian devotion served as a model for the nursing occupation for centuries.

In the midst of religious medicine in the Middle Ages, a small center survived where some Greek culture was retained. The medical school at Salerno was at its zenith at the beginning of the eleventh century, and it urged that medical practitioners should hold some qualifications besides royal touch and magic. However, even physicians at such a medical school found it necessary to avoid persecution by the church by learning theology as well as medicine (Walker, 1955).

Another deviation from the religious culture was Roger Bacon (1214?–1292). In spite of the ecclesiastical discipline and repression to which he had to submit, Roger Bacon stands out as perhaps the first experimental philosopher (Castiglioni, 1958, p. 315). Perceiving the danger of the infiltration of scholasticism into science, he appreciated, as a basis of knowledge, the superiority of observation and experimentation over pure reasoning.

One factor that led the medieval minds to a clearer vision of objective reality was a series of epidemics (Black Death, Sweating Sickness) that hit Europe during the fourteenth century. Though they were ascribed to supernatural causes, such as divine wrath, the epidemics also made people aware of the forces of the social and physical environment, and that awareness led to practical ideas for sanitary legislation (Castiglioni, 1958, p. 363).

But it was difficult for classic Greek science to survive under the stranglehold of the Christian church. As a result, it fled to the Moslem Empire, which was liberal-minded in its attitude toward learning. Moslems extended a welcome to scholars from wherever they came, and classic Greek science was retained there until the Renaissance. The buds of philosophy and science shooting out during the Greek civilization were arrested, but they managed to survive through the Middle Ages behind a Moslem screen.

The Renaisance

Renaissance Social Thought

It is impossible to draw a clear demarcation between the Middle Ages and modern times. Feudalism existed in France until the great revolution of 1789. Nevertheless, three great events—the Renaissance, the geographical discoveries, and the Reformation—each marked a definite transition from the Middle Ages (Abbott, 1918).

The word *Renaissance* signifies the rebirth of the freedom-loving and adventurous thought of humanity, which, during the Middle Ages, had been fettered by religious authority. It began in Italy and initially was a revival of interest in ancient writings.

Two very closely related problems, political unity and the reconciliation of freedom with authority, dominated social thinking during the Renaissance. Political disunity resulted from the breakdown of feudalism and from Renaissance morality. Renaissance morality stemmed from the loss of faith in a universal empire and from Reformation individualism. In the beginning at least, the revolt from the medieval order did not mean the total rejection of authority but rather led to the substitution of one kind of power for another (Chambliss, 1954, p. 318). The general distrust of human reason that prevailed during the Renaissance was partially responsible for the dependence upon authority (Fletcher, 1971). The emergence of the strong nation state, independent of the church, began during the Renaissance.

Renaissance Medicine

With the revival of classical learning, there also came a revival of all the arts. The artists of the Renaissance, Michelangelo (1475–1564), Raphael (1483–1520), Leonardo da Vinci (1452–1519), and Dürer (1471–1528), were fascinated by the beauty of the human form. In order to represent that form faithfully on canvas or in marble, they sought knowledge of the bones, ligaments, and muscles. Some of these artists began to dissect the human body and to make drawings of its inner structure.

Leonardo da Vinci was not only a painter and a sculptor but also an engineer, an architect, a physicist, and a biologist. He was interested in the study of anatomy and acquired a knowledge of the anatomy of the heart and of the blood vessels. He also acclaimed the importance of experimentation as the only way of attaining positive knowledge of the actual world.

Thus, the encyclopedic mind of the Renaissance contained the knowledge, the understanding, the skills, and the appreciation of diverse areas such as science, art, and philosophy. Those fields were viewed as interdependent and supplementary to one another.

So far, we have seen how two fields of science—medicine and sociology—remained embryonic and undifferentiated in the body of theology or philosophy up to the Renaissance. Before we move on to the next stage, that of divergence, mention should be made of the remnants of medical thought contained in theology and philosophy still to be seen in modern society in the form of faith healing. It may be that there are always certain people who resort to nonscientific healing, or that there is a reaction against scientific explanation. For further discussion, see Chapter 8.

DIVERGENCE OF NATURAL SCIENCE AND SOCIAL SCIENCE

Throughout the seventeenth, eighteenth, and nineteenth centuries, the disciplines of the mind continued to evolve and diverge. First, philosophy established itself as being distinct from theology. Second, natural science began to emancipate itself from philosophy. Then sociology was born as a social science independent of social philosophy.

These new disciplines, the natural sciences and sociology, were anxious to develop their separate identities. Sociology as the latecomer was particularly concerned about legitimizing its existence. Consequently, there was a tendency toward divergence of the various disciplines during this period; hence division of knowledge and specialization were maintained between natural and social sciences.

Under these circumstances, sociology and medicine were extremely far apart. With the advent of the term theory, medical scientists were quite optimistic that they could completely control health and illness without the help of other fields such as sociology. On the other hand, sociology considered that health and illness behavior were outside the domain of sociological concern.

The Age of Enlightenment

Most of the European states in the seventeenth century were monarchies of some kind. When the old feudal and ecclesiastical principles disappeared, people sought for security in temporal rulers and accepted their prerogatives. The concept of divine right—the right to rule being derived directly from God, not from the consent of the people—added further weight to the monarchs' claims (Cowie, 1960).

Living in such a social and political environment, social philosophers of the seventeenth century concentrated upon discovering rational relationships between the individual and the government. Emancipated from theology, they did not approach human nature from the perspective or original sin. Instead, they conceived of government as a contract between free-willed individuals and the state, a contract in which individuals gave up certain rights to receive protection from the government (Becker & Barnes, 1961; Fletcher, 1971; Rossides, 1978).

The dawn of scientific liberty was brought about by a number of scientists—Francis Bacon (1561–1626), William Harvey (1578–1657), Johannes Kepler (1571–1630), Galileo (1564–1642), René Descartes (1596–1650), Blaise Pascal (1623–1662), Robert Boyle (1627–1691), and Isaac Newton (1642–1727). As did many others, Descartes had not only a vast knowledge of the mathematical and natural sciences but also of anatomy and physiology. He believed that all the activities of the organism are forms of motion of the smallest particles and that this motion can be submitted to precise physical and mathematical examination. However, he added that these particles were synthesized into a human body from a machine created by God. At that time there still existed a close connection between philosophic and medical studies.

While these philosophic tendencies determined the orientation of medicine in the seventeenth century, the effect of experimental science on medicine was even more remarkable. Galileo affirmed the need for examining facts in the light of criticism and for reproducing known phenomena experimentally in order to ascertain their causes (Butterfield, 1960; Castiglioni, 1958). Harvey dissected some eighty different species of animals before he established the proof of the circulation of the blood. For instance, by observing motions of the heart in animal experiments, he concluded that the heart contracts and forces blood out:

> In the first place, then, when the chest of a living animal is laid open and the capsule

> that immediately surrounds the heart is split up or removed, the organ is seen now to move, now to be at rest;—there is a time when it moves, and a time when it is motionless. . . .
>
> In the motion, and interval in which this is accomplished, three principal circumstances are to be noted:
>
> 1. That the heart is erected, and rises upwards to a point, so that at this time it strikes against the breast and the pulse is felt externally.
>
> 2. That it is everywhere contracted, but more especially towards the sides, so that it looks narrower, relatively longer, more drawn together. The heart of an eel taken out of the body of the animal and placed upon the table or the hand, shows these particulars; . . .
>
> 3. The heart being grasped in the hand, is felt to become harder during its action. Now this hardness proceeds from tension, precisely as when the forearm is grasped, its tendons are perceived to become tense and resilient when the fingers are moved. . . .
>
> From these particulars it appeared evident to me that the motion of the heart consists in a certain universal tension—both contraction in the line of its fibres, and constriction in every sense (Clendening, 1960, pp. 156–157).

The principal characteristics of the seventeenth century are found in the decisive orientation of medicine toward the natural sciences and experimental research, which was determined by the philosophic trends of the time. Medicine followed philosophy because philosophy itself turned to nature.

Birth of Natural Science

The eighteenth century witnessed a series of revolutions in the political, economic, social, and intellectual spheres. The American Revolution of 1775–1783 and the French Revolution of 1789–1795 dealt severe blows to the theory of absolute monarchy. Both these revolutions asserted the equality of human beings and considered individuals to share a common nature, regardless of birth, color, and religion (McManners, 1967).

Scientific ideas were the causes and effects of the political and social events of this era. On one hand, revolutionary idealism found its spiritual origin in the capacity of natural science to adapt the forces of nature to the benefit of humanity. On the other hand, the free atmosphere of politics favored the scientists' rebellion against dogmatism and other forces that restricted human thought. The Industrial Revolution, which was made possible by scientific inventions, changed not only the economic system but the entire social and intellectual climate in Europe.

Establishment of Natural Science

By the Age of Enlightenment, science had gone through two initial stages: the beginning phase, characterized by a minimum of observation and maximum theoretical synthesis as found in the Greek civilization; and the second level, that of an overwhelming, pioneer enthusiasm for objectivity and measurement that began during the Renaissance period (Shryock, 1947, p. 149).

The first part of the eighteenth century saw a partial reversion to speculative synthesis and hence a failure of quantitative procedures due to methodological difficulties. However, in the eighteenth and nineteenth centuries quantitative methodology was revived, this time on a firmer basis.

During the first part of the eighteenth century, the influence of the philosophers predominated (Burtt, 1954). Gottfried Wilhelm Leibnitz (1646–1716), scientist, mathematician, statesman, and philosopher, developed a synthetic philosophy based on the existence of infinitely small and indivisible units, essential parts of all bodies, which constitute the soul. To him, the single atoms were united with each other and with God by a pre-established harmony.

Newton showed that the three laws of motion together with the assumption of universal gravitation were sufficient to explain the movements of planets and heavenly bodies, as well as the behavior of molecules and atoms. Being a devout churchman, Newton added that God was the Maker and the Maintainer of the universe. By this time, however, many people were coming to the conclusion that it was no longer necessary to postulate the existence of divine will. Newton's discoveries were revolutionary in that they destroyed the foundations of divine order on which previous thought had rested.

After Newton, scientists were busy demonstrating the reign of natural law in every department of science: physics, chemistry, botany, physiology, anatomy, microscopy, and the like. It was against this scientific background that eighteenth and nineteenth century physiology and medicine were developing.

Germ Theory of Disease

Among the many discoveries in medicine in this period, the establishment of germ theory started a new medical era. Infection by hostile forms of organisms had been speculated about for a long time. A visual proof was given in 1675 when minute organisms were observed with the microscope by Anton van Leeuwenhoek (1632–1723). Their probable role in disease was demonstrated by others. It was in the nineteenth century that Louis Pasteur (1822–1895) linked microorganisms with the theory of contagion and revealed that germs caused anthrax, chicken pox, cholera, and other diseases (Castiglioni, 1958).

> By studying alcoholic and lactic fermentation, he [Pasteur] concluded that ferments are living cells, that they originate only from cells of the same species, and that fermentation is impossible in their absence. The demonstration proved a death blow to the idea of spontaneous generation, for Pasteur showed that microscopic organisms were introduced by the air. Pasteur's studies in fermentation led him naturally to the study of disease. During the early 1860s, the lucrative silk industry in France was almost completely destroyed by a mysterious disease that infected the silkworms. Pasteur, after extensive study, showed that the disease was caused, not by one identified disease entity, pebrine, but by another as well, flacherie, which affected the intestines of the worm (Dolan & Adams-Smith, 1978, p. 136).

Because of the work of Pasteur and Robert Koch (1843–1910), the idea that infinitely small organisms played a pre-eminent role in producing many diseases rapidly permeated all areas of medicine. The new concept made such an impression that for a while it was believed that the cause of all diseases could be ascribed to microbes alone. Departments of pathology and the clinics were subordinated to the reports of the laboratory, from which were issued the standards for the legislator, the hygienist, the obstetrician, and the surgeon. Microbiology became the center and goal of medical investigations, and its influence was far-reaching (Castiglioni, 1958).

With the development of microbiology, physicians were forced to make changes in their method, their concept of disease, and their plan of treatment. Physicians became preoccupied with laboratory reports rather than with patients as people. Their mission shifted from the care of patients to the cure of diseases. Medicine became a disease-oriented rather than a people-oriented profession. The earlier concern with the nonbiological and environmental context of illness was replaced by the microscopic focus upon bacteria.

Another outgrowth of the germ theory was an effective preventive medicine. Since germ theory focused on the relationship between the individual (the host) and microorganisms (the agent), the first step taken was to eliminate contact by quarantine and other measures. Once the agent causing a disease was isolated, steps could be taken to develop substances that would immunize the individual. As a result, immunization produced dramatic results in the field of public health.

Bacteriological studies contributed to a third important development. With the understanding that bacteria could be carried from one person to another, public health workers endeavored to discover ways to break the chains of contact, such as enforced pasteurization of milk and the purification of public drinking water. The term "pasteurization" was named after Pasteur, who found that wines were spoiled by parasitic growth that could be destroyed by heating the wine for a few moments at a temperature of 50° to 60° centigrade (Major, 1954, p. 831).

These medical advances were significant in reducing the incidence of some diseases. There has been a dramatic decline in death rates from infectious diseases such as typhoid fever, dysentery, diphtheria, whooping cough, and measles (Graham & Reeder, 1972).

The revelations of the new science of microbiology were combined with reforms in medical education. Better premedical training with a greater emphasis on the basic sciences such as biology and physical sciences was adopted in medical schools. This reorganization of medical training resulted in a new orientation among physicians (Flexner, 1910).

Birth of Social Science

By the nineteenth century the stage had been set for the appearance of sociology. The conditions existed for the emergence of a genuine science: (1) thought processes had evolved to the stage where a new field could be identified; and (2) social conditions needed a new perspective.

Evolution of Science out of Philosophy. The increasing success of the natural sciences in producing an empirically provable and useful body of knowledge gave rise to more exacting demands than before for standards of accuracy in any theory about the nature of the world. One new criterion for validity of a theory was empirical movability.

The differentiation of natural sciences from natural philosophy gave impetus to the emergence of social science out of social philosophy. Eighteenth century rationalists and empiricists assumed that social phenomena could be explained in terms of cause-and-effect sequences occurring in society and that general laws could be reached by empirical studies (Bury, 1932; Hughes, H. S., 1958).

Breakdown of Society and the Need for Reconstruction. The old institutions were collapsing one after another during the eighteenth century: traditional authority in the government, sacred authority in the church, established status and privilege among the rural estates, and feudal economy in the agrarian system. Since the breakdown of society was complete, a total social reconstruction was called for. In order to resurrect the entire society, a new body of knowledge about the nature of society itself was needed to serve as a reliable basis for judgment and activity. A science of society was desired by the politicians and social critics (Hughes, H. S., 1958; McManners, 1967).

At the same time, commercial policies that emphasized the accumulation of national wealth, that is, mercantilism, made people aware of the international fabric of trade relations and the links of political societies. The discovery of new lands resulted in the encounter with people of different physical features, which generated a strong demand for a scientific body of knowledge about the nature and interconnections of human societies.

The Development of Sociology. Auguste Comte (1798–1857) is generally acknowledged as the founder of sociology. Comte first conceived of the word *sociology* in 1839. He had intended to name the new science social physics, but he rejected the term because others gave that label to exclusively statistical studies of society. He defined sociology as an empirical science consisting of generalizations derived from observed data about social phenomena.

Comte devised a hierarchy of the sciences based on (1) the order of their historical emergence and development; (2) the order of their dependence upon each other; (3) the decreasing degree of generality of their subject matter; and (4) the increasing degree of modifiability of the facts they study. That hierarchy ordered mathematics at the top, followed by astronomy, chemistry, physics, biology, sociology, and morals.

Comte stated that the hierarchy of sciences reflected the nature of the objective world in a most sketchy and tentative way. He later proposed another kind of order that placed sociology at the top of the hierarchy. To Comte, all knowledge in sciences was human knowledge, and all the sciences have developed in a human society. Since any data of the sciences deal with the phenomena of people and society, all of the sciences are themselves part of the science of society, namely, sociology. It was his conclusion that sociology brings all other sciences together in an overall intellectual human history (Becker & Barnes, 1961; Fletcher, 1971; Rossides, 1978).

Sociology as a Distinct Field. A new science must win contests in order to gain a place beside older, well-established disciplines. The orthodox or pre-existing fields have consolidated a privileged oligarchy and may claim that they have explained all the phenomena of the universe that are worthy of or amenable to scientific investigation. This jealousy of established science was particularly intense with regard to the new-born sociology.

The struggle of sociology for recognition as a science, and especially for its acceptance as an academic discipline, aroused much hostile criticism. Natural scientists felt that the reality of social phenomena was beyond the limits of human comprehension and that no exact laws could be established comparable to those in physical sciences.

In order to form its identity as social *science,* early sociologists were concerned with demarcating a line between themselves and the so-called applied fields. They considered that the scientific process of discovering general laws and the application of that knowledge to concrete situations were two different things. Furthermore, they believed that applied sociology was not possible until principles had been worked out for application to special issues. This did not mean that theories derived should not be applied to problem areas but rather that those applied works were viewed as belonging to the field of social work rather than to sociology per se.

CONVERGENCE OF MEDICINE AND SOCIOLOGY

The process of divergence had been underway for centuries before it finally culminated during the nineteenth century in the emergence of two distinct fields: medical science and sociology. Similarly, the convergence of medicine and sociology into medical sociology did not occur suddenly in the twentieth century. In fact, several routes toward convergence can be discerned during the very time when medicine and sociology were struggling to establish separate identities.

Routes of Convergence Originating in Medicine

Mercantilism and the Concept of Medical Police

Alongside capitalism as an economic system, there developed in seventeenth-century Europe a commercial policy known as mercantilism. The major aim of mercantilism was to secure a nation's supremacy over other states by accumulating precious metals and by exporting the largest possible quantity of products while importing as little as possible (Cowie, 1960; Lipton, 1932; Schumpeter, 1954).

Under mercantilism, labor came to be regarded as an essential factor in generating national wealth. Any loss of productivity due to illness was detrimental to the nation. Thus developed the concept of a national health policy. In order to secure a healthy labor force, it was seen to be the responsibility of the government to take various public health measures, such as controlling communicable diseases and investigating the causes for occupational morbidity and infant mortality (Rosen, 1953, 1958, 1974, 1979).

In Germany, mercantilism engendered an administrative force called the medical police. They administered an early form of social medicine based on the notion that an absolute monarch knew what was best for his people in the sphere of health as well as in all other activities (Frank, 1941; Small, 1909). If the state was envisioned as a social contract entered into by individuals for self-preservation, then people yielded their rights to the state which, in return, secured for its people the greatest health, welfare, and security.

Specifically, the medical police administered such governmental programs as the maintenance and supervision of midwives, the care of orphans, and the appointment of physicians. The medical profession was obliged not only to treat the sick but also to supervise the health of the population. The development of the concept of medical police reflected a pioneer effort to analyze the health problems of an entire society (Rosen, 1974, 1979).

Revolution and Social Medicine

Rapid social change due to political and industrial revolutions imposed much stress and strain upon people during the eighteenth century. Industrialization threw many craft workers and farmers out of work and resulted in poverty, overcrowding, and ill health. Poor working conditions, long hours, child labor, and industrial slums drew the attention of physicians, writers, economists, and public officials (Evans, 1951).

In France during the nineteenth century concerted efforts were made by medical practitioners, historians, radical politicians, and social philosophers to deal with health problems (Charlety, 1931; Cuvillier, 1948). For instance, an outbreak of cholera in Paris in 1831 led social philosophers to establish a free medical clinic. In turn, physicians participated in the various groups dedicated to social change. To investigate health problems created by the rapid social changes, many surveys and statistical analyses were made (Rosen, 1955). They were concerned with social factors related to illness such as the physical and social history of an area, nutrition, housing, customs of the inhabitants, age, sex, and occupation of individuals as well as the degree of social integration (Galdston, 1949).

But at the same time, people were recognizing that the goal of the state and the welfare of the individual were not necessarily identical and that social forces affecting the individual must be investigated separately from the consideration of national welfare. These were the conditions in which the idea of social medicine appeared. The term *social medicine* was introduced by Jules Guérin in 1848, when he appealed to the French medical profession to act for the public good (Guérin, 1848). The role of social factors in health problems was widely recognized, and the idea that "medicine is essentially a social science" was being formulated in Germany (Kroeger, 1937).

In the United States, the roots of social medicine are to be found in public health and organized social work (Duffy, 1968, 1976; Shryock, 1966). In 1910, a section on sociology was formed within the American Public Health Association, an organization of physicians and social workers.

In short, the history of social medicine has largely been the history of social policy and magmatic welfare action. The terms *public health, social hygiene,* and *social medicine* were used interchangeably. The underlying principles were

(1) the health of the individual is a matter of direct societal concern; (2) social factors have crucial impact on health, hence should be investigated; and (3) the promotion of health must be handled socially as well as medically.

It should be noted that while the concept of social medicine was promoted by some (Grotjahn, 1915) during the nineteenth and early twentieth centuries, others were proclaiming the germ theory as the ultimate medical truth, and still others concentrated on formal and theoretical sociology. Max Weber (1864–1920), a German sociologist, demanded a sharp separation between basic and applied science, and between social science and social policy. In short, there were three currents coexisting at that time: (1) bacteriologists were pursuing pure natural science; (2) sociologists were pursuing pure social science; and (3) social policy administrators were pursuing social medicine.

Reactions to the Germ Theory

The dramatic decline in deaths from infectious disease owed a great deal to the germ theory. However, the initial enthusiasm and optimism were followed by the realization that the germ theory alone would not account for all types of illness. Although infectious diseases came under control, little success was seen in the battle against other kinds of maladies such as chronic and mental illnesses. In fact, the decline of morbidity and mortality due to infectious disease served to accentuate the prevalence of other types of illness.

A monolithic germ theory has been challenged by many who emphasize the importance of interrelations among factors such as that between various microorganisms and a host. In 1959 René Dubos (1901–), himself a microbiologist, presented his view that humans live in a symbiotic or partnership relation with microbes and that the destruction of bacteria does not allow people to control disease or nature. Some germs are beneficial to humans, and even pathogenic germs may be functional to human life. He claimed that complete freedom from disease is nothing but a "mirage of health" (Dubos, 1959) and that the process of living means a constant adaptation to an environment filled with good and bad germs.

Psychiatry. A challenge to an exclusively biological (i.e., germ) theory of disease came from early psychiatry (Foucault, 1965; Howells, 1975; Mora, 1975), especially from the work of Sigmund Freud (1856–1939). First, Freud and others demonstrated that certain types of illness were caused psychologically, which rendered a purely mechanistic theory of disease untenable. Second, as the founder of psychoanalysis, Freud insisted on the importance of the subconscious psychic life, which hitherto was disregarded as unscientific. Furthermore, psychodynamic processes were viewed as the cumulative effect of past experiences of the individual as a social being. Freud introduced a component of personality, the superego, and an internalized set of rules and regulations that represent the values and norms of society. Mental illness was viewed as a manifestation of unsolved conflicts between innate biological needs and repressive social demands (Burgess, 1939).

Psychosomatic Medicine. Once a search for psychological causes of illness was underway, not only mental illness such as hysterical paralysis but also a large number of physical disorders (e.g., asthma, gastric ulcers) were discovered to be influenced by psychological factors. Several different perspectives of psychosomatic illness appeared. The first issue of the *Journal of Psychosomatic Medicine* stated that "psychosomatic medicine concerns itself with the psychological approach to general medicine." Others rejected the dichotomy of psychological and physiological components of medicine and maintained the concept of unity—unity of body and mind, and of internal and external environments (Alexander & French, 1948; Dunbar, 1943; Seguin, C., 1950). Disease was viewed as a reaction of the organism as a whole, responding to external and internal stimuli that might threaten its equilibrium. The external environment includes physical and social variables such as social stress (Grinker, 1953; Moss, 1973; Selye, 1956; Wolff, 1953). It is interesting to note that this psychosomatic orientation resembles Hippocrates' view of illness as being related to the total environment surrounding the patient.

Social Epidemiology and the Health Survey. Social epidemiologists concentrated on a search for social factors of illness. They tried to identify social characteristics peculiar to certain segments of the population that were susceptible to some biochemical or biophysical agent causing a specific disease (May, 1958; McMahon, et al. 1960; Rosen, 1958). In order to trace the process of disease causation, epidemiological field work was necessary in addition to laboratory investigation, and so many health surveys were conducted.

Although health surveys were carried out in the seventeenth century as a part of the German medical police administration, the first modern statistical health survey was done in Hagerstown, Maryland, from 1921 to 1924 (Syndenstricker, 1926). Between 1928 and 1931, the Committee on the Costs of Medical Care made a national survey (Commission on Chronic Illness, 1957), followed by another one by the U.S. Public Health Service during 1935 and 1936 (Perrott, Tibbitts, & Britten, 1939). Finally, in 1956, a continuous program of data collection was established by the National Health Act. Similar surveys have taken place in European countries since 1944.

The contribution of health surveys to the birth of medical sociology was twofold. On the one hand, such surveys provided valuable information concerning social correlates of illness and paved a road to sociological theories of health and illness behavior. On the other hand, they helped to establish methodological techniques for data collection and analysis.

Thus, from the seventeenth to the twentieth centuries, medicine has been approaching the field of social science through pragmatic as well as scientific channels. By the twentieth century, medical science was no longer monolithically germ-oriented but was ready to collaborate with social science in the goal of safeguarding the health and welfare of humanity.

Routes of Convergence Originating in Sociology

Although medical sociology as such has been labeled only recently, there are several precursors. First, there is the theoretical tradition of viewing society as analogous to a biological organism. Second, there are methodological contributions to medical sociology such as survey research and demographic techniques that have proved to be useful tools in social epidemiology. Third, on the substantive level, certain studies of communities, organizations, and individuals gave sociological interpretations to health and illness.

Systemic (System Oriented) Theories of Society

Despite its declaration of independence from natural science, sociology was imbued with the organic tradition; this was particularly strong in the work of early sociologists.

Evolutionism. The foundation of Herbert Spencer's (1820–1903) sociological theory was the evolutionary doctrine influenced by the work of Charles Darwin (1809–1882). Societies were viewed as biological organisms and were considered to be subject to the natural law of evolution. Societies and organisms are similar, Spencer maintained, in the following ways: (1) they both differ from inorganic phenomena in that they grow in size; (2) as they grow in size, a differentiation of the systems takes place both in terms of their structures and functions; (3) the differences in size, structure, and function are brought about by the degree of the system's adjustability to its environment; and (4) the systems that survive are the ones that make this adjustment well (Becker & Barnes, 1961; Fletcher, 1971; Rossides, 1978).

Doubts concerning the doctrine of evolutionism had already arisen in the nineteenth century. They grew out of more or less empirical studies testing specific evolutionary hypotheses.

Functionalism. Another systemic (system oriented) approach to society is found in functionalism. In the work of early functionalists, such as Bronislaw Malinowski (1884–1942), we see a biological analogy of human society. Each organ, or part of the system called an organism, performs a function or functions essential for the survival of the organism (Malinowski, 1944, 1948).

Later on, the argument on biological analogy was dropped, but the principle of the interdependence of the parts within a system remained as the core of functionalism. With the systematization of functionalism by Talcott Parsons (1902–) and modification by Robert K. Merton (1910–), this theory was consolidated as one of the basic frameworks for sociological studies. The contents of the theory and its application to medical sociology are described in Chapter 2.

Durkheim's Suicide. For Emile Durkheim (1858–1917), the concept of system integration was crucial. In his classic study of suicide, he investigated the suicide rates of various European countries and made statistical analysis of the relations between the suicide rates and other variables. Having examined biological, psychological, genetic, climatic, and geogaphic factors, and finding them to be unrelated to suicide rates, Durkheim refuted the existing theories of suicide. He proposed a sociological theory of suicide, stating that differential suicide rates are the consequences of variations in the degree and type of social integration.

The substance of Durkheim's study certainly belongs to the sphere of medical sociology. Furthermore, this work is considered a monumental landmark study in which theory and research, and pure and applied sociology are all brought together.

Methodological Contributions to Medical Sociology

Survey Research. The development of nonspeculative, quantitative methodology contributed to the progress of both sociology and medicine. During the first quarter of the twentieth century, sociologists displayed more interest in exact, detailed procedure than in philosophizing. They were influenced by the objective and mathematical methods used by economists and psychologists.

The core of survey research is the study of society through frequency distributions of given dimensions. Generalizations are made on the basis of the covariation and multivariation of codified and quantified variables. Social systems consist of frequency distributions and covariations among measured variables, and there is no synthesis derived from speculation.

With the advent of public opinion polls in the 1940s, survey research methods progressed rapidly. Opinions and attitudes were collected and analyzed along with objective social categories. Some of these surveys included attitudes toward health and illness and self-reported symptoms of physical and mental illnesses. They added the new dimension of subjective perception of illness to the social epidemiology model.

Demography. Demography is the science of vital and social statistics, such as the births, deaths, marriages, etc., of populations. Methodologically, demography has developed various techniques useful in analyzing statistical data. Furthermore, demography deals with substantive areas of medical sociology, namely, mortality and morbidity as related to the social characteristics of the population.

Except for a few isolated cases, the objective study of demographic variables dates only from the seventeenth century. Until the mid-eighteenth century, data were insufficient to support a full-scale analysis. With the advance of registration systems and census-type enumeration, the way was cleared in many countries to begin systematic analysis. With the appearance of Thomas R. Malthus's (1766–1834) *Essays on Population,* demography attained some maturity. Malthus's work was a detailed, organized compilation of existing statistics, bound together by analyses of causes and consequences.

Knowledge of populations is important to private and public authorities, since national power is demonstrated by population size, standard of living, life expectancy, and the like. Demography has shifted its affiliation to various disciplines—to dilettantism in the seventeenth century, political economy in the eighteenth century, economics in the nineteenth century, and to sociology in the twentieth century. About eighty percent of the demography courses offered in American colleges and universities are given by departments of sociology; the others are usually in public health, medicine, economics, geography, biology, and government departments (Thomlinson, 1965).

Substantive Contributions to Medical Sociology

Community Studies. During the decades around the turn of the century, various socioeconomic conditions fostered a closer relationship among social science, medicine, and public health. Rapid industrialization, urbanization, and immigration during this period generated overcrowded, unsanitary living arrangements; unhealthy working conditions; and social and psychological maladjustments associated with social change—all of which required socio-medical investigations (Rosen, 1976).

From about 1914 to the mid-thirties, the Chicago school of sociologists engaged in the study of urban life focusing upon the physical conditions of the city, its people, and their characteristics and life situations, including alcoholism, drug addiction, venereal disease, and mental illness.

At about the same time, a parallel study of an entire community was conducted by Robert and Helen Lynd (1929, 1937) in Indiana. The Middletown study by the Lynds was carried out largely by participant observation, supplemented by the analyses of historical documents and statistical data. The conceptual framework adopted by the Lynds was functionalism, although their hypothesis of full community integration was not verified. They examined the interlocking relations between various social institutions and social stratifications, including the organization of the medical practices and the use of medical services by community members.

Community studies had been made previously by public health practitioners and epidemiologists. The Middletown study is distinguished by the fact that health and illness were treated as a type of social behavior interrelated to the structure and function of society. Hence the scope of analysis was comprehensive and not limited to narrow areas immediately related to public health.

Organizational Studies. As medicine became more specialized and bureaucratized, sociologists' attention began to be drawn to studies of the hospital as a large complex organization (see Chapter 7), of physicians as members of a professional group (see Chapter 6), and of the physician–patient relationship as an interactional unit (see Chapter 5). Various aspects of medical problems were dealt with in already established subfields of sociology such as sociology of occupation, organization, and education.

Parson's Sick Role. Finally, on the level at which individuals are treated as a study unit, there is Talcott Parsons's analysis of the sick role. According to Parsons, a sick person, as a member of a society, is expected to behave in certain ways. He or she is exempt from performing normal tasks but is expected to attempt an early recovery.

The significance of this concept is twofold. First, Parsons showed the relevance of studying illness in sociological contexts instead of in a strictly physiological perspective. Second, in interpreting the behavior of a sick person,

Parsons used a general theoretical framework—functionalism. Thus, health and illness behavior could be studied in relation to broader social structure and processes. The details of Parsonian functionalism and the sick role will be discussed in Chapters 2 and 5.

By this point the concern for a demarcation between sociology and social work was unwarranted. Parsons indicated the possibility and desirability of dealing with health and illness in sociological frameworks that are clearly separated from social policies and ameliorative activities.

Sociology was now ready to work with medical science, and together they produced this new branch, called medical sociology, toward the end of the 1950s. As already described, the convergence was reached through a variety of developments that in turn resulted in the multiphasic nature of this field. Medical sociology is now at a crossroads where various attempts are being made to resolve its identity dilemma. Some are adhering to pure sociology, while others are developing new branches of applied sociology or behavioral science. Rather than a conflict, the contemporary state of affairs is marked by a continuing convergence and by the sociomedical progress of our time.

SUMMARY

In this chapter we have looked at Western civilization at three stages. The first stage of development of medical and social thought ranged from primitive times to the Renaissance. During that period medical and sociological thinking were subsumed under theology for the most part and under philosophy to some extent.

The second stage in the evolution of medical sociology appeared during the seventeenth, eighteenth, and nineteenth centuries and was characterized by the divergence of medicine and sociology into distinct sciences. As newly born disciplines, natural and social sciences were overzealous in protecting their separate identities.

While the stage of differentiation was taking place between the seventeenth and nineteenth century, opposite trends toward convergence also manifested themselves and culminated in the birth of medical sociology in the twentieth century.

Throughout the evolutionary process of thought, passing from theology to philosophy to science, we can discern one persistent characteristic. It is the effort to reach systematic arrangements of a body of facts and to discover general principles that would account for these arrangements. The methods for realizing these goals are different. The truth and principles of being, knowledge, or conduct are explained by divine will in theology, by rational but chiefly speculative means in philosophy, and by observation and experimentation in science. When medicine and sociology emerged as natural and social sciences in the nineteenth century, they were based on general theories—the germ theory of disease for medical matters and the organic theory for social behaviors.

In contrast, the birth of medical sociology was accompanied by a different orientation, that is, a restraint from developing general theoretical frameworks. The multiphasic nature of this new field is a result of the convergence of medical and social sciences from a variety of channels. The diversity as well as the newness of the field has inhibited many researchers and writers from building general conceptual models because they may be thought of as premature ventures. However, without any theoretical guidelines, it is difficult to develop a research design, to interpret research findings, and above all, to establish the discipline of medical sociology as a science. The task of a science, in the mind of this author, is to generate a sort of mental map of how things are put together and work. If health and illness are to be studied as social behaviors, there is no reason why we should not test applicability of existing sociological theories to medical sociology. In the following chapter, major sociological theories are presented as frameworks for examining medico-sociological data.

CHAPTER 2
Sociological Theories

"A theory is a way of making sense" out of what would otherwise be disparate and meaningless empirical findings (Kaplan, 1964). For example, in his classic, 1897 study of suicide, Durkheim (1950) gathered statistical facts and reported that according to his observations, suicide rates were higher among Protestants than among Catholics and were higher for single than for married people. These data raised questions such as, Is suicide hindered or aided by religion or marital status? Is there a common denominator between being Protestant and single? As an answer, and after careful analysis of the data, Durkheim developed the theory that suicide rates are a function of social cohesion. He postulated that social integration, such as is found in Catholicism and marriage, provides psychic support and relieves anxieties and stresses that might eventually result in suicide.

Theory formation, such as this one by Durkheim, is not only an important and distinctive goal of science, but it also is regarded by Kaplan (1964) as the most important activity for human living. To him, our daily experience is not constituted of random happenings; it is a sequence of more or less meaningful events.

> A theory is a way of making sense of a disturbing situation so as to allow us most effectively to bring to bear our repertoire of habits, and even more important, to modify habits or discard them altogether, replacing them by new ones as the situation demands (Kaplan, 1964, p. 295).

In this sense and also according to Kaplan, a habit might involve an implicit belief in a scientific theory simply because we are conditioned to respond in a habitual way as if our response were necessary and universal.

Thus, theories of social and human behavior serve two functions: *understanding* and *prediction.* They illuminate the ways in which seemingly ad hoc events are related to one another in a significant way and foretell what conditions are to be anticipated (Dubin, 1969).

On the other hand, a theory is not limited to only giving anwers; it can also raise new questions. The value of a theory is heuristic, that is, it *stimulates* and provides *guidelines* for further research. To illustrate, many research activities were conducted in state mental hospitals in response to questions stimulated by the labeling theory. This particular theory postulates that mental illness progresses as a reaction to the negative labeling of the patients in these institutions, but of what value is this and other such theories if they do not stimulate research efforts?

One of the basic issues of medical sociology is and has been the lack of a clear demonstration of how social theory can help solve the health problems of humanity. Such a demonstration has been one of the prerequisites demanded by medicine for a merger with sociology. As a natural science, medicine demands a precision and exactness from social theories; medicine wants hard cause-and-effect proof where natural laws are concerned. Then, as an applied science, medicine does anticipate, pragmatically, that a sociological theory may provide guidelines for resolving certain medical problems.

The current status of sociological theories in medical sociology has been jeopardized by such stringent expectations. An inability simply to meet either of these conditions exactly has led many medical sociologists to hesitate before making any theoretical effort. This chapter is intended to help remedy that situation, and it will introduce the three major sociological theories—functionalism, conflict theories, and interactionism—that will be used to interpret existing sociomedical research findings.

These three theoretical frameworks are adopted because they are the most general perspectives in the field and are widely used. Their diversity can be appreciated by a brief interpretation of the basis of social integration: why do selfish and competitive human beings band together as a society? To functionalists, it is *common interest* and need that link people in societal structures. Conflict theorists, on the other hand, assert that it is the *coercion* of losers by winners in a conflict that cement social organization (Adams, 1966). While functionalists and conflict theorists take deterministic orientations, albeit opposite in direction (i.e., consensus versus dissension), interactionists postulate that social order is indeterminate and is constantly *negotiated* between individuals acting in relation to each other. In other words, people try to figure out and manipulate what others are doing, and they adjust their own behavior accordingly.

We cannot, in this book, do justice to each of these theoretical orientations. Nonetheless, we shall introduce the frameworks and their relevance to medical sociology and apply each to major themes in later chapters.

FUNCTIONALISM

Functionalism originated in the physical science orientation of early sociologists. Biological discoveries during the nineteenth century stimulated the social and intellectual climate of those times. The resulting preoccupation with biology and the concept of evolutionism clearly influenced the description of the social order (Buckley, 1967; Fletcher, 1971).

Society was envisioned by Comte as a type of organism with structures and functions analogous to a biological organism. In his *Polity,* he described families as the basic social cells, social forces as the social tissues, the state and city as the social organs, and nations as biological organisms. Spencer, like Comte, also proclaimed that society is like an organism, and he too compared the growth and evolution of biological organisms with societies.

Functionalism as a well-articulated conceptual framework was introduced by Radcliffe-Brown and Malinowski in the twentieth century. These first functional anthropologists shared the organicism of Comte, Spencer, and others. In particular, Malinowski dogmatically asserted a biological analogy. He began his analysis with the basic human needs such as food, shelter, and reproduction. To meet these biological needs, he said people would organize into groups and communities. Then, cultural symbols would be created to regulate such organizations. In turn, the creation of these organizations and culture would give rise to additional and higher-level needs (psychological and cultural) that would have to be met by more elaborate social organizations.

In sum, the extreme forms of organicism of the early functionalists were based on the following assumptions: (1) society, like a biological organism, is a bounded system that is self-regulating and maintains equilibrium; (2) like the human body, society has basic needs that must be fulfilled in order for the system to survive; (3) various parts play certain functions for the survival and equilibrium of society; and (4) certain types of structures must exist to ensure survival and homeostasis of the system.

The evolution of functionalist theory is shown in Talcott Parsons's full-scale systemic (system oriented) theory construction. Parsons completed his task by visualizing an overall system with culture, social structure, personality, and organism comprising its constituent subsystems (Parsons et al., 1961). Among these four subsystems, Parsons introduced the idea of the hierarchy of control of the behavior of the individual. Cultural values regulate the range of variations in the norms (i.e., standards and rules of behavior in a particular social situation) of the social system. These norms, in turn, limit the range of decisions and motives of the personality system. Then, the personality systems maintain control of the behavioral organism. In short, physical behavior is controlled by personality, which is regulated by social norms as defined by cultural values.

The formulations of Parsons's functionalism clearly indicate his view of the role of theory in science (Parsons et al., 1961, p. 32). Parsons considers theory as a vital component of organized scientific knowledge. The concept of a system, in Parsons's view, is also vital to science in that theoretical propositions are scientifically useful to the extent that they are logically integrated.

Robert K. Merton claimed that the search for such grand theoretical schemes as Parsons's is premature because neither the theoretical nor empirical groundwork had been done (Merton, 1948). Comparing sociology with natural science, Merton observed that the general laws of society must wait, just as Einstein's theory could emerge only on the foundation of the cumulative research efforts of Kepler, Newton, Lalace, Gibbs, Maxwell, and Planck (Merton, 1949, p. 47). In the eyes of Merton, Parsons's functionalism was a philosophical system rather than a theory because theory must consist of general orientations toward data. As a solution, Merton proposed theories of a middle range between highly abstract, grand theories and empiricism with its low level of abstraction. Middle-range theories are abstract, yet they are linked with the empirical world and promote the interplay between theory and research.

With this attitude toward theory, Merton modified questionable postulates made by functionalists. He focused his attention on the varied consequences of specified system parts rather than on the determinate integrated system; he replaced theoretical postulates with empirical hypotheses; and he limited his scope to specific areas of social phenomena rather than dealing with society as a whole.

Prevailing Postulates

Prevailing postulates of functional analysis include the concept of a social system, the functional unity of society, the value consensus in society, the universal functionalism, the functional indispensability, and the equilibrium model.

Concept of Social System. Functionalists pictured human society as an organism composed of many parts, all functioning in an integrated way to maintain the whole system just like our brain, heart, lungs, liver, and other organs function to maintain our body.

This biological analogy, called organicism, was rejected by later functionalists, who tried to avoid such speculative and empirically nonverifiable postulates as that there are societal "needs" analogous to biological needs. However, the legacy of the pioneer functionalists remains in the conceptualization of society as a bounded system in which various parts are interrelated. Specifically, a social system is conceived by Talcott Parsons to be a whole that is composed of a plurality of interacting persons who are motivated to optimize gratifications and whose relation to each other is regulated and structured by culturally shared norms and symbols (Parsons, 1951). That interaction between individuals tends to develop certain uniformities over time, and some of those patterns tend to persist. Then, with their orderly and systematic nature, those interacting persons are recognized as a social system. The study of this orderliness or uniformity in the social system is, according to Parsons, sociology. He also defined society as a large-scale, persistent, and self-sufficient system of patterned social interactions.

Functional Unity of Society. Another functionalist formulation is that all parts of the social system work together with internal consistency. This idea of the functional unity of society is described succinctly by Radcliffe-Brown as follows:

> The function of a particular social usage is the contribution it makes to the total social life as the functioning of the total social system. Such a view implies that a social

> system . . . has a certain kind of unity, which we may speak of as functional unity. We may define it as a condition in which all parts of the social system work together with a sufficient degree of harmony or internal consistency (Radcliffe-Brown, 1935, p. 397).

To illustrate, a doctor's function is to prescribe a therapy, while it is the patient's role to obey the doctor's order. If either one does not behave as expected, the social system of the doctor–patient relationship is likely to disintegrate.

Value Consensus. How can we expect everyone to behave so that a social system will be maintained? Functionalists claim that it is the consensus of values that link human beings in society. Consensus is reached not by coercion (Adams, 1966) but by socialization and internalization of a common value system.

From birth until death, human beings constantly learn how to behave according to what is expected of them. Their behavior is largely a product of adherence to standards of society that they have come to accept as their own principles. For example, health and activity are valued highly in our society. The extent to which these values are internalized by individuals is revealed by the large number of people jogging on the streets.

Universal Functionalism. The postulate of functional unity of the social whole results in another assumption, that of universal functionalism. If a social item exists in an ongoing system and the item is functionally integrated, it must make positive contributions to the system. Malinowski (1944, 1948) extended this line of reasoning by stating that each custom, material object, idea, and belief fulfills some vital function.

Merton (1949), on the other hand, postulated that empirical research would reveal a wide range of possibilities, and he claimed that there are some items that are dysfunctional for the system or for parts of the system. Also, some consequences, whether functional or dysfunctional, are recognized as manifest, whereas others are seen as latent. In short, Merton concluded that functional analysis must calculate a net balance of positive, negative, manifest, and latent consequences.

For example, the manifest function of a patient's visit to a doctor's office is to be cured, while the latent function may be to solicit the doctor's sympathy.

Functional Indispensability. Not only are all standardized social or cultural items viewed as having functions, but there are certain functions that are assumed to be indispensable in the sense that unless they are performed, the society or groups will not persist. Furthermore, it is posited that certain cultural or social forms are indispensable for fulfilling these functions.

Parsons elaborated on what he calls "functional prerequisites of society," that is, conditions that must be met by the group if social life is to persist. They are goal attainment, adaptation, integration, and latency. Parsons states that "process in any social system is subject to four independent functional imperatives or 'problems' which must be met adequately if equilibrium and/or continuing existence of the system is to be maintained" (Parsons & Smelser,

1956, p. 16).

A goal is defined as a compromise between the needs of the system and the conditions of the external environment. Furthermore, a social system is likely to have several goals that must be balanced within the system. Thus, *goal attainment* refers to the problem of first establishing priorities among goals and then of mobilizing resources (e.g., personnel and financial assets) to attain various goals.

Adaptation is the process of securing sufficient facilities (e.g., wealth, material resources, and technical means) from the external environment and distributing them throughout the system. The adaptive problem involves properly perceiving and rationally manipulating the environment for the benefit of the system.

The problem of *integration* concerns achieving and maintaining social and emotional solidarity among members of a social group. The integrative function involves formal and informal control of individuals so as to ensure their cooperation in the process of goal attainment.

Latency consists of restoring, maintaining, or creating the energies, motives, and values of the cooperating individuals. It includes the process of socialization by which the values of the society are internalized in the personality of an individual.

Equilibrium Model of Society. Functionalism rests on the notion of feedback, that is, the process by which any system can regulate itself automatically. Using a biological analogy, when you cut your finger, blood vessels around the injured area immediately contract and clotting mechanisms become active. In a similar way, death due to a physician's negligence may be followed by a malpractice suit, which in turn serves to improve the quality of medical care.

Because of this self-maintaining equilibrium model, functionalism has been charged for its inability to account for social change. However, in the last decade, Parsons has become increasingly concerned with social change (Turk & Simpson, 1970), particularly in the realm of evolutionary change (Parsons, 1966).

Evolutionary change is characterized by a differentiation of society. It occurs when a unit of a system that had a single, relatively well-defined place in society is divided into separate units that differ in both structure and functional significance for the wider system. It is assumed that new principles and the mechanisms of integration are established when a system is differentiated and that the adaptive capacity of a differentiated system has increased in relation to the environment.

Criticisms of Functionalism

Functionalism has been criticized by many people and from various angles (Black, 1961; Demerath & Peterson, 1967).

The first basic issue is whether or not the theory corresponds to events in the "real" world. Without some outside linkage between highly abstract concepts and concrete empirical events, it is difficult to assess whether functionalist concepts would be useful in analyzing social phenomena.

Second, when the functionalists claim that a certain item serves to maintain a social system, that claim also leads to the reverse argument, that the item emerged because of its functional indispensability. For instance, the existence of social stratification is explained in the following way: the unequal distribution of wealth arose because it is functional to the survival of society (David & Moore, 1945; Nagel, 1953).

Third, the functionalist assumption of system integration has caused critics to accuse functionalism of being too conservative. The emphasis upon consensus of values, on integration of parts within the system, and on mechanisms for preserving equilibrium does not allow room for explaining social phenomena such as change, deviance, and conflict (Coser, 1956; Dahrendorf, 1958a; Lockwood, 1956; Mills, 1959).

The substantive functionalist image of society and their problems with logic have stimulated both widespread criticisms as well as efforts to establish a correspondence between abstract concepts and the empirical world. It was partly the rejection of Parsonian functionalism that encouraged the emergence of other theoretical perspectives such as conflict theories and interactionism.

Application to Medical Sociology

Society and the Individual

The functional prerequisites and the notion of the evolutionary adaptability of a society provide promising guidelines for comparative analyses of health and illness behaviors in different societies. The specific structural arrangements for meeting the functional prerequisites differ from one society to another and, in the course of time, will change in any given society. In line with functionalist postulates, it is anticipated that societies which have survived throughout history and have evolved into differentiated stages are equipped with an adaptive capacity and therefore are likely to show low rates of mortality and morbidity.

On the individual level, illness is regarded by functionalists as a social behavior. As such, it is determined by the individual's position in relation to others (social status), and what he or she does in this position (role). Certain statuses and roles may be more conducive to illness than others because they can expose the incumbents to physical hazards and can generate stresses.

In Chapters 3 and 4, the distribution of diseases in different societies and in different social statuses such as occupation, social class, and marital status will be interpreted according to functionalist frameworks.

Medicine as a Social System

A social system is divided into subsystems, each of which maintains its integration and is related to the others. Thus, within a society we can distinguish subsystems such as the polity, the economy, family, and medicine. Each of these subsystems is further differentiated into smaller units. For instance, within a broad system of medicine subunits such as a hospital, the American Medical Association (AMA), and a doctor–patient relationship may be identified. It should be noted that the boundaries of subsystems may frequently overlap. Part 2 of this book deals with selected patterns of medical practice as social systems.

The smallest social system consists of two persons, such as found in the doctor–patient relationship (Chapter 5). Viewed from the functionalist perspective, the system of doctor and patient is based on shared values, namely, that health is functional and illness is dysfunctional. Because of this negative perception of illness, the patient is assigned to a subordinate position in relation to the doctor, who performs a positive function in society. An asymmetrical balance of power is operative in the system of doctor and patient.

Physicians as members of the medical profession constitute a larger subsystem, and they have a strong sense of group identity. Chapter 6 examines a social system consisting only of physicians. That system is accorded high status, a fact that is attributed by functionalists (Davis & Moore, 1945) to the ability of physicians to fulfill an indispensable function. Doctors maintain their profession as a closed social system, and in order to demarcate doctors from outsiders, the AMA has established standardized medical education and licensure. The AMA also performs the adaptive function by manipulating the external environment to the benefit of its members, such as the fight against the Medicare and Medicaid bills.

In contrast with physicians, other health practitioners such as dentists, pharmacists, nurses, physician's assistants, chiropractors, and Christian Scientists are all striving to attain professional status (Chapter 8). These allied health groups face a dilemma in their attempt to draw the boundaries of their practice outside of the domination of physicians while at the same time securing a status equal to that of physicians. In the case of chiropractors and Christian Scientists, their avoidance of physicians' encroachment resulted in their being labeled as "irregular" practitioners by the AMA. In contrast, physician's assistants and nurses do not have their own systems clearly delineated, but rather their activities are legitimized by the medical profession.

Another distinguishable medical subsystem, one with a physical boundary, is the hospital, which is discussed in Chapter 7. Various activities seen in the large, complex organization of a modern hospital can be analyzed in terms of their contributions to the survival of the hospital. First, there are medical staff members whose primary role is to cure patients, which is the major goal of the hospital. Second, administrators coordinate the operations of the various parts of the organization. Finally, on the institutional level, a board of trustees oversees the hospital operation in the light of the values and interests of the community.

Medicine Within a Social System

In Part 3 of this book, the focus is shifted from the internal mechanisms of medical subsystems to the external relations between health-related or other subsystems in a community or a society at large. These relations will be analyzed by the following example illustrated by Parsons and Smelser (1956). With some modification these authors identify four sets of presumably specialized subsystems to meet each of the basic system requirements. Thus, the polity is the subsystem whose goal is to maximize the capacity of a society to attain its goals. Economic activity is related to the adaptive function. The integrative function is played by the subsystem of stratification, which rewards good performance by wealth, status, and power, and punishes poor performance by deprivation, thereby fostering solidarity in goal attainment activities. Finally, the value subsystem insures that members of the social system display motives and skills appropriate for performing their roles.

In Chapter 9, the emergence of neighborhood health centers is examined in terms of the polity, the economy, stratification, and value subsystems in a community. Chapter 10 traces the development of the idea of national health insurance as it relates to these four subsystems. As a contrast to American medical delivery practice, which has maintained a relative freedom from third-party interference, Chapter 11 presents examples of socialized medicine in the United Kingdom, the USSR, and the People's Republic of China, in which medical subsystems are subsumed under the polity.

Functionalism offers useful frameworks for identifying units of study and for examining the interrelation of the parts to the whole and among the parts of the system. However, when the theoretical perspective includes only the equilibrium assumption, it tends to overlook stresses and conflicts within the system. In the following section conflict theories are introduced, and their applicability to medical sociology is illustrated.

CONFLICT THEORIES

The debate over consensus versus conflict as the dominant image of society dates back to Socrates and Aristotle. Throughout the history of social thought, these two perspectives appeared more as rivals than as complementary units.

Sociology came into being with the organicism of Comte and Spencer in the nineteenth century. With organismic unity in a society, every part was assumed to be functionally linked to every other part and to allow little margin for conflict. Due to its failure to account for social conflict, however, organicism could hardly maintain its claim that it was a form of scientific theory. In its pursuit of realism, sociology eventually turned toward conflict theories such as those developed by Karl Marx and Georg Simmel.

Conflict theories corrected some of the excesses of organicism and provided missing elements, such as conflict, dissent, deviance, and change. The rather vague, general concepts of organicism were replaced by more compact and concrete terms such as *capitalists* and *ruling class.* The recognition of specific groups that existed as balanced forces sharpened the concept of the social group.

In the meanwhile, as sociology became well established, its interests and attentions became diversified. Instead of studying the *macroscopic* social system or social processes, many sociological theories began to deal with and to emphasize *microscopic* interactions between individuals and particular groups. Late in the nineteenth century, the pendulum swung away from general orientations toward more detailed theories.

After the turn of the twentieth century, however, and with the rise of modern functionalism, the pendulum seemed to swing back to where sociology started in the early nineteenth century. As a rebellion against the atomistic or elementary concerns of social interactionists, functionalists of the twentieth century, headed by Parsons, reformulated their concept of a social system. It was against this background that the contemporary conflict theories emerged in the work of Ralf Dahrendorf and Lewis Coser.

Two distinct models are identified: dialectic and functional conflict theories (Turner, 1978).

Major Postulates

Dialectic Conflict Theories

The major postulates of dialectic conflict theories as developed by Karl Marx and Ralf Dahrendorf consist of conflict endemic in society, dialectic process, historical materialism (Marx), and conflict over authority (Dahrendorf).

Conflict Endemic in Society. While functionalists posit integration and consensus in a social system, conflict theorists view society in a continuous state of conflict. Such conflict is presumed to be generated by the opposed interests that are inherent in the structure of society.

Dialectic Process of Conflict. Not only did they assume ubiquity of conflict, but Marx and Dahrendorf proposed an inevitable dialectic process of conflict.

In ancient Greece dialectic was the art of disputation practiced by the philosophers. A thesis (a positive statement) would be opposed by an antithesis (a negative statement), and through the clash of ideas something new and better, a synthesis, might occur.

Thus, according to dialectic conflict theorists, everything contains its own contradictions in itself. When the contradictory element becomes apparent, a conflict results between the thesis and antithesis. These conflicts then are the driving forces of nature that reach for a new stage: synthesis.

Historical Materialism (Marx). For Marx history is a dialectic process (Bottomore, 1973). It moves by means of the contradictions inherent in social relations, which are based on the material needs of people and the material conditions of life.

First, Marx postulated that economic organization, especially ownership of property, determines the organization of the rest of a society. For Marx, analysis begins with human actions to master nature in the pursuit of a livelihood. The important issue in the establishment of a social system is how the modes of production are organized. Cultural values, beliefs, ideas, and religions are secondary and are ultimately mere reflections of the economic structures of a given society.

> The mode of production of the material means of life, determines, in general, the social, political, and intellectual processes of life. It is not the consciousness of human beings that determines their existence but, conversely, it is their social existence that determines their consciousness (Marx, 1970, pp. 20–21).

Second, Marx assumed that scarcity is omnipresent in nature, and that as a result, people are constantly fighting for scarce commodities. Thus, even if social relations display systematic features, these relations are rife with conflicting interests. In addition, he stressed the fact that social systems generate conflict systematically, not randomly. Therefore, the conflicts that occur most frequently are the ones that concern the distribution of economic resources, and those conflicts polarize society into opposing class interests. As members of the exploited segments become aware of their true collective interests, they begin to question the legitimacy of a system, and they eventually form a revolutionary political organization against the dominant, property-holding class.

Marx conceptualized social change to be the result of inevitable conflict dialectics within various types of institutionalized patterns. Thus, feudalism contained contradictions that eventually gave rise to capitalism. Similarly, the capitalist system contained in itself the seed of its own destruction and would be followed by the emergence of socialism, which in turn would lead to communism.

Marxian dialectic materialism has been criticized from logical, empirical, and ideological angles: (1) social relations are not determined only by economic factors; (2) many societies have not been polarized into two economic classes; (3) conflict does not necessarily lead to social change; and (4) there is a logical inconsistency in the view of a communist society as the final stage of peace and harmony without contradictions.

Conflict Over Authority (Dahrendorf). Although Dahrendorf (1958b, 1959, 1967) also adopts a dialectic approach, he departs from Marx in several ways. First, unlike Marx, Dahrendorf's conceptualization is nonevolutionary in the sense that there is no logical progression within the system. A synthesis is not necessarily an improvement over the previous stage.

Second, the assumption of stability or equilibrium within each stage of synthesis is absent in Dahrendorf's thinking. Instead of the thesis–antithesis–synthesis scheme, he views social groups and societies as engaged in conflict–disintegration–change cycles.

Third, Dahrendorf does not accept economic determinism, and he posits a different basis of conflict than Marx's property ownership. For Dahrendorf, the source of conflict is the legitimate authority and power per se; these are the scarce resources to be fought over.

Dahrendorf assumes that wherever human beings live together, power relations develop between those with varying positions. However, some power relations tend to become legitimized as authority relations in which coercion of some positions by others is accepted. The social order is maintained by this institutionalization of power relations. On the other hand, since power and authority are scarce commodities, groups and individuals fight and compete for them. Thus, power and authority are the major sources of conflict. The resolution of this conflict involves the redistribution of authority, which results in the institutionalization of a new pattern of ruling and ruled roles. Under certain conditions, this reorganized pattern will generate further conflict, and it will again polarize society into two interest groups. Thus, social change is seen as an inevitable outcome of conflict.

The primary criticism of Dahrendorf is phrased in such questions as, How is it possible that conflict emerges from legitimate power relations? How is it that the same structure is conducive to integration as well as to conflict? (Weingart, 1969). Dahrendorf admits that the idea of authority reveals two faces of society: integration and coercion. Authority facilitates the performance of function on behalf of the social system, but it also produces and is a product of conflict. Yet, beneath all these faces, coercion is singled out by some (Adams, 1966) as the pervasive characteristic of social organization in the eyes of Dahrendorf.

Functional Conflict Theories

Functional conflict theory was initially formulated by Georg Simmel (Levine, 1971; Wolff, 1950) in the nineteenth century, and it was later expanded by Lewis Coser in the twentieth century into one of the most comprehensive theories of conflict. While dialectic theorists view society as filled with contradictions and ready to disintegrate, Simmel and Coser, as do many functional sociologists, emphasize that the social order is maintained by some degree of consensus. Major postulates derive from (1) organic analogy, (2) systemic approach, and (3) integrative consequence of conflict.

Organic Analogy. Simmel described social relationships within an organic and systemic context; such relationships are characterized by associative and dissociative processes. These processes are viewed as a reflection of both the instinctual impulses of individuals and the demands made by social groups. Simmel posited that there was an innate hostile impulse as well as an instinct for love and affection among the units of organic wholes.

Having inherited Simmel's organic analogy, Coser equates violence with pain in the human body, and he explains dissent in terms of sickness in the "body social."

Systemic Approach. For dialectic theorists, the causes of conflict are to be found in contradictions or competing interests. In contrast, Coser (1956, 1966), whose primary concern rests with social order, views conflict as arising from decreased legitimacy or consensus over existing social arrangements. Coser specifies the conditions leading to a breakdown of legitimacy and the situations in which people's emotional energies are mobilized to pursue conflict.

Although conflict is perceived to be endemic in a social system, functional conflict theorists do not assume that it will necessarily lead to the breakdown of the system and/or to social change. Simmel recognized that when goals are clearly defined, people are likely to seek for compromise and conciliation to avoid the high cost and unpredictable results of violent conflict. Coser accepts this proposition and further elaborates upon the social structure inhibition to conflict. In short, while Marx concentrated on delineating conditions under which conflict will be violent, Coser's attention is directed to conditions under which conflict will be avoided.

Integrative Consequences of Conflict. Implicit in the theories of Simmel and Coser is the functionalist assumption that conflict is good when it promotes integration based on solidarity, clear authority, functional interdependence, and normative control. These very same characteristics of integration are likely to be denounced by other types of conflict theorists as exploitative and negative.

Simmel and Coser envision conflict as one of the principal mechanisms that operate to preserve the social system. Simmel considered that an overly cooperative, consensual, and integrated society would not show any life process, and he focused his attention upon the process by which conflict promotes solidarity and unification of the "body social." He stated that

> Conflict is thus designed to resolve dualisms; it is a way of achieving some kind of unity, even if it is through the annihilation of one of the conflicting parties. This is roughly parallel to the fact that it is the most violent symptom of a disease which represents the effort of the organism to free itself of disturbances and damages caused by them (Simmel, 1955, p. 13).

Simmel and Coser present integrative functions of conflict as they pertain to the respective conflicting parties and to the social system as a whole. According to Simmel, frequent and mild conflict will serve to allow individuals to release their hostilities and frustrations, thereby preventing the accumulation of ill will. Through this process of interchange of moderate frustrations, the individuals come to grasp a sense of control over their destiny.

In connection with intergroup conflict, Simmel and Coser postulate that conflict will increase the demarcation of boundaries, the centralization of authority, an ideological solidarity, and the suppression of dissent and deviance within each of the conflict parties. In short, intergroup conflict serves to strengthen group integration. Both Simmel and Coser are aware of the potentially malintegrative aspects of despotic centralization and suppression of dissent, but their analysis is skewed toward the integrative consequences of conflict.

With regard to the results of conflict to the social system, frequent but mild conflicts in flexible social structures are assumed to enhance innovation, creativity, adaptability, integration, equilibrium, normative regulation of conflict, balance of power, and value and norm consensus. Also, to the extent that conflict does not contradict the basic values upon which the legitimacy of the system rests, conflict is positively functional to the system in a sense that it increases the system's integration and adaptability.

Application to Medical Sociology

Although conflict theorists posit conflict rather than integration as the predominant characteristic of a social group, they, like the functionalists, conduct their analysis within the framework of a social system. Therefore, the same units of social systems that have been identified for functional analysis will be used for testing postulates proposed by conflict theorists.

Society and the Individual

While functionalists attribute the adaptability of a society to its successful fulfillment of basic system requirements, conflict theorists view adaptability as the degree of success in winning battles against other, weaker groups.

High mortality rates and poor health in underdeveloped countries in the contemporary world are explained by conflict theory as the outcome of exploitation by dominant nations. Similarly, civilized societies have lower mortality and morbidity rates than primitive ones (Chapter 4) because the former have survived through centuries of conflict.

Then, even within a dominant nation, social groups are seen to be in an incessant struggle over power and scarce commodities. The Marxian theory of class conflict appears to be pertinent to the social class differences in health and illness behavior—the poor are sicker than the affluent (Richardson, 1972). Lower-class people are likely to be exposed to physical hazards such as overcrowded living, poor sanitation, and malnutrition, they suffer from sociopsychological stresses that enhance their vulnerability to illness, and they are often deprived of medical care facilities.

This concept of exploitation of the weaker by the dominant group extends beyond social class. It is applicable to racial, ethnic, sexual, and other categories. For instance, higher morbidity rates among women than among men can be interpreted as the consequence of male exploitation of the female.

Conflict can also result from the occupancy of a social position that makes contradictory demands upon the incumbent. A female engineer may suffer the difficulty of satisfying two sets of expectations: behaving like a female and behaving like an engineer.

Medicine as a Social System

While functionalists view the doctor–patient relationship (Chapter 5) as an asymmetrical equilibrium in which a patient is willingly to be subordinate to a doctor, conflict theorists postulate a clash of interests in that relationship. Having rejected Parsons's assumption of value consensus, Freidson (1970) observed that patients have different perspectives than do doctors and that the former do have power resources with which to fight the latter. To illustrate, solo practitioners have to compete among themselves for patients, and hence their behavior is influenced by patients who freely share their lay opinions concerning a solo practitioner's medical competence.

Viewed from a historical perspective, the study of professions and professionalization (Chapter 6) is amenable to conflict theory. Physicians did not always have power or the status of profession. The American Medical Association (AMA) and the Flexner Report (1910) had the effect of distinguishing legitimate physicians from charlatans and quacks. Even after professional status was consolidated, the AMA was always on guard lest the boundary of the profession should be expanded or diluted. One of the effective tactics adopted by the AMA in this regard was to restrict the size of the medical student body so as to maintain an elitist status.

That status is sought by other health practitioners, and their attempts at professionalization (Chapter 8) is viewed by conflict theorists as a zero-sum game in which the gain of professional position by one group results in the loss of status by another. Various health practitioners have been raising their educational standards with the hope of acquiring professional qualification. However, since prestige is a scarce commodity, it may have to be fought for instead of being gained through self-education.

As compared with other social systems such as the doctor–patient relationship and various professions, a hospital as a social system appears to have a more concrete and stable structure bounded by a physical plant. Nevertheless, the analysis of such institutions (Chapter 7) will profit by adopting conflict theories because a modern American hospital has a strife-inducing structure. For instance, a dual-authority system prevails in which the administration and the medical staff operate according to different perspectives. While the relationship between these two segments is symbiotic, the split in authority generates conflict. Also, the extreme division of labor is another feature of the modern hospital that is conducive to intergroup antagonism.

Medicine Within a Social System

Conflict theory can give us some insight into how nontraditional concepts such as a neighborhood health center and national health insurance came into being in this country. Functionalist interpretations are not quite adequate in explaining how the common value orientations of American society (e.g., individualism and capitalism) integrate with the ideas underlying neighborhood health centers and national health insurance (e.g., control of medical practice by nonphysicians and the redistribution of wealth according to need).

The conflict perspective will show that the history of American medicine is a repetition of conflict generation and resolution among many interest groups such as the AMA, organized labor, the government, private insurance companies, civil rights movement supporters, and consumers. The AMA's original policies, that is, fee for service and no third-party interference, have gone through several stages of modification in response to pressures from other groups, and the AMA has finally come to propose its own version of national health insurance.

INTERACTIONISM

Sociology has claimed to be the general science of society, and it has considered the basic unit of analysis to be a social group. It has focused on macro structure and processes, such as system integration, social evolution, class conflict, and the nature of the "body social." The analytical schemes of Comte, Spencer, and others were based on the assumption that *human* attitudes, sentiments, and behaviors were reflections of *societal* needs, conditions, structures, and the like.

Interactionists challenged these assumptions when they undertook systematic analyses of the detailed mechanisms whereby the self came to reflect society. Interactionists study the processes of social interaction and their consequences for the individual and society.

While the origin of interactionism can be traced to the work of William James, Charles Horton Cooley, W. I. Thomas, and many others, it was George Herbert Mead who brought related concepts together into a coherent theory. He linked biological, psychological, and sociological aspects of human beings, as well as social structure, to interactional processes. The Meadian legacy gave rise to three variants of interactionism: role theory, symbolic interactionism (and its derivative, labeling theory), and exchange theory (Kahn, 1964).

The first two variants can be viewed as a continuum—from the highly structured view of interactions found in role theory to the less structured process of symbolic interaction. Exchange theory may be located somewhere in between. An interesting analogy has been made to distinguish the two: theatrical acting as role taking and game playing as symbolic interaction (Turner, 1978, p. 347). While role theorists view individuals in society as actors and actresses in the theater, symbolic interactionists envision people as participants in a game (Biddle & Thomas, 1966; Goffman, 1959). In a theatrical play, interaction is controlled by the script, directors, other players, and the audience, allowing little room for the individual actors and actresses to create their own lines of action. Role theory focuses on the structure of status networks and accompanying expectations as they circumscribe interactions among individuals. In contrast, interaction in a game is fluid and is influenced by the wide range of tactics used by the participants. Symbolic interaction theory concerns the symbolic process by which each player tries to anticipate an opponent's move and to adjust his or her act accordingly.

Despite the difference in emphasis between these two variants of interactionism, they have one thing in common, that is, the *interpretive* approach as distinct from the *normative* orientation of functionalism. Behavior is not assumed to be a product of adherence to normative standards. Instead, it is assumed that the individual interprets the situation and determines his or her behavior accordingly.

Role Theory

Network of Interrelated Positions. For role theorists, society is viewed as a network of interrelated positions or statuses in which individuals enact roles (Biddle & Thomas, 1966; Deutch & Krauss, 1965; Shaw & Costanzo, 1970).

Each position is associated with a set of norms or expectations that specify how the incumbent of that position is to behave. Just as actors and actresses are given defined parts to play and follow a written script, individuals in society occupy clearcut positions and conform to norms.

The main concern of role theorists has been to articulate the relationship between the individual and society—how specific social contexts determine variations in an individual's conduct. Role theory implies that the entire society resembles one big stage play and is structured in terms of statuses and expectations. Although the main thrust of the theory has been restricted to small groups and other micro social units, there are implicit assumptions that the social order is structured by certain basic micro groups and organizations. It is further assumed that the macro structures and processes such as cultural values, social integration, and class conflict can be understood in terms of their constituent micro group mechanisms.

Range of Expectations. According to role theory, players must meet a wide range of expectations. These expectations can be classified into the three sets of demands placed upon actors in a play: the script, other players, and the audience (Turner, 1978, p. 350). Just like actors and actresses must follow the script, individuals in society must learn and conform to norms associated with the position they occupy. Thus, norms prescribe how a doctor, a nurse, or a patient ought to behave in social settings. Since roles are interrelated and players must work with one another, their behavior is modified by the expectations of other players. To illustrate the point, if a nurse discovers that a doctor has forgotten a medication, the former has to remind the latter of the negligence in such a way that the doctor does not lose face. Finally, role players have some audience whom they wish to impress. These audiences can be real or imagined. For instance, the audiences selected by nurses may consist of doctors, patients, other nurses, friends, family members, or Florence Nightingale. In any event, the audience has an impact on the way players behave.

Limited Interpretation of Roles. Actors and actresses in a play bring their unique interpretations of their parts to the stage. In a similar fashion, role theorists acknowledge that role players assess and interpret what is expected of them and have the option to decide how to respond to these expectations (Deutch & Krauss, 1965). For example, it is not so much that patients are ignorant of prescribed behaviors, but that they perceive it to be harmless to disobey doctor's orders.

Dispite this postulate, advocated by role theoriests such as Ralph Turner (1968), the main focus of role theorists has been on how individuals adjust and adapt to the demands of others. In this sense much of our social action is envisaged as orderly and overtly structured.

Role Conflict Viewed as Deviance. Role theorists are cognizant of strain and strife in the social structure. In fact they have defined such concepts as the following: role conflict, which refers to contradictions among expectations (Getzels & Guba, 1954; Merton, 1949; Newcomb, 1950; Parsons, 1951); role strain, which recognizes the impossibility of meeting all expectations (Goode, 1960b); and anomie, which is defined as the lack of clearcut expectations (Merton, 1949). However, it is assumed that potential conflicts become manifest only under unusual circumstances because potentially conflicting roles are usually nonoverlapping and involve different times and contexts (Newcomb, 1950). For instance, the latent role conflict of a man who is a father and a mental patient may be attenuated by the fact that he is not accompanied by his family when visiting a psychiatrist's office.

Symbolic Interactionism

In contrast to role theory, which views human interaction as structured by expectations, symbolic interactionists tend to conceptualize reciprocal social exchange as the strategic adjustments and readjustments of players in a game.

Symbolic Communication. As the term *symbolic interaction* indicates, this theory is concerned with human interaction by means of symbols and gestures. George Herbert Mead claimed that the human mind is superior to that of lower animals because it has the capacity to create and use symbols (e.g., language) to designate objects in the environment. Furthermore, the human ability to agree upon the meaning of vocal and bodily syumbols and gestures (e.g., words, voice inflection, facial expression, bodily stance, and dress) enhances the effectiveness of communication (Mead, 1934; Strauss, 1964).

Stressing the importance of symbols even further, Erving Goffman (1959) views social interaction as a cool and calculating management of impressions and gestures. This means that the crucial aspect of game playing is not the conscientious enactment of the game's requirements nor the consequence of the player's performance. It is the appearance a person gives while discharging the game's requirements that is important. After all, only one's appearance is visible to the opponents. Hence, good bedside manners (e.g., sympathetic tone of voice) are frequently appreciated more by patients than is the technical competence of doctors.

Role Taking. Another component of symbolic interactionism is the human capacity to "take the role of others," that is, to "put oneself in another's place." As Mead noted, humans are able to assume the dispositions, needs, and perspectives of those with whom they interact. By taking the role of others, individuals seek to ascertain the direction in which others are going to act. This information in turn enables the actors to assess the consequences of their actions. Having anticipated what goes on in the minds of others, individuals can covertly rehearse the alternative lines of action they can take toward others, and they can select what appears to be the most strategic course of action (Meltzer, 1964).

This ability to empathize, analyze, and act is a learned process, according to Mead, who delineated the stages in the development of the role-playing self. In the first stage, called "play," the child is only capable of taking on a limited number of roles, such as that of the mother or a teacher. Later, as the child matures biologically and gains experience in role taking, the individual grows competent and can assume the roles of several others who are engaged in some organized activity. Mead called this evolutionary stage a "game." Eventually, the individual learns the sum of the viewpoints and expectations of the social group or community. The attitudes of the group become incorporated into the structure of the self, thereby giving the individual a unity of self.

Tentative Nature of Interaction. Once an action is taken, additional cues or gestures are emitted by others. If these new cues are not consistent with those previously captured or with the imputed roles of others, the individual must modify his or her action of behavior. An actor must repeatedly re-evaluate and redefine the situation. Thus, interaction is seen as an emergent, tentative, negotiated, and frequently unpredictable process rather than as a well-defined structure.

At the macro level, symbolic interactionists consider that society is in a constant state of flux and is rife with potential change. As such, society is viewed as consisting of a pattern that is altered and reconstructed through the interaction of individuals.

Labeling Theory

As an offshoot of symbolic interaction, the labeling theory emerged to explain deviance.

Labeling: Definition of the Situation. The labeling theory is based on the premise that the definition of a situation makes that situation real. Thus, a behavior is deviant to the extent that it is defined and labeled as such by a person who has behaved in a special way and by those who have observed that behavior (Gove, 1975b; Schur, 1971).

One of the most fundamental distinctions made by labeling theorists involves the difference between primary and secondary deviance (Lemert, 1951, 1967). Primary deviance refers to rule breaking that has not provoked public reaction. It is episodic and of little significance. An occasional shoplifting act, speeding without receiving a traffic ticket, or experimental homosexual activity are some example of primary deviance.

Secondary deviance is a behavior that has been stigmatized as deviance by others and has generated a deviant identity in the individual. To labeling theorists, deviance is not the quality of an act but rather is the product of the interaction between a person who commits an act and those who respond to it (Becker, 1963; Erikson, 1962).

Norms and Labeling. Despite the heritage of symbolic interactionism, many labeling formulations present a passive view of an actor controlled by norms. The postulate that deviance is in the eyes of beholder does not preclude that many observers simultaneously preceive an unusual act as deviance. These similarities in perception serve as norms in the labeling process.

These norms also imply a power relation between the labelers and the labeled. First, the more powerful the labeler, the greater the impact upon the labeled. Thus, official labeling (e.g., police arrest, hospitalization) is more likely to affect the individual than is the informal labeling by friends and relatives. Second, it is postulated that the more powerful a person is, the less likely he or she is to be labeled and channeled into a deviant role.

Exchange Theory

Social exchange theory is viewed by some (Rossides, 1978; Shortell, 1972) as a subset of the social interactionist perspective. This is because exchange theory begins with the analysis of micro-level interaction among individuals. However, in the classification of sociological theories (Wagner, 1963), exchange theory has been located in various categories: in a separate and independent niche (Turner, 1978); as a part of functionalism (Demerath & Peterson, 1967; Martindale, 1960); dialectic theory (Turner, 1978); and so on. As Turner (1978) observes, exchange theory is based on a synthesis of diverse theoretical traditions such as utilitarianism, functionalism, conflict theory, and psychological behaviorism as well as interactionism.

Interactional Postulates. Initially, exchange theory focuses upon face-to-face interaction among individuals. The basic tenet of exchange theory, as developed by George Homans (1950, 1961), Peter Blau (1964), and John W. Thibault and H. H. Kelley (1959), states that interaction is a social behavior whereby the individual actions have *cost* and *reward* implications. Here the term *reward* refers to a positive reinforcement in any form that gratifies a person's needs. An individual is motivated to enter social interaction with others if he or she perceives that it will be more rewarding than costly.

In assessing costs and rewards, each actor assumes the perspectives of another to discern the other's needs. In Meadian terms, the individual "takes the role of others." Actors then manipulate symbolic representations of themselves to impress others as if they possess something that is highly desirable. However, people operate under the principle of *reciprocity.* All exchanges are presumed to be carried out so that those who bestow benefits upon others will in turn receive rewards as payment for their service.

From Micro to Macro Analysis. Unlike symbolic interactionists, who concentrate on micro analysis, and functionalists, whose primary concern is with the macro level of social structure, exchange theorists attempt to build a bridge between the two. Having conceptualized simple, direct exchange processes in small-group interactional networks, exchange theorists claim that the same set of principles and laws are applicable to the exchange processes in larger social systems.

Functionalist Assumptions. To explain the link between elementary face-to-face interaction and more complex patterns, exchange theorists use the concept of institutionalization.

At some point in history there are some people who have the "capital" (e.g., food, money, moral code, leadership quality) to provide rewards to others. By investing the capital in some new activities, these people can induce others, through rewards or threats of punishment, to engage in activities that would further increase the rewards for all the participants. Such an organization of activities becomes more efficient when explicit norms and rules regulate exchange relations. Norms regularize exchange relations and eliminate conflict bargaining. This increased efficiency allows greater organization of activities. Such a patterning of social interaction in ways that reduce the possibility for tension, conflict, and deviance is called *institutionalization.*

In line with functionalism, exchange theorists postulate the importance of shared values. Participants in an exchange must be socialized into a common set of values that constitute "fair exchange" in a given situation. However, unlike functionalists, exchange theorists view institutionalization in a much more flexible manner. Definitions of reciprocity are not treated as absolute but are to be worked out in the course of social interaction, which is rife with strain and tension. Furthermore, institutionalized patterns of interaction must ultimately yield returns for the reward-seeking individuals involved.

Dialectic Conflict Elements. Exchange theorists assume that humans have primary needs that frequently are at variance with the rewards provided by social structures. Thus, an inherent dialectic is postulated in the exchange process. The failure to receive expected rewards leads actors to attempt to apply negative sanctions or to retaliate against those who have violated the norm of fair exchange. The more the exchange relations become unbalanced, the greater the possibility for conflict.

Sources of conflict are identified in (1) unequal distribution of valued resources, (2) unbalanced exchange relations, (3) violation of norms of reciprocity, and (4) the inevitable forces of opposition to power.

Application to Medical Sociology

Society and the Individual

Since the focus of interactionism is upon micro social units, except for exchange theory, it is difficult to use this theory in analyzing social phenomena on a societal level. One of the limited areas of application involves the social definition of illness, provided there is a certain degree of consensus. According to labeling theory, society will label illness as a deviance in a consensus that the individual is different and bad.

Although interactionism is not generally applicable to the macro study of societies, one of its variants, role theory, is useful in analyzing human behavior in terms of social status and role (Gordon, 1966). Knowledge of one's identity or social position is a powerful index of behavior, including health and illness behavior. Thus, from a role theory point of view, correspondence may exist between social roles and types of illness. For instance, a corporate executive who is expected to fulfill demanding tasks is likely to suffer from symptoms of stress and exhaustion that may lead to high blood pressure (Chapter 4).

Medicine as a Social System

If we shift our attention from society to smaller medical subsystems, we find a greater use of interactionism. For example, the doctor–patient relationship (Chapter 5) is an ideal example of a small group that can be explained by symbolic interactionism.

If we follow the symbolic interactionism of Mead, we can predict that a patient will have an active voice in structuring the interaction. On the other hand, labeling theory will view the whole process as one in which a doctor labels a client as sick, and the latter simply accepts that situation.

The professional system of physicians (Chapter 6) can be viewed as a network of interactions. At work, informal collegial interaction serves a supervisorial function over their medical practices. Until recently, control of the quality of medical care has been left largely to informal peer group sanctions because of the norm of professional autonomy. Off-work, informal strategic interaction through a local medical society is important to many physicians because it may increase or decrease patient referrals.

The behavior of physicians in referring patients to other physicians has been examined from an exchange theory standpoint of social costs and rewards to the interacting physicians. The possible rewards for the referring physician include procuring high quality treatment for his or her patients and the possibility of return referral; on the other hand, referral may cost the physician additional income. The consultant's reward lies in enhancing his or her professional image as well as increased financial compensation. The cost may be receiving undersirable patients.

Physicians have maintained their elitist status not only by political lobbying but also have used effective labeling and interactional tactics. By labeling themselves "regular" and other health practitioners (e.g., chiropractors) as "irregular," physicians have managed to keep the latter in a subordinate position (Chapter 8). Furthermore, a physician's informal association with an irregular practitioner was sometimes considered to be unethical conduct and could be used to revoke membership in the AMA.

The study of behavior regularities using role theory has been particularly useful for hospitals (Chapter 7). There, the process of recruitment, socialization, and interaction can easily be examined in terms of occupational roles and statuses. In a hospital, that which is left unexplained by role theory may be elucidated by symbolic interactionism. For instance, from the point of view of role theory, a nurse's position is a difficult one because it is subject to two sets of frequently conflicting demands that come from the medical and the administrative staff. On the other hand, from the perspective of symbolic interaction, a nurse who is in close contact with doctors as well as administrators is in a strategic position to manipulate both.

Perhaps the most widely used model of interactionism is the labeling theory as it is applied to mental hospitalization. Labeling theorists claim that many of those who come to be typed as deviant, that is, mentally ill, are *created* through the labeling processes conducted by bureaucratic organizations such as a mental hospital (Goffman, 1961; Hawkins & Tiedeman, 1975).

When persons with minor behavioral symptoms come to a mental hospital, voluntarily or involuntarily, they are likely to perceive themselves as normal people with some difficulties. However, admission procedures, diagnostic sessions, and daily routines in the hospital serve to categorize them with sterotyped labels of mental patients (e.g., schizophrenic, homosexual, neurotic). The setting, the house rules, and the staff treatment press home the fact that the patient is, after all, a mental case.

This labeling process is not limited to mental hospitals but is found in other locales such as long-term hospitals for the physically disabled and the chronically ill, and in nursing homes.

Medicine Within a Social System

Interaction between medical and other social systems can be examined on a micro level through the personal interactions of individuals who have come from different social systems.

For instance, the type of interaction that is crucial to the emergence and survival of neighborhood health centers (Chapter 9) is between the professional medical staff members and the people of the community. While the medical staff represents the upper-middle class and a professional group, the people who use neighborhood health centers are from the working class and nonprofessional groups. Success or failure of the neighborhood health center largely depends upon effective communications between menbers representing these two groups.

As was pointed out earlier, interactionism is not amenable to the study of interrelations between large groups on a societal level. One exception is found in the use of labeling theory to describe the role played by organized medicine. In line with the labeling postulate, the AMA, as a power group, has been successful in providing official definitions and in using labels such as health, illness, and the "American way." For example, when the AMA was opposing public health insurance, they labeled it as an unAmerican practice.

Another way to use interactionism in the macro studies of intergroup dynamics is to observe personal interactions between members of different groups (e.g., doctors and politicians) so that generalizations based on micro units can be extended to macro groups. This is methodologically difficult due to the fact that intergroup interaction is frequently carried out by mediators (e.g., hired lobbyists) rather than by genuine group members.

SUMMARY

In this chapter, three major sociological theories—functionalism, conflict theories, and interactionism—are introduced and their relevance to medical sociology is discussed in relation to the substantive material in the remainder of this book.

Prevailing postulates of functionalism include the following: (1) social events, human behavior, and attitudes are best understood if they are viewed as forming a social system; (2) the component parts of the system make positive contributions to the system, and they work together with an internal consistency because they are guided by commonly shared values; (3) there are certain functions that are indispensable to the survival of the system; and (4) the system has a self-regulating mechanism to maintain its equilibrium.

In contrast to the integrative assumption of functionalism, conflict theorists posit that conflict is endemic in society. There are two schools of conflict theory: dialectic and functional. While the former postulates that any social item or group has in itself its own contradictions, which are the source of conflict, the latter finds that some conflicts have integrative consequences for the system.

In comparison with the normative regulation of behavior assumed by functionalists, interactionists stress the active role played by an individual in interpreting and manipulating social situations. Within the interactional framework, role theory concerns the networks of social positions and their associated expectations, while symbolic interactionism emphasizes the individual's power in affecting interactional processes.

The pertinence of these theories to sociomedical data has been briefly discussed. Using the functionalist approach as a point of departure, society is viewed as a social system that contains subsystems such as medicine, the polity, the economy, and so on. Within the medical subsystem, smaller subunits such as the doctor–patient relationship, the medical profession, and hospitals are identified.

In the remainder of this book, each system and subsystem will first be subjected to functional analysis to test the integrative postulate of functionalism. Then, conflict perspectives will be used to examine the systems when those theories correspond to reality better than functionalism. Finally, micro units for personal interaction will be described within and between the larger social systems, and interactionist interpretations will be attempted.

We often hear that a plan of action is all right *in theory* but it will not work *in practice.* The criticism is valid if it means that a given theory does not provide a solution to a particular case, when that case meets all the conditions specified by the theory. After all, "theory is *of* practice, and must stand or fall with its practicality" (Kaplan, 1964, p. 296). However, this attack on theorizing is unwarranted if it concerns success or failure in an inappropriate application. Doctors do become sick and psychiatrists do commit suicide not because the theory of disease is invalid but rather because of the doctors' inadequacy in applying the theories they preach.

An important criterion for acceptability of a theory is its correspondence with reality. A theory must fit the facts. In the process of testing the validity of a theory, however, there is a danger that a theoretical framework may limit the type of data to be assembled and processed. In order to avoid this abuse of a theory, a wide range of facts must be brought to bear upon the theory. Research findings should not be used only to revise and improve existing theories but also to stimulate new theories (Merton, 1957).

In the following chapters available data will be examined within the frameworks of major sociological theories so that (1) meaningful, coherent, and systematic interpretations can be provided, (2) validity of these theories can be compared, and (3) further research might be stimulated to fill theoretical, methodological, and substantive gaps.

CHAPTER 3

Characteristics of Diseases

In the previous chapters we have established that medical sociology emerged from (1) the medical practitioner's concern about social causes of illness in response to the inadequacy of germ theory; and (2) the sociologist's interest in fitting illness into the general theoretical frameworks of sociology. Thus the quest for sociological causes of diseases is one of the major concerns of medical sociology.

Etiology is important in science because knowledge of the causation of a phenomenon enables us to predict and control the occurrence of the phenomenon. The following two chapters deal with sociological factors that have been associated with the occurrence of diseases. But before we examine research findings on social etiology in Chapter 4, we need to know the characteristics of what we are going to study. The study of the causes of diseases presumes the existence of valid definitions and measurements of health and ill health.

Therefore this chapter begins with official definitions of health and disease from dictionaries and statements of health organizations. Having noted the vagueness of these definitions, we will proceed to operational definitions, namely, statistical measures of normality and abnormality. Despite inherent biases in statistical definitions of health, they are the commonly used instruments in health surveys. Hence, basic concepts in health statistics are briefly introduced.

The second major task of this chapter is to familiarize ourselves with terms used in health surveys to designate and classify various diseases.

Finally, in order to give guidelines for interpreting the data in Chapter 4, conceptual frameworks for causal analysis of diseases are discussed. This chapter closes with a proposal for a synthetic etiological scheme based on existing causal models of diseases.

DEFINITION OF HEALTH AND ILL HEALTH

Definition of Ill Health

Disease Model. The medical view of health places emphasis on detection and alleviation of disease. Since the emergence of germ theory, modern medical practice has leaned toward biological theories in diagnosing symptoms and treating disease. Thus, conditions are defined as diseased when impairment of bodily functioning can be recognized through physical symptoms by physicians who are knowledgeable of biological theories. Disease is seen as a physiological imbalance caused by outside agents (e.g., germs, stress) (Siegler & Osmond, 1974).

However, this disease model has been challenged by those who emphasize the interplay of host, agent, and environment. They advocate the notion that disease can be defined or interpreted not only by physicians as biological conditions but by patients, other people, and by society as a whole as psychological or sociological malfunctioning.

The applicability of the disease model has been debated, especially in the field of psychiatry. The proponents of the disease model in psychiatry (Lewis, 1953) state that behavior which is *socially* inappropriate or deviant does not provide a sufficient basis for its being labeled as mental illness. They claim that pathological criteria, such as those applied in evaluating physical diseases, should be used in diagnosing mental illness. The disease model has proven effective in the case of some psychoactive drugs, whose use has contributed to the decline of mental hospitalization since the mid-1950s.

However, the weakness of this approach lies in the vagueness of the concept of psychiatric pathology. Spitzer and Wilson (1975) note that most psychiatric impairments do not meet the four criteria for a physiological dysfunction: (1) a specific etiology such as a germ, (2) qualitative difference from normal functioning, (3) a demonstrable physical change, and (4) internal physiological process, largely independent of external environment.

In his article, "The Myth of Mental Illness," Thomas Szasz (1960, 1963) contends that, except for particular mental disorders caused by brain dysfunctions, the disease model is irrelevant to psychiatry. He observes that most of the symptoms labeled mental illnesses do not show demonstrable physical lesions but rather are deviations from psychosocial, ethical, or legal norms. For example, Szasz states that

> "excessive repression" or "acting out an unconscious impulse" illustrates the use of the psychological concept for judging (so-called) mental health and illness. The idea that chronic hostility, vengefulness, or divorce are indicative of mental illness would be illustrations of the use of ethical norms. . . . Finally, the widespread psychiatric opinion that a mentally ill person would commit homicide illustrates the use of a legal concept as a norm of mental health (Szasz, 1960, p. 114).

The problem, as Szasz sees it, is the discrepancy between such psychosocial and ethical definitons of mental illness and the biomedical remedies sought in psychiatry, which are assumed to be free from ethical values. Szasz's criticism that the concept of mental illness is confusing and therefore is frequently abused is well taken. However, health and ill health are multidimensional concepts and cannot be specified by either biological or sociocultural factors alone.

Dictionaries define disease as a condition of the living animal or plant body or of one of its parts that impairs the performance of a vital function. Here, the word *vital* needs further clarification; its definition as "existing as a manifestation of life" is not specific enough when considering someone such as Karen Ann Quinlan, who was sustained in a vegetative state by a life-supporting mechanism. Does life mean heartbeat, consciousness, or social interaction?

Disease, Illness, and Sickness. In our daily conversation, terms such as *disease, illness,* and *sickness* are frequently used interchangeably to denote the opposite of health. Because of the multidimensionality of unhealthy states, sociologists have come to attach different meanings to such concepts (Twaddle & Hessler, 1977, p. 97). The term *disease* is used to refer to objective conditions in which the internal functioning of the body as a biological organism is impaired. The diagnosis of a disease is made by correlating the observable symptoms of the body with knowledge of its functioning. Symptoms may or may not be manifest, and they may be objective (a rise in body temperature), or subjective (pain).

Illness is a subjective phenomenon in which individuals perceive themselves as not feeling well and therefore may tend to modify their normal behavior. Experiences with weakness, dizziness, nausea, or anxiety may fall into this category. Illness is usually assumed to be caused by disease, and vice versa. A cancer patient may not feel ill at all until he or she is diagnosed as such by a physician. A person who has lost a job may feel ill without having contracted any disease.

While disease is a physical concept, and illness is a psychological concept, *sickness* is a sociological concept. When a person is defined by others as being unhealthy, his or her social identity shifts to that of a sick person. The incumbent of a sick role is exempt from normal social functioning but must conform to the norms associated with the sick role.

Perspectives on Health

The absence of disease is a necessary but not a sufficient condition for health. The World Health Organization (1946) defines health as "a state of complete physical, mental, and social wellbeing, and not merely the absence of disease and infirmity." Herbert Spencer defined health as the perfect adjustment of an organism to its environment (Fletcher, 1971). It is characteristic of such definitions to give attention to psychic and social variables, including the individual's capacity to operate effectively in his or her environment. A healthy individual is one who can avoid pain, but more positively, a healthy individual has a joyous attitude toward life's challenges.

Among various definitions of health, Schlenger (1976) identified two conceptually distinct dimensions: equilibrium and actualization. The *equilibrium* scale ranges from death through disequilibrium (disease, imbalance) to balance. By *balance* is meant optimal functioning of the body system. Disease results from outside agents (e.g., germs, stress) acting on the physiological system to disrupt its equilibrium.

While the goal of the equilibrium aspect of health is the maintenance of a steady state, the *actualization* component of health refers to the generation of growth and change. It involves effective dealing with the environment by actualizing one's potential. This definition stresses what has become known as positive health, an approach emphasizing activity and growth as seen in the self-care movement and related movements. Here, health is perceived as an asymptote, an ideal on the horizon that can be approached but never reached.

An assessment of health depends on (1) the current state of the equilibrium process, (2) the current state of the actualization process, and (3) the interaction between the two. Thus, one may actualize oneself within limits in the face of terminal illness. It is also possible to reduce the morbidity rate without increasing the feeling of health.

Operational Definition

What is common to many definitions of health is asymptotic, open-ended, or elastic conceptualization. From the viewpoint of measurement of health, open-ended definitions present various problems (Callahan, 1973). Where do we draw a cutting line on the continuum to differentiate good health from ill health?

For operational purposes, a statistical definition has frequently been used as the major device for arriving at norms. Doctors can recognize a disease because the patient deviates from normal values that have been established through observations of normal populations over a period of time.

Official statistics are used to compare the levels of health in various social groups. Statistics such as the death rate and life expectancy in different societies are contrasted so that norms will be derived to distinguish healthy from unhealthy groups, or developed from underdeveloped countries. For instance, we frequently hear that a country has reached a certain stage of civilization because its infant death rate has been reduced to such and such.

To delineate the configuration of the health status of a population, statistical distribution curves have been devised. Allport (1934) demonstrated the applicability of the normal distribution curve (i.e., bell-shaped) to a population when there is no rule for a given behavior, and the adoption of the J-curve in reverse when the population is under a behavioral regulation.

Paterson (1964) extended the analysis further and drew a threshold toward the tail end of Allport's J-curve in reverse to separate the normal from the abnormal. Paterson further postulated that the location of the threshold is determined by the strength of the rule imposed upon the population.

The difficulty in using a statistical definition of normality stems from the assumption that what most people do is normal. Thus, many physical symptoms can be ignored if they are experienced by a large portion of the people. To illustrate, poor eyesight, bad posture, or fatigue due to malnutrition that is exhibited in a poor neighborhood may be considered normal in that environment.

The use of official statistics as definition and measurement of health entails further biases. Problems are aggravated because there is a tendency to accept official statistics as "official," hence legitimate and infallible.

To begin with, there are problems in defining the population to be used in health statistics. For example, division and classification of study populations are not made solely according to objective characteristics but are affected by power relations (Petersen, 1969). While the dominant whites are subdivided into categories by ethnicity, the subordinate groups are likely to be lumped together as nonwhites, Asians, others, and the like. Not only is it true that the definition of a population affects its size but it also skews health statistics, hence invalidating much of the analysis.

In accepting official statistics, care must be taken in interpreting what the figures really mean. Officially recorded illneses indicate reported cases rather than actual illnesses and often include only medically attended incidents. For example, higher rates of schizophrenia in uban than rural areas may be a function of the availability of psychiatric facilities. Also, higher rates of illness among females than males may reflect a stronger tendency among women than men to seek medical care. A more detailed interpretation of these issues will be presented in Chapter 4.

Statistical data may imply cultural value orientations (Opler, 1959). According to Zborowski's (1952) study, there are marked ethnic differences in reaction to pain. While "old Americans" are stoic about pain, Jews and Italians are ready to express their feelings of pain emotionally. In addition, he observed that Italians are concerned with immediate relief from pain, as compared with Jews who show future-oriented anxiety as to the physical implications of the pain. Follow-up studies conducted by others have indicated that Jews are more inclined to use medical facilities for preventive medicine (Linn, 1967; Scheff, 1966a; Segal et al., 1965; Silverman, 1964; Zola, 1966). Cultural variation in the seeking of health care is dealt with in Chapter 5.

Setting aside methodological and interpretive biases, we still must question the validity of statistical figures as measures of health. With advances in technology, what is considered to be normal at one time will be considered abnormal at a later time. Each new device, such as sphygmomanometers or electrocardiographs, that helps physicians determine the presence or absence of diseases, tends to encourage physicians to classify an increasing proportion of the population as unhealthy. Also, diseases that are unknown today will nonetheless be present in a population that is currently thought to be healthy.

MEASUREMENT: BASIC CONCEPTS IN VITAL STATISTICS

In search of satisfactory definitions of health and disease, there has been a great deal of debate between health administrators and researchers. Some even go so far as to maintain that a good definition is not possible or even is unnecessary (Wylie, 1970). Despite this disagreement, certain measurements have been officially used to determine and record community health.

Vital statistics are officially accepted measures of births, deaths, marriages, health, and disease, and are internationally standarized. As so-called maps and milestones of public health, they are used to compare various social groups such as nations, local areas, age groups, social classes, ethnic groups, and the like.

Vital statistics can be obtained systematically in three ways: (1) by registration, which may be defined as the continuous and permanent recording of the occurrence and the characteristics of vital events (births, marriages, deaths), primarily for their value as legal documents and secondarily for their usefulness as a source of statistics; (2) by enumeration, represented by the census of populations and by sickness surveys; and (3) by special returns—notifications of infectious disease, certificates of incapacity for work, abstracts of hospital case records, and the like.

Mortality. Mortality refers to the number of deaths relative to a population in a given time and place. The basis of mortality statistics is the information recorded during the registration of a death. This information includes the date and place of death, the name and usual place of residence of the deceased, his or her sex, age, and occupation, and the cause of death.

The *crude death rate* is calculated by dividing the total number of deaths registered in a given period by the estimated number of the total population. The denominator is usually taken for convenience as the estimated population at the mid-point of the period, which is often a year.

$$\text{Crude death rate for 1980 per 1,000} = \frac{\text{Total deaths, all ages, 1980}}{\text{Estimated population on June 30, 1980}} \times 1{,}000$$

The crude death rate is useful only for gross comparison because it obscures the fact that certain age, sex, ethnic, occupational, and other categories have differing rates of death. From the crude death rate we are not able to determine whether men have a higher mortality rate than women, or whether infants have a higher death rate than adults. In order to make such observations, a *specific rate* for a specific category is computed. For instance, a sex–age specific rate is calculated by dividing the number of deaths of persons in a given sex–age category (e.g., males, aged 50–54) by the number of persons in that group at mid-period.

$$\text{Sex-age specific per 1,000 males, aged 50-54} = \frac{\text{Deaths of males, aged 50-54, 1980}}{\text{Estimated male population, aged 50-54, June 30, 1980}} \times 1{,}000$$

A death rate has little meaning on its own. It is only when comparisons are made that death rates assume significance. For purposes of comparison of death rates, say from one time to another or from area to area, it is important that misleading factors caused by the demographic compositions of the populations (e.g., age and sex) be eliminated. A crude death rate of a population may be relatively high merely because the population has a large proportion of elderly and retired people whose death rates are naturally above average.

The procedure for adjusting the crude death rates to discard the effect of population composition with respect to age and other variables is sometimes called *standardization.* Suppose we want to compare age-standardized mortality rates of various countries, say Japan, relative to that of the United States, which is used as a standard population. Standardization involves (1) applying the age-specific death rates of the Japanese to the age-specific subpopulations of the United States, (2) computing the expected number of deaths that would occur in each age-specific standard population (the United States), (3) summing the deaths, and (4) computing a new overall death rate by dividing the sum of the deaths by the total standard population (the United States).

The *life table* is one form of combining mortality rates of a population at different ages into a single statistical model. In its simplest form, the entire table is generated from age-specific mortality rates and the resulting values are used to measure mortality, survivorship, and life expectation.

The life table shows how a hypothetical cohort of individuals would die off, from birth on, if the cohort were subject to the mortality rates of specified years and time span. The average length of life experienced by this cohort, from the time they were born until they die, is the expectation of life.

One of the advantages of the life table is that it does not reflect the effects of the age distribution of an actual population, and, therefore, it does not require the adoption of a standard population for acceptable comparison.

Morbidity. Morbidity refers to the extent to which a given population is diseased. It can be measured in terms of three units: (1) persons who are ill, (2) the number of spells of illness that are experienced, and (3) the duration of these illnesses.

Morbidity statistics must take several factors into account that do not affect mortality statistics. Unlike death, illness may occur many times to the same person. Its duration can range from hours to years. It may vary in severity from the most trivial to the most serious and from a minimum disability to a lengthy hospitalization.

An important distinction is made in morbidity statistics between incidence and prevalence. *Incidence* refers to the occurrence of new cases of disease within a specified period of time within a specified population. Since it provides information as to how a disease first appears in a population, it is useful when studying the causes of disease.

Prevalence, in contrast, indicates the number of all cases of a disease in a given population during a specific time period disregarding when the disease first attacked a person. A knowledge of prevalence is useful in estimating the magnitude of existing health problems, which in turn help in planning the purchases and distribution of health resources efficiently.

It should be noted that the incidence and prevalence of certain diseases are quite different. For example, chronic disease that is counted in the incidence statistics in one year will be counted again and again in the prevalence studies during succeeding years. Because of this cumulative effect, the prevalence of chronic illness may be higher than its incidence.

An example is venereal disease, whose prevention and therapy have progressed to the extent that both the incidence and prevalence are fairly low among adults. However, among teen-agers who have become sexually liberated without adequate sexual education, the incidence of venereal disease has risen recently. Once they realize that they have contracted such a disease, however, they are likely to rush to the clinics for therapy, which helps keep the prevalence low.

TYPES OF DISEASES

Before examining vital statistics and other health data, one should be familiar with official and nonofficial classifications of diseases. Diseases will be categorized, first in the broad categories of communicable, chronic, and mental (Coe, 1978); and then in relation to the functioning of physiological systems.

Communicable, Chronic, and Mental Diseases

Communicable Diseases. Exposure is an important variable in the analysis of communicable diseases such as diphtheria, dysentery, measles, small pox, typhoid fever, and gonorrhea. Most such illnesses are caused by a variety of microorganisms that become parasites of the human host. A primary method of prevention is to break the chain of transmission, that is, to prevent the carrier from reaching and infecting a new host. Sanitation and immunization represent the first steps in reducing the danger of contact between a disease agent and a noninfected host. Once a host is exposed to the disease bacteria, however, secondary prevention is provided by drugs, particularly antibiotics, to arrest the growth or to actually destroy the disease germs already at work in the body.

Typically, a communicable disease has an incubation period between the time of infection and the time when the first symptoms of the illness appear. If the infected person has a strong internal coping ability or an immunity, the infection may be contained by the body's defenses. If not, and if the body has gone through the automatic tissue responses to the disease germ, the individual will begin to exhibit manifest symptoms at the end of the incubation period. Eventually, the body may repair itself, with or without medical intervention, or the patient may die.

Fortunately, most communicable disease, such as the common cold, are self-limiting in that their effects do not pass beyond a relatively short period of time, which is termed the *disease cycle.* Of course there are some negative exceptions, such as streptococal infections, where the disease can have aftereffects that bring about permanent structural damage.

Chronic Diseases. Chronic diseases include arthritis, cancer, heart disease, rheumatic fever, syphilis, tuberculosis, and others. Most of them are not contagious, and their causes cannot be traced to a single agent as is the case in communicable diseases. For example, many chronic diseases involve the degeneration of tissue and the dysfunction of vital organs. In some cases, however, those conditions are simply due to processes of senescence.

Unlike communicable diseases, the cycle for chronic diseases is not self-limiting, and they are insidiously characterized by chronicity. Even worse, the deterioration of tissue or organ functions usually has made considerable progress by the time the individual actually feels ill. For that reason, the individual rarely fully recovers from a chronic ailment.

In contrast to communicable maladies, chronic diseases do not seem to have simple or singular origins, and that characteristic is the basis for the theory of multiple causation for chronic diseases. This theory has not only led researchers to investigate social variables (particularly the factor of social stress) and physical variables, but their interactions have been examined as well.

Mental Diseases. There is much less consensus on the classification of mental disorders than on the nomenclature of physical diseases. Mental symptoms are frequently subjective in nature and depend on sociocultural norms. In order to reduce unreliability due to varying diagnostic criteria used by clinicians, the American Psychiatric Association set forth the standard diagnostic nomenclature—the *Diagnostic and Statistical Manual of Mental Disorders*—the first edition (DSM-I) having appeared in 1952, the second edition (DSM-II) in 1968, and the third edition (DSM-III) currently being drafted.

Since a large portion of the research data presented in Chapter 4 is based on the DSM-II classification, the DSM-II is explained briefly here. According to this system, mental disorders are classified as follows: mental retardation, organic brain syndromes (psychotic and nonpsychotic), psychoses (schizophrenia, affective psychoses, paranoid states, and others), neuroses, personality disorders, psychophysiologic disorders (psychosomatic), and transient situational distrubances.

From the sociological perspective, an important distinction should be made between organic and functional mental disorders, although there frequently is an overlap between the two. *Organic* disorders are those in which the cause can be attributed to some identifiable physical malfunction such as syphilitic paresis, pellagrous dementia, or bacterial infection of the brain. *Functional* disorders refer to those affecting physiological or psychological functions without a known organic cause or structural change. Care must be taken in studying the symptoms as they can reveal either organic or functional disorders.

An organic brain disorder is a basic mental impairment caused by the actual weakening of brain tissue functions. The resulting syndromes are grouped into psychotic and nonpsychotic disorders according to the severity of the physical impairment. An important category of chronic brain syndromes consists of the mental disorders of old age. They are senile dementia and psychosis with cerebral arteriosclerosis, and they are characterized by symptoms such as confusion, suspicion, a lack of concern for amenities, and the loss of control of bodily functions. Although such disorders often result from organic causes, they are also related to other sociopsychological factors.

In the extreme case, the label of *insanity* is generally given to a psychotic reaction that results in such a gross derangement of mental processes that there is no longer a capacity to perceive reality correctly. Such psychoses can be attributed either to physical conditions (organic brain syndromes), functional conditions (schizophrenia or manic depression), or both.

Schizophrenia includes a group of disorders that are characterized by (1) disturbance of thinking, involving alterations of concept formation, misinterpretations of reality, delusions, or hallucinations; and (2) mood disorder, where ambivalence, constricted or inappropriate emotional responsiveness, or a loss of empathy with others occur.

Manic-depressive psychoses are marked by severe mood swings, such that the patient has periods of manic excitement and euphoria and then periods of extreme despair and depression. Psychotics in this category are classed as the manic type, depressive type, or the circular type, depending upon the dominance of the mood.

Neuroses have anxiety as their chief characteristic. Anxiety may be felt and expressed directly, it may be controlled unconsciously, or it may be channeled into indirect defense mechanisms. In contrast to the psychoses, the neuroses manifest neither gross distortion, misinterpretation of external reality, nor do they result in gross personality disorganization, except in the case of hysterical neurosis.

Psychosomatic disorders are those syndromes that manifest themselves in a physiological malfunction without any apparent organic cause, and as such they are usually purely functional.

Although DSM-II has been in use for ten years, it has been challenged by many psychiatrists who are currently drafting the third version, DSM-III. The basic approach of DSM-III is atheoretical with regard to etiology or pathophysiological process except for well-established cases. This approach is justified in that the inclusion of etiological theories in DSM-III would be an obstacle to its use by clinicians of different theoretical orientations, since DSM-III cannot include all etiological theories. What DSM-III attempts to do is to describe *what* the manifestations of mental disorders are, but not to account for *how* the disturbances come about ("Current DSM-III . . . ," 1978; Spitzer, 1979).

One of the most controversial issues in drafting DSM-III has been the category of neurosis. The term neurosis was eliminated in the earlier draft of DSM-III but was included later. At present there is no consensus as to how to define neurosis. Some clinicians limit the term to its descriptive meaning, whereas others imply specific etiological process. Many psychodynamically oriented psychiatrists think that the exclusion of neurotic disorder is a step backward, throwing out already accumulated psychodynamic knowledge (Spitzer, 1979; Spitzer, Endicott, & Robins, 1975; Spitzer & Wilson, 1975; "Trustees to draft . . . ," 1979).

While this debate is yet to be resolved, many empirical research projects are being conducted to test the validity and reliability of proposed drafts of DSM-III

(Abrams & Taylor, 1976; Fauman, 1977; Hyler & Spitzer, 1978; Spitzer, 1979). A brief explanation of the functioning of the human body and of the diseases associated with physiological systems is useful before looking at the medical terminologies used for the classification of diseases in vital statistics. The body systems have been variously classified depending on how much detail one wishes to include. Following is one list consisting of eight body systems (Davies, 1969; Memmler & Rada, 1970; Sodeman & Sodeman, 1967).

Circulatory System. The circulatory system contains approximately sixty thousand miles of veins, arteries, capillaries, and the like, all of which are connected in some way to the heart. The heart pumps blood to all the body tissues. The blood transports food, oxygen and other needed substances, and it carries away waste materials.

Heart diseases can be classified according to causative and age factors. Congenital heart disease refers to certain abnormalities present at birth. Rheumatic heart disease begins with an attack of rheumatic fever in childhood or youth, whereby bacteria may first involve the walls of the blood vessels, known as the coronary arteries, that supply blood to the muscle of the heart. Degenerative heart disease is common after the age of 45 and is due to deterioration of tissues such as muscles because of the prolonged effects of various disease conditions. High blood pressure, also known as hypertension, may cause an enlargement of the heart if it exists over a period of years, and it may finally cause heart failure.

Nervous System. The main components of the nervous system are the brain, the spinal cord, and the nerves, where the nerves reach every part of the skin's surface, plus all of the muscles, blood vessels, bones, etc. Their basic function is to receive, filter, and to send messages between the various parts of the body and the brain.

Organic disease of the nervous system is associated with permanent or temporary damage of the nervous system tissues or with abnormal mechanisms producing disturbance of function with or without recognizable damage to the nervous tissue.

Stroke (cerebral apoplexy), the most common kind of brain disorder, is a sudden diminution of consciousness, sensation, and voluntary motion caused by the rupture or obstruction of an artery of the brain. Such disorder is more frequent in the presence of artery wall disease, and hence is more common after the age of 40.

Digestive System. The digestive system is divided into two groups of organs: the alimentary canal and the accessory organs. The alimentary canal is a continuous passageway of over thirty feet beginning at the mouth, followed by the pharynx, the esophagus, the stomach, the intestine, and terminating at the anus. The accessory organs, while vitally necessary for the digestive process, are not part of the alimentary canal. They include the liver, the gallbladder, and the pancreas.

Two chief functions of the digestive system are (1) the digestion process, which converts food into a state in which it can be taken into the cells by way of the blood plasma, and (2) absorption, the process by which digested food is transferred to the blood stream.

Cancer frequently attacks parts of the digestive system, such as the throat, the colon, and particularly the stomach. Some people chronically suffer various forms of indigestion and heartburn, which though debilitating is usually not serious. A peptic ulcer is the disintegration and loss of tissues in the mucous membrane, and it can occur in the esophagus, stomach, or duodenum. Peptic ulcers are most frequently found in people between the ages of 30 and 45.

Of the accessory organs, the liver suffers most frequently from cancer or cirrhosis. The latter is a chronic disease, common to alcoholics, in which active liver cells are replaced by inactive scar tissue.

Respiratory System. The respiratory system includes the nasal cavities, the pharynx, the larynx, the tracheae (windpipe) and the lungs. Respiration has two aspects. The first, external respiration, is that which takes place only in the lungs, where oxygen from the outside air enters the blood, and carbon dioxide is taken off from the blood to be breathed into the outside air. The second aspect is called internal respiration, referring to the gas exchange of oxygen and carbon dioxide within the body cells.

In order for the lungs to perform their functions, they must be in constant contact with air, which may contain dust, bacteria, fungi, viruses, and various other noxious agents. For defense against those potentially harmful materials the respiratory tract possesses protective mechanisms such as cleansing, warming, and humidifying ventilated air. Disruption of these mechanisms by internal change or overwhelming attack from outside results in many respiratory diseases.

Some of the major respiratory diseases include influenza, pneumonia, bronchial asthma, emphysema, tuberculosis, and lung cancer.

Urogenital System. The urinary system contains kidneys, ureters, urinary bladder, and urethra, and its function is to remove certain waste products from the blood and to eliminate them from the body. The kidney is a pair of approximately five-inch long organs that filter a very large volume of blood without causing the body to lose too much of its water or other essential materials.

Nephritis means inflammation of the kidney tissue, and it is a result of infection or of certain degenerative changes in the kidney that may occur as a part of a generalized arteriosclerosis (disease of the veins and arteries). Chronic nephritis can lead to a potentially fatal condition known as uremia, which is an accumulation of urinary constituents in the blood. Kidney malfunctions can occur from tuberculosis, tumor, and kidney stones.

The reproductive system contains (1) sex glands or gonads, which produce the sex cells and manufacture hormones; (2) the tubes and passageways for the sex cells; and (3) the accessory organs. Tumor formation may involve the male reproductive organs, most commonly the prostate, and it is quite common in elderly men. Uterine and breast cancers are common in the female. Various forms of venereal diseases affect the reproductive system as well as other systems.

Endocrine System. The endocrine system refers to the scattered organs and glands that produce internal substances known as hormones, which are dispensed to the body through the blood and lymph systems. Hormones regulate many body functions, including growth and food use. The thyroid gland, located in the neck, produces a hormone that regulates the production of body heat and energy. The pituitary gland, located near the brain promotes physical growth and sexual development.

Since those glands are involved with the basic changes in human physiology, a glandular disease can have bizarre consequences. For example, it can result in dwarfs, giants, muscular females, or feminine males.

The glands of the pancreas, located behind the stomach, produce insulin, which is a hormone necessary for normal use of sugar in the body. When the pancreas fails to produce enough insulin, an overabundance of sugar appears, and that condition is called diabetes mellitus.

Musculoskeletal System. The combination of bones, joints, muscles, and related connective tissues is known as the musculoskeletal system. The bones are the frameworks around which the body is constructed. The muscles may be considered as its motive power. The joints allow the bones, powered by the muscles, to have a great variety and range of motion.

The most common type of joint infection is arthritis, which is an inflamation of the joints. There are many kinds of arthritis; a familiar form is rheumatoid arthritis. This condition is a crippling one, characterized by a swelling of the joints. The articular cartilage is gradually destroyed, and the joint cavity develops adhesions to the extent that the joints stiffen and are rendered useless. Gout is another form of arthritis, and it is caused by a disturbance of the body's metabolism such as that resulting in too much uric acid. The overproduced uric acid forms crystals, which are deposited in groups about the joints.

The Skin System. The surface of the body is covered by three main layers of tissues: the epidermis or outer-most layer, the dermis or true skin, and the subcutaneous or under-the-skin layer. Major functions of the skin are (1) the protection of deeper tissues against drying and from an invasion by pathogenic organisms or their toxins; (2) the regulation of the body temperature by dissipating heat to the surrounding air; and (3) the detection of information about the environment by means of the nerve endings, which are profusely distributed in the skin.

Skin diseases, including skin cancer, are usually less serious than other diseases.

Suprasystem Diseases. Diseases that are not localized to a specific body system but affect several systems include degeneration and neoplasm. Degeneration means deterioration of tissues resulting in a lessening in activity and capability to perform their normal functions. Such a degenerative process may be caused by continuous infection, by repeated minor injuries to tissues by poisonous substances, or by the normal wear and tear of life with aging.

Neoplasm means"new growth" and refers to cancer and other types of tumors. Tumors occur everywhere in the body. They are the abnormal growth of new body tissue, and they are both independent of the surrounding body structures and have no beneficial physiological functions. When they have fixed boundaries, do not spread, and their limits can be identified, they are benign. However, when tumor cells break off and spread to other parts of the body, they are malignant. At this point the tumors are called cancerous.

CAUSES OF DISEASES

Causal Analysis

The first step in the understanding of a disease is the classification of symptoms. Noting that many patients show a similar departure from the normal, physicians and other healers develop a concept of a disease. They give the disease a title and classify all these presenting similar symptoms as suffering from that disease.

However, such a concept of disease is nothing but a classification of patients. The next mental process in the understanding of a disease is the consideration of causation. The repeated observation of a sequence of events or circumstances arouses confidence that a particular effect is likely to follow a particular cause.

Throughout history there have been two basic methods by which causal inferences are made: the survey of a large number of cases and controlled experiment.

In the primitive world thousands of concoctions and procedures were tried and certain effective curative medicines and procedures were empirically stumbled upon. Based on the study of these large numbers of cases, primitive healers inferred that certain events or circumstances tended to follow others in time. In addition, prescientific people used experiment. To cure diphtheria, they may have used the blood of a patient who recovered from diphtheria because such blood was considered an acceptable sacrifice to the demon of the disease (Winslow, 1967).

The era of modern medicine opened with an upsurge in interest in the causes of disease, which was brought about by the discovery of micoorganisms as etiological agents. Laboratory experimentation began by taking the inciting agent of disease, manipulating it at will, exposing a susceptible animal to it, and studying the developing changes from the beginning. In 1890 Koch formulated the rules by which the specific causative organisms of infectious disease can be recognized:

> 1. If the parasite is found in every case of a disease and under conditions which conform with the pathological changes and clinical picture.
> 2. If it is not found in any other disease as an accidental and non-pathogenic parasite.
> 3. If after being completely isolated from the body and repeatedly transplanted in pure culture it can reproduce the disease on inoculation; then it cannot have an accidental relation to the disease, but the parasite must be the cause of the disease (Stallybrass, 1931, p. 23).

The discovery of microorganisms as causative agents of disease stimulated large-scale surveys to track down the link between the agent (microorganism), the environment, and the host (human). There are many facts that can be revealed only by the examination of a large collection of individual observations.

Thus the etiology of disease has been pursued by means of experimental and survey methods. However, the knowledge of the etiology of disease is not sufficient for an ideal classification of diseases. This is not surprising since there are certain stringent requirements for establishing a causal relationship between two events, which go beyond simple sharing of some common features.

For instance, from the data indicating a high prevalence of mental illness among lower class people, it may be suspected that membership in the lower class is the cause of mental illness. However, before reaching a conclusion, the first condition for a causal explanation must be met, that is, the cause must precede the effect in time. This requirement is difficult to satisfy in many of the research surveys that deal with respondents only at one time instead of over a period of time. Without tracing life histories, it is not easy to determine whether stresses associated with lower class living have caused mental illnss, or if inadequate social adjustment due to mental illness has caused the person to slide down to the lower class.

The second requirement in a causal analysis is that the observed relationship between the two phenomena is not due to the influence of some third factor that has caused both of them. If the prevalence of mental illness is measured by hospitalization rates, it may be the result of (1) police or social workers' referral of disorderly people to mental hospitals and (2) the greater likelihood of lower rather than middle class people being arrested for antisocial behaviors.

Epidemiology

Epidemiology is the study of the distribution of diseases among various groups of people in different environments. "Epidemiology may be defined as the study of the distribution of a disease or condition in a population and of the factors that influence this distribution" (Lilienfeld, 1957). In this definition, emphasis is placed on the descriptive aspect of observing facts (i.e., Among what types of people and under what conditions are certain types of diseases prevalent?) and the analytical aspect in searching for general laws governing observed facts (i.e., What is the causal link?)

The development of scientific epidemiology during the nineteenth century owes much to two factors. First, the appearance of the germ theory attracted scientific attention to the microorganism as the causal agent of disease. This encouraged the attempt to seek a specific causal microorganism for a particular disease.

Another impetus came from the occurrence of acute epidemics during this period. In 1885 a cholera epidemic killed over 500 people in London in less than ten days. Anxious to discover the source of the epidemic, John Snow compared the ill and the nonill. Through interviewing the family members of the deceased, Snow isolated a single common factor, that is, the Broad Street pump, from which all the victims drank water. Snow had the authorities remove the handle of the cholera-carrying pump, which resulted in an immediate decline in the incidence of cholera (MacMahon & Pugh, 1970).

Many of the early epidemiologists confined their investigation to infectious diseases. Epidemiology was defined, to use the words of Wade Hampton Frost, as "the science of the mass-phenomena of infectious disease" (Maxcy, 1941). However, even then there were some who included noninfectious diseases, such as pellagra, which Goldberger studied starting in 1915. Yet is is probable that Goldberger was assigned to this task because pellagra was considered to be contagious in his day (Terris, 1964).

The essential cause of pellagra was not known and there were two hypotheses available: infection and dietary causation. Goldberger rejected the infectious hypothesis on the ground that while inmates of asylums contracted the disease, none of the nurses and attendants did, despite their close contact with the inmates. Also at the institutions he found that those who subsisted on better diets were exempt from the disease. As for the correlation found between untidyness and pellagra, Goldberger introduced a third factor, apathy, that would explain both untidyness and the eccentricity of the diet he linked to pellagra. Thus, he established poor diet as the cause of pellagra.

During the first half of the twentieth century, virtually all the infectious diseases were brought under control, particularly in the scientifically advanced countries. The change in orientation in epidemiology became manifest. The meaning of epidemiology was broadened from the study of epidemics to the study of all diseases in their usual as well as epidemic occurrences. Seeing that communicable disease evidently conformed to biologic laws and that these processes could be interpreted in terms of their distributions, epidemiologists were enticed to consider that other diseases could be described in a similar fashion (Kark, 1974; Winslow, 1967).

The epidemiological model links three elements: the agent, the environment, and the host (see Figure 3.1). The noxious agents include biological (bacteria, viruses, fungi, etc.), chemical (chemical dusts, gases, etc.), physical (soil, climate, radiation, etc.), nutritional (vitamins, minerals, fats, etc.), and other agents. The environment consists of physical as well as socioeconomic circumstances. The study of the host involves genetic, psychological, and sociological traits of humans.

Figure 3.1: Epidemiological Model

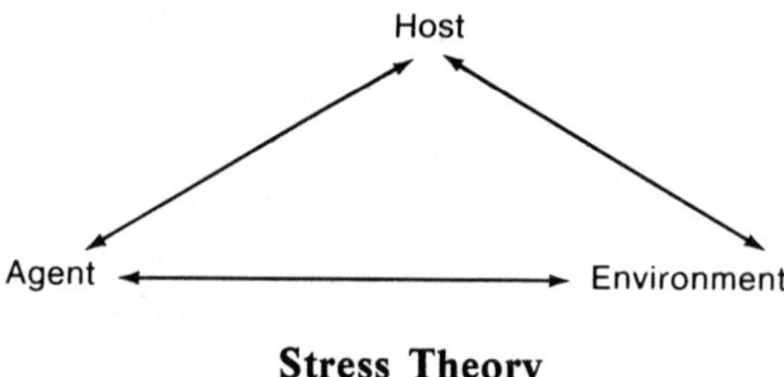

Stress Theory

As is obvious in the above description of the epidemiological model, microbes or germs are *agents* of disease, not its *cause* (Wheeler, 1914). As such, germs can affect only those who are susceptible and whose defense mechanisms have weakened sufficiently. The concept of stress was introduced as the condition that disturbs or interferes with the normal physiological equilibrium of an organism and makes the body vulnerable to disease agents.

The stress theory of disease gained prominence because it became clear that the control of germs does not prevent chronic and mental illnesses. Also, the advances in methods of controlling the physical environment have been accompanied by the creation of new hazards in the environment. Some germs, and even insects, have grown stronger and more resistant to the use of antibiotics. In the meanwhile, new physical hazards, such as air pollution, synthetic food containers, and artificial food coloring, which are suspected of having an adverse effect on humans, have been developed and are in common use. As a result, the distribution of disease agents has become fairly homogeneous in the world. Microbes and other health hazards appear to be ubiquitous in the environment, and they persist in the body without causing obvious harm under ordinary circumstances. Insiduously, they only seem to exert pathological effects when the infected people are under stress, thereby rendering them vulnerable (Dubos, 1965).

Attempts to establish a causal link between stress and illness have been made both by experimental and survey methods. Dating back to Selye's (1956) studies of the effects of stressful stimuli on laboratory animals, there have been hundreds of inventive experiments on human and animal subjects. They demonstrate that both the threat and the actual use of either psychic or physical stressors produce physiological reactions in vital organs, such as increased acidity in the stomach, which might erode the walls of the stomach (Kaplan, 1979).

Experiment is helpful in elucidating the relationship between stress and illness, but it lacks the complexity of a natural situation. Thus, health surveys have been supplemented to derive causal associations between the occurrence of disease and the stresses experienced by people in various social settings.

One of the difficulties in validating the stress theory of disease stems from conceptual ambiguity in defining the term *stress*. *Stress* has been defined either explicitly or implicitly by different investigators: stress as stimulus, response, or mediator (Scott & Howard, 1970).

Stress as a Stimulus

The term *stress* is used by many researchers to refer to stimuli or to stressors such as an electric shock, flood, or the loss of loved ones (Arthur, 1974; Basowitz et al., 1955; Janis, 1958; Kinston & Rosser, 1974; Melick, 1978; Schein, 1957).

The efforts to identify stressors have taken two directions. One is the attempt to locate potential stressors in social structures and processes. On a very general level, society as a whole can be viewed as a stress-inducing environment (e.g., society going through rapid social change). On a more specific level, certain subgroups, social institutions, or organizations may be designated as stressors. Thus, racial minority groups, lower social classes, physically demanding or hazardous jobs, and disorganized families have been identified as potential stressors (Croog, 1970; Dohrenwend & Dohrenwend, 1970; Gross, 1970; Simmons & Wolff, 1954).

The second source of stress is found in life events. It is assumed that a significant change in life is stressful to individuals and is likely to lower their resistence to disease (Brown & Birley, 1968; Dohrenwend & Dohrenwend, 1974c; Hinkle et al., 1952; Rahe, 1974).

The first quantitative measure of life events is the Social Readjustment Ration Scale (SRRS) developed by Holmes, Rahe, and their coworkers (1967). The unique feature of this scale is its inclusion of pleasant as well as unpleasant life events. Stress scores are given as 100 for the death of a spouse, 73 for divorce, 65 for a jail term, 50 for marriage, 47 for the loss of a job, and 13 for a vacation.

These and other researchers utilized this scale in numerous studies and found that increased life-change scores (i.e., clusters of life events) precede the onset of reported illnesses (Gunderson & Rahe, 1974). However, not every researcher found a positive correlation (Jenkins, 1976; Liem & Liem, 1978; Wershow & Reinhart, 1974).

One of the difficulties in using this scale is ambiguity in the interpretation of the results since the scale contains a mixture of pleasant and unpleasant events (Mueller et al., 1977). Some problems, such as depression, appear to be associated primarily with loss events (e.g., loss of a spouse, loss of a job), while schizophrenia (Brown & Birley, 1968), or coronary heart disease (Holmes & Masuda, 1974) are related to life change in general. Ruch (1977) claimed the need to differentiate three dimensions in the concept of life events: (1) the degree of change evoked, (2) the desirability of change, and (3) the life area in which the change occurs.

Apart from the SRRS scale, the study of life events and illness suffer from methodological shortcomings (Brown et al., 1973). Most of the studies are based on retrospective data, which makes it difficult to ascertain the extent of response biases. A person's perception of his or her life situation is likely to be affected by the illness and in turn life events affect a person's threshold of complaint and inclination to adopt the sick role (Campbell et al., 1976; Minter & Kimball, 1978; Palmore & Luikart, 1972; Tessler & Mechanic, 1978).

Even if response biases are controlled, there are other problems in the hypothesis of life events and illness. Stressful life events may affect the individual confounded with other factors (Gersten et al., 1977). Further, potentially stressful events are not necessarily perceived as stressful by everyone (Kaplan, 1979).

Stress as a Response

A second definition of stress is to view it as a response to stimuli. Thus, stress may take the form of hyperventilation, increased blood pressure, or personality disintegration (Cassell, 1970; Fox, 1957; Janis, 1958; Notterman & Trumbull, 1959). Stress is also used to indicate the emotional state accompanying a changing personal or social situation, such as anxiety and frustration (Barrabee & Mehring, 1953; Mechanic & Volkart, 1961).

The definition of what constitutes a stress response has met theoretical and methodological difficulties. On the physiological level, different autonomic measures such as heart beat and skin conductance have yielded different results depending on the measures used and the biological constitutions of the subjects (Lazarus, 1966). To make it worse, there is only a low correlation between subjective reports of stress and physiological stress.

These kinds of difficulties with interpretation and implication have been acknowledged by many researchers. Caudill (1961), among others, has noted that there are divergent consequences of the potentially stressful event, with stress in one system (the physiological, psychological, social, etc.) having ramifications in another system.

Integration of Stress Concepts

One-sided definitions of stress either as stimuli or responses are accompanied by a number of unwarranted assumptions: (1) all difficult situations are stressful; (2) what is perceived as stressful by one person will inevitably be stressful for another; and (3) stressful events must lead to pathological consequences.

Because of such difficulties, attempts have been made to integrate various components of stress.

Levine and Scotch (1970) conceptualized stress as being both stimulus and response. Stress as a stimulus refers to various sources of stress (e.g., family, occupation) to which one is exposed. When the individual is unable to cope with a stressful situation, stress as a response results, which may take the form of mental illness.

In a stress etiological model, Dodge and Martin (1970) presented the following sequence for the origin and deterioration due to stress: social environment, socially induced stress, functional disorder, chronic disease morbidity, and chronic disease mortality. They based their position on the following logic:

- Variation in the sociocultural environment of people govern the nature and types of social structure in which they participate.
- The social structures expose people to different types and degrees of stress (i.e., stress as stimuli).
- When stress is not resolved (due to an inability to cope), functional disorders occur and permanent structural changes of the organs may result in organic disease (i.e., stress as a response).

While they distinguished conceptually between stimulus and response aspects of stress, Dodge and Martin concentrated their research efforts only on the first aspect.

A different approach to a stress model was formulated by House (1974). Reviewing the studies of occupational stress and coronary heart disease, he tried to reach a theoretical integration of the various stress concepts. In his paradigm for stress research, he identified five classes of variables:

- Objective social conditions that are conducive to stress
- Individual perceptions of stress
- Individual responses (physiological, affective, and behavioral) to perceived stress
- More enduring outcomes of perceived stress and responses thereto
- Individual situational conditioning variables that influence the relationships among the four sets of factors

In order to add clarity to the process, Dohrenwend (1961) defined stress as an intervening state that is the internal reaction to stressors. Stress was described by him as that state of the organism which results from the interaction between any antecedent stressor and the mediating force trying to reduce it. These mediating forces are determined by one's social status and social relations.

Exposure–Coping Model

The version of the epidemiological model influenced by the germ theory encourages preventing a host's exposure to an agent (microorganism) by manipulating the environment and by fostering the host's capacity to overpower the agent, such as by immunization. The main thrust of the model is breaking the link between the host and the agent. In contrast, stress theory assumes the inevitability of a host's exposure to an agent, and it concentrates on examining how the individual copes with the agent (hazards), which is viewed as ubiquitous in the environment. According to this theory, one's coping ability decreases, or in other words, one's susceptibility to hazards increases, when one is under stress.

Figure 3.2: Exposure-Coping Model

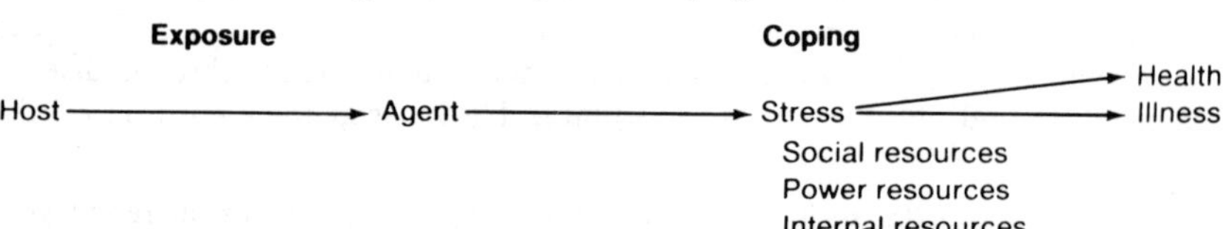

An alternative perspective proposed here is the exposure-coping model, which incorporates concepts from both epidemiological and stress theories (see Figure 3.2). The physiological implications of exposure variables (e.g., physical environment, agent) in the epidemiological model and the psychological connotation attached to stress in the stress theory have been combined. The proposed model *consists of* (1) an individual's socially determined degree of exposure to physical hazards, and (2) his or her socially determined ability to cope with the hazards once exposed.

The manner in which the degree of exposure and the coping ability are determined will be examined in terms of functional, conflict, and interactionist perspectives.

Functionalist Perspectives

Functionalism assumes a social system in which the component units perform their functions for the maintenance of the system. Each unit has a unique function to play, which entails unique activity levels, and hence results in unique exposure to hazards.

Simplistically stated, boys and girls constitute social units. Traditionally the boy's role has been defined to be task-oriented, which tends to expose him to more accident-inducing hazards than in the case of a girl. In the same vein, differential mortality and morbidity rates among social groups such as race, social class, sex, and age can be perceived as functions of differential exposure to hazards, which in turn are determined by the differential roles prescribed by society.

Functionalists further assume that certain positions in any society are more important functionally than others, and that the more important ones require special skills for their performance (Davis & Moore, 1945).

The model of functional importance suggests that there are distinguishing stresses that are unique to social positions. Statuses of functional importance are likely to demand a greater degree of competence, responsibility, and alertness than other positions. All of these generate more stress. The prevalence of high blood pressure in top executives fits this model.

However, there is another side of the coin: incumbents of functionally important positions are rewarded both psychologically and financially. Functionalists (Davis & Moore, 1945) argue that, without these rewards, people would not be induced to enter demanding professions such as that of medical doctor. From this it is possible to deduce the following hypothesis: functionally trivial positions generate more stress because the incumbents suffer from the threats of subsistence as well as from low self-esteem. That logic has been used by some analysts to explain the correlation between the female sex and high rates of mental illness.

In short, the degree of exposure to stress-inducing situations can be exlained by functionalists in terms of the importance attached to social positions.

According to that same perspective, once people find themselves in certain statuses, they must cope with the stresses that are characteristic of the role. Their coping ability can be affected by the extent to which individuals are integrated into the role configurations of society. By controlling other factors, such as heredity and personality, individuals will find it easier to cope with specific role stresses if they are not torn between conflicting values and norms.

Another aspect of the coping variable in the functionalist framework relates to the adaptation of a social system to the external environment. A society can persist only if it can mobilize its facilities and resources efficiently to cope with external challenges. Differential mortality and morbidity rates among countries and social groups may be a reflection of differential ability to adapt to the environment.

Conflict Perspectives

The crux of conflict theories is that conflict is the result of the pursuit of incompatible goals and scarce commodities. These theories also assert that the extent to which one group obtains its goals will determine the degree to which the opposing group must fail to obtain those same goals. The inevitable existence of structural incompatibilities, the inherent dysfunctional aspects of fundamental social structures (e.g., authority structures), and the existence of inequalities in power, material comforts, and other desired rewards—all of these factors lead to the idea that conflict is inherent in society.

It is the loser in the power struggle who is exposed to physical hazards. High rates of mortality in the lower classes, racial minorities, and in the underdeveloped countries may be explained as a result of their exposure to physical hazards, such as bacteria in an unsanitary environment, or uncontrolled heat and cold, because they have been squeezed out of a better environment by their opponents.

Losers in a conflict are also deprived of resources by which to remedy their life environment. They lack material resources to buy nutritional food to strengthen their bodies so as to cope with and work against hazards or to obtain medical services for preventive or therapeutic purposes. They also suffer from a sense of powerlessness, which reduces their ability to cope with hazards. Low utilization rates of medical facilities among lower class people are in part the result of their apathy.

Another aspect of conflict theories concerns social change. Change implies readjustment to new environments that may offer values and norms which are different from those of the previous stage. Although change is omnipresent in social life, some people or groups are more transient than others. Mobile groups, therefore, are more exposed to stressors than are sedentary groups. Mobility includes geographical, occupational, social class, and various other changes. The studies of immigration, acculturation, and mental illness all assume that the mobile have a greater exposure to potentially stressful situations.

In dealing with mobility issues, there is a question of selectivity. That is, the type of people who frequently move around might have been originally maladjusted. Possibly those who cannot form satisfactory social relations are the ones who move to another city or another country, or who drift into disorganized neighborhoods. This selectivity in mobility can account for the deficiency in coping ability among some of the modern day urban nomads.

Conflict may also promote either adaptation or basic system change. The oppressed group may develop a mechanism of adaptation to the plight, they may negotiate with the dominant group for an improvement through a compromise, or they may decide to rebel against the oppressor and hope to bring about a structural change in society. An example of the last alternative is seen in the Chinese communist revolution, which resulted in a dramatic improvement of the nation's health status as compared with that of the prerevolutionary period (see Chapter 11). Whichever coping method is adopted, human behavior is viewed by conflict theorists as arising from the process of conflict rather than from the integrative mechanism of a social system.

Interactionist Perspectives

Shifting the focus of attention from social structure and group conflicts, the interactionists concentrate upon interactional situations that occur among individuals. Either as actors on the stage or players in a game, individuals are seen to attempt to manipulate the situation by taking the roles of others, while simultaneously straining to present themselves advantageously. The situation becomes real only to the extent that one defines it as such. Thus, individuals are ill, regardless of their symptoms, if they perceive that others have labeled them as ill.

In negotiating for one's identity in the process of symbolic interaction, one is also generally drawn into power struggles. In a theatrical play, there are heroes and bystanders. In a game there are winners and losers. Similarly, in labeling processes there are some people who label others. The basic position of labeling theorists is that the more powerful a person is, the more likely he or she will be able to label others as well as to avoid being channeled into a deviant role. For instance, a lower class person who demonstrates disorderly behavior is more likely to be sent to a public mental hospital than is a middle class person.

According to the interactionist framework, then, the exposure-to-stress variable consists of the vulnerability of the individual to being labeled as sick. This vulnerability is determined by the extent of one's power. However, interactionists envision that power is derived from a wide range of sources including one's appearance and personality.

They contend that the ability to cope with stress develops, like various other social interactional skills, during the process of interacting with others who are significant to the individual. The individual learns to take the roles of others, to examine the situation objectively, and to decide upon the most strategic action. For example, a child who is labeled as having a cold and is exempt from going to school may start having a running nose. A person who is diagnosed as being chronically ill is likely to act "sick" all the time.

The ability to cope with hazards can be hampered when roles are ambiguously defined or incompatible with one another. Individuals will be at a loss as to what to expect and how to behave. Since they cannot define the situation, and since there is no one to emulate, they do not know how to cope with the resultant stress. A good illustration of this is the development of schizophrenia by children who are caught in a bind, love and hatred shown by their mothers.

Finally, social isolation impairs one's coping ability because of (1) the lack of group support during stressful situations, and (2) the degeneration of the ability to assess social situations accurately. To use the expression of Cooley (1902), human nature seems to "decay in isolation." High rates of schizophrenia have been reported for those who dwell in the social isolation of rooming houses.

To sum up, the exposure–coping model views the disease process as beginning with the exposure of a host to a disease agent. The degree of exposure is affected by the extent of (1) the host's integration into the social structural or interactional system, and of (2) his or her power position in the process of conflict. Once exposed to hazards, the coping ability of the host will determine the outcome, either health or illness. This coping ability is influenced by the host's access to power resources (e.g., money, power, or status), social relational resources (e.g., group support), and internal resources (e.g., value orientation).

SUMMARY

This chapter has provided the definitions, measurements, and theoretical frameworks that are necessary for interpreting the data on social causes of disease presented in Chapter 4.

Etymologically the word *disease* means discomfort or a reversal of "ease." It refers to the sensations of the sufferer. However, physicians use the word differently. To them disease means a departure from the normal state of health, of which pain is only one of the indications. In fact, traditionally physicians tended to detach themselves from the psychological aspect of disease and concentrate on the objective, biophysical functioning of human organisms.

Thus, the term *disease* means different things to doctors, patients, and healthy people. The dictionary definitions of health and disease are inclined to be open-ended and elastic without a clear demarcation as to where health ends and illness begins. For the practical purpose of assessing the health status of various individuals and groups, a statistical measure of normality has been adopted. According to this method, people are defined to be healthy if they do not deviate from the behavior patterns of the majority of a given population. Thus, in health surveys those subjects who check off more than a specific number of items of physical symptoms are labeled as ill. In official statistics countries whose mortality rates are higher than a certain limit are classified as "unhealthy" or even as "underdeveloped."

The acceptance of a statistical definition of health entails serious problems that should be kept in mind in interpreting health statistics and surveys. Nevertheless, because of expediency and standardizability, statistical measures are widely used and sometimes are the only data available for etiological analyses. Therefore, basic concepts and indices used in vital statistics are introduced in this chapter.

Having defined and measured the state of disease in general, the chapter proceeds to the classification of diseases. This section is included in this chapter for two reasons. First, it is necessary to familiarize the readers with the terminologies designating various types of diseases that will be discussed in the next chapter. Second, classification of diseases has been the first step in understanding disease, which must precede the search for causes. This chapter contains a broad typology of communicable, chronic, and mental diseases as well as a classification of disease related to the functioning of physiological systems.

Finally, conceptual models for etiological analysis are examined so as to facilitate meaningful interpretation of the data in the next chapter. The epidemiological model is based on the interactions among three components: the host, the agent, and the environment. When the germ theory was dominant, the link between a host and an agent (microorganism) was emphasized as crucial for the occurrence of disease. The environment was seen as a mediator to expedite or circumvent the contact of the host with the disease agent.

When infectious diseases were brought under control, attention shifted to other sources of disease than microbes and to the manner in which a host responds to the onslaughts of agents. According to stress theory, a host is vulnerable to these attacks when he or she is under stress.

In the pursuit of a social etiology of disease, two variables are extracted from the prevailing etiological models (germ theory, epidemiology, and stress theory) to construct an alternative framework. The disease process is conceptualized in two stages: (1) exposure to disease-inducing agent, and (2) failure to cope with that agent. The exposure–coping model is then decribed in terms of the major sociological theories. The degree to which an individual is exposed to noxious agents and the level of his or her ability to cope with the hazards are explained in terms of the host's position in functional social structures, conflicting social processes, and in symbolic interactional processes.

We are now equipped with the instruments—(1) the definition, measurement, and classification of diseases, and (2) the conceptual models for causal analysis—necessary to embark on an examination of the social causes of diseases.

CHAPTER 4

The Sociological Correlates of Diseases

Now that we have all the instruments ready for a causal analysis of sociological predictors of diseases, we will examine health statistics and survey data.

Available data are classified into the following units of analysis from macro to micro levels: (1) society, (2) community, (3) institution, and (4) status. The structure and process in these social units will be examined to discover how they affect the degree of the individual's exposure to disease agents and his or her ability to cope with them.

Society as a unit of analysis is dealt with from the perspectives of historical and cross-national comparisons of health status. The community-level inquiry refers to the rural–urban contrast from the structural angle and to studies of urbanization and migration as processes. Available data on institutions concentrate on the structure and dynamics of the family. Prevalent among studies of social statuses are those of race, age, sex, marital status, and social class as they relate to stress-inducing structures and the stressful processes caused by life events, status incongruence, status mobility, etc.

It should be noted that most of the investigations included in this chapter concern cross-sectional distributions of diseases among different social categories rather than longitudinal and controlled experiments. Causal inference is being made on correlational data, which must be interpreted cautiously. Many studies do not meet requirements for establishing causality, and all we are able to report are the sociological correlates rather than the etiology of disease.

The substance of this chapter coincides with that of the field traditionally labled social epidemiology. The major objective here is to synthesize empirical findings and generalizations hitherto gathered in social epidemiology and to fashion these data into more general theoretical perspectives.

The problems encountered in this endeavor are twofold. On the one hand, sociological research in medicine is still underdeveloped and does not offer enough materials to choose from in developing models. On the other hand, sociological theories are quite abstract and cannot easily be made to fit medical data. While we cannot resolve these difficulties at this stage of development in medical sociology, we will attempt to evaluate the theoretical frameworks in terms of the power and efficiency of their explanations. This evaluation will also aid us in recognizing and highlighting neglected areas where future research can provide the missing links in sociological explanations of health and illness.

It must be kept in mind that the studies of disease described in this chapter are incomplete and fragmentary. In certain instances, interpretations or even speculations by this author will be used in an effort to integrate some of the disparate research findings. The interpretations and the etiological implications that this author offers should be viewed as tentative formulations and as an attempt to provide a systematic theoretical integration. This position is taken despite the claims by some medical sociologists that the present state of epidemiological knowledge makes such an endeavor premature.

This chapter is not intended as a review and catalog of all the available literature, which in any case is frequently methodologically invalid and contradictory. Rather, certain works have been selected to present attempts at developing sociological interpretations and analytical frameworks.

SOCIETY: PREINDUSTRIAL VERSUS MODERN

Can culture determine the amount or kind of illness in a society? Are some societies sick, or at least, sicker than others?

Apart from speculation, the main difficulty with a rigorous test of this hypothesis concerning the cultural determination of disease is that of obtaining accurate statistics on disease incidence in various societies. It is difficult enough to eliminate biases in statistics gathered in the United States, not to mention the inaccessibility or nonavailability of figures from other countries.

Even if statistics are available, they are of a questionable nature because cultural variation in symptomatology and in the reactions to them tend to make a standardized quantification in cross-cultural studies invalid.

In addition to methodological difficulties, there are more intrinsic issues in that variations within a society may be greater than differences between societies. Except for relatively homogeneous primitive societies, it is nearly impossible to ascertain any general traits of complex and heterogeneous modern societies. It is true that there have been many anthropological studies concerning cross-cultural comparisons of psychiatric symptomatologies in preindustralized societies. However, due to the above-mentioned difficulties in comparing primitive as well as modern societies, this chapter will be limited to standard vital statistical measurements such as mortality and morbidity of preindustrial and modern societies.

From Ancient to Modern Societies

A summary of gains in human longevity from ancient to modern times is presented in Table 4.1.

Life expectancies in antiquity are at best very inaccurate because data bearing on them are the results of research on available records, tombstones,

Table 4.1:
Life Expectancy from Antiquity to Modern Times

Time and place	*Life expectancy at birth (in years)*
Early Iron and Bronze Age—Greece[1]	18.0
2000 years ago—Rome[1]	22.0
Middle Ages—England[1]	33.0
1687-1691—Breslau[1]	33.5
Before 1789—Massachusetts, New Hampshire[1]	35.5
1838-1854—England and Wales[1]	40.9
1900-1902—United States[1]	49.2
1946—United States[2]	66.7
1960—United States[2]	69.7
1970—United States[2]	70.9
1975—United States[2]	72.5

Sources: [1] Data quoted in L. Dublin, et al., *Length of Life: A Study of the Life Table* (New York: The Ronald Press, 1949).

[2] U.S. Department of Commerce, *Statistical Abstract of the United States, 1960, 1970, 1975* (Washington, D.C.: U.S. Government Printing Office, 1960, 1970, 1975).

and physical remains. A cautious conclusion that can be drawn from these results is that, in antiquity, an average length of life may have been somewhere between 20 and 30 years (Dublin et al., 1949).

From the time of the Roman Empire to the latter part of the seventeenth century, the basis for estimates is meager. Records concerning the inheritance of property were used by Russell (1948), and he found an average length of life of about 33 years in England during the Middle Ages. Based on the geneological records for men in the ruling classes of Europe in the Renaissance, Peller (1944) found 30 years to be the average length of life. The first scientific computation by Halley of the mean length of life in Breslau was 33.5 years toward the end of the seventeenth century (Dublin et al., 1949).

Through the seventeenth and eighteenth centuries, life expectancies steadily increased. Hollingsworth (1965), who traced the legitimate offspring of British royal families for six centuries, indicated that life expectancy more than doubled between the fourteenth and eighteenth centuries. An expectancy of 24 years for males and 33 years for females from 1330 to 1479 grew to 55 years for males and 70 years for females during the period of 1880 to 1954. It should be noted, however, that life expectancy at birth in eighteenth-century Europe and America was still relatively short: 25 years in parts of Philadelphia in the 1780s; 35.5 years in Massachusetts and New Hampshire before 1789; and 28.2 years in different parts of France before 1789 (Dawson, 1898). Up to the beginning of the nineteenth century, an average life of 35 to 40 years may have been common in various localities among the civilized nations (Dublin et al., 1949).

It was as late as the twentieth century when the falling death rate became manifest. This tendency first became apparent in Sweden, the Netherlands, and Denmark shortly after 1850. Before the end of the nineteenth century, the mortality data for England and Wales, Scotland, France, Germany, and Italy indicates that there was a definite rise in life expectancy (reaching 51 years) and that life expectancy was rising at an increasing rate (Smith, 1948).

After 1900, declining mortality and the extension of life expectancy characterized most of Europe, Australia, New Zealand, the United States, and Canada. In all these highly developed countries, the upward trend in life expectancy continued till the second half of the twentieth century, at which time the mortality rate began to level off.

In the mid-twentieth century the average length of life in the United States was about 62 years for males and 66 years for females (see Table 4.2). Sweden, in 1931–1935, showed corresponding figures of 63 years for males and 65 years for females, and they had an average of greater than 60 years as early as 1921–1925. England and Wales did not reach the 60-year level for males until 1937. The best record for longevity was established by New Zealand where, in 1934–1938, the average length of life for males was 65 years and 68 years for females.

The contrasts between the developed and underdeveloped countries are great in the twentieth century. As late as 1931, India had an average length of life of less than 27 years, a figure that is only 5 years greater than that estimated for ancient Rome by Karl Pearson (Dublin et al., 1949). Egypt in the decade

Table 4.2:
Life Expectancy in the Mid-Twentieth Century

Country	*Year*	*Life expectancy at birth (in years)* *Male*	*Female*
United States	1939–1941	61.6	65.9
Sweden	1931-1935	63.2	65.3
England and Wales	1930–1932	58.7	62.9
New Zealand	1934-1938	65.5	68.5
India	1921-1931	26.9	26.6
	1941-1950	32.5	31.7
Egypt	1927-1937	30.0	31.5
Chile	1939–1942	40.7	43.1

Source: United Nations, *Demographic Yearbook, 1948* (New York, 1948).

1927–1937 did little better than India, with an average length of life of 30 years for males and 32 years for females. The record of Chile in 1939–1942, with an average length of life of 41 years for males and 43 years for females, was practically at the level for the United States in the middle of the last century.

It has only been since the mid-twentieth century that developing nations began to experience declining mortality and the extension of life expectancy. Relatively underdeveloped countries with high death rates now have the opportunity to decrease their mortality rates much more rapidly than did the developed nations.

Comparisons of the increase in life expectancy during the twentieth century indicate an annual gain of under .30 years for males in such countries as South Africa (white population), Canada, the United States, Israel, Denmark, Germany, Norway, Sweden, Scotland, Australia, and New Zealand. The rates of increase have been slightly higher in other countries. The most spectacular annual increases, of over .66 years, have taken place in developing nations such as Egypt, Barbados, El Salvador, Ceylon, the Republic of Korea, West Malasia, the Philippines, the Rhuku Islands, and Albania. Rapid gains in life expectancy from an extremely low starting point in these places began to appear after the end of World War II. For example, Egypt registered a life expectancy of 35.6 years for males and 41.5 for females in 1937; by 1960, it showed an annual increase of .69 and .54 years, respectively (United Nations, 1948–1976).

Contemporary Preindustrial and Industrial Societies

The dramatic increase in life expectancy began to take place in the early twentieth century for highly developed countries and in the mid-twentieth century for developing nations. It has yet to occur in the underdeveloped countries. Therefore, the contrasts in the current records for longevity between the preindustrial and industrial countries are as great as those between the ancient and modern nations.

Mortality. Crude death rates in the 1970s for developing and underdeveloped countries are still significantly higher than those in the developed countries (United Nations, 1976). In developed countries the rates are 8.9 per 1,000 population for the United States, 7.3 for Canada, 8.7 for Switzerland, 9.9 for Italy; in developing and underdeveloped countries the rates are 15.8 for Burma, 14.4 for India, 10.8 for Thailand, 14.4 for Rhodesia, and 22.5 for the Central African Republic.

Life Expectancy. Likewise, life expectancy at birth is considerably lower in Asian and African countries. It is 48.6 years for males and 51.5 for females in Burma; 41.9 years for males and 40.6 years for females in India; and 33.0 years for males and 36.0 years for females in the Central African Republic. In contrast, rates in developed countries are 68.7 years for males and 76.5 years for females in the United States; 69.3 years for males and 76.4 years for females in Canada; and 72.1 years for males and 77.7 years for females in Sweden.

Infant Mortality. Infant mortality, which is death in the first year of life, is regarded as a sensitive indicator of death. Infant mortality is the major component of life expectancy rates since the decline in the crude death rate has occurred at the earliest stages of life.

International differences in infant mortality are shown in Table 4.3. Interpretation of this table is facilitated by using a measuring stick suggested by Chandrasekhar (1972); low rates are those below 35 deaths per 1,000 live births, moderate rates are between 35 and 75, high rates are between 75 and 125, and very high rates, above 125. Until recently, still higher rates were found. In the first two decades of the twentieth century, the annual infant mortality rates for India varied between 195 and 243. By the 1960s, the Indian infant mortality rates had declined to about one-half of the 1901–1920 level, although they are still relatively high. Low rates are found in Australia, New Zealand, Japan, Denmark, Switzerland, Finland, and the Netherlands; the lowest rate of all is in Sweden (8.7). The United States registered 15.1 in 1976. Infant mortality rates in underdeveloped and developing countries during 1970–1975 were 195.0–300.0 for Burma, 122.0 for India, 122.0 for Rhodesia, 190.0 for the Central Africa Republic, and 100.4 for Egypt.

Causes of Death. In most underdeveloped countries, the prevailing causes of death are infectious and parasitic diseases, partly because few live long enough to develop chronic or degenerative diseases.

According to the World Health Statistics Annual, mortality rates from infectious disease per 100,000 population are as follows (also see Table 4.4): typhoid fever—5.1 in Mexico; dysentery—5.4 in Mexico; enteritis and diarrhea—6.2 in Egypt, 277.9 in the South African black population, and 107.4 in Mexico; tuberculosis—7.0 in Egypt, 45.4 in the South African black population, 14.7 in Mexico, and 13.7 in Singapore; measles—25.2 in black Africa. Except for tuberculosis in Japan, Italy, and Spain, infectious diseases have almost vanished from the developed countries.

Influenza and pneumonia have much higher rates of occurrence in underdeveloped countries than in developed countries, except in the tropical climates. However, highly developed countries such as Japan, white South Africa, Italy, and Spain have more than one-third, and Canada, the United States, and Sweden have more than one-half of their total deaths attributed to circulatory disease. Particularly prevalent are ischemic heart disease and cerebrovascular diseases. Another major cause for death in developed countries is malignant neoplasm; that factor is not very important in developing or underdeveloped countries.

Although both live in the same geographical areas, the white and black populations in South Africa have vastly different mortality patterns. The whites show the characteristics of the developed societies and have a low crude death rate, low infant mortality, high life expectancy, and high prevalence of heart diseases and malignant neoplasms; the black population is characterized by the traits of underdeveloped countries, namely, high death rate and high prevalence of infectious diseases.

Table 4.3
Death Rate, Infant Mortality, and Life Expectancy for Selected Countries, 1951-1976

Country	*Year*	*Death rate*	*Infant mortality*	*Year*	*Life expectancy at birth (in years)*	
					Male	*Female*
United States	1976	8.9	15.1	1975	68.7	76.5
Argentina	1970	9.4	59.0	1970-75	65.2	71.4
Brazil	1970-75	8.8	---	1960-70	57.6	61.0
Canada	1975	7.3	15.0	1970-72	69.3	76.4
USSR	1975	9.3	27.7	1971-72	64.0	74.0
Burma	1970-75	15.8	195.0-300.0	1970-75	48.6	51.5
India	1974	14.4	122.0	1951-60	41.9	40.6
Japan	1975	6.4	10.1	1974	71.2	76.3
Thailand	1970-75	10.8	26.3	1960	53.6	58.7
Italy	1975	9.9	20.7	1970-72	69.0	74.9
Spain	1976	8.0	12.0	1970	69.7	75.0
Sweden	1976	11.0	8.7	1971-75	72.1	77.7
Portugal	1974	11.0	37.9	1974	65.3	72.0
Switzerland	1975	8.7	10.7	1968-73	70.3	76.2
Rhodesia	1970-75	14.4	122.0	1970-75	49.8	53.3
Central Africa Republic	1970-75	22.5	190.0	1959-60	33.0	36.0
Egypt	1974	12.4	100.4	1960	51.6	53.8

Notes: *Death rate Number of deaths per 1,000 population.*
Infant mortality rate: Number of deaths during the first year of life per 1,000 live births.

Source: United Nations, *Demographic Yearbook, 1976* (New York, 1976).

Table 4.4: Causes and Rates of Death for Selected Countries, 1973–1976

Cause of death	*U.S., 1975*	*Sweden, 1976*	*Italy, 1973*	*Spain, 1974*	*S.Africa, 1973*	*Japan, 1976*	*Egypt, 1973*	*S.Africa, (black) 1973*	*Mexico, 1973*	*Singapore 1976*
Typhoid fever	0.0	-	-	-	-	0.0	1.5	-	5.1	-
Dysentery	0.0	-	-	-	-	0.0	0.0	-	5.4	0.1
Enteritis	0.9	0.2	-	-	6.8	2.3	6.2	277.9	107.4	2.9
Tuberculosis	1.2	2.0	5.3	7.5	-	8.1	7.0	45.4	14.7	13.7
Measles	0.0	-	-	-	-	0.2	2.3	25.2	4.8	0.1
Neoplasm	174.0	241.8	196.5	143.8	135.1	131.1	20.8	98.5	38.7	100.0
Diabetes	16.5	19.2	23.6	18.0	7.7	8.2	6.7	11.7	14.3	14.7
Hypertensive disease	8.1	4.2	28.0	6.9	16.6	17.6	34.5	41.7	3.9	11.8
Ischemic heart disease	301.7	386.3	150.3	67.2	205.1	39.7	19.0	87.5	20.7	64.6
Cerebrovascular disease	91.1	119.8	134.0	141.5	99.5	154.5	7.1	115.6	24.9	62.6
Pneumonia	23.5	28.5	33.0	37.2	47.5	26.6	40.8	174.5	111.0	43.9
Cirrhosis of liver	14.8	12.9	32.3	22.3	13.2	13.8	11.0	15.1	21.2	7.2

Note: *Death rate: Number of deaths per 100,000 population.*

Source: World Health Organization, *World Health Statistics Annual, 1977–1978* (Geneva, 1977–1978).

The United States from 1900 to 1976

Mortality. The age-adjusted death rate in the United States was 17.8 per 1,000 in 1900. It declined slowly and regularly until 1936 with the exception of 1918, which was the year of the great influenza epidemic. Then, beginning in 1937, the death rate dropped more rapidly because of the introduction of sulfa and antibiotic drugs and their availability on the civilian market. This decline lasted until 1954, and then the death rate leveled off. The rate has been relatively stable since 1954 except for fluctuations associated for the most part with epidemics of influenza.

The gap between the crude death rate and the age-adjusted death rate (the rate adjusted to the age composition of the 1940 population) has widened since 1940. The rapid decrease in the age-adjusted death rate relative to the decrease in the crude death rate resulted primarily from the increasing proportion of older people in the population.

Figure 4.1:
Age-Adjusted Death Rate, United States, by Sex and Color, 1900-197

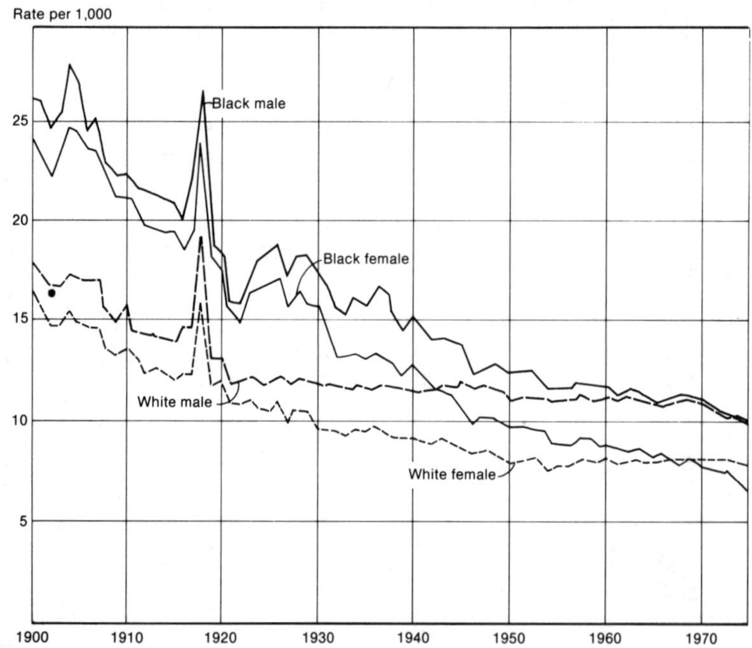

Note: *Death rate: Number of deaths per 1,000 population.*

Sources: U.S. Department of Commerce, *Historical Statistics of the United States* (Washington, D.C.: U.S. Government Printing Office, 1975).

U.S. Department of Commerce, *Statistical Abstract of the United States* (Washington, D.C.: U.S. Government Printing Office, 1977).

The age-adjusted death rate decreased 60.1 percent from 1900 to 1970, when the rates were 17.8 and 7.1, respectively (see Figure 4.1). However, the decrease in the crude death rate was only 44.8 percent, and the values were 17.2 and 9.5 for those same years.

The age-adjusted death rates have declined for all four age–color groups (i.e., white males, white females, black males, and black females), but the rates of change differ. For both white (70.2 percent) and nonwhite (71.6 percent) females, the percentages of decrease in the death rate are greater than the corresponding decrease for white (51.6 percent) and nonwhite (57.1 percent) males. Females started with a lower death rate than males in 1900, and their rate decreased faster than that of the males.

Throughout the period of 1900–1976, whites have maintained a lower age-adjusted death rate than nonwhites. However, the mortality/color ratio (obtained by dividing the age-adjusted death rate for nonwhites by the corresponding rate for whites) decreased from 1.58 in 1900 to 1.44 in 1970. It would be incorrect to conclude from this, however, that the racial gap in mortality has been reduced significantly (U.S. DHEW, 1973b). The reduction is in part attributable to the changing structure of the population.

Infant Mortality. There was a rapid decline in infant mortality that lasted until 1955. Then, the rate began to level off until about 1966, but after 1966 the rate of decrease began to accelerate again (see Table 4.5). While the total death rate in 1970 was about one-half that of 1920, the infant mortality rate in 1970 was less than a quarter.

The decrease in infant mortality since 1915 has been spectacular. Among whites, the rate dropped from 98.6 in 1915 to 17.8 in 1970. Among nonwhites during the same period, the decrease was from 181.2 to 30.9. Until 1966, infant mortality rates declined more rapidly for the whites than for nonwhites, but after 1966 the rates for nonwhites began to drop faster. By 1977 the rates had converged somewhat.

Life Expectancy. During the period from 1900 to 1975, life expectancy at birth has risen from 46.3 for males and 48.3 for females to 68.7 for males and 76.5 for females. Racial and sexual differences in the extension of life expectancy are worth noting (see Table 4.6). Life expectancy in the 1970s is higher for females than for males and for whites than for blacks. However, gains in life expectancy in the past 70 years is greater for blacks than for whites, and within the racial groups, females gained more than males in life expectancy. Note, however, that life expectancy at age 70 has not changed much. Between 1900 and 1970 it was extended from 9.0 years to 10.5 years for white males, and from 9.6 years to 13.6 years for white females. It appears that technology to conquer senility and old age diseases has not progressed as fast as medical advancements dealing with diseases of younger people.

Causes of Death. In 1900, three infectious conditions—influenza and pneumonia, tuberculosis, and gastroenteritis—led the list of causes of death, and they accounted for 31.4 percent of all deaths (see Table 4.7). The three cardiovascular-renal conditions—diseases of the heart, cerebral hemorrhage, and chronic nephritis—constituted only 18.9 percent of the total deaths.

Table 4.5:
Infant Mortality, United States, by Color, 1915-1976

	Infant Mortality		
Year	*Total*	*Whites*	*Nonwhites*
1915	99.9	98.6	181.2
1920	85.8	82.1	131.7
1930	64.6	60.1	99.9
1940	47.0	43.2	73.8
1950	29.2	26.8	44.5
1960	26.0	22.9	43.2
1970	20.0	17.8	30.9
1975	16.1	14.2	24.2
1976	15.2	13.3	23.5

Note: *Infant mortality rate:*
Number of deaths during the first year of life per 1,000 live births.

Sources: U.S. Department of Commerce, *Statistical Abstract of the United States, 1977* (Washington, D.C. U.S. Government Printing Office, 1977).

U.S. Department of Commerce, *Historical Statistics of the United States* (Washington, D.C.: U.S. Government Printing Office, 1975).

Table 4.6:
Life Expectancy, United States, by Sex and Color, 1900-1976

	Life Expectancy at birth (in years)								
		Total			*Whites*			*Nonwhites*	
Year	*Total*	*Male*	*Female*	*Total*	*Male*	*Female*	*Total*	*Male*	*Female*
1900	47.3	46.3	48.3	47.6	46.6	48.7	33.0	32.5	33.5
1910	50.0	48.4	51.8	50.3	48.6	52.0	35.6	33.8	37.5
1920	54.1	53.6	54.6	54.9	54.4	55.6	45.3	45.4	45.2
1930	59.7	58.1	61.6	61.4	59.7	63.5	48.1	47.3	49.2
1940	62.9	60.8	65.2	64.2	62.1	66.6	53.1	51.5	54.9
1950	68.2	65.6	71.1	69.1	66.5	72.2	60.8	59.1	62.9
1960	69.7	66.6	73.1	70.6	67.4	74.1	63.6	61.1	66.3
1970	70.9	67.1	74.8	71.7	68.0	75.6	65.3	61.3	69.4
1975	72.5	68.7	76.5	73.2	68.9	76.6	67.0	62.9	71.3

Sources: U.S. Department of Commerce, *Statistical Abstract of the United States, 1977* (Washington, D.C.: U.S. Government Printing Office, 1977).

U.S. Department of Commerce, *Historical Statistics of the United States* (Washington, D.C.: U.S. Government Printing Office, 1975).

Table 4.7:
The Ten Leading Causes of Death, United States, 1900 and 1975

Rank	*Cause of death*	*Rate per 100,000*	*Percent of all deaths*
	1900		
	All causes	1,719.1	100.0
1.	Influenza and pneumonia	202.2	11.8
2.	Tuberculosis	194.4	11.3
3.	Gastroenteritis	142.7	8.3
4.	Diseases of heart	137.4	8.0
5.	Cerebral hemorrhage	106.9	6.2
6.	Chronic nephritis	81.0	4.7
7.	Accidents, total	72.3	4.2
8.	Malignant neoplasms	64.0	3.7
9.	Certain diseases of early infancy	62.6	3.6
10.	Diphtheria	40.3	2.3
	1975		
	All causes	896.1	100.0
1.	Diseases of heart	339.0	37.8
2.	Malignant neoplasms	174.4	19.5
3.	Cerebrovascular disease	91.8	10.2
4.	Accidents, total	47.6	5.3
5.	Influenza and pneumonia	27.0	3.0
6.	Diabetes mellitus	16.8	1.9
7.	Cirrhosis of liver	15.1	1.7
8.	Arteriosclerosis	13.7	1.5
9.	Certain diseases of early infancy	12.6	1.4
10.	Suicide	12.6	1.4

Source. U.S. Department of Commerce, *Statistical Abstract of the United States, 1900, 1975* (Washington, D.C.: U.S. Government Printing Office, 1900, 1975).

In marked contrast to 1900, the leading causes of death in 1975 were three chronic conditions—diseases of the heart, malignant neoplasms, and cerebrovascular diseases—to which 67.5 percent of the total deaths were attributed. Tuberculosis, gastroenteritis, and diphtheria disappeared from the list of the first ten causes of death, and each accounted for less than 1 percent of all deaths by 1975.

Aside from the general trend of age-adjusted death rates for the total population, there have been steady decreases since 1900 for the following leading causes of death: tuberculosis, gastroenteritis, diphtheria, influenza and pneumonia, and cerebrovascular diseases. Among the other causes for this decrease, the age-adjusted death rate from malignant neoplasms has steadily increased from 1900 to 1975. The mortality rate for diseases of the heart rose from 1900 until 1950 but has declined ever since. Mortality rates for diabetes mellitus and cirrhosis of the liver have fluctuated within a relatively narrow range during this century (see Figure 4.2).

In examining the changes in the distribution of diseases, disorders can be classified into three categories: declining, increasing, and persisting.

Among diseases that were once common and have all but disappeared are infectious diseases such as tuberculosis, syphilis, typhoid fever, diphtheria, whooping cough, measles, and gastroenteritis.

An example of a new epidemic is malignant neoplasm. As measured by age-adjusted death rates, the increases between 1900 and 1975 in mortality from malignant neoplasms amounts to 58 percent.

Persistent diseases can be divided into two types: those with and those without drastic changes in death rates since the beginning of the century. Persistent diseases with drastic changes in death rate include diseases of the heart, cerebrovascular diseases, and influenza and pneumonia. The age-adjusted death rate for diseases of the heart increased 65 percent between 1900 and 1950, but it decreased by 25.5 percent between 1950 and 1975, from the rate of 298.7 to 222.5 per 100,000 in 1975. As for cerebrovascular diseases, there was a 59 percent decline in the age-adjusted death rate between 1900 and 1975, reaching the rate of 54.7 per 100,000 in 1975. The mortality rate from influenza and pneumonia dropped 91 percent from 1900 to 1975, although the rates were stablized during 1950–1969.

Among those diseases that have kept comparatively low but persistent death rates without much fluctuation over time are diabetes mellitus and cirrhosis of the liver.

Aging Population. All these above-mentioned factors—the decrease in infant mortality, the stretch in life expectancy, and the control of contagious diseases—plus the lowering of the fertility rate over the years have resulted in producing an aging of the population.

In 1900, in the United States, there were only 3.1 million persons aged 65 and over. Today, there are over 20 million, of whom about one-third are 75 or older. Those in this age category (65 and over) are increasing by 300,000 to 400,000 per year with an anticipated figure of about 29 million by the year 2000. What is even more striking is the growing proportion of senior citizens. In

Figure 4.2:
Age-Adjusted Death Rate, United States, by Cause, 1900-1975

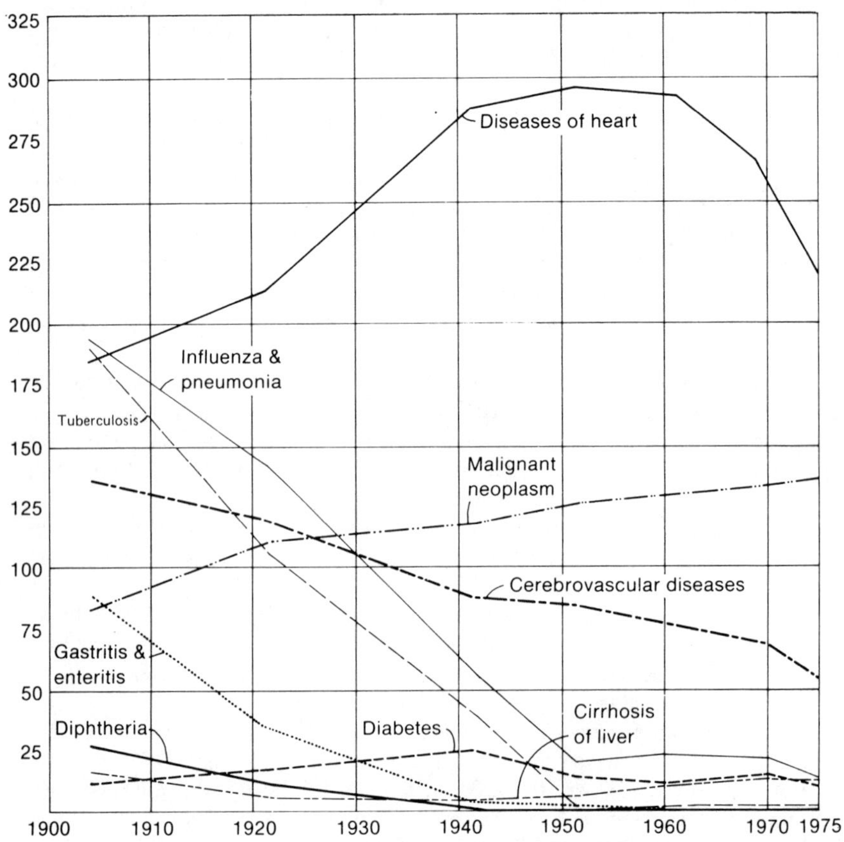

Notes: *Death rate: Number of deaths per 100,000 population.*

Age-adjusted rate: Based on the age distribution of the total population of the United States Census, April 1940.

Sources: For 1900-1904, 1920-1924, 1940-1944: U.S. National Center for Health Statistics, *Vital Statistics—Special Reports,* vol. 43 (Washington, D.C.: U.S. Government Printing Office, 1956).

For 1950-1954, 1960-1964, 1969: U.S. Department of Health, Education, and Welfare, *Mortality Trends for Leading Causes of Death, U.S.—1950-1969* (DHEW Publication No. (HRA) 74-1853) (Washington, D.C.: U.S. Government Printing Office, 1974).

For 1975: U.S. National Center for Health Statistics, *Monthly Vital Statistics Report for the United States. Annual Summary for the United States, 1975* (Washington, D.C.: U.S. Government Printing Office, 1975).

1900 only about 4 percent of the total U.S. population was 65 or over. By 1970, they constituted 9.7 percent and by 2020 it is projected that 13.4 percent will be in this age group. In other words, one in every eight will be a senior citizen (U.S. Department of Commerce, Bureau of Census, 1970; U.S. DHEW, 1971).

Interpretation

From the preceding data we can make the following generalizations about the distribution of health in various societies. From ancient to modern societies, historical trends are characterized by (1) declining death rates; (2) particularly a declining infant mortality rate; hence, (3) an increased life expectancy; (4) decreasing death rates due to infectious diseases; and (5) increasing death rates due to cancer and heart diseases (Omran, 1974)

Such changes began to appear earlier in societies and groups that had better technological and material resources than those with lesser resources. In other words, technologically developed countries and dominant groups in the world have experienced greater degrees of change in the directions stated above than the underdeveloped countries or minority groups in society.

Direct Causes of Mortality

The human being, as a physical and physiological unit, has probably changed but little since remote antiquity. How then can we account for such changes in the distribution of disease? Preindustrialized societies suffered from three major causes of mortality: famine, epidemics, and high infant mortality (Wrigley, 1969).

Famine. In preindustrialized societies, and even as late as the mid-nineteenth century in Europe, chronic food shortages were common. In Ireland in the 1840s several hundred thousand people died of starvation.

Short of famine, malnutrition resulted from a continual insufficiency of food, especially grievous with regard to adequate supplies of complete protein. At present, people in underdeveloped countries do not actually starve to death, but many of them are victims of malnutrition. They have enough food to keep them alive and working, but not enough to stay healthy and function efficiently. Malnutrition weakens people and lowers their ability to cope with infection.

Epidemics. A great pestilence was described by Marcus Aurelius in the second century, and Procopius wrote of a great pandemic—Justian's Plague—that undermined the health of the known world from 542 to 590. The plague was probably the greatest single impetus in the decline of the Roman Empire, reducing the population by 40 to 50 percent, hence reducing the size of the army.

During the seven crusades of 1096–1270, the Christian army suffered more from epidemics than from Saracen blades. In 1343 the Black Death is said to have killed 25 million people, a quarter of the population of Europe. Gowen (1907) described the scene as follows:

> In the fourteenth century [there were] more pestilences and peculiar epidemics than have ever been known at any other time. Not to mention the famine which, in the second decade of the century, strewed the roads with the dead, and caused imprisoned thieves to devour one another, nor the severe scourges of some of the more common diseases, such as measles and smallpox, there were probably twenty visits of the plague in various parts of Europe (Gowen, 1907, p. 2).

Even in the seventeenth century Europe was not free from the threat of epidemics. The plague killed one-fifth of the inhabitants of London in 1603 (Kastenbaum & Aisenberg, 1972).

Infant Mortality. During the sixteenth and seventeenth centuries one out of every five babies of British aristocrats would die before attaining one year of age. Similarly, infant mortality rates were fully one fourth of all births in a wealthy urban parish in England in the late sixteenth century (Goldscheider, 1971). During the first half of the twentieth century, infant mortality rates were in the region of from 300 to 500 per 1,000 live births in most of Africa (Chandrasekhar, 1959).

Mortality in the first year of life reveals the great vulnerability of infants to environmental forces. Trends in infant mortality rates generally reflect the progress that a society has made in controlling the various causes of death. In underdeveloped countries, the main causes for infant mortality are nutritional disorders and infections. An infant's diet is often markedly inadequate, and as a result, undernutrition and malnutrition are widespread. Malnutrition also contributes largely to childhood deaths from infection. Weakened children are little able to resist measles and pneumonia in the winter and gastroenteritis and diarrhea in the summer.

Sociological Interpretation

The disappearance of famine, epidemics, and high infant mortality from modern, developed societies can be interpreted from the three perspectives of sociological theories as they explain exposure and coping variables.

Functionalist Perspective. From the functionalist viewpoint society is able to survive because of its capacity: (1) to manipulate the physical environment and to minimize its exposure to hazards, and (2) to maximize its coping ability once exposed to hazards. Modern industrial and differentiated societies are viewed by functionalists as more evolved systems than primitive, undifferentiated peasant societies because each differentiated substructure is assumed to have an increased adaptive capacity for performing its function as compared to the performance of that function in the previous structure.

Accordingly, famine or malnutrition are attributed to the low technological adaptability of preindustrialized societies as demonstrated by their low agricultural productivity and inadequate transportation systems to redistribute food from one locale to another. The functionalist concept of interrelatedness of parts within a system further explains how famine affects every part of the social system. Famine is accompanied by pestilence and many other symptoms of social disorganization, which are stressful to the inhabitants.

With regard to epidemics, exposure to disease-carrying germs has been limited by various public health and sanitary measures that try to break the contact between the host and microorganismic agents. These public health measures are more effective, according to functionalists, only when (1) society as a whole accepts the importance of sanitation for a healthy life, and (2) health, economic, and political institutions collaborate in their pursuit of sanitation. Functionalists assume the existence of an integrated social system as in the Roman Empire with elaborate public health programs.

The significant reduction in infant mortality during the early part of this century was made possible by controlling diarrhea and enteritis by means of the wide use of sanitary measures to protect the quality of water, milk, and other foods. Much of the improvement after 1966 came about as a result of substantially better control of influenza and pneumonia, asphyxia, birth injuries and problems associated with immaturity, and gastrointestinal diseases of the newborn. The rates of death from congenital anomalies remain almost unchanged.

Thus, the increasing ability to cope with hazards can be explained in functional terms. A well-integrated society with rising standards of living can provide its members with good nutrition and thus an increasing resistence to infection. The benefits derived from medical discoveries have been made available to the general public in the form of immunization, antibiotic drugs, and other therapies. Infectious diseases have been brought under control as a result of an integrated support of societal values, medical discoveries, technological development, improving living standards, and a general rise in social welfare (Goldscheider, 1971; Wrigley, 1969).

Conflict Perspective. While the functionalists describe social change as a process of adaptation to a disturbance of the system's equilibrium, conflict theorists posit that change is inherent in societies which are in constant struggle for scarce commodities. For instance, famine and malnutrition may be interpreted as consequences of the power struggle in which the stronger groups monopolized food, better land, technology, and other resources. Conflict implicit in social structure becomes manifest in dealing with crisis situations. Thus, unable to trace the source of epidemics in the physical environment, people in some places thought that the Jews had poisoned the world and therefore they killed Jews. In other places blame was put on the deformed, who were driven out of their communities (Hollingsworth & Hollingsworth, 1971).

Conflict theorists do not accept the functionalist premise that technological development, material advancement, and the ensuing benefits are used for the welfare of the entire society. Instead, they assume that the stronger groups monopolize all the profits and further exploit the weaker groups.

During the early stages of industrialization the proletariat lived in overcrowded areas filled with physical hazards such as inadequate ventilation, high temperatures, poor lighting, and insufficient bathing facilities. Capitalists, on the other hand, enjoyed all the advantages accruing from industrialization including sanitary living conditions and nutritious diets.

The differential distribution of disease in contemporary South Africa is amenable to a conflict explanation. While the white population enjoys good health, the black natives are still subject to the diseases characteristic of underdeveloped societies. The contrasting prevalence of diseases in adjacent neighborhoods is due to extreme social differentiation whereby only the politically dominant whites secure the benefits of industrial expansion. The native population is segregated in overcrowded, unsanitary urban areas, and remains at a bare subsistence level without good public health provisions.

In the United States, racial differences in mortality and morbidity have also been great. The nonwhites have lived in the least healthy portions of large cities and have been exposed to physical hazards. Malnutrition and a substandard level of existence have drained them of their physical resistence against diseases. Their coping ability is reduced further by the inaccessibility to advanced medical technology and health measures (Krause, 1977).

The conflict perspective thus elucidates the mechanisms under which disorders such as the venereal disases, low birth weight, and infant mortality cluster in certain social groups. The failure to control preventable diseases is attributed to the unequal distribution of power and resources among various social groups, which makes the overall administration of public health difficult.

Interactionist Perspective. Since the interactionist perspective deals with person-to-person transactions, it is difficult to apply it to the analyses of societal structures and processes. Within its limited utility, interactionism may account for the differential prevalence of diseases related to the type of personal interaction commonly practiced in societies.

From the interactionist viewpoint, a peasant society provides a better environment for the individual's mental health than do industrialized societies. Rural societies characterized by intimate social interaction, homogeneity in population, and simple role structures are less likely to generate stress for individuals. This may partially explain the rise in death rates due to stress-related diseases such as heart ailments and cancer that occur in industrial societies. It should be remembered, however, that many chronic diseases occur in the later years of one's life. Primitive people, who more generally experienced a peasant lifestyle, did not live long enough to suffer from these diseases.

For study units smaller than society, including the community, the institution, and social status, there are more detailed data available than crude overall mortality rates. Many studies have been conducted to discover social variables related to diseases, mainly chronic and mental diseases. These types of diseases are concentrated on because (1) communicable diseases have been virtually controlled, and (2) chronic and mental illnesses are more likely than communicable diseases to be associated with socially induced stresses. Between the two types of diseases, attention has been focused more upon mental than physical (chronic) diseases as a proper domain of sociological research.

COMMUNITY: RURAL VERSUS URBAN

Comparisons of illness at the community level differ from those at the societal level because communities tend to be more homogeneous. Communities are likely to contain people from the same race with the same national origin, who speak the same language, and who share a culture.

The search for an etiology of disease in city life was apparently "inaugurated by the indictment of civilization itself" (Leacock, 1957, p. 310) with the romantic idealization of Rousseau's fast disappearing Natural Man. The city was blamed for being the source of stress because of its malintegration, complexity, anonymity, competitiveness of industrialized life, and many other ills, all long before the advent of smog and clogged freeways (Altman, 1975).

Chronic Illness. Urban living has been associated with medical problems such as high blood pressure, apoplexia, hypertension, and a higher morbidity rate due to cardiovascular disease (Powles, 1973; Scotch & Geiger, 1963; Stamler et al., 1967b), although there are some exceptional findings (Kasl & Hamburg, 1975).

Tyroler and Cassel (1964) note that rates of death by coronary heart disease increased during 1950–1960 as urbanization progressed in a rural country. When comparing generations of once rural mountaineers engaged in industrial work, Cassel and Tyroler (1961) found that the second generation was better prepared for the situation and had less illness than the first generation. In another study whose data were controlled for cigarette smoking, the lung cancer rate was found to be higher among the farmers who had migrated to the cities than it was among lifelong urban dwellers (Haenszel et al.,1962). Similarly, an association has been suggested between a high mortality from tuberculosis and migration from rural to urban life. It was found that the tuberculosis mortality rate increased during relocations of Navaho and Sioux Indians within the same climate and geographical area (Dubos & Dubos, 1952).

These studies indicate that the degree of unpreparedness to new and unfamiliar situations is in itself a measure of stress.

Mental Illness. Using New York State statistics, Malzberg (1936a,b,c, 1943) concluded that there was an upward trend in mental illness for those who moved from rural to urban areas, but the trend was far slighter than previously feared. Higher urban hospitalization rates for mental illness are reported by many (Dayton, 1949; Jaco, 1960), but there are also other studies indicating no difference by urbanicity (Lemert, 1948; Lin, 1953). Recent reviews of the evidence on the urban–rural comparison (Dohrenwend & Dohrenwend, 1974a; Srole et al., 1962) suggest that the differences in rates are, at most, very small.

Several attempts have been made to interpret these rather inconsistent findings about the rural–urban differences in the incidence of mental illness. In accordance with functionalist perspectives, the question was raised that rather than urbanization itself, perhaps the degree of social integration in the community is the crucial factor and a potential source of stress. Therefore, various types of city or rural areas were examined. For example, Hyde and others (1944) found a high rate of stress in disorganized rural communities and densely populated communities. Kasl and Hamburg (1975) identified high stress areas in the urban environment, which were assessed by danger from crime, unsafe neighborhoods, poor facilities in neighborhoods, dissatisfaction with dwellings, and crowdedness. They found that the residents in high stress areas perceived their neighborhood as subjectively stressful but that this perception was not significantly associated with mental health.

Faris and Dunham (1939), on the other hand, hypothesized a selectivity of urban migrants, that is, people who are already disturbed tend to "drift" into the city. They examined the ecological distribution of migration and mental illness indexes and noted that schizophrenia was associated with the mobility characteristics of the city, that is, a high percentage of hotel and rooming-house dwellers.

Following Faris and Dunham, many ecological studies were conducted. Most of them (Dunham, 1947; Freedman, 1950; Queen, 1940; Schroeder, 1942; Tietze el al., 1942) corroborated the findings that the rates of hospitalized schizophrenics are highest near the centers of large cities. These areas are commonly characterized as economically poor, socially disorganized, and highly mobile. In contrast, however, the rates of manic-depressive hospitalizations are not systematically related to the residential areas.

There are also studies that do not support the drift hypothesis (Clausen & Kohn, 1954; Hollingshead & Redlich, 1954, 1958; Lapouse et al., 1956). For instance, some researchers (Hollingshead & Redlich, 1958; Lapouse et al., 1956) reported that in terms of occupation, neurotic and schizophrenic patients were more upwardly mobile than the control subjects and further that geographic mobility had little to do with mental illness.

Having failed to prove the selectivity and drift hypotheses, some raised the question that migration to the city itself may be the cause of mental disorders. With a few exceptions (Freedman, 1950; Jaco, 1960), many studies (Locke et al., 1960; Malzberg, 1936a,b) showed a strong correlation between mobility and mental illness even after they controlled other factors such as color, sex, and age (Lazarus et al., 1963; Malzberg & Lee, 1956).

The above studies do not provide a basis for conclusions since ecological distributions as epidemiological indicators have not been demonstrated. Rural–urban differences may be the result of statistical artifacts. Dohrenwend and Dohrenwend (1974a) have reviewed studies of the prevalence of psychiatric disorder for both treated and untreated populations. In two out of the five studies reviewed for untreated populations the rate of prevalence in rural areas was higher than in urban areas, while in the remaining three studies the reverse was true. A tentative conclusion is that the rates of untreated schizophrenia are equal in rural and urban areas. The rates of treated schizophrenia are simply the rates of annual first admissions and as such, they are only approximation of the actual incidence of this illness.

It is possible that the duration of schizophrenia is much greater in rural areas than in urban areas, thus inflating the rural prevalence rate to match the urban rate. However, it seems more likely that utilization patterns differ: in rural areas schizophrenics are less likely to receive treatment.

INSTITUTION: FAMILY

Among the various kinds of institutions in society, the family has been singled out for the etiological study of disease. This is not because the family is the greatest stressor in society but rather because family life, through its intimate relations, is seen as having compelling influences upon the behavior of its members. Precise knowledge of the structure and an insight into the relationship between the members of a family is essential to an understanding of the origin and perpetuation of illness, and in the case of therapy, the family should be considered as a unit of treatment.

The family can be viewed, in the functionalist framework, as an integrated system of interpersonal relationships existing within itself and in its relation to the community. On the other hand, it may be conceptualized as a dynamic process of symbolic interaction. For conflict theorists the family as an institution appears to be in a moving equilibrium in which family members are constantly generating and resolving conflicts among themselves.

Because of the importance of the influence of the family upon each of its members, this institution has deservedly been examined as a potential source of stress. Croog (1970) identified several sources of stress: (1) family forms and structures inducing comparative stresses (e.g., the extended versus nuclear family), (2) a skewed structure due to the breakup of the family, (3) value conflict, (4) role conflict, (5) life cycle, and (6) interpersonal relations.

Chronic Illness. The etiological study of the family involves the issue of biological versus sociological inheritance of disease. It is frequently mentioned that a certain illness "runs in the family." What appears to be a genetic inheritance on the surface, however, is frequently related to social factors such as dietary (Barrows et al., 1978) and feeding patterns peculiar to an individual family that are followed by successive generations.

In line with the above reasoning, associations have been found between breast cancer and breast feeding (Levin et al., 1962; Vorherr et al., 1978), hypertension and a salty diet (Graham, 1963; Michell, 1978; Morgan et al., 1978), and gastric cancer and a special diet (Graham & Lilienfeld, 1958; Wynder et al., 1977). Another disease that has stimulated sociological interest is the cancer of the uterine cervix. This problem has been associated with female hygiene practices (Dorn, 1954; Kennaway, 1948), circumcision (Wynder et al., 1954), sexual behaviors such as the frequency of coitus (Jones et al., 1958; Terris & Calmann, 1960), the age at which coitus began (Jones et al., 1958; Wynder et al., 1954), and marital status (Maliphant, 1949).

Although the family has been studied as a source of stress, few studies have been made regarding the direct relationship between chronic illness and the family as a stressor. Among the few is the study by Metzer and others (1977), who tested the general hypothesis that conflict and deprivation experienced in the family in early life have sustained effects on health that can be detected much later in life. Specifically, parental deprivation (i.e., the number of years lived without one or both parents during childhood) and conflicting expectations by parents were examined for their association with the incidence of chronic diseases. Their data did not substantiate the hypothesis.

Mental Illness. Most childhood schizophrenia studies have been focused on the family as a symbolic interaction system. There, the child is exposed to stresses generated in familial, marital, or generational conflicts. If the child is torn between conflicting affections and loyalties and incompatible demands, he or she is not able to develop the capacity to relate effectively with others and to cope with stresses.

The etiology of childhood schizophrenia was first explored in the notion that a father or mother was pathogenic. For example, the father of a schizophrenic child is said to be weak and passive and remain aloof from the child (Lidz et al., 1957; Richard & Tillman, 1950). Occasionally the father overtly rejects the child and is cruel to him or her. The mother is unstable (Friedlander, 1945; Gerald & Siegel, 1950; Lidz and Lidz, 1949) in that she is domineering, aggressive, hostile, while possessively overprotective and indulgent (Lidz & Lidz, 1949). In short, the parental authority structure that may be associated with childhood schizophrenia is unstable and inconsistent (Clausen & Kohn, 1960; Kohn & Clausen, 1956; Myers & Roberts, 1959).

Parental inconsistency can manifest itself in many dimensions. It may take the form of love versus hatred or may appear in the sphere of basic value orientations. Bateson et al. (1956) introduced the notion of a "double bind" experienced by schizophrenic children. An example of this concept occurs when a male child is placed in a situation where he is punished either for responding to the mother lovingly or for being neutral or aloof. A loving response can generate anxiety in the mother concerning social disapproval of mother–son intimacy; or, when there is no response, she worries that she is not a loving mother. In the double bind situation, a mother offers inducements for a particular kind of behavior, and at the same time, she punishes or discourages the logical outcome of such inducements. Along this same line, other researchers (Cleveland & Longaker, 1957) have examined contradictory demands placed by parents upon children, such as those of dependence versus self-reliance.

Childhood schizophrenia is also associated with marital problems of parents. In this case, usually because of parental incompatibility (Lidz & Lidz, 1949), there is a marital schism (Lidz et al., 1957). As a result, the conjugal interaction lacks reciprocity and turns into demands and defiance. A marriage that is practically an emotional divorce, that is filled with unhappiness (Richard & Tillman, 1950; Tietze, 1949), strife, and conflict (Gerald & Siegle, 1950), has been held responsible for the advent of schizophrenia in the child. Children are torn between conflicting attachments and loyalties.

Since it is the interaction system that produces the schizophrenic child, attention has gradually shifted to the family as a whole instead of individuals such as the father or mother, or dyads as in the double bind hypothesis. A current research direction is toward devising a theoretical system for describing the family as an integrated unit with particular emphasis on the family communication system (Reiss, 1976). All of these studies seem to indicate that children become schizophrenic if there is conflict in their family interactions.

From the conflict perspective, however, *any* family is a social process that is filled with conflicts, while it maintains a dynamic equilibrium. Viewed in this way, the question arises, To what extent does the schizophrenic family differ from normal families?

Jacob (1975) evaluated 57 direct observational studies that compared family interactions in schizophrenic and normal families in terms of the amount of conflict, the dominance patterns, the exhibition of affection, and the clarity of communication. Methodological difficulties arose from cross-study differences in the diagnostic status of experimental groups, measurement techniques, types of analysis, and the demographic factors. When he compared the various substantive findings, Jacob noticed a considerable inconsistency, a lack of generalizability, and only nonsignificant variations. In sum, he concluded that these studies, although based on a potentially sound methodological strategy, had not yet isolated family patterns that reliably differentiate the disturbed from the normal families.

STATUS

From the perspective of functionalism, status is a social position within the social structure, and each incumbent is expected to perform certain functions so that society will remain an integral unit. When varying importance is attached to these functions, different amounts of stress will be generated for the incumbents of a given status. Conflict theorists, on the other hand, conceive of status groups as being involved in an incessant struggle for scarce commodities, which generates stresses. In the framework of symbolic interactionism, everyone brings certain symbolic attributes of his or her status into the interactional setting where symbols are exchanged and interpreted. Stresses arising from this process of interaction are partially determined by the status of the interactor.

Statuses that have been associated by many researchers with chronic and mental illnesses include (1) racial, ethnic, and religious groups, (2) age status, (3) sex status, (4) marital status, and (5) socioeconomic status.

Racial, Ethnic, and Religious Groups

People whose social statuses are based on race, ethnicity, or religion usually share certain characteristics of genetics, diet, hygiene, education, and customs. Because of inbreeding (McKusick, 1978) or shared experience, members of racial, ethnic, or religious groups, in all likelihood, experience similar amount of exposure to hazards and are alike in their coping abilities. The major concern in this area of study has been to differentiate three types of correlates of diseases: (1) genetic and hereditary factors, (2) customs that affect human organisms directly (e.g., diet), and (3) social experiences that induce unique stress (e.g., poverty and inadequate education).

Chronic Illness

Race. To begin with, the mortality rate for nonwhites is higher than that for whites at each age level (Reid & Lee, 1977; Reid et al., 1977). In particular, the infant mortality rate is higher for blacks than for whites (Kovar, 1977). Another noticeable trend is that since the late 1950s mortality rates for young (the age groups between 15 and 44) nonwhite males have shown significant increases. This was attributed by Dennis (1977) to growing social stress caused by rapid social changes affecting blacks in the last twenty years, such as migration from a rural to an urban setting, changes in shape and structure of the family, transformation of age structure, occupational mobility, and increased opportunities in socioeconomic and political spheres.

More specifically, while mortality rates from chronic noninfectious and degenerative diseases are generally higher in whites than in nonwhites (Seltzer et al., 1974), there are certain diseases (e.g., diabetes mellitus, hypertensive diseases, and vascular lesions of the central nervous system) that have afflicted blacks more frequently. Also, cancer mortality in blacks has shown a striking rise in the last twenty years. In 1950 the black cancer mortality rate was 2 percent lower while by 1967 it was 18 percent higher than the white cancer mortality rate (White, 1977). Further, mortality rates from infectious diseases relating to childbirth and diseases of infancy (Chabot et al., 1975) are greater among nonwhites (Malina, 1973).

A great deal of attention has been given to the racial difference in mortality rates in hypertensive diseases. Blacks of both sexes have a significantly higher prevalence of hypertensive heart disease, hypertension, and high blood pressure (HDFP, 1977; Syme et al., 1974; Wilber, 1977). Various hypotheses have been proposed and tested in an effort to explain racial sensitivity to hypertension.

From hereditary perspectives, some argue that blacks are genetically different from whites in their predisposition to hypertension (Lennard & Glock, 1957; McDonough et al., 1964; Nichaman et al., 1962). In support of this genetic hypothesis, Schachter and others (Schacter, Lachin, & Wimberly, 1976) found that black newborns had higher heart rate levels during sleep than white newborns among urban dwellers of the upper and middle classes as well as of the lower class (Schachter et al., 1976).

Supporters of the diet hypothesis claim that blacks have dietary patterns that increase their susceptibility to hypertension (Stamler et al., 1960). However, in some studies hypertension was not related to obesity (Boyle et al., 1967) or with salt and fat intake (Henry & Cassel, 1969) among blacks, although the correlation was found among whites (Boyle et al., 1967).

Viewed from the perspective of conflict theories, blacks occupy the stressful roles of a racial minority and a low social class. Harburg and others (1970, 1973) found that a greater proportion of blacks living in what they defined as high stress census tracts showed higher blood pressure than blacks in low stress census tracts.

Combining racial and social class variables, many researchers found that for both whites and blacks the rate of hypertension tended to be inversely related to education and occupation (Gordon & Devine, 1966; Keil et al., 1977; Oaks et al., 1973; Syme et al., 1974; Yabura, 1977). Social class, however, does not fully account for the racial difference. Regardless of education (HDFP, 1977), occupation, or class (Howard & Holman, 1970), blacks are found to have a higher rate of hypertension than whites, suggesting the relevance of the genetic or racial discrimination hypotheses. Yet, for both races, laborers have the greatest mortality from hypertension (Howard & Holman, 1970). In this case, socioeconomic explanations seem to be pertinent.

Ethnicity and Religion. Comparing the populations of Utah and Nevada, Fuchs (1974) attributed the lower mortality rate in Utah to the lifestyle of Mormons, namely, no drinking, no smoking, and a regulated, spiritual life (Lyon et al., 1976). A fatty diet and heart diseases have been linked by many (Epstein et al., 1957; Epstein, 1971; Kahn et al., 1969; McDonough et al., 1965; Morris, 1964; Krehl, 1977) who found that Jews have a higher prevalence of coronary artery disease and that they also have higher serum cholesterol levels than Italians do. Irish American males are found to have higher coronary death rates than do Japanese Americans (Matsumoto, 1970), Chinese Americans, and American Indians. The fact that ethnic groups of the higher socioeconomic statuses have the highest incidence of heart disease reminds us that their diet is rich in animal fat (Barrows et al., 1978; Toor et al., 1960).

Various population studies have alleged that southern Italian and eastern European Jewish populations have higher than average rates of diabetes (Opler, 1967). Opler also noted that in both cultural groups, the mothers' nurturing and cooking abilities are seen as important in maintaining health as well as in practicing ritualistic dietary excellence.

Finally a mention should be made about the patterns of cardiovascular and cerebrovascular diseases among persons of Japanese descent. Many researchers (Gordon, 1957; Marmot & Syme, 1976; Winkelstein et al., 1975) have observed that the Japanese in Japan had the lowest death rates from coronary heart disease, followed by Hawaiian-Japanese, the U.S. mainland Japanese, and the Caucasians. On the other hand, the deaths from vascular lesions of the central nervous system (stroke) have shown an inverse gradient among these groups of people. Hypotheses have been proposed and tested that acculturation into the American way of life (e.g., diet, method of stress management) is a significant determinant of coronary heart disease but the results are not conclusive yet.

Mental Illness

Race. Ever since the days of slavery, diverse hypotheses have been offered suggesting that racial factors play an important etiological role in accounting for perceived racial differences in rates of mental illness.

Census data show that rates for nonwhites hospitalized in mental institutions have consistently been higher than those for whites since 1950 (Redick & Johnson, 1974; Warheit et al., 1975). On the other hand, of the eight studies reviewed by Dohrenwend nd Dohrenwend (1969), four reported higher rates for blacks and the other four, lower rates. Fischer (1969) and Crawford and others (1960), after comprehensive reviews of the epidemiological literature, concluded that there is no evidence in support of black–white differences in rates of mental disorder.

The seemingly contradictory findings indicate that a relationship between race and mental illness, if in fact it does exist, must be complex in nature. Among various efforts to disentangle this complexity, three distinct types of interpretation are discernible.

First, there are attempts made to arrive at direct causal relations between race and mental illness. Some (Fried, 1969) affirm that the evidence plainly shows that serious mental disorder is indeed more common among blacks. According to the conflict theory model, blacks as racial subordinates are more frequently exposed to stresses than whites, for example, stresses due to migration, marital disruption, forced residential relocation, unemployment, and poverty (McAdoo, 1977). Also, the traditional image of blacks with negative self-identification is derived from the theoretical underpinnings of Cooley and Mead—that individual self-attitudes are a function of reflected appraisals by others. However, recent studies show that blacks do not necessarily have low self-esteem or are psychologically maladjusted. The portrait of blacks as passive recipients of self-destructive communications about themselves has been challenged and replaced by one of resilient and self-motivated individuals (Taylor, 1976).

Second, a large number of research projects have been carried out to demonstrate that race and mental illness are not directly related, but that other factors intervene, such as age, sex, socioeconomic status (Carr & Krause, 1978; Warheit et al., 1975) and goal-striving stress (Kleiner & Parker, 1966). Thus, what is crucial for mental disorder is not being black but being poor or having high aspirations without the means to realize them.

Third, the societal reaction theory of symbolic interactionism leads to the postulate that racial minorities, because of their low status and powerlessness, would be more likely than whites to be labeled insane and hospitalized. Except for a few studies, such as Jaco's (1960), that include admission to private as well as public institutions, most surveys have been confined to public institutions and reveal much higher rates for nonwhites (Cannon & Locke, 1977; Crawford et al., 1960; Malzberg, 1940, 1963; Rose & Stub, 1955). The black–white admission rate differential is partially attributable to the fact that the tolerance of blacks for deviance is lower than that of whites. When individuals show unusual behavior blacks are much more quickly committed to hospitals by social agencies than are whites (Andrew, 1968; Calnek, 1970; Dunham, 1965), or adjudicated as incompetent by the court (Cannon & Locke, 1977; Wenger & Fletcher, 1969). Once committed, blacks are likely to be labeled as psychotic, schizophrenic, and paranoid; while whites are diagnosed as depressive (Cannon & Locke, 1977).

Having reviewed the literature on race and mental illness, during the period 1966 to late 1970, See and Miller (1973) note an overall movement away from comparative research of black versus white. Blacks and other racial minorities are studied more and more without comparison to whites. For instance, the differential incidence of depression is attributed to technological and social change among southern blacks (Warheit et al., 1973) and to a sense of blocked opportunities among Mexican Americans and black females in the southwestern cities (Quesada et al., 1978). This tendency is partly the consequence of the racial movements of the 1960s to establish racial identity and racial culture. On the other hand, it is also due to the fact that variations among blacks in terms of socioeconomic status and other factors have grown so large that direct etiological analysis of race and mental illness is meaningless.

Ethnicity and Religion. Direct association between ethnic and religious status and mental disorder has also been subject to methodological criticisms. There are many intervening variables that make the ethnic differential in mental illness spurious. For example, when data on age, education, and socioeconomic status were controlled, the association between ethnic and religious status and mental health became small (Freeman & Kassebaum, 1960; Nunnally, 1959; Srole et al., 1962).

Another factor that makes ethnic differences in hospitalization rates invalid is the differential utilization rates. Jaco (1959) found that Mexican Americans are less frequently treated for psychoses than Anglo Americans, and Madsen (1973) claims that Mexican Americans seldom seek treatment for mental illness. Viewing mental illness as a result of witchcraft, they consider it more terrifying to enter a hospital away from home than to suffer from the illness.

From the viewpoints of functionalism and interactionism, societal integration is beneficial for all members because they can secure social support when they are caught in stressful situations. Furthermore, in an integrated society people can predict the behaviors of others, thereby reducing the stresses caused by unexpected conduct. Durkheim (1950) pointed out, however, that too much integration leads to negative consequences. Also, a tightly knit society is more likely to discourage individuals from spontaneous expressions of aggression. Such an individual must then cope with the stress internally rather than have the option to act overtly.

These contrasts are exemplified by study results which point out that the Irish show high rates for psychopathy, overaggression, and alcoholism, while the Jews have a high risk of psychoneurosis (Leighton, Clausen, & Wilson, 1957; Roberts & Myers, 1954; Rose & Stub, 1955). There seems to be a difference in culturally prescribed methods of coping with stress. While the Irish have a high tolerance for alcohol as means of tension relaxation, psychopathy and alcoholism are taboos to the Jews, who consequently turn stress inward.

Another study showed that among the Hutterites (Eaton & Weil, 1954), there are few cases of schizophrenia, but there are a great deal of manic-depressive reactions with predominantly depressive symptoms. In contrast with the functionalist model, these symptoms are most likely to be found in an integrated society whose members have a strong need to live up to social expectations. The Hutterites fit that mold since they are integrated by a strict religion. Everything is owned in the name of their church, and the group comes before the individual. Aggressive or antisocial impulses must be repressed.

Japanese Americans are another group that has maintained a collective orientation, and they too have a cultural style that controls overt expressions. Their family and ethnic community integration have had a cushioning effect against mental illness that has in turn resulted in low hospitalization rates (Kitano, 1969). However, comparing Japanese Canadians and Mennonites, both of whom have expression-controlling cultures, with the Italian Canadians, who have an expression-releasing style, Kurokawa (1969) found that those in the controlled culture are more likely to show psychosomatic symptoms than are the voluble Italians (Maykovich, 1972).

Age Status

The mortality patterns vary strikingly with age. For all groups, the death rate is relatively high in the first year of life, and it decreases rapidly to a minimum at around age 10 or 11 years. It then proceeds to mount—slowly with added years until about 45 or 50, and then it rises at an accelerating pace for all but the last few years.

Leading causes for infant mortality are influenza and pneumonia, congenital anomalities, infectious and parasitic diseases (particularly enteritis), and accidents. Accidents are the most important causes for deaths between the ages of 1 and 35.

In the age-group 35–44, major cardiovascular diseases (particularly diseases of the heart) and malignant neoplasms become the most prevalent causes of death, and they remain so throughout the rest of the life span. Around age 50, cerebrovascular disease is a very prominent cause of death. Diabetes mellitus and cirrhosis of the liver are also associated with aging.

Certain types of mental disorders are also related to age–sociopathic conditions typical of adolescence, schizophrenia in early adulthood, affective and psychophysiological disorders in middle adulthood, chronic addiction and involutional disorders in later maturity, and cerebral arteriosclerosis and senile dementia in old age.

Age is not only a biological phenomenon, it also represents a social status characterized by its unique sequence of functions and stresses. Developmental studies of individuals as they pass through age-epochs have become a method of organizing and relating their life cycles with the frequency and types of stresses to which they are exposed, as well as to their reactions to them (Jaco, 1970). This effort is supported by existing epidemiological studies in which many of the diseases are more frequent during certain stages of the life cycle than others.

However, longitudinal studies that continue through the life cycle and that have adequate research controls of the subjects are accompanied by many methodological difficulties. Besides all of the usual problems, such as sheer cost, there is the unscheduled death of some of the subjects, which makes them immune to chronic illness. Therefore many of the age-related data are derived from cross-sectional rather than cohort studies. In other words, a comparison of young and old deals with two sets of people: those who are currently young and those who are currently old, rather than one group of subjects who have grown from youth to old age.

Despite the importance of the age factor as a biosocial determinant of one's health status, this subject is not pursued in this section. This is partly because characteristics of age groups overlap those of other social statuses and institutions discussed in this chapter. To illustrate, (1) the health of preschool children is likely to be affected by socialization practices in the family; (2) the adult male role is primarily determined by the sex role and occupational position.

The Aged and Diseases. Because of the aging of the American population, civil rights movements directed toward the aged as a minority, Medicare legislation, and a host of other factors, there has been a recent upsurge of interest in gerontology. The study of social gerontology has so increased in scope and importance among both medical and social scientists that it has almost been established as an independent subfield, separate from medical sociology. Hence, an extensive review of a vastly growing literature (Binstock & Shanas, 1977; Birren & Schaie, 1977; Finch & Hayflick, 1977) is beyond the limited scope of this book. Only a cursory examination will be made of the relationship between old age and chronic or mental illnesses.

Diseases associated with advanced age include hardening of the arteries, senility, strokes, and mental disorders. Apart from biological wear and tear of bodily tissues and organs accompanying aging, stress has been singled out by many investigators as a vital determinant of the diseases of the elderly (Eisdorfer & Wilke, 1977). Stress may accelerate the aging process or it may result in disease, which increases the speed of physical deterioration. Stress may also impair the coping ability of the human organism. Much of the gerontological research in conjunction with stress has tended to focus upon life crises (loss of loved ones) and transitions (child leaving home, retirement, relocation).

Transitions in life have been explained by the disengagement theory of aging (Cumming & Henry, 1961), which stems from the functionalist perspective (Davis & Moore, 1945). The major premises of this theory are that (1) a process of withdrawal of aging individuals and society from each other is inevitable; (2) the transfer of power from the older to the younger, better qualified members of society is necessary to maintain social stability and functioning; and (3) the disengaged person is able to make an adjustment to the aging process, free from the stresses of the preretirement role, by recognizing his or her reduced ability and assuming a new social role that is more self-centered.

A seemingly contrasting theory, activity theory (Havighurst, 1963), on the other hand, postulates a positive relationship between activity and life satisfaction. It posits that successful aging is attained if the elderly person continues to engage in activities. But activity theory shares the same functionalist assumption of the disengagement theory—that older persons judge themselves according to commonly shared social values, namely, activity. To the extent that they fail to live up to these norms, they suffer from stress.

From a different standpoint, that of conflict theory, the assumption of value consensus is replaced by the notion of power struggle. The aged are viewed as a powerless minority group, deprived of class, status, and power (Streib, 1977). The dominant young and middle-aged groups have forced the elderly people out of occupations (forced retirement) and other social activities. Therefore, the only way for the aged to enjoy life satisfaction is to develop age-specific subcultures with distinct group identity and further organize themselves into political pressure groups to counteract the younger generation.

The struggle against the dominant young group involves not only a political power contest but also psychological warfare against the negative stereotyping of the aged. Society has labeled older persons with negative images—senile, rigid, sexless, poor, ugly, incapable, useless, inferior, etc. (Atchley, 1972; Palmore, 1971). In line with the labeling theory, the end result of these invidious stereotypes is that elderly persons come to develop negative self-concepts. They must confront not only the fact of biological decline but also cope with being relegated to an inferior social status (Rosow, 1967, 1974).

Research findings so far have yielded contradictory results with regard to the validity of these theories of aging. It is obvious that the field of social gerontology is still in the formative stage and awaits the accumulation of an extensive body of research.

Sex Status

Women live longer than men and have lower mortality rates for most causes of death. Nevertheless, women report more physical and mental illness than men, have more days of disability, and utilize physicians and hospital services at higher rates than do men.

The apparent contradiction between mortality and morbidity data has led many investigators to seek for sociocultural interpretations. Having surveyed existing writings, Nathanson (1975) extrapolated three major explanatory schemes that can be cast into our three theoretical frameworks.

First, from the functionalist perspective of role integration, it can be postulated that the sick role is adopted readily when it is compatible with other roles one has to perform. In other words, the sick role is more compatible with women's other role responsibilities than it is with men's, which implies that women's roles are relatively undemanding, giving them ample time to be sick.

This hypothesis has been reformulated by Rivkin (1972) to be tested among women; Rivkin proposed that those with a large number of functionally important roles are unlikely to adopt the sick role. Based on data from the World Health Organization/National Collaboration Study of medical care utilization, collected in Baltimore, Maryland, in 1968–1969, the hypothesis was supported to the extent that lower morbidity rates were found among married women, who presumably have more role obligations than single women, and lower sickness rates were found among gainfully employed than nonemployed women. Also, women with demanding role obligations (e.g., having children and no spouse, or having children and working) were found to report fewer days of disability with self-treatment at home but have a greater tendency to get into the medical care system for faster recovery.

Another supporting survey for this explanatory model comes from Moriyama and others (1971). Their survey indicates that since 1950 the male rate of heart diseases has leveled off, while the female rate (for ages 35 to 54 years) is rising along with the increase in female employment (Johnson, 1977).

Pursuing their research on sex differences in role obligations, Gove and Hughes (1979) note the important link between role characteristics and type of illness. They suggest that women are obliged to perform nurturing tasks, such as caring for others, that may interfere with their ability to care for themselves. Such obligations may result in minor forms of physical disabilities in reaction to psychological distress and also in poor mental health. In other words, the higher rates of morbidity reported for women reflect the higher rates of mild forms of physical illness among women rather than of the chronic diseases that are the leading causes of death.

In terms of the conflict theory, women would be assumed to have more illness than men because their assigned social roles as sexual subordinates are more stressful.

Gove and Tudor (1973, 1977) contend that the status of women in modern industrial societies is more conducive to stress than that of men. First, housewives who are fettered to domesticity have no alternative sources of gratification. Second, in comparison to man's work, housework is unskilled and of low prestige. Third, even at work women's jobs are of low esteem and psychologically unrewarding. Finally, role expectations for women are diffuse and unstructured, thereby producing anxiety and stress. They also note that sex differences in rates of mental illness appear only among the married, not the singles, because the woman's role in marriage is more stressful than that of a single woman.

Gove and Tudor's work has been criticized on methodological grounds (Cooperstock & Parnell, 1976; Dohrenwend & Dohrenwend, 1974b) as well as substantive grounds (Warheit et al., 1976). Methodologically, Gove and Tudor's conception of mental illness is based only upon functional psychoses, not on other diagnostic psychiatric categories such as personality disorders and alcoholic psychosis, where the rates for males exceed those for females. Hence the higher rate of mental illness among women is an artifact of their method.

Even apart from methodological issues, the conflict–stress hypothesis does not stand up well against other data. For instance, women with a large number of role obligations are expected to experience more role conflict and strain than other women, but as discussed above, they have lower rates of illness (Rivkin, 1972).

A third explanatory model for the sex differential in morbidity is based on the labeling theory. According to this view, women report more illness than men because it is culturally more acceptable for them to be ill. Broverman and others (1970) reported that concepts of mental health among psychiatrists, psychologists, and social workers differ for men and women, paralleling traditional sex role stereotypes. Women are less stigmatized than men for complaining about symptoms of illness and for seeking medical care.

According to Phillips's (1964) study, identical behavior patterns symptomatic of various mental illnesses were rejected more strongly when the patient was identified as a man than as a woman. Phillips and Segal (1969) further demonstrated that among men and women with similar physical symptoms, women report more psychological distress and are more likely to seek medical help.

However, attempts to replicate Phillips's findings have shown inconsistent results (Gove & Tudor, 1973; Nathanson, 1975; Tudor et al., 1977). Disputes over the validity of the labeling interpretation have led to a series of methodological investigations on response biases. Gove, Clancy, Geerken, and others (Clancy & Gove, 1974; Gove & Geerken, 1977) empirically researched the impact of biases such as the tendency for yea-saying or nay-saying, the perception of the desirability of a given trait, and the need for social approval. When these biases were controlled, the sex difference in mental illness not only did not diminish, but increased. Thus they concluded that the sex difference is not an artifact of response bias and rejected the labeling theory of mental illness.

Wary of the debate on the applicability of these explanatory models to overall rates of mental illness in a limited time and place, Dohrenwend and Dohrenwend (1976, 1977) stressed the importance of the specification of conditions under which certain types of illness appear. They found that (1) there are no consistent sex differences in rates of functional psychoses; (2) the rates for manic-depressive psychosis are generally higher among women; (3) the rates for neurosis are consistently higher for women regardless of time and place; and (4) the rates of personality disorders are consistently higher for men regardless of time and place. Dohrenwend and Dohrenwend suggested the existence of common denominators: (1) depressive symptomatology underlying the neurosis and manic-depressive psychosis among women, and (2) irresponsible and antisocial behaviors underlying male personality disorders.

Unlike other variables, such as socioeconomic status or family, sex is an independent variable that contains clear-cut categories and is free from definitional problems. Therefore the consideration of sex differences in studies of mental disorder has been pursued fairly vigorously both theoretically and methodologically. However, sex status does not operate in a vacuum. The association between sex and disease must be examined in relation to other variables such as marital status, employment, lifestyle, and number of children (Johnson, 1977).

Marital Status

Going back to Durkheim, the status of the divorced and the unmarried has been associated with unhappiness, distress, psychoses, or suicide rather than with freedom or peace of mind. Reports dating back to the middle of the nineteenth century have shown a persistent relationship between marital status and mental health (Adler, 1953; Carter & Glick, 1976; Farina et al., 1963; Gaudet & Watson, 1935; Gove, 1972a; Jaco, 1960; Malzberg, 1940; Odegaard, 1946; Radloff, 1975; Retherford, 1975; Rose & Stub, 1955; Turner, 1972; Verbrugge, 1979). Researchers have used different instruments to measure mental health such as self-assessment of psychological well-being (Bradburn & Caplovitz, 1965; Gurin et al., 1960; Pearlin & Johnson, 1977), prognosis and duration of confinement in mental hospitals (Farina et al., 1963; Mason et al., 1960; Turner et al., 1970), suicide rates (Durkheim, 1950; Gibbs & Martin, 1964; Gove, 1972b), and the psychological stress component associated with marital status (Dodge & Martin, 1970; Geerken & Gove, 1974; Gove, 1973).

The overall conclusion is that the rate of mental disorder is highest among the divorced, lowest among the married, and intermediate among single and widowed.

Competing interpretations can be broadly classified into four categories. The first is based on the functionalist premise that there is a commonly held value that attaches importance to marriage. Thus, the single who remains single is considered to be deviant from the social norms (Lee, 1974; Udry, 1974) and therefore experiences psychological distress. Conversely, marriage offers individuals security and social support. This argument is not very convincing these days when the proportion of the unmarrieid is increasing. There are even studies (Renne, 1971; Zalokar, 1960) which indicate that divorced people are healthier, happier, and less isolated than the unhappily married. Another facet associated with marital status is the life style. Nonmarried people are more likely to adopt life styles with high health risks such as drinking, smoking, and irregular eating (Verbrugge, 1979).

A second interpretation pertains to the formerly married. It states that the very transition from marriage to singleness is the source of stress (Bachrach, 1975). The formerly married have the difficult task of readjusting to new role definitions. Self-concept, social networks, lifestyles, and other activities have to be changed to fit the new role of a nonmarried. It is these demands that generate psychological disturbances.

Third, it has been suggested that the psychological disorders of the nonmarried are a cause of their marital status rather than a consequence of it. According to this view, those who remain single, widowed, or divorced may include a large portion of individuals who are too maladjusted for marriage. This is because marriage requires a certain amount of initiative as well as the ability to provide a home, good health, social skills, and personality integration (Farina et al., 1963; Garfield & Sundland, 1966; Odegaard, 1946; Turner et al., 1970). In support of the selection hypothesis, Turner and Gartrell (1978) presented data indicating that there is nothing about marriage per se that results in mental illness. Rather, the relationship between marital status and mental disorder arises as a consequence of conditions within individuals, namely, social competence. The more ineffective an individual is, the less likely he or she is to find a marital partner and the more likely he or she is to be mentally disturbed.

The fourth interpretation is to envision the correspondence of marital status and mental health as a reflection of persistent life strains shaped by social and economic structural arrangements. Pearlin and Johnson (1977) postulated and validated that nonmarried people are both more exposed and more vulnerable than the married to three stressful conditions of life, namely, economic hardship, social isolation, and parental responsibility (Verbrugge, 1979).

Instead of accepting the validity of a direct relationship between marital status and mental disorder, some researchers began to examine interactive effects of more than one status upon the incidence of mental illness. They assume that a certain configuration of statuses is culturally prescribed as functional to societal integration. For instance, there are commonly accepted combinations of marital status, age, and sex. The status of a 16-year-old married male is ambivalent. He is expected to play an adult role, which tends to isolate him from his unmarried age-peers. Yet he is not accepted as a mature adult. Such status incongruence sets a person off as being deviant, and it tends to isolate him from meaningful social interaction. The absence of stable and durable social relations is conducive to mental disturbances. This hypothesis concerning status incongruence and mental illness was supported by Martin (1976), although his data are quite old (1933).

Another example of status inconsistency has to do with marital status compared with socioeconomic status. Gove and Tudor (Gove, 1972a,b; Gove & Tudor, 1973) suggested that the housewife's role ambivalence and inconsistency account for her higher rates of mental disorder. Meile and others (1976) studied the interactive effect of marital and socioeconomic statuses upon the mental health of married women. They conjectured that the structural features of the stress, which are associated with marital status, are related to the socioeconomic status of married women. Lower class married women tend to concentrate their efforts on their role of motherhood (Bell, 1971), placing less emphasis upon the roles of wife and companion to their husbands (Komarovsky, 1964). Although motherhood is central to them, they view it as a source of problems (Langner & Michael, 1963; Veroff & Feld, 1970). On the other hand, middle class married women play many roles—they are mothers, wives, working women, and members of social organizations. Opportunities for gratification outside the marital role increases with socioeconomic status. Women with a better education may have challenging career opportunities or they may be more active in volunteer associations (Booth, 1972).

Consequently, Meile and others (1976) hypothesized that the marital role is more stressful for lower class women than for middle class women. They found a statistically significant interaction effect between marital status and educational attainment upon mental disorder. This relationship persisted even after age and employment status were taken into consideration. Among women of lower educational attainment, the married showed more disorder than the never married. Among women with a high school or higher education, no significant differences in mental disorder were found that related to the marital status of the subjects.

Finally, another example of an interaction effect is found in Geerken and Gove's (1974) study of race, sex, marital status, and mortality. They began with the traditional assumption that blacks are likely to have matrifocal families. Then, in comparison with the black female, who is the dominant figure in the family, the black male is more exposed to the stresses that result from racial discrimination, menial and low income occupations, and powerlessness in the family. In contrast with this, the white female has lower status and less power in occupational and other social spheres than the white male. Geerken and Gove found no sharp difference in the mortality rates in the marital roles of blacks and whites. However, their hypotheses were supported by the fact that marriage is better for the white man than for the black man, and better for the black woman than for the white woman. That is, the mortality rate is lower for white married men than for black married men, and lower for black married women than for white married women.

The association between social structure such as marital status and mental disorder has been acknowledged by many sociologists, epidemiologists, and other investigators. Although there is relatively little research aimed directly at understanding how this relationship arises, at least four major explanatory models are available. In addition, in recent years research efforts have been directed toward finding an interactive effect of marital status.

Socioeconomic Status

Generations of sociologists have attempted to demonstrate a link between social class and human behavior, including rates of sickness. Among the various categories and units of analysis, socioeconomic status has attracted the greatest attention from researchers, who have tried to explain why lower class people are more likely to suffer from illness than middle class people.

Chronic Illness

Despite the multiplicity of methods and the varigated populations in the studies reviewed, Antonovosky (1967a) reached his "inescapable" conclusion that economic status influences one's chances of staying alive. Almost without exception, the evidence shows that the classes clearly differ in their mortality rates. Antonovosky also noted that the trend toward the closing of the class differences in mortality rates, apparent in the earlier decades of this century, has since been slowed.

Although the control of infectious disease has narrowed the gap in the degree of class exposure to germs, there are still other factors that are more likely to expose the lower class than the middle class to stress (Antonovosky, 1967b). Those in the lower strata experience more unpleasant events due to their economic and cultural poverty (Myers & Roberts, 1959). They are also less equipped than middle class individuals to cope with stress because they lack adequate, durable interpersonal relations and social support (Myers et al., 1974; Syme & Berkman, 1976). To make matters worse, the poor are less inclined than the affluent to receive what few medical services they have in their neighborhood because of (1) financial difficulties, (2) the "culture of poverty," which inhibits their use of medical care (see Chapter 5), and (3) the medical subculture, which is prejudiced against lower class clients (Dutton, 1978).

Lower economic class status has been associated with high blood pressure, hypertension ("Cardiac . . . ," 1967; Dawber et al., 1967; Gordon & Devine, 1966; Guralnick, 1963b; Lilienfeld, 1956; McDonough et al., 1964; Skinner et al., 1966; Taylor et al., 1966), and with lung, stomach, and esophageal cancer (Graham et al., 1960), although coronary artery diseases ("Register . . . ," 1951) are found more often in higher social classes.

Specifically, the relation of socioeconomic status and occupation to coronary disease incidence and mortality has been widely studied. Through comprehensive reviews of the literature, Jenkins (1971, 1976) observed conflicting directions in the results and interpreted that the social stratum most vulnerable to coronary disease may be different at varying periods of a nation's evolution from agrarian to industrialized society. Early in the process of urbanization and industrialization, the upper socioeconomic classes are at an elevated risk of coronary diseases whereas toward the end of the process, the lower economic classes have higher risk.

In general, Jenkins (1976) found that demographic indicators are not consistent predictors of coronary risk. For example, occupation per se shows unstable relations with coronary diseases. However, studies of the health-related aspects of lifestyle associated with occupation show promise in demonstrating a relationship between social class and coronary disease. It is typically found that the way of life characteristic to an occupation contributes to coronary risk above and beyond the physical labor involved in the job itself (Keys, 1970).

Those in occupations that involve greater stress indicate a higher susceptibility to heart disease (Guralnick, 1963a). Such occupations include that of air traffic controllers (Dougherty, 1967), military people in basic training (Weiner et al., 1957), first-line supervisors (Dunn et al., 1962), and comparable activities that involve visible responsibilities (Brod, 1971; Friedman et al., 1958; Friedman & Roseman, 1959; Russek, 1959). The key components of occupational stress are job dissatisfaction, work overload, and responsibility.

Coronary heart disease, when associated with job dissatisfaction, is keyed to working conditions—such as tediousness, lack of recognition, impoverished interpersonal relations, and other poor working conditions (Jenkins, 1971a,b; Medalie et al., 1973; Sales & House, 1971)—with their correlate: low self-esteem. This relationship is more pronounced among the middle-aged or older white-collar males than it is among blue-collar or younger workers. These findings can be interpreted as a result of the combined effect of aspiration and opportunity (Kleiner & Parker, 1966). First, there are those such as young workers who aspire to a better occupational future and who perceive their opportunity for attaining the goal to be high. Second, there are low ranking employees, e.g., blue-collar workers, who have low aspiration. These two types of people are less likely to be distressed by the current unpleasant jobs than those who have been ambitious but whose opportunities have been blocked, for example the middle-aged or older white-collar males.

Job pressure is also generated by workloads that exceed one's capability, time, or resources. The association between heart disease and work overload, which has been assessed both objectively and subjectively, has been established by many (French et al., 1965).

Assuming responsibility for the safety and welfare of known individuals is more likely to cause stress than taking responsibility for impersonal objects such as budgets and equipment (Marks, 1967). Occupations which involve that kind of stress-inducing responsibility have been associated with coronary heart disease (Montoye et al., 1967; Russek, 1962).

Kitagawa and Hauser (1973) pointed out that both occupation and income usually change with advancing age, which raises mortality risk. They recommended education as the better indicator of socioeconomic status and reported an inverse relation between mortality from arteriosclerotic heart disease and level of education.

Some research attention has been focused on social mobility and status incongruity as stressors rather than on socioeconomic status. Status incongruity is defined as a discrepancy in an individual's ratings on various components of social class, such as level of education, occupation, income, quality of house, and organizational membership. An example would be a highly educated person with low income. This inconsistency is believed to result in more frequent tensions and conflicts.

The association of social mobility and status incongruity with coronary disease has yielded conflicting evidence (Caplan, 1971; Horan & Gray, 1974; Jenkins, 1971b; Shekells, 1976). Jenkins (1976) concluded that social mobility and status inconsistency may be conditional predictors valid only in certain places and eras, only for certain aspects of coronary disease, or only in conjunction with other variables.

Mental Illness

As far as total prevalence is concerned, lower social class is associated with a higher rate of mental disorder. Many studies have derived their data from hospital admission records and army rejection lists (Adler et al., 1952; Clark, 1949; Frumkin, 1955; Hepple, 1946; Rowntree et al., 1945; Srole et al., 1962). Of greater significance, and ever since the classic study of Faris and Dunham (1939), innumerable researchers have established an inverse relationship between socioeconomic status and schizophrenic disorder; and those results, in turn, have been reviewed by many in the field (Dohrenwend & Dohrenwend, 1969; Kohn, 1968; Mishler & Scotch, 1963; Roman & Trice, 1967).

However, there are certain types of psychological impairments, such as manic depression, that are associated more with higher socioeconomic strata (Hollingshead & Redlich, 1953, 1954; Myers & Schaffer, 1954; Redlich et al., 1953; Roberts & Myers, 1954).

Why do lower class people have more mental problems? Etiological hypotheses can be divided into two types: (1) the causation hypothesis, which suggests that lower class life causes mental disorder (Dohrenwend & Dohrenwend, 1969; Langner & Michael, 1963; Wheaton, 1978), and (2) the selection-drift hypothesis, which proposes that the mentally disturbed move into or are forced into lower social classes. Each of these hypotheses will now be discussed in detail.

Social Causation Hypothesis. The causation hypothesis will be viewed from three perspectives: economic insecurity, social reaction, and coping ability.

1. Economic Insecurity. According to the causation hypothesis, members of the lower class are exposed to stress because of their economic deprivation (Lapouse et al., 1956; Rushing, 1969). Leavy and Freedman (1956) found that psychoneurotic patients express their fears in economic terms, either as threats to subsistence or threats to self-esteem. Periods of economic decline have been linked with enhanced emotional disturbances (Bakke, 1940; Brenner, 1973; Hollingshead & Redlich, 1958; Neff, 1968), and, specifically, with increased rates of admission to mental hospitals (Brenner, 1973; Draughon, 1975; Malzberg, 1959).

From the interactionist perspective, economic insecurity becomes crucial when individuals, regardless of the actual level in class structure, perceive that their status is deprived in relation to others. That sense of relative deprivation has been associated with higher hospitalization rates (Tuckman & Kleiner, 1962).

Economic deprivation not only generates stress for subsistence but also results in a psychological stress that affects one's self-esteem. In this case, the functionalist argument holds that there are culturally prescribed goals such as material success, and the failure to achieve comparative success brings disappointment to the individual (Clark, 1949; Jaco, 1960; Merton, 1949; Odegaard, 1956). In turn, Kasl and French (1962) suggested that there are links between the skill level required on the job and the worker's self-concept, which can influence rates of physical and mental illnesses. Neurotic behavior has been accounted for in terms of blocked aspiration and resulting disparagement (Jaco, 1960; Leavy & Freedman, 1956; Srole et al., 1962).

At this level of analysis the issue is no longer a question of social class; rather, it is the identification of the class that is most susceptible to stresses arising from achievement versus aspiration discrepancies. Kardiner and Ovesey (1951) found in their study of blacks that striving for achievement was an important etiological factor in middle class, but not lower class, psychopathology. Hollingshead, Ellis, and Kirby (1954) discovered that the mentally ill, both in the lower and middle classes, showed large discrepancies between achievements and aspirations in the fields of education and occupation. Still, Myers and Roberts (1959) found a large disparity between ambition and accomplishment among only the middle class patients, and there was none among those from the lower class.

In his intensive sociopsychological study of the schizophrenic type, Weinberg (1952, 1967) found that the inability of such patients to assess their own limitations and/or the limitations of a given situation was in itself a contributing factor to their subsequent breakdowns. Similar findings have been reported by many (Hinkle & Wolff, 1957; Sewell & Haller, 1959).

Pursuing the same line of reasoning, Kleiner and Parker (1966) developed a formula to measure goal-striving stress. They assumed that the amount of stress generated by discrepancies between achievement and aspiration will differ depending on the centrality of the goal for the individual, that is, the importance he or she attaches to reaching the goal. Here, if a person is far from the set goal, he or she can drop the goal easily; near-success tends to generate the most stress. In Kleiner and Parker's study, goal-striving stress was found to be higher for the mentally ill than for normal people.

2. Social Reaction. Interactionists emphasize the process by which people come to be perceived as mentally disordered, and then concentrate on what happens to those people after they are so labeled. The social causation hypothesis states that individuals with more resources are better able to control their fates and hence to resist legal coercion that would lead to hospitalization. Available evidence appears to support the contention that patients committed by the courts are more apt to have fewer socioeconomic resources than patients who enter voluntarily (Gove & Fain, 1977; Linsky, 1970; Rushing, 1971; Rushing & Esco, 1969). After being hospitalized, those from lower social classes are less likely to receive therapeutic treatment and will stay institutionalized longer than middle class patients. In the eyes of interactionists, social class is important not because of its role in producing the initially deviant behavior but because its real pathogenic force is the way it affects people's perception of deviance and their reaction to that behavior.

However, results from the above quoted studies do not deny the role of psychiatric status in the hospitalization process. Most of the committed patients are indeed seriously ill rather than merely labeled as such. Rather than accepting or rejecting the labeling perspective completely, Rushing (1978) supports a theory of conjoined impacts, namely, that the effect of status resources varies depending on the severity of the psychiatric symptoms and the level of behavioral deviance. In other words, lower class people are more likely to be labeled as mentally ill if they show severe symptoms of disorders that are socially disruptive.

3. Coping Ability. It has been argued that resources to cope with stress are unevenly distributed in social classes (Liem & Liem, 1978). Langner and Michael (1963) reported that at any given level of stress, people with lower class positions are more likely to be mentally disturbed than those having higher positions. The implication here is that class difference has an influence on how effectively people can cope with stress.

Lower class people cope with stress less effectively because the type of stress they experienced is not apt to be altered by individual action. At the same time, they also have little money or power to employ in coping with stress (Langner & Michael, 1963).

Kohn (1972) delved further into the nature of subjectively perceived reality for the lower class. He noted that conditions of life experienced by lower class people foster limited and confined conceptions of social reality, which impair their ability to cope resourcefully with stress. Their fearful, fatalistic, and conformist attitudes destroy their ability to cope with the type of stress that requires flexibility and a perceptive understanding of social complexity. Langner and Michael (1963) assume that such values, beliefs, and behavior styles of the lower class originate early in the person's socialization experience and exert a continuing influence.

This supports Kadushin's (1964) view that social classes do not differ so much in becoming ill as they do in feeling ill. He claims that people in the lower economic class are more likely to feel sick than those in the middle class because the former have fatalistic attitudes and therefore do not avail themselves of medical care services.

It should be noted, however, that the health care utilization patterns among social classes have changed significantly since the mid-1960s when Medicare and Medicaid were enacted. Several studies indicate that when an illness is present, there is no significant difference in the use of physician services among various income-groups. When an illness is not present and if free care is available, lower income people are more likely than others to visit physicians

(Bellin & Geiger, 1972; Bice, Eichhorn, & Fox, 1972; Galvin & Fan, 1975; Monteiro, 1973; Sparer & Okada, 1974).

The coping ability of individuals in the lower class is further weakened by a lack of group support. They participate less in institutions of the *larger society* and have less durable human relations than do middle class people (Dohrenwend & Dohrenwend, 1969). However, that opinion has been rebutted by others (Lewis, 1966), who claim that the culture of poverty is a rational adaptation to social reality and that the evolving culture is built upon the institutions unique to the lower class.

Social Drift Hypothesis. In comparison with the social causation hypothesis, the social drift hypothesis explains mental disturbance in terms of the individual rather than the social class. It is not the characteristics of the lower classes that makes people mentally ill, but rather it is the mentally disturbed that tend to move into the lower classes (Harkey et al., 1976; Rushing, 1969).

The mentally ill are inept in fitting into the class hierarchy, with the exception of the lowest ranking positions. Among schizophrenics, intergenerational downward mobility was noted by some (Dunham, 1965), and a lag in upward mobility was reported by others (Turner & Wagenfeld, 1967), although some found no significant mobility (Goldberg & Morrison, 1963).

Hare (1956) reported that the distribution of schizophrenic cases in family settings did not differ significantly from a random distribution, but schizophrenics out of family settings were concentrated in areas of cities that had single dwelling units. Schizophrenics seem to move out of family contexts because of personality disorders, relocating themselves in lower social class areas (Hare, 1956). Dunham (1965) explained that, among those who left the parental home, some developed a shcizophrenic condition that prevented them from realizing their goals and forced them into the lower social class.

The drift hypothesis was further expanded to include the combined effect of mobility and region (Eaton, 1974; Kohn, 1968). In rural areas the child tends to follow the father's occupation as a farmer. In urban areas the child has to leave home and enter the cold, impersonal environment of a competitive, occupational world. The social drift hypothesis is applicable to these urban children. This partly explains why an inverse relation between social class and mental disorder was found in most of the urban studies and seldom in the rural studies (Eaton, 1974).

As an explanation for the inverse relation between social class and mental illness, intergenerational downward mobility was supported by some (Jaco, 1959; Langner & Michael, 1963; Morris, 1959), and rejected by others (Clausen & Kohn, 1959; Hollingshead & Redlich, 1954; Lapouse et al., 1956; Tietze et al., 1942). Still others found relations between upward mobility and mental illness (Hollingshead & Redlich, 1954; Hollingshead, Ellis, & Kirby, 1954).

After a detailed review of the evidence, Kohn (1968) was led to conclude that downward mobility does not provide a sufficient explanation, while Kleiner and Parker (1969) decided that mobility itself, whether upward or downward, reflects the anomie situation and hence induces stress. Using data from a panel study, Lee (1976) evaluated the causal priority between socioeconomic status and psychiatric disorder and suggested that the social causation hypothesis is more plausible than the social drift hypothesis.

Overview

For decades sociologists have attempted to explain an overall inverse relation between social class and psychological dysfunction. Through the analysis of such relations, conceptual models have grown to be so sophisticated that social class is now viewed not only as an independent variable but also as an intervening and even as a dependent variable (Antonovosky, 1967a,b; Dohrenwend & Dohrenwend, 1969; House, 1974). Feedback interactions (Britt, 1975) between social class and psychological impairment are also being taken into account in such models.

Other researchers concerned themselves with the dimensionality of socioeconomic status. That status is frequently measured by an index that takes into account occupation, education, income, and in some instances, ethnicity. By so doing, the postulate of unidimensionality of status is rejected, and it is assumed that each component status variable has a more or less independent and additive effect (Hollingshead & Redlich, 1958; Meile & Haese, 1969; Srole et al., 1962).

In contrast, some writers have held that there is a nonvertical dimension to status, one of consistency. For these researchers, individuals occupy a number of social positions that vary in the magnitudes of status and power. When there is a lack of consistency across status indicators (e.g., high scores on education as compared to low scores on occupational status), it leads to stress that may manifest itself in mental disorders (Baldwin, Floyd, & McSeveney, 1975; Geschwender, 1967; Gibbs & Martin, 1965; Jackson, 1962; Lenski, 1954).

Despite all of the above efforts, a detailed examination of their results clearly shows that the stability of the relationship between socioeconomic status and mental disorder is open to question (Kleiner & Parker, 1963). There are some who found no communality (Clausen & Kohn, 1960), and there are others who noted curvilinear relations (Jaco, 1960; Parker et al., 1962). A review of much of the literature led Rushing (1969) to theorize about two patterns: (1) a discrete relationship (the lowest class having a higher illness rate than all others, but little difference in the rates for the other classes); or (2) a continuous relationship, with the illness rates systematically increasing as class status dropped, but with a disproportionate expansion for the lowest class.

There are some who take the "cart before the horse" approach (Mechanic, 1972c), insisting that the effort to establish the relationship between social class and mental disorder logically precedes the need to explain such a correspondence. In other words, first determine that the two are indeed related; then proceed to talk about their relationship.

SUMMARY

This chapter begins with descriptions of the distributions of health and illness in various societies in time and space. Standard demographic variables such as age and sex are shown in their relation to mortality and morbidity. General conclusions are derived: (1) mortality rates decreased significantly as society progressed from the preindustrial to the modern industrial state; and (2) preindustrial societies are characterized by high morbidity and mortality rates of communicable disease, while industrialized societies suffer from high rates of chronic and mental illnesses.

For the unit of analysis smaller than society, there are more detailed research data available than mortality rates based on simple classification of demographic variables. Thus the social factors of physical and mental dysfunctioning are reviewed for social organizations at various levels, ranging from community, institution (family), and social statuses (race, age, sex, marital status, and socioeconomic status).

The validity and reliability of the findings have not been established, which makes any overall generalizations and interpretations tenuous. Characteristically, the instability and inconsistency of research results stem from a relative deficiency in the following: (1) standardization in definitions, diagnosis, and measurements; (2) representativeness of the sample; (3) control of response biases; and (4) control over other variables such as the availability and utilization of medical facilities.

Therefore, when reading research findings, the first problem is to determine whether the relationship is real or only a methodological artifact. When the result is accepted as real (Kleiner & Parker, 1971), the next task is to interpret the correlation by seeing if it meets the conditions for causal inference: (1) Do social structure or process cause illness? (2) Does illness cause a change in one's membership in social groups? (3) Are there any other factors that influence the relationship between social group and mobility?

In the presence of conflicting research findings, various methodological and substantive interpretations have been proposed.

The first methodological interpretation pertains to response biases. In other words, high morbidity rates are due to the fact that some people are more likely than others to report illness or to be labeled as sick. This is argued from the perspective of the labeling theory. Thus, women are more inclined than men to complain about physical symptoms and to seek medical care because they are culturally expected to be the weaker sex. According to the labeling theory, the less powerful are more likely than the powerful to be channeled into a sick role; therefore lower class people are more prone than middle class individuals to be committed to mental hospitals.

The second methodological insight is the possibility that the relationship between social group and morbidity is a spurious one. Much attention has been focused upon determining whether or not racial difference in illness rates is a function of socioeconomic status rather than race per se. Also, the association between sex and morbidity has been obscured by other variables such as education, marital status, age, and employment. Another much investigated issue involves the availability of medical services and utilization patterns. In this regard it is suspected that lower rates of mental illness in rural areas may reflect the scarcity of psychiatric facilities rather than the fact that rural people are healthier than urban people.

Once methodological biases are assumed to be controlled, efforts are shifted to explaining the correspondence of social group with morbidity. Social groups can be divided into two types: ascribed and achieved. The ascribed status group includes sex, race, and the like, of which membership is ascribed to the individual by birth and rarely can be changed. The achieved status group is one that individuals can attain by their efforts, such as socioeconomic status, marital status, and urban or rural community living.

In the case of the ascribed statuses, the first consideration is to evaluate the weight of genetics. High rates of hypertension among blacks and high morbidity rates of women can be explained in part by hereditary and biological conditions of blacks and females. That part which cannot be accounted for biologically, has been subjected to sociological analysis. Accordingly, high morbidity rates among females and blacks have been attributed to stresses associated with subordinate group membership.

In dealing with achieved status groups, three explanatory themes are suggested. The first is the causal hypothesis, that a particular social group is susceptible to stress which affects the health of its membership. For example, the statuses of the unmarried, the lower class, or the urbanites are viewed as inherently stressful.

The second hypothesis states that health status lets people drift into certain social groups rather than that the social group induces illness. To illustrate, physical or mental illness incapacitates the individual and leads him or her to move down to the lower class. Also, sick people are likely to be less fit for marriage and so more likely to remain single.

The third approach is to view the mobility into or out of social groups as stressful in itself, disposing the movers to higher risks of illness. Urban migrants, the divorced, and occupationally mobile people are subject to stresses by mobility.

One of the implications of the review in this chapter is that contributions to the etiology of diseases originating in different levels of social organizations are interlocked and must be examined holistically rather than separately. The relationship of social categories to individual physical and psychological functioning can be viewed as an aspect of the more general relationship of social structure and process to individual behavior. Although in principle this larger issue has a place in epidemiological inquiry, few examples of research paying explicit attention to it can be found in the literature.

The fundamental obstacle to a conceptually integrated theory lies in the fact that different levels of social organization may have unique internal structure and dynamics that must be retained in an attempt to describe their interrelations. Nevertheless, a start has been made toward delineating multiple levels of analysis, aided by the integration of diverse bodies of existing research. More well-designed, large-scale research with theoretical foundations is needed to consolidate available findings and to resolve inconsistencies.

PART 2
Medicine as a Social System

CHAPTER 5

The Physician–Patient Relationship

In Part 1 of this book we described three sociological perspectives and used them to examine the emergence of medical sociology and the social etiology of diseases.

In Part 2, various aspects of medical practice will be discussed. Our analysis begins with the postulate that medicine is a social system whose component parts are interrelated and in equilibrium. Next, this systemic assumption is subjected to the opposite view, that medical practice consists of conflicting process or symbolic bargaining dynamics. The physician–patient relationship is the most basic unit in medicine. Every medical activity involves at least two parties, the healer and the sick or, in a broader sense, the medical corps and the public. In essence, the organization of medicine can be reduced to the manifold, dyadic relations between these two groups (Marti-Ibanez, 1960).

Traditionally, the physician–patient encounter was cemented by the public's "sacred trust" (Harris, 1966) in medicine. In recent years, however, there has been an erosion in the physician–patient relationship (Haug, 1976), which is evidenced by an upsurge in the number of malpractice suits and by doctor's strikes. The medical profession is now being scrutinized by demanding consumers who are dissatisfied with the quality and cost of their medical care.

In the face of this growing crisis, a study of the interaction between doctor and patient is important not only because of the pragmatic necessity to evaluate this situation, but also because of the significance it has for an understanding of the basic nature of the medical delivery system. To that end, the interdependence of the sick and the healer will be examined historically and systematically according to (1) the doctor–patient relations that existed before medical practice attained the status of a profession; (2) the manner in which physicians, as members of a profession, approached and were being approached by their patients during the period of medical domination; and (3) the type of associations that are fermenting now that the status and power of the medical profession has been challenged by various social forces.

THE PHYSICIAN–PATIENT RELATIONSHIP IN HISTORY

Primitive Medicine

Historically, cultural values have tended to stress the priorities of a theological institution over all others, including the practice of healing. As described in Chapter 1, early medicine was practiced within a rigid, pantheistic framework. In primitive medicine, the origins of disease were attributed to natural causes, human action (human manipulation of an evil spirit), or supernatural forces (punishment by an evil spirit for violation of a taboo) (Hallowell, 1935). Thus, disease was treated by dealing with the evil spirit, and the priestly healer claimed to have influence over the spirit that had entered the sick person. The healers in the prescientific era were believed to have been chosen by the gods. They not only treated the individual patient for illness and injury, but played leading roles in all tribal ceremonies and in all supplications for rain, grain, game, or victory in war.

The relationship between the priest-healer and patient can be viewed as a well-integrated social system. The patient's confidence in the practitioner was based on the religious belief that the art of medicine was taught by the gods, thereby lending great divine power to the healer, irrespective of the medical technology. The patient was also bound to the healing practitioner by social norms because certain illnesses were looked upon as punishments for socially disapproved behavior, and the priest-healer had the power to sanction the patient. Being subordinate to the healer, the patients surrendered themselves willingly to any treatment the healer chose to provide (Ackerknecht, 1942; Corlett, 1935; Maddox, 1923).

However, the functionalist assumption of stability in the healer–patient relationship is not warranted since the status of a healer was never secure. Even as a tribal chief, that position could be usurped by someone else who could win the contest for chieftainship. A tribal chief could also lose the office after repeated failure in bringing rain or a good harvest.

If we examine the healer–patient relationship from the symbolic interaction viewpoint, we may see that it was characterized by the healer's management of the cues provided by the patient. Having perceived the fear and pain of the patient, the healing practitioner must authenticate himself or herself with the aid of rituals, clothing, tone of voice, and other symbols. Technically, the healer had very little to offer to the patient, and that minimal offering was derived from pure empiricism. The rest was a placebo effect provoked by the healer's ability to impress the patient with an imaginery supernatural power.

Greek Medicine

The basis for the doctor–patient relationship was described as *philia* or "friendship" by Greek philosophers such as Socrates, Plato, and Aristotle. Thus, rather than the provision of technical help, diagnosis, and therapy, the relationship between doctor and patient was considered to be one of friendship. For Plato, the aim of friendship was the perfection of human nature—therefore of the nature of the universe—through the expression of the individualities of friends (Entralgo, 1969).

The functionalist perspective can be identified in the Greek's belief that the *physis* (nature) of an individual human being was related to the natural order, both directly (through procreation, nutrition, breathing, etc.) and through society—the *polis.* In other words, the individual is the component member and the doctor–patient relationship is a subunit of the larger system of the society or of the universe. Such a view, however, could lead to varying degrees of stress to the social order in the relation between the individual and the cosmos. For instance, a Hippocratic physician felt friendly to patients as siblings sharing the common filial relation of all humanity, while Plato's ideal healer found a bond with patients as members of the human community—the *polis.*

The social system of the doctor–patient relationship was ultimately based on the religious and mythological outlook that resulted from the worship of the gods Apollo and Asclepius. Greek patients' confidence in the art of healing and in the particular doctor who was treating them, was built upon their trust in the gods of medicine. This confidence in a doctor constituted the patients' contribution to the friendship.

On the part of doctors, friendship for the patient consisted of a correct combination of *philanthropia* (love of humanity) and *philantechnica* (love of the art of healing). Doctors' love of technical knowledge would allow them to help the patients' own natural tendency to get well and to assist them to reach for the perfection of the human being (health, harmony) as embodied in the individuals.

Thus, the Greek doctor–patient relationship was maintained by the commonly shared religio-medical value of friendship. Friendship assumed an equalitarian and reciprocal relationship, and it provided an effective communication. The art of healing was improved by communication between the doctor and patient, and it expedited the individualized diagnosis and treatment for every patient. The doctor entered into a discourse and then treated a sick person as a friend, not as a subordinate. Finally, the functionalist premise of an integrated system was carried out by Aristotle's advice to abandon a person with an incurable disease because he or she would never again be capable of *philia.*

We can draw a parallel with the modern practice of psychiatry. Successful psychotherapy is based on a reciprocal relationship between doctor and patient. Therapists must have the capacity to convey concern for their patients' welfare as well as have healing abilities. On the other hand, in order to receive a favorable therapeutic response patients must show good adaptive ability and heightened susceptibility to methods of healing such as are found in primitive medicine and faith healing (Frank, 1973).

However, this functionalist view of the social system has a built-in source of instability. The ability of Greek doctors to cure illness was delimited by the religious belief that inexorable forces existed in nature and that some diseases were mortal or incurable. In order to gain the confidence and friendship of patients, the technical insufficiency of the doctors had to be supplemented by their interactional manipulation of the doctor–patient relationship. First of all, they had to have an "appearance" that would gain the patients' trust. They had to present themselves as: (1) serious and diligent, (2) sharp, decisive, and stubborn to opposition, (3) composed, self-controlled, and artless, (4) decently and cleanly dressed as well as discretely perfumed, and (5) caring for and sympathetic with the patient. (Entralgo, 1969).

In addition to their appearance, the doctors needed to engage in verbal persuasion to win the patients' confidence. Good doctors, according to Plato, would not prescribe for their patients until they had first convinced them that the treatment would be effective or at least was the best available.

Friendship in a therapeutic relation was the Greek philosopher's ideal, but that was not always realized in practice. A struggle between patient and doctor is manifest in the Hippocratic corpus. Doctors complained about the nonprofessional criteria that people used to select their physicians, and patients were criticized for insisting on their own remedies (Jones, 1943). Patients sometimes viewed a physician as a potential danger, to be consulted cautiously. No legal mechanisms existed in classical Greece whereby the injured patient or his or her relatives could seek legal redress. The only penalty for malpractice was that of ill repute (Amundsen, 1977).

An even further degradation of the ideals of friendship in ancient Greece was exhibited when the slaves and the poor needed medical treatment. Verbal communication from a doctor in those cases was reduced to a minimum. Individualization of treatment was also minimal, and slaves were all treated alike and with only a crude and purely quantitative appraisal. It resembled a veterinary service for people. In time, servants of physicians acquired a knowledge of medicine by obeying and observing their masters, and they became the doctors for the slaves.

Medicine in the Middle Ages

The central value of medieval society was the belief in the absolute and infinite power of God, who created the world. It was God's will that certain diseases were cured and others were mortal. Medicine was only necessary for those illnesses that were meant by God to be curable.

Thus, the physicians' duty was primarily religious. They were morally and socially obliged to care for their patients' bodily and spiritual welfare. The doctors' duty was to think of their patients' souls before considering medicine for their bodies. When doctors visited sick persons, their first responsibility was to make the patients confess their sins because the patients' bad conscience might have caused and even could aggravate the disease. Confession was important not merely for the benefit of the patients' soul, it was also practical for avoiding the possibility that the doctors could be accused of malpractice in case the illness worsened (Castiglioni, 1958; Talbot, 1967).

Rather than an art of healing or a technical science, medieval medicine was a charitable office practiced by the monk-physician. In the name of Christian love of humanity, it was believed that the practice of religion alone had a supernatural effect which made natural remedies unnecessary. Medical technique consisted of empirical therapy, Christian charity, and supernatural beliefs in miracles.

In theory, medieval society admitted medical *philia* in the form of Christian love, and medicine was held in high esteem with the physician enjoying the patients' confidence. In reality, however, there was a gradual process of legal rationalism with a contractual slant that revealed a latent conflict in the doctor–patient relationship. Medical *philia* was mistrusted enough to be subjected to the authority of written law. For instance, before undertaking treatment, physicians had to agree on their fees and deposits. If a patient died, the doctor had no right to any fee (Entralgo, 1969).

The functionalist assumption of social integration is challenged by the existence of a class difference in medieval medical care. The poorer classes received medical care in the hospitals, which were inadequately equipped, while wealthier patients received more personal care in their homes through doctors' visits.

While medicine was subsumed under religious authority, it could borrow power from the latter in authenticating its performance or establishing an alibi for a lack of performance. If a patient died, it could be attributed to God's will, provided that the doctor had conformed to the prescribed norms of conduct. Technical deficiency did not upset a patient's confidence in the doctor so long as the behavior of both the patient and the doctor was governed by religious principles. In that way, patients with diseases that were considered terminal and who were beyond the realm of the art of healing died happy.

From the Renaissance until the Early Twentieth Century

Beginning with the Renaissance, European societies gradually emancipated themselves from the domination of the theological structure that had persisted for centuries. The desire of the liberated persons was that they be allowed to earn their living exclusively through the use of the potentialities and resources inherent in their own nature, and they wanted nothing from the supernatural. People came to be conceived of not merely as pieces of cosmic reality but as having a natural reality capable of developing a personality. Friendship or philanthropy was based on love of a person for his or her own sake, not because of the part he or she played in the world. Any human relationship, including that of the physician and patient, no longer needed the gods as intermediary agents.

However, in order for medicine to become separate from the sanction of the theological institution, physicians were obliged to establish foundations of their own that would provide the norms of behavior for themselves and their patients. And the only logical foundation for a medical profession, if it sought autonomy, was scientific technology and the ability to show concrete results of medical therapy to the public.

The Seventeenth and Eighteenth Centuries. As will be pointed out in Chapter 6, there was a wide discrepancy between scientific accomplishment and medical practice during the seventeenth and eighteenth centuries. While science was flourishing in the academies, universities were producing philosophizing academicians who could not adopt or even adapt themselves to any of the new techniques.

In the seventeenth century, Molière ridiculed the doctors of Europe as being pompous asses (Haggard, 1934; Hall, 1977). Doctors were caricatured in laces and frills in the eighteenth century, and the manners and customs of those times were characterized by a strong class distinction and by elaborate etiquette. The dress of the fashionable doctor of England in those days was suitable for an aristocrat: he wore a red coat, satin breeches, silk stockings, buckled shoes, a powdered wig, and a three-cornered hat (Clendening, 1960).

These physicians were hiding their technical incompetence under the cover of aristocratic respectability. The real question was whether or not the physicians could inspire the patients' confidence in their medical skill. The answer was negative, and that was not only supported by the satirists' attacks on the empty grandiloquence of the physicians, but by the prevalence of quackery in those days. In other words, what the public saw and some might have admired in the doctors was not their medical technique, but their polished manners. It was easy for the quacks to imitate doctors because all that the charlatan needed were an equal ostentation, snobbery, and effrontery.

But the frippery of fashion adopted by physicians did not take them a long way up the ladder of social leadership. In time of pestilence, people did not turn to the physicians for protection, but rather they turned in hope to the priests. While the priests retained social leadership and were shaping the beliefs, customs, and behaviors of people, the physicians were left in the seclusion of the sick rooms.

From the Late Nineteenth to the Early Twentieth Centuries. The public finally gained confidence in medicine in the latter half of the nineteenth century when scientific medical research began to show concrete results.

However, the love and pursuit of technical knowledge led the doctors' interests astray, and they became attracted to problems of physical diagnosis. The hospital patient was viewed both as a scientifically cognizable and modifiable object and as an unknown individual. In those days, only the destitute used the hospital because it was known that hospital patients were used for medical research. In anticipation of such a reception, patients usually arrived at the hospital with confidence and resignation. They knew that they would receive excellent diagnoses because the hospital doctors were usually the best in the country. However, they also knew that the treatment would sometimes be limited by the meager hospital resources and that they would receive careful autopsies if they should die. The patients submissively handed themselves over: "Here is my body, do what you like with it" (Abel-Smith, 1964; Entralgo, 1969).

In private practice for the middle class, the family doctor knew the patient as a friend. Here, the doctor–patient relationship was more of a friendship.

By the turn of the century, physicians established the status of the medical profession and thereby monopolized the healing techniques. They enjoyed a professional autonomy that was unhampered by other institutions such as a church or the government. The physician–patient relationship was governed by the disease model, which was characterized by impersonality and complete submission of the patient to the physician.

THE PHYSICIAN–PATIENT RELATIONSHIP TODAY

Medical Care Utilization

Before we begin our discussion of the doctor–patient relationship in contemporary American society, we should examine the factors that prompt individuals to enter the therapeutic relationship. According to the disease model, people seek medical care because they suffer from physical symptoms of dysfunctioning. However, there are other factors that encourage or deter people in utilizing health care facilities. As Mechanic and Volkart (1961) noted, illness behavior is "the way in which symptoms are perceived, evaluated and acted upon by a person who recognizes some pain, discomfort or other signs of organic malfunction."

Suchman's Five Stages of Illness

More specifically, Suchman (1965b) distinguished five stages of illness experience as (1) the symptom experience, (2) the assumption of the sick role, (3) medical care contact, (4) the dependent-patient role, and (5) recovery and rehabilitation.

The individual's perception that "something is wrong" is the beginning of the process of illness behavior. The person recognizes some physical change in daily bodily functioning. Reactions to the perceived symptoms range from (1) denial of disorder, or (2) delay in assessment of the condition, to (3) acknowledgment of the onset of illness.

If the symptoms are severe or persistent, the individual is likely to enter the second stage whereby he or she assumes a sick role. Here, being sick has social implications. The sick person is informally excused by family members and friends from performing regular duties but is expected to seek medical care so as to expedite recovery. Some people resort to professional help immediately, while others try various self-remedies.

When the sick person decides to accept professional assistance, he or she is in the third stage of Suchman's model, medical care contact. However, the initial encounter with a physician may or may not result in a professional validation of the sick role. The doctor may diagnose the person as well and reject the client's sick-role claim. At this point, the client may discontinue the sick role or go "shopping" for another doctor who legitimates the sick role.

If an agreement is reached between patient and physician that treatment is necessary, the fourth stage begins. Now, the patient is expected to be dependent upon the physician and faithfully follow the medical regimen. Some patients rebel against the regimentation and "go shopping" for other practitioners for possible alternatives. Others may enjoy the secondary gain of the sick role, that is, exemption from normal obligations and so attempt to prolong this stage of the dependent-patient role.

When patient and physician cooperate in a therapeutic relationship and if the therapy is effective, the person arrives at the final stage of recovery and rehabilitation.

Of course, an illness experience may not go through all these stages. Certain stages may be skipped as in the case of an acute, unexpected heart failure, whereby the first stage is immediately followed by the fourth stage. Also the duration of each stage varies depending upon both individual and social factors.

Determinants of Health Care Utilization

In recent years special attention has been focused by investigators upon the first three stages of Suchman's model. They constitute the pretherapeutic stage in which individuals make decisions as to whether or not they should utilize health care services. The upsurge of interest in the determinants of medical care utilization is partly due to the changing social climate in which health has come to be considered a right rather than a privilege. Equity in health services is defined as the state in which the utilization of medical care is determined by the severity of illness, and not by socioeconomic factors (Anderson, Kravits, & Anderson, 1975).

A large number of studies of health-seeking behavior have been conducted, and many reviews and classifications of determinants have appeared (Aday & Anderson, 1975; Aday & Eichhorn, 1972; Anderson et al., 1972; Bice, 1969; Brook, 1974; Hulka et al., 1972; McKinlay, 1972). There are some who emphasize certain factors as overriding predictors of medical utilization. For instance, many researchers take the sociopsychological perspective, claiming that unless the individual is psychologically ready to take action, the decision to seek health care will not be made (Becker & Maiman, 1975; Maiman & Becker, 1974). Furthermore, the perception of symptoms and the motivation to seek medical care are functions of learning and attitude formation (Becker, 1974, 1979; Becker et al., 1977; Rosenstock, 1969, 1974; Suchman, 1964; Zola, 1966). Such a medical predisposition also reflects the psychological and cultural makeup of racial and ethnic groups (Coburn & Pope, 1974; Moody & Gray, 1972; Rosenstock, 1969; Suchman, 1964; Zborowski, 1952).

Some of the critics of the sociopsychological perspective stress intragroup differences in value orientations, while others maintain that the basic value placed on good health does not vary significantly among social or racial groups (Bullough, 1972; Coburn & Pope, 1974; Dodge et al., 1970).

At any rate, the opponents of the motivational interpretation of health service utilization hold that availability and accessibility of health care facilities are more important than ideology or outlook (Aday & Eichhorn, 1972; Goering & Coe, 1970; Himes, 1974; Okada & Sparer, 1976; Rainwater, 1969; Riessman, 1974; Wan & Gray, 1978).

In contrast to the above single-factor approach, others have juxtaposed cultural variables against economic factors (Berkanovic & Reeder, 1974). Still others have developed comprehensive classifications of variables and their impact upon health care utilization (Anderson, Kravits, & Anderson, 1975; Berki & Kobashigawa, 1976; Wan & Soifer, 1974). For instance, McKinlay (1972) identified six approaches: economic, sociodemographic, geographic, sociopsychological, sociocultural, and organizational.

Anderson-Newman Model

Anderson and Newman (1973) delineated a framework of health care utilization that takes into account both societal and individual factors. Since it is a comprehensive scheme, it is presented here in detail. Anderson and Newman posited that the individual decision to visit physicians or clinics is affected by societal determinants of utilization both directly and through the health services systems.

On the individual level there are three components: *predisposing, enabling,* and *need* or *the level of illness* factors. The predisposing, and the most immediate, cause for seeking health care is the perception of symptoms of illness. Assuming the presence of physical malfunctioning, the individuals do not necessarily rush to the doctor's office. They may not have the means to enable them to utilize health services. Enabling conditions are measured by (1) family resources such as income, health insurance coverage, and the accessibility to physicians, and (2) community health facilities and health-promoting values. Even though individuals suffering from illness are financially capable of utilizing medical facilities that are readily available in the community, they do not always go to doctors. Some wait until the symptoms become intolerable, and others try self-medication.

The medical care predisposition of individuals is associated with (1) demographic factors (age, sex, marital status, past illness, etc.), (2) social structural variables (education, race, occupation, family size, etc.), and (3) beliefs (attitudes toward health and health services, knowledge about disease, etc.).

Individuals' predisposition and ability to use health care services are also influenced, according to Anderson and Newman, by the nature of the national health services system. How medical care is financed (private versus national health insurance, etc.) and organized (solo versus group practice, etc.) have a bearing upon the readiness with which patients utilize services.

On the societal level Anderson and Newman list technology and norms as the main predictors of health care utilization. For instance, the changes in the treatment of the mentally ill reflect the shifts in social norms and medical technology. These people were chained when the public thought they were dangerous and incurable. Along with the development of drug therapy and social values that cherish human dignity, mental patients came to be treated more and more as outpatients rather than being detained in mental hospitals.

The significant contribution of Anderson and Newman is in providing typological refinement to a causal model of health care utilization. Empirical assessment of the model has been attempted at the national level (Anderson, Kravits, & Anderson, 1975; Wolinsky, 1978) and the international level (Kohn & White, 1976).

The analytical model of predisposing, enabling, and need components of health care utilization was applied to the data in the national study of health services utilization conducted by the Center for Health Administration Studies and the National Opinion Research Center of the University of Chicago in 1971, as well as three earlier national studies examining changes in health care utilization, expenditures, and methods of payment over twenty years. The results are summarized in the book *Equity in Health Services,* edited by Anderson, Kravits, and Anderson (1975). Information was collected not only from families but also from physicians, clinics, hospitals, insuring organizations, and employers. Types of health care utilization are compared by the degree of discretion exercised by the individual. Discretion here means the individual's free choice and judgment, not affected by the decision of the providers of medical care or by the nature of the illness itself. Discretion is found to be the highest for dental care, the lowest for hospitalization, and intermediate for physician service.

Among the *predisposing* variables, age is related to length of hospital stay. In conformity with the existing literature (Anderson & Anderson, 1979; Galvin & Fan, 1975; Monteiro, 1973; Wan & Soifer, 1974), older people are more likely to stay in hospitals longer than others, but this is largely attributable to higher illness levels among the older people. Age is also associated with utilization of dental care because the younger age groups receive more dental care, regardless of the severity of pain involved.

Race has marked impact on health care utilization, particularly on physician service and dental care, which require more discretion on the part of the individual users than hospitalization does. The utilization rate is lower for nonwhites than for whites even when the effects of income, education, and place of residence are controlled.

For the population as a whole, attitudes and beliefs show little bearing on health care use, except for dental care, which is highly discretionary in nature. In other words, individuals with positive attitudes toward health care are not any more inclined to use health services than are those with negative beliefs. This is in sharp contrast to research findings such as the one by Suchman (1965b), which indicates a strong relationship between individual orientation toward modern medicine and health-seeking behavior.

Despite repeated reports (Anderson & Anderson, 1972; Wan & Soifer, 1974) showing higher morbidity and health care utilization rates among females, sex in this 1971 University of Chicago study shows virtually no relationship to health care use, after the effects of other variables are eliminated.

As for *enabling* variables, having a regular source of care induces more frequent visits to physicians. Income, independent of education, was also an important predictor of physician use before the enactment of Medicare and Medicaid. However, by 1970 the extent of comprehensiveness of third-party coverage became a crucial factor, encouraging health care utilization. This is in line with other research findings (Anderson & Anderson, 1979; Bellin & Geiger, 1972; Bice, Eichhorn, & Fox, 1972; Galvin & Fan, 1975; Monteiro, 1973; Sparer & Okada, 1974).

In comparison to other variables, *need* proved to be by far the most important predictor of health care utilization behavior as reported in *Equity in Health Services.* Strong associations are found between disability days and worry about health, and the use of hospital care; between the severity of the diagnosis and physician visits; and between dental problem symptoms and dentist contacts.

Discrepancies are found, however, between subjective and objective assessments of illness levels among blacks. When a subjective measure is used, blacks are less likely to report illness symptoms and the need for medical care than whites. On the other hand, blacks who see physicians and dentists are diagnosed as suffering from more serious illnesses than whites. Thus, the association between the predisposing variables (attitudes and beliefs concerning health) and health care utilization appears to be validated for blacks. This supports Suchman's (1965b) theory that preventive medicine is largely a white middle class concept.

In summary, it is concluded that most of the predisposing variables, especially attitudes and beliefs, were found to have weak predictive values for health care utilization. The most important determinant was the need variable (illness level) in conjunction with the enabling variables.

Using the data from the 1971, 1972, and 1973 National Health Interview Surveys, Wolinsky (1978) also found that most of the explained variances in health care utilization are attributable to the illness-morbidity characteristics. Sociocultural factors (predisposing and enabling variables) are substantially unrelated to the utilization pattern. This result shows how little is known about the causal nexus, particularly sociocultural genesis, of health care utilization behavior. Nevertheless, every theoretical and empirical effort brings us one step closer to understanding illness behavior.

Other Studies of Health Care Utilization

Many studies of illness behavior have been restricted to the first three stages of Suchman's model, centering around the determinants of access to utilization of health care.

There are a few studies, however, that attempt to examine the link among all of Suchman's five stages. For instance, Aday and Anderson (1974) modified Anderson and Newman's 1973 model by adding another variable, consumer satisfaction, to the causal network of health care utilization as determined by predisposing, enabling, and need characteristics. Utilization and satisfaction are conceptualized as a reciprocal causative relationship. Wolinsky (1978), on the other hand, postulated a delayed, or time-lagged, effect of utilization and satisfaction. He also added another component, attitude toward alternatives, to the present health care delivery system.

Shortell and others (1977) studied the relationship among access to health services, utilization, continuity of care, quality of care, and patient satisfaction. This model is composed of three sets of health system variables: (1) *input variables* (patient characteristics such as age, sex, and family size, and health care provider characteristics such as professional qualification and speciality); (2) *process variables* (access to care, utilization of services, continity of care, and physician performance); and (3) *outcome variables* (patient satisfction and objective health status of the patient).

Studying hypertension patients, the study by Shortell and others reported significant differences in health care delivery between group and private practices. In prepaid group practice, as opposed to private practice, a greater degree of homogeneity of providers exists in terms of professional qualifications and physician specialty. Thus, patients' satisfaction was more likely to be affected by their perceived access to care than professional qualifications of the physicians. Particularly, patients in poor health and those from large families expressed having great difficulty with access to services in group practice. Thus, improving access to care will lead to patient satisfaction, but not necessarily increase the volume of utilization. No significant relationship was found between perceived accessibility to care and the actual frequency of visits. In contrast, in private practice, provider characteristics (professional qualifications) were a more important determinant of quality of care than patient characteristics.

Despite various methodological difficulties, recent studies, such as those discussed in this section, indicate efforts to develop what Merton (1957) called a "theory of middle range" as a prelude to a more comprehensive theory of health care delivery systems.

The Physician–Patient Relationship

An understanding of utilization patterns is important because it frequently affects the doctor–patient relationship. Various forces that have led the patients to seek medical care will also generate different expectations toward physicians. For example, lower class patients who score low on predisposing and enabling factors but high on illness levels may be anxious to have an instantaneous cure. On the other hand, women who are highly predisposed to visiting doctors for minor symptoms may expect to receive sympathy rather than a technical cure from physicians.

Thus, the doctor–patient relationship cannot be understood by the disease model alone. Patients do not simply represent disease entities but reflect social value, structure, and processes (Bloom & Wilson, 1972; Blum, 1960). In this section the social system of the therapeutic relationship will be examined from our three sociological perspectives (Cartwright, 1967; Fabrega, 1974; Gordon et al., 1968).

The Functional Perspective

Parsons has developed a comprehensive theory that defines the structure of the social system composed of the physician and the patient. As a functionalist, Parsons envisions the doctor–patient relationship as a subsystem of the larger social system, one that shares the central values of the society as a whole. In other words, both doctors and patients bring commonly accepted societal values into a therapeutic relationship.

Definition of Illness. The functionalist definitions of illness stems from two basic assumptions (Parsons, 1951, p. 27). First, a social framework cannot be structured so that it is radically incompatible with the functioning of individuals both as biological organisms and as personalities. Second, in turn, the survival of a social system depends upon support from the component individuals, who are capable and psychologically motivated to act in accordance with the requirements of their roles in the system.

Viewed in this way, illness is considered as dysfunctional to the social system because it incapacitates individuals and dilutes their effective performance of social roles. There are, of course, certain uncontrollable illnesses. But the functional interest of a society lies in the minimization of illness (Parsons, 1972, 1975).

The Sick Role. "Being sick" constitutes a social role, that is, the sick role (Parsons, 1951, p. 436). There is a set of institutionalized expectations plus corresponding sentiments and sanctions for patients. First, a sick person is exempt from normal social role responsibilities. This exemption requires legitimation by the physician so as to prohibit malingering. In achievement-oriented societies, one may use illness to justify failure to fulfill socially prescribed role obligations. Cole and Lejeure (1972) tested this hypothesis and found that (1) many welfare mothers accept the dominant cultural view that being on welfare symbolizes a personal failure, and that (2) those mothers tend to play the sick role to legitimize their self-defined failure.

The second characteristic of the sick role, according to Parsons, is the institutionalized definition that sick people cannot be expected to become well by acts of decision or will. They are not held responsible for having incurred their conditions. This norm, however, has been repudiated for certain types of illness, such as chronic illness (Kassebaum & Baumann, 1972), mental illness, and addictive illness. Chronically ill patients tend to show a sense of guilt because of the prolonged state of financial and social incapacities. Mental and addictive illnesses tend to be stigmatized because of the social sentiment that this type of illness can be avoided by an act of the will.

The third element in the sick role is the understanding that the state of being ill is undesirable and carries with it the obligation to want to become well. This assumption does not work in the case of malingering. If illness brings a secondary gratification such as staying away from school or work, the sick person will find illness desirable and may wish to prolong the state. During World War II the soldiers who wished to avoid further combat readily accepted the attribution that they were suffering from mental breakdowns (Glass, 1958).

The fourth closely related element is the obligation to seek technically competent help and to cooperate with a physician to achieve a quick recovery. However, as discussed above, the help-seeking behavior is determined not only by the magnitude of the illness symptoms but by other social factors. People are more likely to take action for symptoms that disrupt usual functioning of other roles (Hennes, 1972). As discussed in Chapter 4, some claim that women are more likely than men to seek health care because women play less crucial roles in society.

There is also a tendency to deny symptoms. Particularly in the sphere of mental illness, the patients and their family members are reluctant to recognize the source of the patients' difficulty as psychiatric illness. They try to normalize the situation by viewing the problem as a physical condition, fatigue, or a reflection of the patient's personality (Schwartz, 1957; Yallow et al., 1955).

Denial processes are also seen in the face of discomforting evidence of permanent disability, terminal illness, or even death (Davis, 1963; Friedman et al., 1963).

As for the compliance aspect of the sick role, it has been shown that the majority of the patients perceive a "good patient" to be one who (1) has trust and confidence in the doctor, (2) is cooperative and obedient to orders, and (3) is respectful, considerate, and not demanding (Mechanic, 1968a, Suchman, 1965a; Tagliacozzo & Mauksch, 1972).

Compliance also affects the status of hospital patients. In that environment, the position of a patient resembles that of a customer in a market or of an employee of an organization (Parsons, 1957, p. 115). The patient receives services for which he or she pays and in return is subject to supervision and control by the hospital authorities. The patient is socialized to cooperate with therapeutic agencies and to make an effort to get well. Many studies (Denzin, 1968; Denzin & Spitzer, 1968) indicate that a cooperative patient is likely to be given a favorable prognosis, may receive more hours of therapy, and will usually remain in the hospital a shorter length of time.

The Physician's Role. Now that their occupation has attained the status of a profession (for a discussion of this historical process, see Chapter 6), physicians are expected to behave in certain ways so that their professional autonomy and competence will not be endangered. Parsons characterized such physicians' roles by four qualities: (1) universalistic, (2) functionally specific, (3) affectively neutral, and (4) collectivity oriented.

The universalistic norm requires physicians to treat patients according to scientific and medical standards without being prejudiced by personal or social considerations. Next, the functional specificity of physicians' role concerns their ability to differentiate themselves as medical specialists from their predecessors, the priest-healers and monk-physicians. Physicians are expected to limit their activities to what is strictly "medical" and not to extend their services to religious, political, or personal counsel.

Then, in order to safeguard professional objectivity, physicians must maintain an affective neutrality when dealing with patients. They should understand the patient's feelings and show sympathy, but they must not become emotionally involved.

Finally, as professionals, physicians must transcend self-interest and must work for the welfare of humanity and society. They should treat the patients according to the patients' needs and the health standards of the community, all the while remaining free from self-orientations toward profit or esteem.

Therapeutic Relation. The functionalist assumption of equilibrium (Henderson, 1935) does not necessarily lead to a symmetric reciprocity in the social system of doctor and patient. On the contrary, the asymmetry of the therapeutic relation can be deduced from the functionalist definition of illness and of the physician's role.

Since illness is conceived as dysfunctional to society, a patient, by definition, is assigned to a low status. Conversely, a physician's role in restoring health is given the highest functional importance and the power therefrom. A physician's power is derived from the monopoly of a technique that is vital not only to the individual patient but also to society as a whole. Thus, in a therapeutic situation, the physician establishes the rules of behavior, and the patient is assumed to comply with them passively.

Physicians not only represent the medical profession, but they are integral to the dominant cultural values. In comparison to patients, who have been defined as social deviants, physicians symbolize the well and the normal, and they act as social control agents. Their job is to make sure that the deviants relearn and play normal roles again.

Thus, physicians, as professionals and as social control agents, play dominant roles in the asymmetric therapeutic relation. That skewness is further elaborated by Parsons and Fox (1952) when they parallel the doctor–patient relationship to the childhood socialization process. The physician's role is analogous to the parental task of wearning dependent children into independent adults. Just as in dealing with helpless children, therapists are supportive and permissive in the beginning of the treatment and allow the patients to lean on them. However, the therapists keep the relationship asymmetric by refusing to reciprocate with emotional responsiveness. Furthermore, they control the patients' behavior by manipulating rewards, such as by showing approval for doing "the right thing," that is, following the medical regimen.

Subcultural Variation. The functionalist assumption of value consensus in the Parsonian model suffers when it has to deal with subcultural variation. A constant striving for good health and seeking for scientific medical care are characteristic of the white middle class in the United States, but they are not necessarily shared by other racial or ethnic groups. Some ethnic minority groups even misunderstand a major fraction of the terms used by doctors (Samora et al., 1961; Shuval, 1970).

A great deal of research has been devoted to the basic problem of fitting modern Western health care into the widely varying traditional framework of non-Western beliefs and conduct (Paul, 1955). For example, hallucinatory experiences are accepted without any anxiety or condemnation in some nonliterate societies. In those extreme cases, the fact of the hallucination per se is seldom disturbing, although its contents may attract public attention. Sometimes those experiences are interpreted as the revelation of a divine will (Wallace, 1959). In Western society, however, with its emphasis on rationality and control, hallucination is commonly taken as a grave sign of psychosis.

Another difficulty in the functionalist concept of normality lies in subcultural definitions of illness. Certain conditions may be prevalent within a group and are therefore considered as the normal state, such as diarrhea, sweating, and coughing among some Mexican Americans in the southwest United States (Clark, 1959). This does not mean that the condition is considered good, but rather that it is natural and inevitable, and hence it is ignored as being of little consequence.

Thus, many of the symptoms in such groups exist without being defined as characteristics of an illness, and therefore, the victims never reach the doctor's office. When they do acknowledge disease symptoms, they are likely to expect diagnosis and treatment that are different from what Western physicians would provide. When a doctor and patient of such diverse value orientations and expectations come in contact, the Parsonian model of functional interdependence is not likely to be achieved (Leighton & Leighton, 1945; Mead, 1953; Paul, 1955; Saunders, 1954).

Even among Westerners, there are wide ethnic variations in medical predisposition and response to physicians' diagnosis of symptoms (e.g., pain, swelling, bleeding). For that reason, doctors who are members of certain ethnic groups practice predominantly in areas where members of their own ethnic group reside (Elesh & Schollert, 1972; Lieberson, 1958). When such doctors can frame medical explanations in a manner consistent with their patients' culture, then they can make their patients more receptive to treatment (Shuval, 1970).

Among the various ethnic groups in the United States, Italians, Jews, and the Irish have been compared by many researchers. Zborowski (1952) found that Jewish and Italian patients tend to respond to pain in an emotional fashion and may even exaggerate their pain. In contrast, "old Americans" are more stoic and objective, and the Irish frequently go so far as to deny pain. Then, although their reaction to pain is similar, there is a difference between Italians and Jews in their attitude toward pain in that Italians are oriented to the present as compared to Jews' concern for the future. Italians are primarily concerned with seeking immediate relief from pain, and they are relatively satisfied when relief is obtained. In contrast, Jews worry about the causes and consequences of their pain with respect to how it relates to their future health and welfare.

Zborowski examined child-rearing practices that might account for such ethnic variation in dealing with pain. He reported that both Italian and Jewish mothers tend to show overprotective and overconcerned attitudes toward a child's health, and they constantly warn their children not to catch cold, not to become injured, and the like. The child's complaints about pain or discomforts are quickly responded to with sympathy, concern, and help by these parents. The child seems to learn to pay attention to every physical symptom and to look for sympathy. Jewish mothers are especially apprehensive about a slight deviation from the normal state as being a sign of illness.

Other researchers have found similar tendencies when they compared Italians and Jews. Having examined the records of army inductees, Croog (1961) observed that Italians and Jews reported the greatest number of symptoms. Higher rates of utilization of medical facilities for preventive or therapeutic purposes are found among the Jews than either Protestants or Catholics (Linn, 1967; Scheff, 1966a; Segal et al., 1965; Silverman, 1964; Suchman, 1964, 1965a; Zola, 1966). There have also been experimental laboratory studies that corroborated the above results by differentiating the ethnic groups in their reactions to pain such as that induced by electric shocks (Sternbach & Tursky, 1965).

Whatever the basis is for the formation of a subculture group, its values do diverge from the dominant values of the society. The Parsonian model of a homeostatic therapeutic relationship is unlikely to be seen when a patient representing such subcultural values first encounters a physician, who is apt to be a white middle class male.

The Conflict Perspectives

Professional versus Lay Perspectives. By definition, a conflict perspective of the physician–patient relation will emphasize the differences of interests between the professional healers and their lay customers. Based on his empirical research findings, Freidson (1960, 1970) challenged the Parsonian conceptualization of the sick role as being deficient on three major counts. First, the Parsonian model decribes how a physician and patient should behave normatively rather than how they do behave in reality. Second, the definition of the sick role is derived primarily from the physician's perspective and ignores the patient's point of view. Finally, Parsons is accused of overlooking conflict in human relationships.

While Parsons assumes that the individual has internalized social value and norms, Freidson rejects the notion of psychological internalization. Instead, he draws attention to the social structure in which doctors and patients are located. He claims that these structural variables will influence whether the individual will behave normatively or not. For instance, solo and group practices generate different types of pressure upon physicians, presures that will affect the likelihood of physicians complying with a medical regimen such as doing the proper amount of laboratory testing, referring patients to specialists, and following norms for the prescription of medication requested by patients.

According to Freidson, the doctor–patient relationship is most effectively analyzed within the framework of a clash of perspectives. Unlike Parsons, Freidson does not view patients as passively acquiescing to professional authority but rather evaluating and making demands upon the professionals.

Patients' Views of Physicians. Many empirical studies support Freidson's postulates. According to Mechanic's (1964) study, a "good" doctor is predominantly preceived as someone who (1) is competent and qualified, (2) takes personal interest in patients, and (3) behaves in a friendly and sympathetic manner. The doctor's personal interest in his or her patients is assessed by (1) caring about the patients and their problems, (2) giving patients sufficient time, (3) following up after treatment by calling the patients or asking the patients to call back, (4) behaving respectfully and sympathetically, and (5) listening to the patients and hearing them out. The criteria for choosing family doctors as reported by mothers are the doctors' willingness to make house calls and the accessibility to doctors and to their offices.

Thus, when patients visit physicians, they bring with them such expectations about the physicians' roles. Four-fifths of the respondents in Mechanic's study agreed that it is essential that a doctor be a friend and an advisor, and two-thirds concurred that a doctor's job has a spiritual side to it. The stereotyped feature of the physician's role is that of a general advisor and helper. Silver (1963) found that people prefer to describe and view all of their problems in a physical-medical framework rather than in a behavioral-emotional one. Even when they have emotional problems, patients would rather seek help from physicians instead of going to psychologists or psychiatrists. Physicians are expected to deal with patients' emotional problems, whether they wish to or not.

The extent to which doctors can meet these expectations as friends and priests affects whether patients return to them and even whether the patients conform to their prescribed treatments (Bloom, 1963; Davis, 1968). In Mechanic's study, 72 percent of the respondents had changed, at some time, the doctors or clinics used by their families. The most frequently reported reason was that the doctors failed to provide proper treatment required in the situation. Mechanic interpreted that such a claim by patients did not indicate an objective evaluation of technical competence, but rather it showed the doctors' failure to meet the patients' expectations, possibly in not explaining the procedures and assumptions in the treatment. In fact, when evaluating a doctor's expertise, patients frequently use such cues as presenting oneself with confidence and authority or offering rapid diagnosis and treatment plans. Persons who change doctors seem to complain more about the doctors' lack of personal interest and attention than they do about their medical qualifications. Only a quarter of Mechanic's sample agreed that doctors' personal manners are not important.

In short, patients seek not only adequate medical care, but also sympathetic emotional support from the physician (Clyne, 1961; Cobb, 1954; McKinlay, 1977). A physician's image is that of a "kindly, thoughtful, warm person who is deeply interested in and committed to the welfare of the individual patient" (Hughes, 1958).

Doctors' Views of Patients. The physicians, on the other hand, since they are trained in the science of medicine, prefer to deal with clear physical symptoms rather than the general psychological needs of their patients (Coombs, 1978). That technical proficiency on which their efforts rest is likely to be a barrier to a sympathetic understanding of the patients as human beings. In particular, advanced specialization in modern medicine may make them unable or unwilling to regard the patients as full social beings. Concern for the patients by specialists may be narrowed to the point that the patients are treated as organisms. In addition, the professional value of affective neutrality will further detach the doctors from the patients' desire for personal attention.

How is this affected by the structure of medical practice? There is a fantasy that situations may be different and better in foreign countries. Particularly, the British health care system is said to be a haven for general practice. The United Kingdom has a tradition of family doctors who are concerned with the wider family and community ramifications of illness and who pay close attention to the patients' family and general welfare. The National Health Service has made a concerted attempt to maintain the structure of such primary care through its system of general practice, while the United States has no mechanism to keep physicians in primary medical care.

Comparing the two systems, Mechanic (1972a) found that the British general practitioners spend much time on house calls, while American counterparts rarely visit patients at home. The latter actually do a great deal of telephone consultation. Further, in conformity with the stereotypical contrast of

American versus British general practitioners, the former use diagnostic facilities excessively, which is often considered a reflection of scientific rigor, while the British doctors do less laboratory work.

However, contrary to general belief, Mechanic's data support the notion that American doctors are more socially oriented to medical care (e.g., believing it proper for patients to consult with doctors for the family's financial troubles, disobedience of children, and marital problems) than their British counterparts. Also, the latter showed greater dissatisfaction and frustration (Mechanic, 1970), partly due to the heavy workload which the British general practitioners have to carry. In Great Britain, patients are registered with a general practitioner, who by contract has to be available or produce a deputy at all times. Since payment is on a capitation system, there is little incentive for additional patient visits. Also, the British general practitioners' work is narrowly defined, which accentuates the disparity between the scientific orientation of medical school and their daily routine, and this makes them feel isolated from the mainstream of medicine. However, their dissatisfaction might have been exaggerated by the political dispute over remuneration and terms of service that was going on at the time of Mechanic's survey in 1966 (Mechanic & Faich, 1970).

At any rate, British general practitioners have their own source of dissatisfaction, which prohibits them from realizing the ideal of the socially oriented family doctor.

Therapeutic Relation. Unlike Parsons, who notes the asymmetry in the therapeutic relation, Freidson identifies a symmetry based on clashes of lay versus professional referral systems. For the public, there is a control over professional practice by means of the lay referral system. In the process of recognizing symptoms, defining the nature of the problems, deciding to seek a medical care, and in selecting a particular physician, the patient will consult with other lay people such as friends and family members. The lay referral system can determine the survival of the profession as well as the career and success of a particular physician.

In Mechanic's (1964) study, 34 percent of the responding mothers chose their physicians through the recommendations of friends or neighbors; 20 percent followed referral by another doctor or someone in the health field; and 16 percent chose the physician because of office accessibility.

For the average person, even after consultation with a professional practitioner has begun, the lay referral system still exerts an influence upon the behavior of the new patient. The patients discuss with other lay people the behavior of their physicians and the treatment prescribed in order to ascertain whether or not they are receiving proper attention. The patients often communicate their expectations to the doctors, and they subtly attempt to influence how the doctors will deal with them. The first visit to a practitioner is often tentative, and continued consultation with lay people will partly determine whether a patient will go back to that doctor for further treatment or in the event of a future problem (Ben-Sira, 1976; Hayes-Bautista, 1976; Kasteler et al., 1976; Larson & Rootman, 1976).

Sometimes clients' evaluations of physicians' performance coincide fairly closely to professional evaluations (Kisch & Reeder, 1969). However, whether clients' technical rating of doctors is done objectively or subjectively, physicians have to compete not only with their colleagues but also with the quacks who attract patients. Quacks, especially those who are more attuned to the psychological needs of patients, have perspectives closer to those of the patients than do the physicians (Cobb, 1954). Many patients who are dissatisfied with a physician will turn to the quack because there they will be received with sympathy (Bernard, 1965).

In Freidson's words, "whether their motive be to heal the patient or to survive professionally," physicians will feel pressure to accept or manipulate lay expectations and may make concessions such as administering a harmless placebo or giving up unpopular drugs. Recent controversy over laetrile illustrates the physicians' dilemma in dealing with patients' request for a special therapy. Laetrile is a drug extracted from the apricot pit and is proclaimed to be an anticancer vitamin. Without scientific evidence for its effectiveness, people are demanding that they be allowed to have the substance. While the Food and Drug Administration considers the drug illegal and has banned its importation, many states have passed laws allowing physicians to administer laetrile. Physicians facing terminal cancer patients are under conflicting pressures to conform to the dying patients' requests, to obey the law, to follow professional ethics, etc. (Baker et al., 1976; Crile, 1976; Crippen, 1976; Dipalma, 1977; Gray, C., 1977; Shulman, 1977).

Professional control over clients will be discussed in detail in Chapter 6. Briefly, medical education and licensure differentiate physicians from quacks, who are accorded a low status. Patients who seek scientific treatment are directed to physicians and away from the cultists. Organized medicine controls the supply of physicians, and it also serves to retain the elitist position and the charismatic aura of the physician.

In selecting a physician, the professional referral system counteracts the lay system. When the physician chosen through the lay referral system cannot handle the problem, it becomes his or her function, not that of the patient, to refer the patient to another practitioner. The patient may try to find a specialist, but due to lack of sufficient technical knowledge, he or she eventually has to rely on the professional referral system. At this point, it is the physician who decides whether or not to give service to the patient.

In the eyes of Freidson, the doctor–patient relationship assumes a fundamental symmetry built upon a process of bargaining between the two interest groups. Much of the medical decision-making involves uncertainty. For instance, when physicians cannot find causes, they can try further diagnostic tests, or they may assume that the symptoms are clinically trivial and may decide to wait for further development. Such a decision-making process, however, is not free from social pressures. The clients' power by means of malpractice suits has led many physicians to be overly cautious, whereby they may try all available tests to protect themselves.

Social Class Conflict. When professionals and clients are recruited from different social classes, they represent conflicting cultures: the medical subculture of the white middle class health practitioners versus the culture of poverty held by lower class patients.

The organization through which health services are delivered embodies the culture of medicine (Levine, Scotch, & Vlasak, 1969) with its emphasis on high technology and mass-produced, ultra-specialized care. This medical subculture is accentuated in public health facilities (hospital outpatient departments, emergency rooms, public clinics), which are used by the poor rather than in the private facilities (physicians in solo or group practice), utilized by the middle and upper income groups. The public institutions are characterized by a dehumanizing atmosphere with impersonal, brusque, and even insulting personnel moving around busily in the crowd (Dutton, 1978).

The alienation of indigent patients from the health care delivery system is further aggravated by the prejudice of white middle class professionals. It has been shown that the treatment given depends on the social characteristics of the patients, that is, perceived social worth of the patients. Treating certain types of people is considered "dirty work" by health workers. If the minority group members perceive that the psychological cost of using such services is too high, they are likely to eschew the service (Anderson & Sheatsley, 1967; Berkanovic & Reeder, 1974; Duff & Hollingshead, 1968; Miller, 1973).

The responsibility for the alienation of patients lies also with the cultural backgrounds of the patients. Lower class people have psychological inhibitions induced by the struggle for life. Poverty does not allow the poor to indulge in complaining about minor physical symptoms when their subsistence is at stake. Also, adversity tends to make the indigent fatalistic and less inclined to seek medical care.

For lower class people, motivation arises from the need to exist today, and current life crises override any consideration of future health and welfare (Geiger, 1967a, Horton, 1967; Koos, 1954; Osofsky, 1968; Rosenblatt & Suchman, 1964; Stoeckle & Candib, 1969). Their lives have not taught them that the future is worth waiting for (Davis, 1946), and they have seldom received a reward for deferring gratification. It is difficult for them to continue to return to the clinic for medication or therapy when they are afraid of losing their jobs because of frequent sick leaves.

In the classic study of class differences in the perception of illness, Koos (1954) presented a list of medically important symptoms, for example, loss of appetite and persistent backache, and he asked the respondents to report whether each symptom warranted the attention of a physician. For each symptom listed, the higher status respondents were uniformly more likely to report a need for medical attention than the lower status respondents. Other studies (Apple, 1960; Gordon, 1966; Mechanic, 1962a,b; Suchman, 1964, 1965a) also indicate that the recognition of symptoms and the search for physician care are considered more important by higher class than lower class respondents.

This may be due in part to the fact that when the middle class physician treats the lower class patient, the conversation across classes is likely to be discordant. They do not speak the same language, and they differ in the assumptions made behind the words. However, McKinlay (1975) finds fault with the physicians' imputation of patient ignorance as the barrier to effective communication. His study demonstrates that physicians consistently and markedly underestimate the level of word comprehension of all the lower working-class respondents.

Another source for the medical communication gap between the classes lies in self-expression and introspection, which lower class people tend to lack. This is particularly crucial in psychiatric therapy. Lower class patients tend to conceive of illness solely in somatic terms because they lack the habit of introspection as well as the conceptual tools needed to abstract and objectify elements of their mental life (Frank, 1973; Hollingshead & Redlich, 1958; Kadushin, 1969; Overall & Aronson, 1963). The necessary flows of discussion and information are hampered by inarticulate patients who expect the therapist to assume an active medical role.

Since they are aware of their lack of articulation, lower class patients are inclined to mistrust and fear the authority figure. They are likely to be evasive or to take mutely accepting postures. When exposed to such a patient, a middle class physician frequently makes a moral judgment and tends to view the disadvantaged person as morally bad or inferior. That attitude leads to the assumption that if patients ordered their lives differently, their health would be better.

This class conflict between doctors and patients has been interpreted by the Marxian sociologists (Navarro, 1978a; Waitzkin & Waterman, 1974) as a reflection of the broader economic processes of a capitalist society. The helpless position of the sick is the source of exploitation by physicians who, in turn, are governed by the capitalistic principle of profit motivation. For further elaboration, see the politics of health care in Chapter 10.

Other Sources of Conflict. In addition to the conflicts outlined above between the professional helper versus the lay client and between the middle versus lower social classes, there are other, more personal or situational sources of conflict.

For patients, an illness is the most significant thing in the world at the time, and they are likely to react to it with fear as threatening their overall well-being. In contrast, physicians see a patient and his or her symptoms as one among many daily encounters. Physicians are also trained to concentrate upon identifiable disease symptoms without being distracted by a patient's diffuse complaints about his or her lives (Mechanic, 1976; Tessler & Mechanic, 1978).

Second, the patient's role is hopefully a temporary one, as compared to the physician's role, which is a lifelong professional commitment. For a physician, a therapeutic situation is a normal and an agreeable state of affairs instead of a threatening, traumatic experience.

Third a patient's role is involuntary, ill-prepared, and reluctantly assumed in contrast to a physician's role, which has been chosen voluntarily and for which there has been extensive preparation.

Without adding any of the economic conflict from the medical marketplace, we can appreciate Freidson's approach to the doctor–patient relationship as a functional clash of perspectives. So far, conflicts have been resolved through negotiations and bargaining without major crisis. The assumption has been made that since it is a matter of human life, the patient's sacred trust in the physician will not disappear. Thus, conflict has been studied from the perspective of the functionalist conflict model rather than the dialectic conflict model. In the former model, conflict is viewed as contributive rather than disruptive to the functional integration of the social system. In recent years, however, the potentiality for open battles has revealed itself in the form of patients' malpractice suits and physicians' strikes (see Chapter 6). The relationship between doctor and patient, professional and lay people, and medicine and society are undergoing structural changes that may be better understood by using the dialectic conflict theory.

The Interactive Perspective

Definition of Illness. Though the structural analysis of the doctor–patient relationship has led Freidson to a conflict perspective, he also articulates the basic premises underlying the interactionist theory, particularly the branch called labeling theory.

The social reaction approach is explicit in Freidson's definition of illness as a social deviation. He goes a step beyond Parsons in arguing that medicine not only legitimizes a sick role but in fact creates illness as an official, social role (Freidson, 1970). In the course of acquiring professional autonomy and by controlling the evaluation of therapeutic work, medicine has established its exclusive right to determine what constitutes illness. Lay people may have their own ideas about illness, but the officially sanctioned definition of illness is the one provided by the medical profession. In that way, medicine creates the social possibilities for acting sick.

This tendency is well demonstrated by the recent warnings against iatrogenesis and medicalization of society. Iatrogenesis refers to harm induced inadvertently by a physician or the treatment process. Illich (1976) distinguished three types of iatrogenesis: clinical, social, and structural. Clinical iatrogenesis, which results in injury or sickness, is caused by a physician's misjudgment, ignorance, or imcompetence, such as using improper surgical procedures or overmedication. Social iatrogenesis refers to retaining patients in the sick role and legitimatizing their exemption from other responsibilities.

On a broader scale social iatrogenesis coincides with what Zola (1975) has called the medicalization of society, that is, defining social problems such as crime and delinquency more and more in terms of disease and illness. Alcoholism, drug addiction, hyperactive behavior of children, or the violence of adults are viewed not as crime or delinquency but as illness, for which medical therapies are prescribed. The impact of this medicalization of society is pervasive. By defining a problem as medical, we tend to attribute causes and solutions of complex social problems to the individual rather than to the social system. It diverts our attention from the malaise in the structure of society and depoliticizes political protest and dissent (Conrad, 1975; Kitterie, 1971; Zola, 1975).

Finally, Illich states that the power of a medical bureaucracy has caused structural iatrogenesis in which health professionals have destroyed the potential of people to deal with their human vulnerability and uniqueness in a personal and autonomous way. Since the medical profession defines what health is and how it should be achieved and maintained, lay people have no margin to exercise their own initiatives.

Through the use of labeling theory, Freidson classifies types of illnesses according to social reactions. The notion of legitimacy is central to eliciting various societal responses. Freidson distinguishes three degrees of legitimacy. First, there is conditional legitimacy, in which the deviant is temporarily exempted from normal obligations and gains some privileges, provided he or she seeks help to return to normalcy as soon as possible. This is close to the Parsonian sick role, and it is associated with acute illnesses, such as with a cold as a minor deviation and with pneumonia as a serious case. Second, unconditional legitimacy exists where the deviant is exempt permanently from normal obligations and obtains special privileges because of the helpless nature imputed to the condition. Certain types of chronic or terminal illness belong to this category, pockmarks , as a minor case and cancer as a serious deviation.

Finally, certain illnesses are viewed as illegitimate and the deviant is stigmatized. As far as the ideology of the contemporary medical profession is concerned, there is no illness that is illegitimate in the sense that humans are not held responsible for their illnesses. In practice, however, certain illnesses are labeled as stigma, such as stammering for a minor case and epilepsy for a serious case. The deviant is free from some normal obligations by virtue of deviance, but this illegitimate sick role spoils his or her identity.

Labeling Theory of Disease. The labeling perspective does not view the sick person as someone who is suffering from physical or mental dysfunction, but instead as someone who has become publicly labeled mentally or physically ill and who is self-labeled as deviant in conformity with societal reaction. A basic tenet here is that the act of labeling will severly stigmatize the person and cause him or her to be excluded from a normal role.

An early study of Phillips (1963) on reaction to seeking psychiatric help supports this position. He described housewives exhibiting various forms of disturbed behavior (i.e., that of a normal individual, a phobic compulsive, a simple schizophrenic, a depressed neurotic, and a paranoid schizophrenic) combined with different forms of help-seeking behavior. He found that individuals exhibiting identical behavior were increasingly rejected if they were described as seeking no help, consulting a priest, a physician, a psychiatrist, or entering a mental hospital.

Whether or not certain symptoms are defined as illness is based on their prevalence within a given group, that is, the frequency with which the illness occurs and the relative familiarity that the average member of the group has with the symptoms. Any symptom in a group that is deviant from the normal is likely to be discredited as a sign of illness (Mechanic, 1978). However, as pointed out in Chapter 2, individuals are not influenced by the general public but only are affected by those whose opinions are important to them. Their behaviors are affected by their efforts to accommodate the real or imagined expectations of "significant others."

From the symbolic interactionist perspective, the labeling process contains the elements of bargaining and of power relations, which are central to all social interaction. To what extent do social factors influence society's response to deviant acts, and therefore, how might they influence the response of decision makers? Prominant among these contingencies are the type, degree, amount, and visibility of the deviant act, the power and social distance of the deviant individual in relation to the agents of control, and the availability of alternative roles (Scheff, 1966b).

Resources favor the avoidance of labeling while a lack of resources influences the possibility of false labeling. The more marginal the person's societal attributes, such as socioeconomic status, race, age, and sex, the greater the likelihood of being channeled into a deviant role. The evidence that those in the lower classes are more likely to be treated for mental illness, particularly in mental hospitals (Hollingshead & Redlich, 1958; Kohn, 1968; Rushing, 1969) is consistent with the societal reaction explanation. The greater the individual's social or familial resources, the greater the opportunity to avoid hospitalization (Linsky, 1970; Rushing, 1971) since interested family members will be able to insure and manipulate the medical and legal professions to prevent hospitalization.

On the other hand, the greater "importance" of a person may lead to greater intolerance of deviance. For instance, men are rejected more strongly than women for exhibiting deviant behaviors (Phillips, 1964). It is less permissible for men to be sick or have other problems than for women.

Thus, in essence, the labeling perspective views the deviant as someone who is victimized. Reviewing the available evidence, however, Gove (1975a) claims that there is little evidence of victimization. To begin with, the evidence shows that a substantial majority have a serious disorder quite apart from any societal reaction. Furthermore, contrary to the labeling hypothesis, individuals without social resources are likely to postpone psychiatric treatment. It is those with the most resources who are likely to enter the role of the mentally ill. On the part of the community there is a tendency to delay attribution of mental illness until the situation becomes intolerable. Even after prospective patients are brought into contact with public officials, they are screened instead of being automatically committed to hospitals.

Doctor–Patient Relationship. As conflict theoreticians have pointed out, physicians and patients operate with quite different assumptions, and they have conflicting value orientations. Thus, their interactive processes can be viewed as negotiations, exchanges, and bargaining to reach a mutually acceptable label for the patient (Katz et al., 1963).

Since imputation of a deviant character inevitably requires some exercise of power, and since the physician labels the patient as deviant, the physician must gain control over the patient. However, due to their inadequate medical information, patients cannot appreciate the real power of the physician's technical expertise (Pratt et al., 1957; Samora et al., 1961). Therefore, as Goffman (1959) emphasized in his discussion of "performers," doctors must plan their "performance" in light of the patient's orientations, if they are to inspire the patient's confidence in them and, hence, exercise their therapeutic skills.

Frank (1973) claims that all psychotherapeutic techniques are attempts to heal through persuasion. Shamans in primitive cultures, faith healers of Western cultures, and psychiatrists of contemporary societies use similar methods of persuasion to bring about changes in the thinking and behavior of patients. Frank states that

> Treatment always involves a personal relationship between healer and sufferer. Certain types of therapy rely primarily on the healer's ability to mobilize healing forces in the sufferer by psychological means. These forms of treatment may be generically termed psychotherapy (Frank, 1973, p. 1).

Much of the influence doctors have on patients is nonspecific and rests on their ability to present themselves as authority figures. The study of such suggestive influences has been designated as the study of the placebo effect (Beecher, 1959; Liberman, 1962; Schacher & Singer, 1962). Shapiro (1959, p. 299) defined it as a psychological, physiological, or psychophysical effect of any medication or treatment with therapeutic intent, which is independent of the pharmacological effect of the medication.

As Shapiro (1959) noted, until recently the history of medical treatment has been for the most part the history of the placebo effect. Medications such as dung from crocodiles, geese, or sheep; blood from bats, frogs, and turtles; and oils from ants, wolves, spiders, and earthworms, are effective only when patients are convinced of the technical competence of doctors. This is partially accomplished by the manner in which doctors present themselves to the patients, that is, attire, speech, and behavior. Even now, placebo effects are not only reported as contributing to a patient's recovery but also have manifest side effects such as drowsiness, headache, nervousness, and nausea (Beecher, 1959; Honigfeld, 1964; Schacter & Singer, 1962; Wolf, 1959). However, systematic comparisons of laboratory experiments indicate methodological deficiencies in placebo studies, and they do not lead to a definitive conclusion (Liberman, 1962).

During the initial phase of an illness, the patient presents symptoms to the physician in an unorganized manner. We all have pains and aches, and a variety of symptoms occur commonly. Then, through a negotiation between doctor and patient, the patient settles down to a more organized illness phase (Balint, 1957). Scheff (1974) suggested that something similar to plea bargaining occurs in psychiatric diagnoses even though it is pursued on a much less conscious or deliberate basis. The doctors have definite ideas concerning how patients should behave when ill, and they subtly induce each patient to have the kind of illness they consider appropriate to the situation. As Scheff pointed out, the fact that a therapist has greater power than a client in determining what eventually may be a shared definition of the situation is implicit in this process (Lemert, 1962).

From the perspective of symbolic interactionism, the patient–therapist interaction is determined not by objective physical symptoms of illness but by the manner in which the patient presents himself or herself. Research findings

(Denzin, 1968; Denzin & Spitzer, 1968; Rosenham, 1973) indicate that if patients present themselves as accepting the psychiatric line by (1) recognizing their illness, (2) showing insight into their illness, (3) showing trust and faith in the therapist, and (4) being willing to give up their rights in the outside world; then they will (1) be given more favorable initial prognoses, (2) receive more hours of personal therapy, and (3) remain in the hospital a shorter length of time than others.

Once labeled, correctly or incorrectly, the individual is likely to proceed on a career of chronic deviance (Scheff, 1966b, p. 88). The effect of labeling is so pervasive that it tends to be irreversible for the individual. This leads to the reorganization of social roles and attitudes around deviance—what Lemert has termed secondary deviation.

This labeling process is well demonstrated by Rosenham's (1973) experiment to test whether or not the sane can be distinguished from the insane. Eight sane people, including psychologists, a psychiatrist, a pediatrician, a painter, and a housewife, gained secret admission to twelve different mental hospitals. All that they had to do to be admitted was to complain about hearing vague voices and words sounding like "empty," "hollow," and "thud." Once admitted with a diagnosis of schizophrenia, they behaved thereafter normally and rationally so as to expedite their release. However, despite this public display of sanity, the meanings of the pseudopatients' behaviors were consistently interpreted in accordance with the label of schizophrenia. In the hospital environment characterized by segregation of staff from patient and by depersonalization and mortification of patients, the pseudopatients had little chance to convince the staff members of their sanity. Once branded schizophrenic, they could not erase the mark. When they were eventually discharged, it was with a diagnosis of schizophrenia "in remission."

Hospitalization. The sick role is defined not only from the physician's point of view, but also by a host of others, such as nurses, attendants, and lay associates. This is particularly true in the case of hospitalized patients.

In Goffman's terms, the mental hospital is a "total institution." The key fact of the total institution is "the handling of many human needs by the bureaucratic organization of whole blocks of people" (Goffman, 1961, p. 6). The central features of total institutions are that (1) all aspects of life are conducted in the same place and under a single authority; (2) all the coparticipants live their lives in one place and are treated alike; (3) all daily activities are prearranged and supervised; (4) the activities are intended to fulfill the official aims of the institution; and (5) all phases of the activities in the institutions are insulated from the outside world (Goffman, 1961, p. 6).

Total institutions are both residential communities and bureaucratic mechanisms that have a mission and a goal to carry out. The hospital staff operates on the assumption that before the patients can be cured, they must admit their wrongdoings. With moral judgment injected into the therapeutic process, the patients are stripped of their social identities and are made to return to a state of infantile innocence so that they can be resocialized into normal adult roles. This is an "assault upon the self" of the patient.

The "career of mortification" begins with the admission procedure by which old identities are replaced by a new uniform identity kit provided by the institution. Total institutions disrupt self-determination, autonomy, and freedom of action. One's autonomy is weakened by such specific obligations as having to write home one letter a week or having to refrain from expressing sullenness. The patient has to conform to these rules lest a violation of the rules be diagnosed as a psychiatric symptom. Since many of the statements inmates make are discounted as mere symptoms, they have a hard time making themselves understood and getting the things they need.

In this environment, Goffman argues that the patients eventually come to accept the hospital's definition of themselves as mentally ill. When this process is complete, the patients come to be convinced that they are sick, act sick, and thus are incapable of operating effectively in normal roles outside the hospital. In short, patients become sicker as they stay in the hospital. In fact, the public perception of the total institution such as the homes for the aged is so negative that, as Tobin and Lieberman (1976) noted, prospective residents suffer from preadmission effects—disorientation, withdrawal, apathy, depression—as soon as they make application for admission.

However, the concept of the total institution has been criticized from various angles. Having reviewed the available evidence, Gove (1975a) suggests that the career of mortification is not a common reaction to the modern mental hospital. For example, Karmel (1970) examined patients at the New Jersey State Hospital at the time of their admission and again four weeks later. She did not find debilitating effects that could be measured by a loss of self-esteem and a loss of social identity. Several interpretations have been offered that give us an insight into the staff–inmate relationship in the total institution.

In conformity with the sick role conceptualization, Karmel explained that patients view hospital procedure as therapeutic, and they accept it without resentment. Karmel also postulated that the inmates do not consider the hospital staff as significant others and they assume their hospitalization to be only temporary.

What happens to institutionalized chronic mental patients? Over the years, do the patients finally surrender to the labeling process and consider themselves as deviants? According to Karmel's (1970) study, the patients eventually lost their normal social identity, but they did not acquire a new identity based on a deviant role. This is explained by the absence of conditions at the state hospital for developing a deviant subculture: (1) close interaction among deviants, (2) homogeneity in age and sex, (3) organization of deviants, and (4) leadership.

In analyzing the concept of institutionalism, Townsend (1976) distinguished two important dimensions: behavioral conformity to institutional norms, and psychological conversion of one's self-concept so as to fit into the sick role. Townsend claims that the empirical evidence supports only the behavioral, but not the psychological, aspect of conformity. Patients follow the institutional orders by manipulating the impressions they make, but they do not generally think of themselves as mentally ill.

Another criticism of the total institution has been made from the angle of preconditions of the patients prior to admission. Wing (1967) noted that schizophrenic patients who become long-term hospital residents tend to be selected from those who do not have strong ties with the community, family, or work and are vulnerable because of age, poverty, etc. Comparing nursing home patients who deteriorate rapidly and those who survive in the new environment, Tobin and Lieberman (1976) found that the latter were better adjusted to community living than the former before they came to the institutions. In other words, these critics argue that institutionalism—measured by apathy about life outside the hospital—is not entirely the consequence of institutionalization but is affected by conditions of the patients prior to their admission.

Despite these criticisms, there are important implications of the labeling approach. First, the labeling theory serves to correct the bias of the medical model of disease, which is exclusively based on biological and genetic factors. According to the social reaction hypothesis, what matters is not the nature of the physical symptoms but the manner in which these symptoms are perceived by society. This formulation has sensitized researchers to the importance of social interactional aspects of illness that had been neglected in the medical model.

Second, Goffman's description of asylums stimulated many other researchers to investigate various types of total institutions. They highlighted the adverse effects of institutionalism in the long-term hospitals for mental or chronic illnesses. Partly as a consequence of this and also because of the advent of new drugs that shortened the period of hospitalization, the movement toward community mental health appeared, which relies on treating patients in the natural community environment rather than in the bureaucratic total institution. This topic is followed up in Chapter 7.

Synthetic Model

So far we have compared three sociological interpretations of the doctor–patient relationship, that is, whether it should be viewed as a functionally integrated system, conflicting dynamics, or a labeling process. In the face of these traditionally divergent concepts, there have been some synthesizing efforts. One of the more systematic formulations was attempted by Lefton and Rosengren (1966). They identify two client (or patient) characteristics that are salient to the analysis of the client–organization and the client–practitioner relationships: lateral and longitudinal.

The lateral orientation toward a client refers to the institution's interest in the client's "biological space," that is, whether the organization (or the practitioner) is concerned with only a limited aspect, such as a physical illness, of the client as a person, or whether it has a more extended interest in the client as a socially functioning individual. For instance, a short-term general hospital is likely to show a limited interest in a specific physical aspect of the patient, while the psychiatric hospital is involved with the overall social, psychological, and physical functioning of the patient.

The second characteristic of the client relevant to the organization is the longitudinal or "biographical time" element, that is, the duration of the organizational relation with the client. The span of time ranges from a highly truncated one in the emergency room of a general hospital to an almost indeterminant duration in a long-term psychiatric or chronic illness hospital.

Based on the two dimensions of orientations to clients, four types of organizations can be differentiated, as shown in Table 5.1. These four types have different kinds of problems of control. In utilizing the client as the analytical point of departure for examining organizational dynamics, Lefton and Rosengren distinguish two modes of client compliance: conformity and commitment. With respect to conformity, a client's adherence to rules of conduct is the key issue, while in the case of commitment, the client's endorsement of the ideology of the institution is the focal problem. These modes of compliance pose different problems in each of the four types of client–practitioner relationship.

The greater the sphere of the organization's interest in the client (i.e., the laterality), the greater the areas of the client's conformity expected by the organization. The client's compliance in all these areas is of serious concern to such an organization. In contrast, those institutions with minimal lateral interest in their clients demand a client's conformity only in limited areas. Thus, the patient in a general hospital is expected only to follow instructions pertaining to physical therapy. Conversely, every aspect of the behavior of a psychiatric patient is monitored lest it should deviate from the norms.

With respect to the time dimension, the long-term institution needs to operate on a different mode of patient compliance. Since such an institution must have control over the client for a longer period of time, which may extend beyond the period of institutionalization, the exercise of mere coercion is not effective. The institution must inspire a patient's commitment to the institutional goal. The patient must come to believe in the moral goodness of the therapeutic procedures.

In sum, Lefton and Rosengren describes the doctor–patient relationship as the four combinations of positive and negative conformity and commitment, and they are determined by the types of illness, that is, acute versus chronic and physical versus mental.

This section began by examining the factors that induce individuals to enter into therapeutic relationships with physicians. Determinants of health care utilization are found to include sociocultural variables and are not limited to the presence of physical symptoms, as is proclaimed by the disease model.

Thus, the patient enters the therapeutic unit not as a disease entity but as a social agent interacting with the physician. Three explanatory models of the client–practitioner encounter have been compared: (1) the functionalist view of the association as an asymmetrically integrated system, (2) the conflict perspective of perceiving it as a clash of interests, and (3) the interactionist approach to it as a labeling process.

In an effort to synthesize these divergent orientations, however, the disease model is reintroduced. This model assumes that, after all, the type of illness determines the sociocultural nature of the doctor–patient relationship.

NEW DIRECTIONS IN THE PHYSICIAN–PATIENT RELATIONSHIP

Despite attempts to analyze the doctor–patient relationship from various

Table 5.1:
The Client–Organization Relationship

	Biological Interest: Orientation toward clients		*Compliance Problems*	
Example	*Lateral (Social space)*	*Longitudinal (Social time)*	*Conformity*	*Commitment*
Acute general hospital	–	–	No	No
TB hospital, rehabilitation hospital, public health department	–	+	No	Yes
Short-term therapeutic psychiatric hospital	+	–	Yes	No
Long-term therapeutic hospital	+	+	Yes	Yes

Notes: *The plus sign indicates presence of biological interest.*
The minus sign indicates absence of biological interest.

Source: Mark Lefton and W. R. Rosengren, "Organizations and Clients: Lateral and Longitudinal Dimensions," *American Sociological Review* 31 (1966):806–807.

perspectives—functional, conflict, and interactional—most researchers have clearly recognized the power lodged in the physician. The status of any profession is distinguished by its primary characteristic of autonomy, that is, the right to determine work activity on the basis of professional judgment. The public grant of autonomy to physicians has presumably been founded on the client's implicit acceptance of the professional's technical expertise and service orientation, even though this consent has frequently been based on fear, ignorance, or habit.

However, the whole fabric of social relations has been rapidly changing in the past twenty years. Patients are redefining their status from that of client to one of consumer (Bashshur et al., 1967; Campbell, 1971; Hochbaum, 1969; Thursz, 1970). From the perspective of labeling theory, we can expect differential behavior on the parts of perceivers and perceived, depending on the labels used. In the client–practitioner relationship, clients deliver themselves into the hands of the professionals who in turn are the sole decision makers regarding the nature of the services to be delivered. In comparison, the consumer–provider relationship allows the purchasers of services to be guided by caveat emptor and hence to have considerable bargaining power.

Patient power has been imputed in such areas as doctor-shopping (Kasteler et al., 1976), noncompliance behavior, and autonomous decision-making on the part of patients. Haug and Lavin (1978) differentiated two types of patients who exert pressure on physicians: *demanding* patients who insist on additional services or treatment, expect attention at unusual hours, present vague complaints, and are never satisfied, and *challenging* patients who fail to accept the authority of the physician as given, and wish to make decisions on their own with respect to treatment.

Possible sources of patient power have been inferred in various ways. Some explain that the problems patients bring to doctors are different from those of previous decades. Unlike the acute illnesses of the past, many chronic illnesses in contemporary society allow patients not to conform to the physicians' prescriptions because of the lack of urgency (Zola & Miller, 1971).

Others (Freidson, 1975a; Haug, 1975) claim that consumers have gained greater medical knowledge by virtue of widespread public health education. With this knowledge, the public expect accountability on the part of the medical professional.

Another explanation for the increase of patient power is derived from public dissatisfaction with bureaucratic medicine. The impersonality of modern medical practice is not conducive to the patients' trusting acceptance of doctors' orders (Freidson, 1973; Mechanic, 1976). Also, from the organizational perspective, the payment method has been held responsible for varying patient influence. Some report that persons who pay directly for medical services value and accept them more readily without a challenge than those in a prepaid plan (Haug, 1976). Members of prepaid medical plans are in a better position to bargain for power (Freidson, 1960). However, there are others who have found no significant relationship between the financial arrangement of medical practice and the extent of patient power (Haug & Lavin, 1978; Tessler & Mechanic, 1975).

Whatever the impetus, when patients started shopping around and scrutinizing the marketplace of health care, they made several important discoveries: (1) not only are doctors not always right, but they also make negligent mistakes, and (2) patients can take actions against such malpractice. Unlike the purchase of a defective commodity, the patients often cannot undo the physical damage, but they can gain financial compensation through legal suits. The malpractice issue, which had been gathering momentum for a decade, exploded in 1975. A California bumper sticker read: "Feel sick? Call your lawyer" ("Again, a slowdown," 1976). The crises of the consumer revolt by means of malpractice suits have brought a new phase to the doctor–patient relationship, an open conflict for power.

The Extent of the Malpractice Crisis

> A girl who became a quadraplegic after having radiation therapy for cancer six years ago was awarded $7.6 million in damages Wednesday in San Francisco Superior Court.
>
> It was believed to be the largest malpractice award in California history ("Jury awards . . . ," 1978).

Precise statistics on malpractice insurance, claims, awards, and settlements are almost impossible to gather since state laws, regulations, and experiences differ widely. Also, an immense amount of coverage in the mass media gives the public an exaggerated impression rather than accurate figures. Among the few studies, those made by the Secretary's Commission on Medical Malpractice (hereafter referred to as the Commission) (U.S. DHEW, 1973a), the National Association of Insurance Commissioners (NAIC), and the Industry's Insurance Service Office (ISO) represent attempts at nationwide data collection (NAIC, 1976).

Until 1974, with the exception of 1969 and 1970 when premium jumped 198 percent, the rise in malpractice insurance premiums was fairly consistent and followed the rise in national health care and other expenditures.

But, for 1974 and 1975, the ISO, which acts as the actuarial advisor for insurance companies, recommended increases of 50 and 170 percent respectively for hospitals, and 53 and 170 percent respectively for physicians and surgeons. In 1975, the Argonaut Insurance Company, which was carrying most of the malpractice insurance, requested a 197 percent increase in premiums in New York state and 274 percent in California. This triggered the doctors' strikes. Anesthesiologists in San Francisco's 12 private hospitals boycotted on May 1, 1975. The strike spread quickly to nearby areas. All non-emergency surgery was immediately postponed at the affected hospitals. The dozen institutions laid off 3,000 employees during the first two weeks of the month as occupancy rates dropped suddenly. No death due to a lack of proper treatment was reported, but patient care was endangered by the lack of workers. The strike had the full support of the San Francisco Medical Society, as other physicians were also hit with similarly steep insurance premium increases ("The doctors' revolt," 1975; "Malpractice . . . ," 1975; "When doctors went out . . . ," 1975).

However, this explosion of premium rates was caused by the insurance industry's pessimistic anticipations of future losses rather than by any actual dramatic increase in malpractice claims and settlements. Total premiums paid by all health care providers are now estimated to have been around $1 billion in 1975. The sum is great, but it actually constitutes less than one percent of all health care expenditures. According to a survey based on reports from physicians, the median premium in 1976 was $3,000, which represented no more than three percent of gross receipts and about eight percent of tax deductive professional expenses (Owens, 1976). Premiums vary greatly by geography and type of practice. In New York they ranged from $470 to $19,880 (American Medical Association, 1976).

According to the Commission's report (U.S. DHEW, 1973a), the relative differences in rates by type of practice in 1972 are as follows: against the base rate of 1.00 for physicians who do not perform or ordinarily assist in surgery, 3.00 is the rate for those who perform major surgery or assist with major surgery on patients other than their own, 4.0 is the rate for cardiac surgeons, otolaryngologists, etc., and 5.00 is the rate for anesthesiologists, neurosurgeons, obstetric-gynecologists, otolarygological plastic surgeons, and plastic surgeons, etc. According to the survey in 1976 (Owens, 1976), median premiums were $1,750 for general practitioners, $1,300 for pediatricians, $1,500 for internists, $6,000 for general surgeons, and $7,500 for obstetric-gynecological specialists.

Despite newspaper stories of spectacular settlements, most people who experience some mistreatment do not resort to malpractice suits. A survey prepared for the Commission showed that (1) lawyers refused the majority of potential cases (88 percent) because they either saw no adequate basis for liability or the potential award and fee were too small; (2) most claim actions were resolved out of court by mutual agreement; and (3) less than one out of every 1,000 claims paid was for $1 million or more and three-fourths of the incidents were closed with less than $10,000 paid. A similar picture was reported in a more recent survey from the ISO.

Causes for Malpractice Suits

Poor Doctor–Patient Relationship. The malpractice problem had been growing for a long time, but it was largely neglected until insurance premiums leaped. In the past, the malpractice suit was considered to be a symptom of a "deteriorating doctor–patient relationship" (Blum, 1957; Somers & Somers, 1961). In a later study (U.S. DHEW, 1973a) the Commission also identified the same cause, although it also described other factors such as technical failures. In Blum's (1957) study, two-thirds of the suing patients reported that their doctors could have prevented the suits simply by discussing the matter with them in a plain and candid manner.

Most of the patient dissatisfaction involves a hospital setting. The institutionalized patient is shifted from an active social role to a compliant one whereby the smallest details of living are dictated by strangers. When the enforced passivity and subordination are combined with an impersonal atmosphere, the combination tends to foster frustration and resentment and to intensify the patient's discontent with the treatment (Bernzweig, 1966).

In addition to organizational and contextual elements, there are personality and psychological factors that influence the physician–patient relationship. Profiles have been constructed of both the type of patient and physician who are likely to be parties to a suit. According to Blum (1957), most suits grow from the interaction of a "suit-prone doctor" and a "suit-prone" patient.

The suit-prone patients do not sue primarily for financial gain but are generally angry with the doctors and sue to punish them. Such patients have been described as highly emotional, unconsciously fearful of illness and death, and hence anxious for emotional support. On the other hand, they have underlying suspicions about the technical skills of the attending physicians since they are paranoid and psychoneurotic. In order to compensate for such underlying anxiety, the suit-prone patients overtly display an unreasonable belief in the physicians and medicine, and they openly declare that the doctors can cure any disease. They have a sense of inferiority yet are sensitive to any treatment regimen that appears to be unimportant. They are uncooperative, demanding, belligerant, dogmatic, and quick to blame (Bernzweig, 1966; Blum, 1957; Hershey, 1972).

In contrast, the suit-prone doctors have been characterized by their antipathy and indifference to the emotional needs of their patients. Even when sensing emotional anxieties, they maintain a posture of aloofness and display disdain for any responsibilities for the trivial psychological aspects of patients. This may be due to their preoccupation with their own images as successful scientists rather than as practitioners. Such doctors tend to regard patients as backward children who are too stupid to comprehend medical explanations (Blum, 1957).

Such have been the stereotypical descriptions of the so-called suit-prone personalities. However, these personalities existed prior to the 1970s, when only a few of them entered into law suits. In fact, it used to be difficult, in the usual practice of medicine, for patient dissatisfaction to be expressed in a way that would produce any change in the medical system (Notkin & Notkin, 1970). What then is the new impetus prompting dissatisfied patients to take action that may destroy the career of a physician? The answer may be found in the new era of consumerism.

The Consumer Revolt. The consumer revolt can be seen at various stages in various settings. Reeder (1972) regards "consumerism" as a "social movement" in contemporary society because it is a shared perspective of a large number of people, and it offers a redefinition of traditional social relations. In the past patients simply dropped out of the relation or were passively accommodating to the physician. Now they unite and confront the professionals with charges (Sorenson, 1974).

Professional autonomy is challenged by patients on the following grounds (Haug & Sussman, 1969): (1) inadequacy of professional expertise, (2) lip service to professional altruism, (3) a defective and insufficient organizational delivery system for their service, and (4) the encroachment of professional power into a nonprofessional domain of life.

The consumers' revolts are manifest everywhere. At the university, students deny the expertise and good will of their educators. Poverty groups claim that they know about community needs better than social workers. In the health field, the consumer movement was stimulated by the OEO-sponsored neighborhood health centers (Sparer et al., 1970). Thanks to the encouragement of officialdom, the trend toward consumer control of the neighborhood health center has been promoted (see Chapter 9).

Another area in which the patient has revolted concerns the breadth of professional prerogative, what Lefton and Rosengren (1966) called the lateral dimension. Covert pressure groups formed (Roth, 1963) that implicitly rejected a physician's expertise and judgment by imposing their presumably shared definition of the right moment for hospital discharge. In other situations, patients organized themselves to resist and to prevent the hospital from meddling with their social security, disability, or welfare income (Pilati, 1969). A flurry of legal action centered at the New York Medical College Center for Chronic Diseases drew public attention to the rights of patients in non-mental institutions, a situation which hitherto had been largely ignored. Several dozen patients refused to sign over their Social Security checks (usually $75 to $125) to the Department of Social Services, after which they would receive the $15 monthly allowance. After months of legal maneuvering, the Judge finally issued an order stating that patients who withheld their checks could not be harrassed or intimidated. This was the first major thrust for patients' rights at a public institution.

As consumers of medical services, patients no longer accept the doctors' authority blindly, and they critically evaluate the quality of medical care. They are increasingly insistent on recompense for negligence or malpractice. The consumer-rights movement in the health field is further accelerated by the consumer's unrealistic expectations of what medical intervention can, in fact, produce. Scientific and technological advances, together with material affluence in the United States, has generated a "push-button" mentality (Enos & Sultan 1977, p. 352). The patients push a button to obtain a miracle cure. If that fails, they will push another button to call a lawyer to resolve their disappointment.

Defects in the Medical Delivery System. Deficiencies in the medical profession that have given rise to the malpractice suits are manifold, and most of them will be discussed in the following chapters.

The ideal of professional autonomy has placed the responsibility for the control of quality in the hands of the physicians. As will be pointed out in Chapter 7, current mechanisms for supervising and auditing medical care are clearly inadequate.

Proposals to improve that control through the Professional Standards Review Organization (PSRO) system had been fought by physicians (Gosfield, 1975). To illustrate the low quality in medical care, the Commission's study of two hospitals revealed that 7.5 percent of the hospital admissions resulted in medical injury, and of those, more than 20 percent were due to negligence. Yet, instead of 500 claims that could have been made, only 31 malpractice suits were filed (U.S. DHEW, 1973a, p. 24). According to a congressional report,

2.4 million unnecessary operations were performed in 1974 ("How to protect . . . ," 1977). In a massive five-year study conducted by the Cornell University Medical College, 24 percent of the patients who were initially told they needed elective (non-emergency) surgery really did not need it. This was determined when patients saw another surgeon for second opinion (McCarthy & Widmer, 1974). Makofsky (1977) has estimated that approximately 5 percent of all practicing physicians are unfit for practice because of ignorance of drug side-effects, mental illness, and so on, and 30,000 Americans die annually from faulty drug prescriptions.

In other words, as Schwartz (1976) states, the basic cause of the malpractice crisis is indeed malpractice, that is, poor medical care.

However, the above figures do not necessarily imply that poor medical quality is more prevalent now than in the past. In earlier days sickness was on the whole accepted as a usual and expected thing. Adverse results of treatment were likely to be regarded as the natural outcome of disease or attributed to the will of God. Advances in medical technology, however, increased the complexity of health care and brought about new risks of injury. As the potency of drugs increased, so did the potential hazards of using them. Lacking an appreciation of the complexity and hazards of modern medicine, patients underestimate the inherent risks and assume negligence when the outcome is not satisfactory.

Another feature that affects the doctor–patient relationship and that has undergone various changes is the struture of medical practice. Unlike the classic model of a solo practice, the meeting of a physician and a patient is now likely to be held in a bureaucratic organizational context. As a result, patients are discontent with impersonal care sometimes associated with bureaucracy, while the physicians' behavior is constrained by the administrative needs of this new business format (Mechanic, 1976).

The professional ideal of providing service has been skewed by the changes to the organization of medicine (Mechanic, 1976). Like others in a competitive society, physicians organized themselves around their common interests so as to maintain and to enhance their privileged status. While the public was awarding the highest occupational prestige to physicians, they may have felt jealous and resentful toward their doctors (Enos & Sultan, 1977; Krause, 1977; Navarro, 1976).

Another aspect of the structural change is seen in the shift from curative to preventive medicine (Reeder, 1972). Curative medicine, such as emergency care, implies a seller's market because the provider of the medical service has full control over the situation. Preventive medicine represents a buyer's market because the client has to be persuaded to use a particular type of medical service. Here, the client also has the power to choose the providers.

Although malpractice concerns primarily doctors and patients, it involves many other parties, of which lawyers and insurance people are particularly important.

Responses to the Malpractice Crisis

Legal Issues. Doctors allege that lawyers are responsible for generating the large number of malpractice suits. They attack both the size of contingency fees and the very practice of collecting contingency fees. They criticize the judicial system, judges, juries, and state laws by claiming that the system was made by lawyers for lawyers (Somers, 1977). Apart from these general accusations, there are specific legal issues that are crucial to malpractice suits.

First of all, implementation of the *res ipsa loquitur* doctrine (i.e., "the thing speaks for itself") has been widely considered to be a cause of the problem (Krafchek, 1975; New York, 1976; U.S. DHEW, 1973a). Under this doctrine, a jury may be allowed, in appropriate circumstances, to find that a physician has been negligent on the basis of circumstantial evidence. This is done without expert medical testimony, which establishes the standards of professional care in the community and evaluates the conduct of the physician against those standards. This doctrine eliminates one of the strongest safeguards that the physician has against unwarranted professional liability suits.

There is an opposing view, however, that the abolition of the *res ipsa loquitur* doctrine would only require additional expert testimony where it is not really needed, would lead to increased trial costs, and still would not produce favorable results for the physician (New York, 1976, p. 34).

The matter of informed consent has also been viewed as contributing to the malpractice problem. Alleged lack of consent may make the physician a frequent target for malpractice claims whenever a bad result occurs. Since the gist of the action does not involve negligent treatment but negligence in explaining the hazards to the patient, it has become attractive to those lawyers who seek new theories of liability against physicians. Of course, the doctrine of informed consent is not *merely* a legal device. It is an ethical part of modern medical practice, which will be elaborated upon in Chapter 12.

Some of the legal procedures that have been associated with malpractice suits are mentioned above. However, there are contradictory evidence and interpretations concerning the exact effects of these legal mechanisms upon the prevalence of malpractice suits and the costs of malpractice insurance (Schwartz, 1976).

Insurance Issues. In addition to the lawyers, the insurance companies have also been the target of attacks by physicians who accuse them of making large profits on the malpractice premiums.

Until recently, insurance companies could charge low premiums, invest those funds, and possibly earn considerable income before any actual payment because there was usually a long time between the filing of the claim and the actual settlement (New York, 1976). With the decline of the stock market of the sixties and early seventies, and the resulting recession, many of the insurance companies experienced financial difficulties. Furthermore, the insurance market became exceedingly risky because of the long duration of time covered by malpractice settlements, the rapidly growing size of the awards, and the increasing number of claims. According to the Commission's reports (U.S. DHEW, 1973a), on the average only half are closed within 18 months and 10 percent remain open 6½ years after they are opened. By 1975, commercial insurance companies in New York and other states even decided not to handle malpractice insurance.

Thus, while there may have been high insurance company profits in the past, the hike in premiums in 1975 reflected the increase in actual payments and the insurers' fear of the risky market situation rather than any profit motive (Schwartz, 1976).

State Legislation. The first reponses to the malpractice crisis were erratic, semi-hysterical, superficial, and took the form of volumes of state legislation. Virtually all states had passed some new type of malpractice laws by the end of 1976.

Much of these actions were taken hastily and without factual information to substantiate their rationale. The primary concern of the new laws was to reduce the liability of the physician defendants by assuring the availability of insurance and by keeping the premiums down. Some of the legislation was of dubious constitutional nature and sacrificed the equity of the patient. With their political and financial power, the medical profession tried to restore the old equilibrium in which physicians could control patients. Few attempts were made to change the characteristics of the medical delivery system that had generated the suits.

The first wave of state legislation made sure that malpractice insurance was available by forcing joint underwriting pools among all of the companies that offered personal injury liability insurance and by establishing physician- and/or hospital-owned insurance associations.

The second series of state actions involved tort law changes that were designed to reduce the number of claims, lessen liability, expedite settlements, and improve the physician defendant's position in suits. For instance, time limitations were set, beyond which delayed discovery of injuries could not be brought up for action. Also, arbitrary ceilings on the amount of recovery were set in some states irrespective of the severity of the injury. The constitutionality of these restrictions was challenged by many authorities, and in some cases they were declared unconstitutional by the State's Supreme Court.

The third device was to set up a screening panel to expedite the handling of claims and to settle the issue before it reached the trial stage. This move was intended to prevent the sensational publicity that is detrimental to the physician's reputation as well as to forestall expensive court trials.

Gradually, the initial shock subsided, and later legislation became more balanced and constructive. Nevertheless, most of the legal changes were designed to assuage the physicians and resulted in the curtailment of the existing rights of patients (Somers, 1977).

Quality Control. Finally, some states began to show an awareness of the fact that the malpractice problem did not arise entirely from shortcomings in the legal or insurance systems, but that the root of the problem was in medical practice itself.

As a result, substantial steps were taken by several states toward the prevention of malpractice claims through a quality control of the medical delivery system. These measures can be divided into three categories (Somers, 1977). The first category refers to the mandatory reporting of claims and/or financial recoveries to insurance companies and to a state medical licensing or review board for investigation. Based on these reports the fitness of the physician is reviewed and proper sanctions are taken.

Second, the disciplinary power of licensing boards was expanded to include professional incompetence as a new ground for suspension or revocation of a license. Some states have created new evaluation boards consisting of both physicians and lay people. The boards investigate each suspected misconduct, and they are empowered to take disciplinary action.

Finally, some states have provisions that require continuing professional education, and those laws are used either as the necessary requirement for periodic relicensing or as a disciplinary measure to rehabilitate "impaired" physicians.

Interestingly enough, medical societies supported, or at least did not oppose, most of this new legislation. It appears that the malpractice crisis shook the traditional professional system to such an extent that physicians came to realize the necessity for structural changes. On the other hand, their willingness to undertake such changes may be due, at least in part, to their fear of a more complete revolution, that is, socialized medicine. Fear of governmental intervention has generated more individual and organized attempts to raise practicing standards and discipline than ever before (*American Medical News,* 1976; *Medical World News,* 1975). The traditional public posture of "the doctor knows best" has been abandoned. Instead, we see professional organizations publicly acknowledging the reality of incompetence and negligence and even urging public officials to assume more disciplinary authority over the profession.

Future Alternatives

The malpractice crisis destroyed the traditional picture of "a distant and peer-responsible professional and a humble, ministered-to client" (Haug & Sussman, 1969). The patient as consumer appears to be more sophisticated and aware of his or her needs than ever before, as evidenced by the prevalence of doctor-shopping (Kasteler et al., 1976). Clients are highly critical of professionals who do not understand those they are supposed to serve, who are elitists, and who are unwilling to accept an accountability to the consumers.

Yet, the exact direction for the future doctor–patient relationship is difficult to assess. The first possibility is consumer triumph and deprofessionalization of the physicians. The scope of professional power and autonomy will be progressively curtailed, which in turn will lower the status of the profession. Consumer representation on hospital boards, prepaid medical care plans, community medical centers, and the like will change the professional into a mere technician.

On the other hand, the technical expertise of physicians that make them life-savers can never be underestimated by society. The physicians' power may become limited in social, political, and other areas, but it may become focused in a narrow range that will actually serve to intensify their importance (Haug & Sussman, 1969). The modal pattern of professional response to the consumer challenge has been cooption. In this way, the professionals educate the dissident consumers into the special organization knowledge of the profession. By being allowed to participate in professional circles, consumers will come to accept the professional rationale. Cooption assumes that the clients are in reality ignorant and uninformed. Thus, the profession can preserve its authority and autonomy at the expense of sharing a small portion of its power with consumers. In this connection, see Chapter 9 for a discussion of consumer participation in policy decision-making in the neighborhood health centers.

The third alternative is the appearance of the third-party mediation. It may take the form of using a mediator (Reeder, 1972) who will settle differences between professionals and clients. On a larger scale, it may lead to a national health insurance. Some people (Schwartz, 1976) advocate this as the only reasonable solution to the malpractice crisis. They assert that the provision of comprehensive medical care would inhibit patients from suing, and that quality control and disciplining measures could be built into the national health insurance system (for detailed discussion of this topic, see Chapter 10).

In whichever direction the medical delivery system is moving, the functionalist equilibrium of the traditional medical profession has broken down, and the current condition should be viewed as a process of power struggle among the professionals, the clients, and the government. We can anticipate, however, that some stability will be reached with a new equilibrium, sooner or later.

SUMMARY

Before physicians consolidated their status and established the power of their profession, their authority had to be derived from sources other than medical technology. From primitive days until the end of the Middle Ages, physicians were sheltered in theological institutions, and their power over patients was based on religious faith. The physician–patient relationship in those days was fairly close to the functional model of a social system. Value consensus was found in the religious doctrines that were endorsed by doctors and patients.

When medicine declared its independence from theology after the Renaissance, it had to build its own foundations from which to win the patients' confidence in medicine per se. But though science was making advances during the seventeenth and the eighteenth centuries, medical practitioners were not availing themselves of that new technology. They simply continued to administer primitive medieval cures. Patients were impressed by the aristocratic manners with which doctors presented themselves, but they had little faith in the technical effectiveness of such physicians.

Then, during the early part of the nineteenth century, progress was made in medical science, but it was accompanied by disputes and conflicts among medical practitioners who held different perspectives. The public was confused and felt abandoned by the medical profession, and they turned to quacks who offered sure and instantaneous remedies.

It was only during the early twentieth century that medicine achieved the status of a profession, and that consolidation was based solely upon its monopoly of medical technology. Patients gained confidence in the technical expertise of physicians, who in turn began to view patients as disease entities rather than as whole persons.

From the functionalist perspective, the doctor–patient relationship today is viewed as a social system that is integrated on the consensus of values. This system shares the central values prevailing in the society at large, namely, the importance of health for individuals so that they may perform social functions. In this respect, illness is regarded as socially dysfunctional, and a sick person must conform to certain institutionalized expectations.

The functionalist premise of value consensus has been criticized from the perspectives of conflict theory. For instance, Freidson conceives of the therapeutic relationship as a social process by which clashes of incompatible interests of two groups are resolved through negotiation and bargaining. Unlike Parsons, who emphasizes compliance in patient behavior, Freidson draws attention to the client control of the profession through the lay referral system.

The genesis as well as the resolution of such conflicts can be studied in terms of social structural variables on the macro level, but it is also important to consider relations in small-scale groups. This micro perspective is found among the various formulations of the interactionist theory, in particular, the labeling theory. According to this theory, the medical profession "creates" illness as an official social role. Specifically, the severity of the physical symptoms are not nearly as important as the type of social reactions generated by the symptoms. Once a person is labeled as mentally ill for minor deviations, it is difficult for him or her to recover an original, unsullied identity.

Finally, there is one major factor that underlies all three sociological interpretations of the doctor–patient relationship, and that is the type of illness. The Parsonian sick role is applicable only to some types of illness. Conflict in a therapeutic situation is more manifest in dealing with certain illnesses than for others. Thus, the type of illness serves to specify the conditions under which a particular sociological framework can be used effectively.

A new era of strain in the doctor–patient relationship reached recognizable proportions in the 1950s, and conflicts centering around an upsurge in malpractice suits are continuing to erupt. Actually, malpractice suits are not new phenomena, and in the past were explained away as a sign of a deteriorated doctor–patient relationship. Articulation of patient malcontent through legal action on a massive level has been facilitated in recent years by a type of social movement called consumerism. Patients have redefined their status from that of clients to that of consumers. As a consumer, the patient examines and evaluates physicians, whose status has also been redefined and who are now perceived as providers of health services. In the medical marketplace as well as in other professional–client relations, consumers found many faults with providers, and they began to organize themselves and to take action to change the structure of the relations. The future direction is not definite, but at least there does not seem to be a possibility of a recourse to the traditional relationship in which the authoritarian professional ministers to the humble client.

This chapter has examined the vicissitudes of the doctor–patient encounter throughout history. This dyadic relationship is a reflection of broader social mechanisms by which the medical profession transacts with other groups in society. Physicians gained the sacred trust of patients only when the former attained the status of a profession with a monopoly on medical technology and autonomy over their practice. In the next chapter we will focus our attention upon the wax and wane of the medical profession.

CHAPTER 6
Physicians: The Medical Profession

Professionals, particularly physicians, have long been placed on a very high pedestal in our society. In almost all studies of occupational prestige in the United States, physicians receive top ratings. They form an elite group. This chapter deals with the medical profession as a social system. Physicians, wherever they are found—in the hospital, in the clinic, or in private offices—are distinguished from the rest of society by their professional characteristics, which tend to generate honor, respect, and prestige. This chapter examines how physicians gained the status and power of a profession, how they have maintained that position, and whether they can retain or increase their power in the future.

From the functionalist perspective, such social and economic status as held by physicians is warranted because they perform the most crucial function of all, maintaining the survival of humanity and society. Furthermore, only a limited number of people have the capacity to endure difficult, extended, and rigorous training. As a consequence, the ensuing reward must be large enough to motivate them to enter the field (Davis & Moore, 1945).

The elitism in the profession of physicians, however, has not persisted throughout history. For the most part, physicians were subordinate to religious, political, and other social power groups. Physicians had to organize themselves as members of a profession, which was possible only after they had sufficiently advanced their technology. In this respect, the rise and fall of the status of physicians is more easily understood within a conflict theory framework. Physicians as a status group are in a continuous struggle for power against other status groups. Thus, their future is not guaranteed by the functionalist assumption concerning the functional importance of medicine but is threatened by the power of other interest groups.

Turning to the interactionist perspective, we are alerted to numerous symbols and symbolic interactions reinforcing the physician's status. The elevated status of doctors is emphasized throughout medical school by their white uniform, the exclusivity of the medical language, as well as by the unspoken power derived from the public's confidence in the physician's superior knowledge.

This chapter concerns the following four topics: (1) development of the profession—how doctors have come to identify themselves as a professional group; (2) medical school—how new members are socialized into the profession of physicians; (3) organized medicine—how the status and power of the medical profession were consolidated and have been protected against trespassers; and (4) medical practice—how individual physicians maintain professional autonomy in a variety of work settings.

THE MEDICAL PROFESSION

Characteristics of the Profession

In comparison to other occupations in all industrialized countries, the prestige of the physician is quite high. To exemplify that point further, in the United States it appears that the medical profession is the prototype upon which all would-be healing professions as well as other professions model themselves (Hughes, E. C., 1958).

Functionalist Perspective. The study of professions has been conducted predominantly within the functionalist framework. To begin with, the functionalist theory of profession stresses two strategic attributes for explaining any profession's position and function in society (Goode, 1957), namely, technical competence and functional importance to society. Thus a profession is conceived of as an occupation that (1) applies a systematic body of knowledge to problems that (2) are highly relevant to central values of the society (Carr-Saunders & Wilson, 1933; Davis & Moore, 1945).

A corollary to the above is the assumption that professionals are accorded high statuses because only a limited number of people are capable of acquiring the particular specialized skills through a prolonged period of training. However, the professional's high degree of learned competence creates special problems of social control in that lay people cannot realistically judge the performance of the professional. As a consequence, bureaucratic supervision and judgment by the customer, which are two of the most common forms of control, are not applicable to the profession. The dilemma is supposedly resolved by a strong emphasis on the professional's individual self-control, supplemented by collegial surveillance.

Second, a profession, which is a collection of individuals, is viewed by functionalists as an element of social structure. Goode (1957) aptly called it a community within a community. As a community and a social system, a profession meets the following functional prerequisites.

1. Latency. The boundaries of a profession are reasonably clear, though it should be noted that they are not physical or geographical, but social. A profession does not produce future generations biologically, yet it does so on a social level through its control of the recruitment and socialization of its members.

As a rule members of a profession maintain values in common, speak the same language, which is only partially understood by outsiders, and therefore are bound by a sense of identity. Among the values shared by medical professionals in particular is other-orientation, that is, the offering of a service to the public at large. According to functionalists (Parsons, 1951), this value system is designed to prevent exploitation of vulnerable lay people by the professional, who monopolizes a specialized technique.

2. Integration. A profession has power over its members by defining the roles for each member and by sanctioning those who deviate from the professional norms. In order to insure that professional autonomy remains inviolate from external interference, a profession must socialize its members to acquire not only the required technical competence but a firm commitment to the values and norms of the profession. Among examples of unprofessional medical conduct is the advertisement of one's practice. This is because advertising presumes the client's ability to evaluate medicine and also violates the service orientation of the profession.

3. Adaptation. A profession fights against outside forces that threaten the existence of the community. Adaptive techniques used in the medical profession include, but are not limited to, licensing and mandate. With licensure, the medical profession sets up formal mechanisms to protect itself from invaders. The profession claims the right to practice on the basis of the special knowledge gained during the training period. Mandate refers to the right of the profession to declare the standards or goals to which the public should aspire. The definition of good health standards or good health practices are determined by the medical profession, and the public is expected to accept them.

4. Goal Attainment. A profession owes its very existence to commonly agreed-upon goals, around which its activities are organized. Medicine has agreed that illness and disease are social objects toward which its services are to be directed. The goal of physicians is to cure, control, or eliminate disease, and not to make any other utilization of the object. While illness and disease are sometimes used in teaching institutions as learning tools, this activity is still part of the professional goal, that is, medical care.

Conflict Perspective. Contrary to functionalist arguments, conflict theorists suggest that professions are not static and integrated institutions but rather are in constant struggle to win and maintain the title of profession. Doctors won the contest over quacks and charlatans during the early part of this century by establishing licensure and mandate, which enabled them to monopolize advanced medical technology. Ever since that time physicians have been on constant guard lest their professional power should be eroded by the public, government, and other health practitioners. The part played by the American Medical Association in fighting against the Medicare and Medicaid bills demonstrates how physicians can form a united front against third-party intervention.

In addition to the external struggle for survival, the medical profession must live with constant internal conflict. The medical profession is not a group of persons sharing the same title and values. Rather, it contains "moving, shifting, growing, splitting, and assimilating bodies of persons" (Bucher & Strauss, 1961, p. 325) held together at one point in time by a common name or label. Within the same profession there are many values and interests, which tend to become patterned and shared. Coalitions or segments develop and organize in order to oppose older, entrenched groups and further their own interests. Viewed from this angle, Bucher and Strauss (1961) stated that professions are like social movements.

Thus, according to the conflict theorists, the profession is the process of tension, growth, and change (Bucher, 1972; Bucher & Strauss, 1961). Sources of conflicts are both internal and external, that is, power contests (1) within specialized segments among those holding the title of M.D., such as general practitioners versus specialists; (2) physicians in relation to other healers such as chiropractors; and (3) medicine versus other occupations and institutions such as the government, insurance companies, and organized labor. Research indicates, however, that the most conflict exists among doctors themselves rather than between doctors and other professional groups (Georgopoulos & Mann, 1962).

The inevitability of conflict can be inferred from the assumption of a zero-sum game (Goode, 1961)—one in which there is a limited supply of power and income available. As one group rises, another must decline. Since professionalization is characteristic of an industrialized society, many occupational groups are aspiring to reach professional status. Struggle is unavoidable since as one group reaches for a higher place, other groups react so as to maintain their positions.

Interactionist Perspective. As functionalists claim, the technical competence of the physician rests on a body of systematic scientific theory. However, in the actual application of this knowledge, other less rationalized elements play an important role. The "art" of medicine includes the use of interpersonal relations in the healing process.

The interactionist perspective is also valid in distinguishing between objective expertise and social recognition of it (Gerver & Bensman, 1954). Because of the complexity of the technological field and the ignorance of the public, mere possession of a skill does not automatically grant a person the title of expert. Claims for recognition as an expert must be accompanied by the social visibility of that particular skill. In a situation where symbolic expression of reality is emphasized, the attainment of expert status becomes equated with successful manipulation of symbols, such as manners of speech, physical appearance, and display of diplomas.

In short, there is ambiguity concerning the concrete meaning of the ultimate values of the profession, such as "expertise in a particular field." The public image of the profession influences not only the general public but the professionals' behavior as well.

Ambivalence Hypothesis. Thus far, the physicians' high status has been attributed by functionalists to their possession of technical competence, by conflict theorists to their winning the power contest, and by symbolic interactionists to their manipulation of symbols.

In contrast to these interpretations, Cohn (1960) proposed an ambivalence hypothesis, which explains the physician's exalted position in terms of human irrationality. According to Cohn, social judgments are self-contradictory or ambivalent. Thus in American culture there are two fundamentally opposed, though dynamically related, value scales. One is labeled social stratification; it rank-orders people according to their economic success. The other is charismatic distinction; it honors a personal quality of leadership arousing special popular loyalty or enthusiasm. Physicians can command eminence because they excel in performance judged from both angles, that is, they are financially successful, and they also play the altruistic role of priests.

The Historical Roots of the Medical Profession

Despite the many claims of scientific excellence, functional importance, or charismatic distinction that the medical profession makes at the present time, medical authority is not the de jure nor de facto (in functionalist terms) property of the profession. One may even recall that there were periods in the past when healing practitioners did not occupy a position of stability, let alone a professional status. It was not until the latter part of the nineteenth century that physicians acquired enough technique and knowledge to validate the authority they had previously sought unsuccessfully. As L. J. Henderson so aptly put it, until around 1910 or 1912 a patient had as good a chance of recovery by not seeing a doctor as otherwise (Freidson, 1979).

Before the Middle Ages. In primitive societies witch doctors attempted to support their occupational status by asserting that the efficacy of their work was based on the knowledge gained through apprenticeship. They assumed special "professional" mannerisms such as peculiar dress and speech to set themselves off from everyday lay people. A witch doctor might enjoy a position of high authority in one society while in others, the position a witch doctor occupied was extremely low.

In ancient Greece, medicine was considered to be secret knowledge shared by a relatively small number of families believed to be descendents of Asclepius. Each such family comprised a guild to transmit medical knowledge from father to son. During the time of Hippocrates in the fifth century B.C., the number of doctors had to be increased, which necessitated the adoption of outsiders into the family to practice medicine. The Hippocratic oath was primarily the contract between a master and pupil, and between an adoptive father and the adopted son. In addition, the Hippocratic oath was an oath to the gods to lead a pure and dignified life and preserve "professional" standards (Sigerist, 1960). Thus, Greek healers constituted an unstable and defensive occupation. They were drawn together into clusters of apprentices around the masters, and each cluster jealously guarded its secrets from one another.

It appears that before the Middle Ages there was no clear identity attached to physicians except in the most general way. Throughout the centuries, healers varied markedly both in practicing groups and in their training and skills. Medicine was not a recognized occupation, if measured by the criteria of an occupation commanding exclusive competence that is publicly acknowledged (Freidson, 1975b).

The Middle Ages. Many of the physicians during the Middle Ages were clerics and so were members of a powerful organization, the Church. The Church, however, objected to their ministers engaging in medicine, particularly in the area of surgery (Sigerist, 1960).

Gradually, the guild system, the workers' association, came into existence. During the thirteenth century, the guilds became self-governing bodies and in many cities gained political power. They began setting working hours, wages, and prices to exclude competition. As a consequence, they created a monopoly surrounding their craft so that no one could exercise these skills outside the guild (Sigerist, 1960).

Precise steps toward the mastery of crafts were thus cultivated within the guild. In order to become surgeons, individuals entered the guild as apprentices. After two to three years they were awarded certificates to practice as journeyworkers for four to six years. If they desired to become masters, they were required to pass strict examinations. However, surgery was at a low social level during this period. Surgeons in most places were at the same time barbers or keepers of bathhouses. It was not uncommon to see surgeons joining other guilds such as that of blacksmiths when there were too few to form their own guild.

The guild served to consolidate public identity of occupational groups. Another source for fostering an occupational identity for the physician was the medieval university, which created definite and distinct administrative standards for conferring the title "doctor" (Warbasse, 1970). The physicians organized themselves, and their licensing body became the medical faculty of the universities. Nevertheless, the chancellor of the university who conferred the license was usually a cleric representing the pope.

Guild and university physicians began to form elite groups with clients restricted to nobility and the wealthy. But even the elite could not bind themselves to clients who sought other healers as well. Equipped with a meager level of technology, the physicians could not generate widespread public confidence in their practice. As a result, neither university nor guild alone was sufficient to establish the physician's exclusive monopoly over the healing technique (Freidson, 1975b).

From the Renaissance to the Nineteenth Century. Historically, cultural values tended to stress the priorities of theological institutions, including pantheism, over those of professional medical care. Physicians practicing in such a setting could effectively direct negative sanctions for their lack of competence to other sources such as "god's will." Gradually as physicians became disengaged from the controls of the theological institution, they were obliged to create a professional institution as their own protection; from its outset, it stressed scientific methods and direct observation as the basis for expertise.

With the reinstatement of cultural values formulated during the Renaissance, the professional medical institution attempted to establish autonomy from the Church. Concerns about the nature of secular existence and a pursuit of a scientific rationale were its marked characteristics. Through the foundation of human anatomy, the Renaissance contributed to the development of scientific medicine. However, it would be many years before this influence had any effect upon the professionalization of medicine.

In fact, the impact of the Middle Ages upon medicine was far-reaching beyond the Renaissance. For example, during the seventeenth century a great amount of scientific progress was made, but none of it salvaged medical practices from very poor conditions. The reason for this paradox lay in the universities, which still clung to their medieval traditions and failed to adapt themselves to the new scientific methods. Doctors from these universities could discuss texts but were unable to apply the new scientific methods. Since virtually all scientific research requires apparatus of one kind or another, new institutions, the academies, began to flourish from the 1600s throughout Europe. While medical science began to blossom in the academies, universities were training unqualified practitioners (Sigerist, 1960).

Meanwhile, the social structure and prevalent values of the eighteenth century (i.e., mercantilism) placed a premium on the physician's practice as a technological system of production. Specialization and scientific orientation in medicine were viewed as being the most efficient. Thus, the direct and technological aspect of medical practice came to be highly prized. Quackery as an instantaneous therapy appealed to the sense of efficacy of a technological society where scientific medicine failed to give an immediate solution.

The tide began to turn in the nineteenth century with the appearance of a medical body of expertise based on the germ theory and the successful scientific treatment of epidemics by vaccination. Such contributions enabled medicine to gradually establish itself as a profession, claiming a monopoly of expertise and social worth.

The American Medical Scene. Toward the end of the eighteenth century and into the beginning of the nineteenth century, the development of medicine in the United States steadily followed the pattern started in Europe. Medical schools were founded from 1765 onward and their curricula were as advanced as those in many European universities.

During the nineteenth century, however, the climate began to change. The enormous expansion to the western frontier was accompanied by an even more explosive need for medical services. Hundreds of medical schools were founded to meet the demand, but many of them were poorly equipped and gave inadequate training. As their educated, scientific treatments of choice, physicians continued to offer the remedies of bleeding and purging because they believed that all illnesses resulted from tension in the blood vessels.

Mass distaste for such therapies and awareness of their ineffectiveness led to the support of a variety of more palatable healing movements, such as alcohol and patent medicines. Under these circumstances neither guilds nor licensing laws insured a monopoly of medical practice to any single group of healers (Packard, 1963).

In addition to the low technological level (which made the public mistrust the physician), there was another cause for the mushrooming of folk medicine and quackery. That was the ideology of equalitarianism, which stated that no one should be prevented by medical licensing laws from the freedom to practice medicine. On the frontier, virtually anyone could practice healing in some way or another. Also, anyone who was desirous of obtaining a degree could easily receive one from the proprietary schools (Bonner, 1957; Young, 1961).

Only toward the end of the nineteenth century did physicians begin to consolidate their status as a profession. There were two basic channels that led to the professionalization of medicine: medical education and organized medicine. Differentiation from quasiprofessional institutions and their practices was achieved by controlling the quality of medical practice in a closed educational system and by establishing an authority base—the American Medical Association.

MEDICAL EDUCATION

The Development of the Medical School

During the colonial days a few medical practitioners came from abroad as medical immigrants, a few were sent abroad to study medicine, and some were products of the apprenticeship system.

The first medical school in the United States was established in Philadelphia in 1765 by John Morgan, who had completed his medical education abroad (Carson, 1869). Two years after the medical school was created, the trustees decided to confer degrees in medicine with the following requirements:

> For a Bachelor's Degree in Physic:—
>
> Each shall attend at least one course of lectures in Anatomy, Materia Medica, Chemistry, the Theory and Practice of Physic, and one course of Clinical lectures, and shall attend to the practice of the Pennsylvania Hospital for one year; and may then be admitted to a public examination for a Bachelor's Degree in Physic; . . .
>
> Qualifications for a Doctor's Degree in Physic:—
>
> It is required for this Degree that at least three years shall have intervened from the time of taking the Bachelor's Degree, and that the candidate be full 24 years of age, and that he shall write and defend a Thesis publicly in the College (Norris, 1866, pp. 61–63).

Beginning in the 1800s, proprietary schools were developed. They were mostly inadequate, and their graduates were ill trained. Before the Revolutionary War, there were 3,500 practicing physicians, but only 400 of them had bona fide medical degrees (O'Malley, 1970). The educational process that awarded those degrees was deficient. People who could not even write often entered medical school, and others were literally dragged off the streets for a medical education that was available to anyone who could pay the tuition (Norwood, 1971).

Following the Civil War, the stage was set for social and economic change. Industrialization and urbanization helped improve conditions, and these developments were responsible for creating large individual fortunes, which could be used for medical science. As a result, the second half of the nineteenth century was a period of massive and revolutionary improvement in medical research and education. Physicians trained in Germany actively supported this reform movement, and medical education from 1850 to 1920 was greatly influenced by German medical science. During this same period (1880–1890), the germ theory of disease appeared and revolutionalized medical thought.

An important landmark was the Flexner Report (Flexner, 1910). Commissioned by the Carnegie Foundation and published in 1910, it was an assessment of medical education. The report disclosed disgraceful conditions in all but a few medical schools. Its major thrust was to recommend that medical education (1) should be based upon the rapidly developing biomedical sciences, which necessitated the affiliation of medical schools with universities; and (2) should be related to extensive hospital clinical experience combined with laboratory work. The report concluded that many of the proprietary medical schools could no longer serve a useful purpose and should be discontinued.

The impact of the Flexner Report was far reaching. First of all, it served to institutionalize the accreditation process and to formalize the procedures for licensing the medical practitioner. During the three decades following the Flexner Report, the standardization of medical education was secured.

Next, the Report helped to enhance scientific performance, and that resulted in the transformation of medical schools into research enclaves. It also brought the plight of the medical school to the attention of the federal government. As a result, there was a massive infusion of federal funds over the years that helped to raise the average medical school income. However, such federal funding reinforced the tendency for medical schools to concentrate on research of the biology and chemistry of disease. This had its drawbacks since it geared students toward specialization, leaving only a few in general practice (Perlstadt, 1972).

There was also an expansion of biomedical research due to the increasing federal funds, which resulted in the autonomy of departments. This happened because it was the strength of the individual members and of the departments themselves that secured research grants rather than the medical school as a whole. As a result, medical schools began to resemble a loose federation of independent departments, where each turned inward and concentrated upon its own specialized field (Sheps & Seipp, 1972).

The Flexner Report had a third major impact in that it affected the recruitment procedure and eventually only those with high MCAT (Medical College Admission Test) science scores were admitted to medical schools. Supported by the rationale of quality control, this restrictive policy reduced the number of medical students. This tendency was reinforced by the effect of the depression years when many physicians were not fully employed. The influence of the concern for jobs and income generated during this period persisted, especially on the part of organized medicine. It was not until 1967 that the Board of Trustees of the American Medical Association oficially adopted a public position that advocated the expansion of medical schools (Sheps & Seipp, 1972).

Whether it was through the direct or indirect influence of the Flexner Report, the medical elite became firmly established. The admission criteria of GPA (grade point average) and MCAT scores tended to be biased against racial minority and lower class students who had not been formally trained in white middle class schools. Moreover, the anticipation of a lengthy medical education discouraged economically handicapped students from entering the medical profession. Consequently, the medical profession became a closed system consisting of white middle class or upper middle class males.

Furthermore, in order to ensure that the door of the medical profession would remain closed except for a select few, organized medicine played an active part in political power contests against various other interest groups. This subject will be elaborated upon in the next section.

During the latter half of the 1960s, however, medical schools were exposed to the voice of the minorities through civil rights movements. Although only a minority of students were activists, they were able to work through various student organizations, and with that power, they fought for the provision of health services to the underprivileged. The social concern they manifested had an important effect on policy making in many medical schools. They brought to the surface the need for a reassessment of the relevance of medical education. They discovered that there was a fundamental alienation between the medical establishment and the society that it was supposed to serve. The intrusion of these outside forces made medical schools sensitive to the limitations of the "self-contained approach," which had been adopted since the Flexner Report.

New directions for medical education have been discussed both inside and outside medical schools during the past decade, and some new policies have already been adopted.

The crux of all phases of the reorganization of medical education is the democratization of opportunities to receive medical care and to join the medical profession. First of all, there has been an increase in the number of medical schools. During the 1960s, there was a very substantial impetus toward the creation of additional facilities as well as support for medical students. A variety of scholarships and loan funds were made available to equalize the opportunities for everyone. In 1969–1970, 58 percent of all medical students received loans to defray part of their expenses (Sheps & Seipp, 1972), compared with 11 percent in 1957–1958. While 41 percent of all medical students in 1969–1970 were awarded scholarships, only 10 percent had scholarships in 1957–1958.

The sex, racial, and ethnic barriers to entry into the medical profession have been relaxed in recent years. Active recruitment of minority members has been conducted at the high school level. The traditional admission criteria of MCAT and GPA scores are being seriously re-evaluated (Burke, 1977; Fredericks & Mundy, 1976; Rhoads et al., 1974). Furthermore, the image of the medical school as a lengthy process without financial reward is being changed. By 1970, some medical schools had started or were ready to initiate programs to reduce the calendar years needed for the completion of the M.D. (Barbee & Dinham, 1977).

Second, a change in curriculum has been urged to shift the focus from biomedical research in the laboratory to people in the community. More humanizing educational experiences are advocated in which problems are discussed in social and ethical terms as well as in biological terms. For instance, throughout the first four years of the program at Brown University, students attend bimonthly evening seminars with university faculty to discuss topics of broad interest such as religion, drama, astronomy, medical ethics, and socioeconomic problems (Hamolsky, 1972). In 1969 a project was initiated by the American Sociological Association to review behavioral science programs in nine major medical schools. It was found that anthropology, psychology, and sociology were becoming integral parts of their educational curricula (Wexler, 1976).

In addition, onto the traditional three-legged model of teaching, research, and patient care, a fourth leg—community service—has been attached (Sheps et al., 1965). It has been recommended that medical schools make their experience and skills readily available to the communities where they function. Throughout the nation there is a growing network of medical school–community hospital affiliations (Somers, 1972a).

If all these proposed changes in medical schools are carried out completely, their impact upon the medical profession will be as great as that of the Flexner Report. The future medical profession will extend its (1) membership from the white elite to minorities, (2) service from the hospital laboratory to the community, and (3) concern from disease to the human aspects of patients.

However, change has been slow. Few if any schools in Lippard's survey (1972) have been willing to declare that henceforth they will be devoted to turning out family physicians or that their major research effort will be in community needs for health care. Also, few physicians desire to work in poverty programs on a full-time basis (Fredericks, Mundy, & Kosa, 1974).

Further, there are many indications of resistance to such changes in the medical profession, among white male students, and even among racial minority physicians. For instance, the School of Medicine at the University of California, Davis, with its special admission program assigning a quota for minority students, is reported to have had little impact thus far on minority health care in its community. There is a tendency for minority doctors to enter the white mainstream of medicine instead of returning to the minority community (Mendel, 1978).

It has taken decades to build the medical profession; that empire is not likely to be dissolved overnight. There is also much speculation that the liberalism of the 1960s is only temporary. It is still too early to tell what type of practice most doctors under the new curriculum will enter.

The Sociology of Medical Education

Along with the consolidation of medical education and medical professionalization, sociologists' attention began to be directed toward medical schools, though interest in the attitudes of medical students was not new. An entire body of psychological measurements had been collected on such students, particularly with respect to their occupational interests. For the most part, however, the emphasis of such research during the early nineteenth century was on the individual characteristics, aptitudes, and intellectual characteristics because at that time the school as a research object was conceived of as being secondary to the student (Bloom, 1965).

At about the end of World War II, sociologists were brought into the medical picture for the first time, and they undertook the task of analyzing the medical school as an environmental setting for learning. During the 1950s many systematic research projects were initiated at various medical schools. These activities by behavioral scientists centered around the process of socialization of the physician's role: (1) From where and how are the students recruited into the system? (2) Through what social processes do students come to acquire professional values? (3) What are the contents of these values?

Medical School Recruitment

According to the functionalist theory of stratification (Davis & Moore, 1945), only a limited number of people are intellectually capable, psychologically equipped, and sufficiently persistent to pursue a highly skilled occupation, especially where almost endlessly dedicated study is required. As if to validate this assumption, the medical school had traditionally adopted the MCAT and GPA scores as major criteria for admission. These standards had the effect of screening out applicants from lower social classes, racial minorities, and females (Waldman, 1977). The prevailing social attitudes until the mid-twentieth century were that blacks and females were intellectually inferior to white males, and thus were not suitable for the medical profession.

Minority Enrollment. While blacks constituted 11.1 percent of the slightly more than 200 million Americans, they made up 2.8 percent of the medical student body enrolled in 1969–1970, and they represented only 2 percent of all active physicians (in the fields of medicine and osteopathy) in 1970. From the 1968–1969 school year to that of 1969–1970, there was about a one-third increase in the number of black medical students (from 782 to 1042). By 1977–1978, the proportion of black students rose to 6.0 percent of total enrollment ("Medical education . . . ," 1978). It should be noted, however, that as recently as 1955–1956, 32 of the 82 medical schools were still exclusively white (Curtis, 1971; Reitzes, 1958). Therefore, by 1970 more than half of the black students entered predominantly white schools for the first time (Gordon & Dubé, 1976; U.S. DHEW, 1975).

Due to the myth of intellectual superiority of whites, separate medical schools were built for the blacks after the Civil War in response to the need to provide health services to emancipated blacks. During the latter part of the nineteenth century, the new black physicians applied for membership in the American Medical Association. Their rejection was quick and final, and so they formed an all-black medical society. The AMA justified its rejection, stating that the quality of the black medical school was so inferior that even the graduates of Howard and Meharry universities, which were the two major black-only schools, would not be admitted as students to the average white medical school by conventional measures such as MCAT (Reitzes, 1958).

Along with the racial minorities, women have also fared poorly throughout history in their pursuit of a medical education. The first American medical school was also the one to initiate the tradition of barring women from a medical degree (Lopate, 1968). That sexist attitude worsened when, around the second decade of the nineteenth century, women also began to be further separated from the labor force due to industrialization. However, that era also produced some wealthy benefactors, and women's medical colleges were opened. Toward the end of the nineteenth century, some medical schools reluctantly became coeducational, and in 1915, women were finally admitted to the American Medical Association. At the same time, however, a small and enterprising group established the women's association (American Medical Women's Association).

Percentages of women in the total medical student enrollment have increased from 4.4 percent in 1929–1930 to 9.0 percent in 1969–1970, and to 18.0 percent in 1974–1975, and as high as 23.4 percent by 1977–1978 ("Medical Education . . . ," 1978). The number of female applicants as well as the number of enrollments has slowly but steadily increased. In particular, the past five years have seen a remarkable leap. The acceptance rate for women applicants is 40 percent, similar to that for men (39.2 percent). A recent study by Weinberg and Rodney (1973) showed that although the performance of women in their first year or two of medical school was slightly but consistently lower, their overall academic performance was equal to that of the men by their senior year.

The significant rise in minority enrollment in the 1970s can be interpreted more accurately as the result of power conflicts rather than by a sudden change in the intellect of the minorities. During the 1960s, racial and sexual minority groups gained power by means of militant tactics. They used that power to demand equality of opportunity and a change in admission criteria. As a result, an affirmative action program was adopted that favored certain minority students but kept many qualified members of other minorities as well as white male applicants out of medical school.

Affirmative action produced many dissatisfied white male applicants, who charged that the program constituted reverse discrimination. The most dramatic case is the recent Supreme Court suit of Bakke versus the Regents of the University of California. Having been rejected for admission, Allan Bakke, a white male, sued the University of California medical school at Davis. The school had reserved 16 of its 100 seats for blacks, Chicanos, and Asian Americans. The basic issue was whether the 1964 Civil Rights Law prohibiting racial discrimination applied to the white majority when it is discriminated against as a result of affirmative action programs.

The Supreme Court opened the doors of the UC Davis Medical School to Allan Bakke but said that other whites still can be excluded from the nation's colleges under the admission policies designed to give an advantage to minorities. Over all, the Supreme Court took a middle-of-the-road position, neither excluding race as a consideration nor making race the only criterion in the admission procedure ("Bakke case . . . ," 1978; "In wake of Bakke case . . . ," 1978).

Career Decision. Traditionally, there has been a great deal of occupational inheritance in the medical profession. Many students, as noted by Becker and others (1972) and more recently by Baird (1975), tend to be recruited from the higher socioeconomic groups. More than half of all medical students are from professional, proprietary, or managerial family backgrounds, although a significant proportion of contemporary students do report financial problems (Coombs, 1978; Fredericks & Mundy, 1976).

Furthermore, many medical students come from doctor's families (Bourgeois, 1975; Coombs, 1978; Hall, 1948). Their fathers and uncles and friends of their families are physicians, which shows the importance of family socialization. Future doctors are indoctrinated from childhood to the glories of the medical career, for example, the remarkable challenge of medical science and the opportunity to serve and help humanity. They are given encouragement, advice, and the proper guidance to steer them along the road to the profession without wasting time.

A possible outcome of this family socialization is that a substantial portion of the medical students make their career decision at a very young age (Bourgeois, 1975; Coombs, 1978; Thielens, 1957). According to the classic study of Rogoff (1957), slightly over one-half of the entering students first considered a medical career before the age of 14 or 15. As a whole, Rogoff indicated that 74 percent of those students whose fathers or other relatives were physicians but only 40 percent of other students first thought of a medical career at an early age. In particular, when the move up to the status of a physician also meant a considerable leap up the social ladder from a lower economic class, the presence of an uncle or cousin who was a physician had a significant effect on arousing an early interest in medicine. An early career choice seems to be more typical in medicine than in other professions such as jurisprudence (Thielens, 1957).

Of course, an early interest was not necessarily followed by an immediate commitment to a medical career. Actually, few students in Rogoff's study made their decision to pursue a medical career much before they reached college age. Those who began to consider the medical profession at a younger age, but did not make the final decision at that time, obviously had a long period for contemplation. For example, if they were sons of doctors, they may have struggled to develop their own identity before making their decision.

It appears that the more contact one has with physicians in and near the family, the earlier appears the interest in medicine; a great deal of thought has been given to the career decision by the time of college entrance. That lead time appears to be of crucial importance in medical training, which is a long, cumulative process. Latecomers may be at a great disadvantage in competing with the early joiners, who have steadily begun working toward the goal by studying appropriate subjects such as biology and chemistry (Sheps & Seipp, 1972). It should be noted, however, that there are recent studies (Fredericks & Mundy, 1976; Gough & Hall, 1977) which indicate that those from medical families and/or upper social classes are not significantly different from their classmates on premedical scholastic achievement, MCAT scores, or academic and clinical performances in medical schools.

The importance of family socialization toward the medical career has been pronounced among women. During the nineteenth century, women who went to medical schools were of middle class or upper middle class background, and they frequently had fathers or husbands already in that field. Many women studied for a medical degree so that they could become partners with their fathers or husbands. Even now, parental support is an important motive for women to enter medical school. In Cartwright's studies (1971, 1972a,b), over one-half of the female medical students reported parental approval of educational achievement as the most important incentive for their career decision. Thus, female students are recruited from the upper crust of our society, and they have parents who are professionally oriented. However, this does not necessarily support the hypothesis that women come from more affluent family backgrounds than men (Gordon & Johnson, 1977).

In contrast, black students are likely to have no role model at home. Many of them come from families of skilled or unskilled working-class background. As compared with successful, achievement-oriented professional fathers of white students, black students have witnessed their fathers suffering from financial instability (Curtis, 1971).

At the age of 14, it is unlikely that many lower class black children can seriously think about a medical career. They are seldom exposed to physicians in the family, and they are usually expected to go to work as soon as possible. A medical education is not only expensive, but it also takes a long time without any remuneration. Furthermore, lower class black students are not likely to pass the admission tests, which are based on white middle class cultural standards.

Career Motivation. Many classical studies on white male students (Becker et al., 1961; Bloom, 1973) have reported idealistic reasons for entering a medical career, such as intrinsic medical interest and the ability to help patients. Wage and hours were seldom considered. This is in conformity with the dominant social values, which assign to the role of a healer technical competence and altruism.

However, when asked to estimate their average income and social prestige, medical students indicate that they are certainly cognizant of the privileged status of the medical profession (Leerman, 1978; Thielens, 1957). In more recent studies, particularly among students from lower class backgrounds, success values, such as social prestige and economic opportunity, are acknowledged as reasons for going into medicine (Colombotos, 1969b). For racial minority groups, the status of the physician serves as the admission ticket into the upper social class (Curtis, 1971).

For female medical students, economic motive is rarely seen, since most of them come from financially secure backgrounds (Johnson & Hutchings, 1966; Stafford, 1966). A woman's entrance into the medical profession is seldom a rise in socioeconomic status because many of them would have been able to marry into their parents' social class group. For women, the central motivation is described as the desire for personal independence, an individual identity, self-discovery, self-expression, and the like (Cartwright, 1972a,b). Comparing male and female medical students, McGrath and Zimet (1977) found that females rated themselves higher than males on self-confidence, autonomy, and aggression.

Selection of Medical Specialty. Again, most studies about career selection have been concerned with white male students.

According to these studies, some students know their specialization upon their entrance into medical school, others may intend to go into general medicine and then change their minds, while a sizable number enter school undecided. For the undecided group of students, the medical school education seems to have an affect on their choice of specialization (Becker et al., 1961; Glaser, 1959; Hammond et al., 1959; Kandel, 1960; Kendall & Selvin, 1957). Although the medical school itself does not seem to produce a firm choice of specialty, it does offer a stable criteria for choosing one (Becker et al., 1961), and it provides an opportunity for medical specialists to recruit students (Bucher & Strauss, 1961). Through the early years of a medical education, students come to realize that the body of knowledge required to perform general practice is too extensive to be mastered in a short time (Kendall & Selvin, 1957; Magraw, 1975; Miller, 1970).

More positive reasons for choosing specialization over general practice are reported in earlier studies (Beale & Kriesberg, 1959; Calahan et al., 1957), such as (1) intellectual challenge, (2) attractiveness of the subject matter, (3) certainty of benefits to patients, (4) comprehensiveness of the specialty, and (5) preference for the type of patients associated with that specialty. The least-often mentioned reasons for choosing a specialty are shorter hours and higher fees.

Awareness of the higher status and social attractiveness in a specialty has begun to appear more frequently in recent studies. For instance, Fishman and Zimel (1972) report that surgery is seen as having the highest status, although the lowest social attractiveness, and that general practice is seen as the opposite of surgery.

Since World War II, the general trend in the field of medicine has been toward specialization. In 1945, 80 percent of all physicians reported themselves to be general practitioners, as compared to only 20 percent in 1967 and 18.6 percent in 1972. A more recent tendency is for the internists and pediatricians to practice general medicine (Martin, 1972).

Many students oscillate in their career choice (Rogoff, 1957) and are affected by such factors as background, economic status, ability, personality, and experiential factors (Otis et al., 1975). Mitchell (1975) developed a conceptual model for career decisions, describing the process in which students seek an optimum match between the career alternatives open to them and their own preferences and life circumstances.

When minority students seek an optimum balance, they are likely to find only a limited number of alternatives available to them. Similarly, students from the lower socioeconomic or rural backgrounds that have financial difficulties tend to prefer general practice because they feel that specialization takes more time and expense (Gray, L., 1977).

Female students tend to select medical fields where sex and professional roles are relatively compatible (Davidson, 1977; Kosa & Coker, 1965; Quadagno, 1976). They try to reduce conflict centering around the entrepreneurial role and to avoid free competition with men. They are apt to choose the fields that are traditionally considered as female specialities, such as pediatrics, gynecology, public health, and psychiatry (McGrath & Zimat, 1977; U.S. DHEW, 1975).

In sum, the functionalist assumption that people who go into the medical profession are limited to a few with special intellectual ability has never been validated even among white male students. Yet, this assumption has been endorsed by the public view that medicine is an elitist profession. The membership of the profession has been limited until recently to the select few, underrepresented by racial, sexual, economic, and other minorities. Medicine basically has been a conservative profession in both philosophical and political senses.

Socialization at Medical School

Medical school generally ("Medical education . . . ," 1978) begins with two years of basic sciences, including anatomy, physiology, biochemistry, pharmacology, microbiology, pathology, and behavioral sciences. During this period there is hardly any clinical experience except a course dealing with physical examinations and some practice in making diagnoses. This preclinical education is completed by successfully passing an examination administered by the National Board of Medical Examiners.

The second two years are devoted to clinical training, wherein students are rotated among the various medical and surgical specialty departments. During these years students work under the supervision of interns, residents, and medical school faculty. Upon passing the second section of the National Board Examination, normally at the end of the clinical years, students are graduated with the M.D. degree.

From the societal perspective, a medical school is an organizational enterprise to replenish the supply of physicians. It functions as the basic institution for initiating and conveying the body of shared and transmitted knowledge, skills, ideas, values, and standards to its future graduates.

In addition to teaching new skills and values, the medical school as a socialization agency can control the behavior of students by setting the standards they will be expected to follow as members of the profession.

Furthermore, the medical school serves to keep the profession a closed system by protecting it from outsiders. Admission and graduation are controlled by the medical school so that only those who have gone through its process of socialization, the "rite of passage," can join the profession.

Structurally, as a complex organization, the medical school engages staff members to perform various functions besides teaching, such as patient care and research. While it is possible to carry out research and patient care without teaching, medical instruction cannot be performed properly without research and patient care. Therefore, the whole process requires a great deal of administration, and each member of the medical staff may participate in all of these functions (Becker et al., 1961; Coombs, 1978).

Specifically, clinical faculty members are not only practicing physicians, but also they teach and supervise the work of resident physicians and interns, they have administrative responsibilities for their wards, and they must teach the medical students as well. This means that the undergraduate students are at the bottom of the totem pole and are outranked in experience, responsibility, and access to the faculty by a hierarchy of other learners. They have a further handicap—they are the only ones without the legal authority to practice medicine. Thus, medical socialization has been viewed as an extension of childhood socialization by Olmstead and Pacet (1969) because both medical and childhood socialization processes emphasize normative control of behaviors, give power to the socializers, and place the socializees in a dependent status.

Given this formal structure of the medical school, the socialization process will be examined from functional, conflict, and interaction perspectives.

Functional Perspective. The functionalist assumption of system integration by means of socialization is implied in the work of Columbia University researchers such as Robert K. Merton (1957).

They view the status of medical students as that of "student-physician" or physician-in-training. The basic premise is that students and faculty members share common values and goals. The student body is perceived as a "little society" within the larger system, and its function is to facilitate the overall socialization process, which is the goal of the system.

This little society is a tightly regulated student group, and it exerts a significant force to help mold the attitudes of doctors-in-training by (1) serving as the communication network between school and the individual students, (2) clarifying the standards and messages transmitted from the higher ranks, and above all, by (3) controlling student behavior based on norms mutually held by students and the faculty.

Some of the values, norms, and attitudes learned by students in the mid-1950s are designated by the Columbia University researchers as the increased preference for specialization, self-identification as doctors, and skill at maintaining objectivity and coping with uncertainty as they advance in medical training.

Conflict Perspective. In contrast to the Columbia group, the Chicago school, with researchers such as Howard S. Becker, sees conflicts of interest rather than commonly shared goals between the superordinate and subordinate groups. For instance,

> There is a significant disparity between the assumptions students and faculty make about the place of the four years of undergraduate training in a medical career. The faculty think it only the beginning of a lifetime of training, but the students think it is, at least, the end of one important phase of their training. These varying assumptions underlie some of the more specific disagreements between faculty and students, the existence of which indicates clearly that students do exercise some autonomy in setting the direction of their academic effort (Becker et al., 1961, p. 344).

As the title of Becker's book, *Boys in White,* indicates, a student is a "boy" who is required to prove himself worthy. Students are in a deliberately contained subordinate position, and they are separated from the faculty by a high social barrier. The generalized feeling of subordination coloring students' view of their relations with faculty is expressed in Becker's field notes as follows:

> A faculty member had done something the students resented very much, something that emphasized his power over them. I sat and listened to a discussion of what they could do about this. One of the students said, "One thing you have to understand is that most of us here will put up with just about anything if we really have to in order to get through. We've spent too much time getting this far to start being crusaders about something like that" (Becker et al., 1961, p. 281).

In order to cope with this subordinate status and provide themselves with a measure of autonomy from authoritative demands, students develop group cohesion in a "secret society." Unlike the little society described above, this secret society has its own values and goals, which contradict those enforced by the faculty. As members of this secret society, the students "play it cool" by presenting cooperative acquiescence to the faculty, while in their secret world they are highly critical of institutional goals.

The sources of conflict that create this covert culture are identified in the structure of the medical school as well as in the contents of the medical education (Becker et al., 1961). A student's subordinate position in the hierarchy is accentuated by the open forum for learning. Faculty members quiz the students in public on diagnosis and prognosis, and a student may be humiliated before fellow students. A staff physician may ask any question derived from long clinical experience, far beyond what is in the textbook. The student may resent the faculty member as being capricious, yet feels the necessity of making a good impression on the instructor.

As a subordinate group, the students support each other against their common antagonist by becoming "test-wise" and by exchanging information concerning how much and what kind of studying is appropriate. This development of study norms is the result of the first-year students' perception of heavy work loads and their desperation to try to master everything (Coombs, 1978).

Apart from these structural conflicts, there tend to be basic value disparities between students and the faculty (Bloom, 1973; Coombs, 1978). The goal of medical education is to integrate effectively the roles of "healer" and "scientist" in the future physician. Yet, each group, the faculty and student, stresses one role and sees the other as an obstacle. While the faculty emphasizes the academic values of gaining knowledge for its own sake and of fostering basic competence, students are anxious to have practical healing experience. Students fail to see a role model in the faculty and view them as uninterested in the human and service aspects of medicine. The faculty, on the other hand, regard students as mediocre, antiacademic, and too pragmatic.

However, among medical students in the 1950s, (Bloom, 1973) or even in the late 1960s (Coombs, 1978), an open rebellion was rarely observed. Instead, conflict manifested itself in a defensive type of withdrawal behavior on both sides. For example, passive hostility was exhibited by the students, while the faculty members adhered to their narrow definition of competence.

Neither Functional nor Conflict Views. Rather than debating which interpretation, functional or conflict, is more valid for the typical process of socialization at a medical school, Bloom noted that the sources of variation could be attributed to the types of school (Bloom, 1965), the faculty, and the students (Bloom, 1973).

First of all, the school studied by the Columbia group is a private, Ivy League type in which the students are able to obtain more personalized instruction, while the educational setting observed by the Chicago team is a large public school.

Second, a certain number of students with dissenting ideas can set the tone for the whole medical school. In the 1950s, their influence seems to have been limited to their own school, but later, in the 1960s, collective effort grew strong enough to affect the whole structure of medical education.

Third, the faculty's attitudes toward students tend to be divided. While the basic science faculty may view students as inferior, the voluntary and part-time clinical faculty seem to be divided into authoritarian and equalitarian orientations (Coombs, 1978).

There are other studies that have shown the student–faculty relationship as being neither integrative nor divisive. For example, Bloom (1973) found an amorphous and unstable situation where a clear and definable character of student culture was absent. Others (Coombs, 1978; Huntington, 1957; Nathanson, 1975) observed a gradual increase in the professional image and identity of the future doctors as the students progressed through school.

Interactionism. Instead of a one-way process toward integration or dissension, Shuval (1975) viewed professional socialization as a two-directional process in which the students are constantly pushed forward into the professional role as well as backward into the "boy's" role. Socializers include not only physicians, but nurses, patients, and above all, peers. Medical socialization is a process of adapting to a "looking-glass self" by playing the role of others and by responding to the expectations of those of significance.

Miller (1970) considered the social structure of medical school as a network of relationships made up of social exchanges. By a social exchange, Miller meant that the recipient of something valuable incurs an obligation to reciprocate to the benefactor with something of equal value. For instance, interns begin their year with little idea of what is expected of them. Hence, the interns accept subordination to the residents because the former has to depend on the latter's experience and expertise. Interns do not have direct access to the physician and must learn the "ropes" first. This is a prerequisite for negotiations to obtain the expert opinion of residents. Students, interns and residents define the situation, set goals for themselves, and negotiate for privileges.

The interactionist approach to medical school is not limited to the above researchers. As a matter of fact, Becker's *Boys in White* is guided by a variant of symbolic interaction theory. Becker stressed manipulative aspects of human behavior, and he viewed them as processes in which the individuals shape and control their conduct by taking into account the expectations of others with whom they interact.

The analogy of game-playing is well illustrated in Becker's description of the process by which first-year students get information on what and how to study. After the initial shock of the study load, first-year students come to realize that they cannot possibly master everything. The crucial issue becomes ascertaining what the faculty expects them to learn, that is, what will be tested for. However, individual students do not make a direct approach to the faculty since they belong to a student team in opposition to the faculty team.

> In many instances, the stars of the student team (those who get the most information) are fraternity men. With their greater social ease, they do not hesitate to argue in class with a professor or complain to him about examination questions, and the class learns more about an instructor's perspective on his subject (Becker et al., 1961, p. 180).

Becker's symbolic interactionism has been criticized (Levinson, 1967) for disregarding the relevance of psychodynamic factors in socialization and for focusing only upon unified, conscious, and widely-held perspectives. Levinson compared different observations about medical students' first experiences with dissection and autopsy. For instance, Fox (1957) reported that students were emotionally moved and troubled by the experience. In trying to find a balance of detachment and concern, they had to go through various forms of ego defense (e.g., dreams) to cope with fantasies and anxieties evoked by the experience. In contrast, Becker viewed the dissecting and autopsy experience as having a simple, rational significance upon students. After a brief initial disturbance, he assumed that students sweep aside those inappropriate feelings and fantasies as nonprofessional and barriers to their pursuit of technical competence. For Becker, feelings and other nonrational processes are incidental, and an effective adaptation is made by rational beliefs and actions.

Minority Students. As discussed above, students learn as much from other students as from their classroom lectures or from the physician-teachers. The student culture interprets the messages coming from the upper echelons. It protects them from the common enemy, and it provides them with information as to how to negotiate for power and knowledge. Furthermore, to be a medical student is not merely to study and to be taught. One also has to participate in the myriad ways of the life of an intricately formed world that has clinical, residential, recreational, and familial facets (Coombs, 1978).

If this is the social climate of a medical school, what happens to a student who is not integrated into the student group, be it a little society or secret society?

For women and minority students, unless they have extremely outgoing personalities, the years at medical school can be long and lonesome. They have few members of their own groups as classmates, and they are excluded from the dominant student culture.

In relation to the faculty members, research findings indicate that minority students in the traditional medical school feel that their performance is being singled out. The faculty expectations of them are higher than for others. Their errors are more easily noticed and remembered, and every failure is attributed to their minority status (Lopate, 1968).

Among the students, there are both overt and subtle discriminations. Some white male students openly and intentionally try to annoy or anger minority members by belittling them or showing hostility. Covertly, the culture of medical schools is similar to a fraternity or a man's club where women and minorities are stereotyped or excluded (Bourne & Wikler, 1978; Campbell, 1973).

Structurally, minority students have been on the lowest rung of the ladder and are alienated from the informal social networks of the medical school. They not only suffer psychological discomforts, but they are at a disadvantage in learning medical skills.

Contents of Socialization. Through the processes of conflict, negotiation, and concession, as well as positive identification with the physician-teacher, medical students are expected to learn medical skills and medical values.

Medical skills range from taking blood pressure to performing a dissection and autopsy. For beginning students, even touching the body of another person for a physical examination can be quite traumatic (Coombs, 1978). In most of the sociological literature, this aspect of socialization is assumed to be adequately carried out. However, there are some (Morehead, Donaldson, & Burt, 1964; Rhee, 1977; Ross & Duff, 1978) who noted that there is only a slight correlation between performance at medical school and the quality of practice in later years. The conditions under which one practices are frequently more important than the totality of knowledge that one acquires at school. Also, due to rapid technological advances, the information one learns in school may have little relevance to the situation in later years.

Regarding the socialization of medical values, there is greater doubt as to whether or not the medical school is successful in attaining that goal. The professional value placed on the interaction with patients and the welfare of the patient as a whole human being is not well inculcated at school (Adler & Shuval, 1978; Peterson et al., 1956). The students' awareness of the bureaucratic basis for contemporary medical practice is revealed by their attaching greater importance to the status component (i.e., place in the organization) than to human relations or scientific areas (i.e., research, knowledge) of the occupational role (Adler & Shuval, 1978).

Among the important social values transmitted at medical school are a tolerance for uncertainty and a detached concern (Fox, 1957). From the stereotypical belief in the infallibility of medical technique, the students come to learn to cope with uncertainty, the inability of medical science to cure all diseases, and their own inadequacy to master all the techniques.

Through clinical experience (Miller, 1970), the students learn to keep an emotional distance from patients and to take a universalistic rather than a particularistic attitude. For instance, despite a large portion of curriculum time devoted to the anatomy laboratory, Coombs (1978) noted that not a single hour is set aside to discuss the emotional impact of the cadaver dissection upon the students. This omission produces future doctors who are inclined to suppress the emotional aspect of patient care. This detachment has been viewed as cynicism by some (Christie & Merton, 1958; Eron, 1955). They consider that students have grown less idealistic and have lost interest in patients as persons but instead see them as an embodiment of disease entities. As compared with others, such as college students, business executives, and lobbyists, medical students seem to be more callous in the face of death and suffering.

Becker and others (1961) look at the issue of cynicism versus idealism from a different perspective. They claim that the students' conception of the doctor's role becomes more specific and less stereotyped as they advance in school. Such realistic and detached concern cultivated during school years will have positive implications for later practice such as in helping patients achieve a "good death." They also refer to the fact that students are not in a position to do very much in the face of suffering and death. They are constantly being tested by the faculty, who ignore the humanitarian aspect of medicine. As a result, they become realistic about the situation, and they try to learn only specific techniques while at school with the hope that they can put their idealism into effect later (Fox, 1957; Reinhardt & Gray, 1972). To support this interpretation, Gray and others (1965) found that when students graduate from school, relieved from social constraints on idealism, their cynicism tends to give way to a more informed idealism.

It should be also noted that some researchers (Juan et al., 1974) found no change in social values taking place during medical school years.

Overview

As we have seen, medical education has come a long way. From the one-to-one apprenticeship system and from proprietary schools "dragging illiterates off the streets," medical education has undergone a revolutionary change. The Flexner Report of 1910 was the turning point of that change toward professionalization. The quality of medical schools was standardized, and the medical profession was consolidated as a self-contained, closed system. The goal of the medical school was defined as the development of technical competence in students to cure disease by means of basic biomedical research. The functionalist assumption was supported by the public, who felt whatever this medical elite did was best for the rest of society because they knew all the answers to the questions of illness.

After about half a century of peace and complaiscence, the medical school and medical profession as a whole have come under severe attack by outside forces. During the 1960s the elitism and intellectualism of the profession were criticized to such an extent that the professional system could no longer remain self-contained. Sixty years after the publication of the Flexner Report, the Carnegie Foundation for the Advancement of Teaching, the same body that supported the Flexner study, established a commission to re-evaluate the whole medical educational system (Carnegie Commission, 1970). The major thrust of this report lay in relaxing the boundary between the medical profession and the rest of society. Nevertheless, there are signs to indicate that the liberalism of the 1960s might have been a temporary phenomenon which had little impact on the institutionalized process of medical education (Coombs, 1978). Some studies in the 1970s (Coe, Pepper, & Mattis, 1977; Goldman & Ebbert, 1973) have revealed increasing conservatism among entering students and graduating seniors as well as among physicians. However, other observers claim that medical students have become more open-minded, egalitarian, and idealistic in the 1970s than they were in the 1960s (Fox, 1974a; Rezler, 1974). In short, there is evidence of change in medical education but the magnitude of the change is difficult to measure.

ORGANIZED MEDICINE

In addition to the important function played by medical education, a parallel role played by organized medicine has been crucial in establishing and maintaining the status and power of the medical profession in this country. The American Medical Association (AMA) has served as the gatekeeper of the profession, preventing harmful external forces from reaching its members.

From the functionalist perspective, the AMA can be viewed as a social system that is enclosed by (1) another larger system consisting of all holders of the M.D. degree, (2) a still larger system of health practitioners in general, and finally, (3) the total society as a system. The positions and functions of the AMA can be examined in terms of these larger systems as well as of the component members of the association. From this perspective, the authority vested in the AMA to set standards of quality for medical practice will be accepted as a socially desirable function of the professional organization.

On the other hand, the activities of the AMA may be interpreted as the process of conflict resolution among various interest groups. The AMA must deal with internal conflict among its members, while coping with outside pressures coming from the non-AMA physicians, other healing practitioners, and nonmedical social institutions and groups. Naturally, the professional organization is concerned with protecting and advancing the socioeconomic interests of its members. Thus, the AMA's restriction on the number of graduates of medical schools, and hence on the number of physicians, is a powerful tactic for preserving physician's elitist position.

Development of the AMA

Prior to 1932. In 1847, some 250 physicians, representing medical societies and schools in 22 states, met in Philadelphia to found a national society, the American Medical Association (AMA). Its objective, stated with a functionalist tenor was that of "promoting the science and art of medicine, and the establishment of public health," that is, the advancement of the central goals of society (Welch, 1964). Its efforts were directed toward raising and maintaining the standards of medical practice in order to gain the confidence of the public. The first elected president of the AMA said in his opening speech that "the medical profession had become corrupt and degenerate to the forfeiture of its social position" (Means, 1961), and he espoused the cause of "cleaning of one's own house."

From the viewpoint of conflict theorists, the AMA was merely trying to gain control over the practice of medicine by eliminating its competitors, the unlicensed and untrained healing practitioners. This was accomplished by obtaining favorable legislation from respective state governments to curb unlicensed practitioners.

During the early days, the AMA was not a well-integrated system, and it had to contend with the resistence of various states that were against uniform standards and any kind of interference by governmental bodies. The spirit of equalitarianism and free enterprise was behind their argument, "If all religious sects are to be tolerated, why not all medical sects as well?" (Shryock, 1947, p. 262). The consequence of this internal conflict was a further decline in the status of physicians and the concomitant rise of quackery.

It was not until the development of the germ theory toward the end of the nineteenth century that the AMA began to consolidate its position. A survey of medical education initiated by the AMA in 1901 marked the beginning of a successful 30-year campaign to raise medical school standards. The AMA was instrumental in bringing about the Flexner Report (1910) and in implementing its recommendations. The necessary pronounced improvement in educational quality resulted in a sharp reduction in the number of medical schools and students. This substantial restriction on the supply of physicians was an unintended by-product of the positive function played by the AMA to ameliorate the deplorable conditions of medical training that had existed up to the turn of the century (Rayack, 1967).

After the Depression Years. During the 1930s, the AMA altered its target from amelioration to restrictionism. The depression hit the physicians hard, and between 1929 and 1932, their income fell almost 40 percent (Rayack, 1967). The AMA's desire to retain high economic status in the competitive market was disguised by the functional pretense for the need of professional "birth control." To that end, the Association persisted in its position that there was an oversupply of physicians, and it claimed that the excess practitioners would tend to introduce excessive economic competition, elevate medical costs, and cause a decline in standards.

The AMA achieved professional "birth control" by exerting pressure upon the medical schools to curtail their enrollment. This method was effective because the very existence of the medical schools depended on the AMA's approval of their academic standards. Within two years after the AMA's announcement of that policy, there was a 74 percent decline in the number of applicants to medical schools (Rayack, 1967).

During World War II, however, the necessity for the total mobilization of resources and the sharply increased demands for physicians by the armed forces caused the AMA to suspend its policy of curbing medical school admissions.

After the war, the need for medical services continued to increase, but the inadequacy of existing facilities set an upper limit to the number of students who could be enrolled. Hence, it was not necessary for the AMA to apply pressure to medical schools. Instead, the AMA focused its efforts upon opposing the provision of federal aid to medical education. Through public pronouncement that there was no shortage of physicians and by the use of political lobbying tactics (1946–1960), the AMA was able to maintain its restrictionist policy.

In short, prior to the depression years, the AMA's rôle in raising medical standards was functional to the goal of society, even though that position led to a decrease in the number of physicians. Since the depression years, however, the AMA has become more concerned with advancing its self-interests which do not always coincide with societal demands. In studying the latter period, a conflict perspective will be more fruitful than the functionalist model.

Structure and Membership of the AMA

Organizational Structure. The AMA is a national association composed of state and county societies. To be eligible for membership in the AMA, a physician must first be a member of the appropriate county medical society. Each county society sets its own qualifications for membership. In principle, all "reputable and ethical" licensed M.D.s are eligible, but ambiguity in the meaning of those terms allows arbitrariness in the admission practices of each county in dealing with extraneous factors such as race, ethnicity, or religion (Freeborn & Darsky, 1974; Lieberson, 1958).

Representatives to the state assembly are elected by a direct vote of the county society members. These delegates select the state officer, and they elect the state representatives to the national House of Delegates. The latter group elects the president and the other AMA officers, including the Board of Trustees. The Board of Trustees is charged with implementing the policies approved by the House, and in general, it manages the association when the House is not in session. The House meets twice a year to discuss and formulate policy on a wide range of topics. Members of the House are elected from the state societies on the basis of one delegate per 1,000 active AMA members in each area.

This hierarchical structure is dominated by a comparatively small group of people by virtue of the nominating procedures and indirect representation. Election to office in the state societies is controlled by the county officers because they make nominations to a committee appointed by the state officers. National officers are elected from the nominees who are approved by state officers and screened by the national organization. Thus, the Board of Trustees, the policy-making organ of the AMA, is virtually free of rank-and-file pressures, making it difficult for an organized opposition to develop.

Membership. At the end of 1847, the AMA had 426 members. One hundred years later, just after World War II, it had 132,224 members, and that roster included almost all but the black physicians in the United States. By 1963, it had grown to over 200,000 members.

Does organized medicine accurately reflect the collective will of the medical profession as the official spokesperson for medicine (Rayack, 1967)? Is the AMA truly the voice of American medicine (Burrow, 1963)? Or is it an "autocracy" that avoids open elections and hesitates to debate policy for fear of a disagreement (Markovits, 1963)? The AMA denies that it is a self-perpetuating minority and asserts that it represents over two-thirds of all of the "eligible" physicians. However, this same figure really constitutes only one-third of all the physicians in the United States, which means that fully one-third of the physicians do not even belong to the county societies (Twaddle & Hessler, 1977). Nonmembers include (1) those who have retired, who have not satisfied local residence requirements, or who have violated the AMA code of ethics; (2) those who do not need the benefits of membership (employees of the government, the armed forces, research agencies, or universities); and (3) those who are not acceptable (opponents of AMA policies, racial and ethnic minorities, or foreign doctors). It was only in 1964 that the AMA voted to be opposed to racial discrimination by local medical societies. Each year the number of black physicians in the AMA is increasing, but there still exists resistance to black membership in certain areas (Curtis, 1971).

During the controversy over Medicare legislation, the AMA lost a significant number of its members, who formed alternative organizations such as Physicians for Social Responsibility and the Medical Committee for Human Rights.

Since medical practice requires an enormous amount of time, the active members of the AMA tend to be those who have time to spare for medical politics: (1) old or semi-retired physicians, (2) specialists with well-established practices who can turn their patients over to assistants or partners, (3) physicians with exceptionally lucrative practices or an independent income, and (4) physicians who are too devoted to the cause of the AMA to worry about their own practices.

Despite the AMA's demonstrated unity against pressures, it is far from a monolithic organization. Internally it is a house divided. First, there are conflicts between private practitioners and academic or administrative physicians, between general practitioners and specialists, and among the specialists themselves. The diversity and discrepancy of specific interests of various subgroups (Smith, 1958) within the profession lead to an internal struggle, where each faction is vying for power to influence policies for the benefit of its own segment. For instance, even the general acceptance of germ theory was delayed by a long and bitter conflict among members with different theoretical approaches.

The second source of conflict is a divided loyalty to the profession and to the organization in which physicians are teamed together as employees (Ben-David, 1958). Organizational values are frequently antithetical to those of a profession. For instance, as a scientist a physician may want to request an expensive medical instrument, while as an employee of a hospital he may be encouraged to forego the expenditure for organizational cost efficiency.

The third cause of internal struggle is found in opposing political views. Conservative segments tend to include surgeons and the general or family practitioners, while the liberals are represented by such subgroups as the

American Academy of Pediatrics (Goldman, 1974). The liberals have headed the fight against elitism, sexism, and racism in the AMA.

Despite those internal conflicts, the AMA has preserved a fairly united front. Revolts against the leadership of the AMA should not be construed as indicative of general discontent with the politics of organized medicine. The solid integration of the AMA is due to (1) the autocratic structure of the organization, (2) a general apathy of the membership, (3) the policy of the *Journal of the American Medical Association* not to print dissenting opinions, and (4) the majority support that the private physicians give to AMA policy on socioeconomic issues.

The AMA as the Gatekeeper for the Profession

In order to maintain the status and power of the medical profession, the AMA formulated in the mid-1930s the following basic principles: (1) all aspects of medical care and medical practice should be controlled by the medical profession, and no third-party interference should be allowed; and (2) patients should be free to choose any qualified physician, but they should bear the cost of care, if at all possible (Lasagna, 1963; Means, 1953).

Over the years, these policies have been threatened both by internal and external influences. The AMA's maintenance tasks include its surveillance of members to prevent their deviation from professional values as well as its control over outsiders so that they do not intrude into professional territory.

Control over Physicians. Local societies used to serve as a means of ensuring professional behavior on the part of their members. That which was defined "unprofessional" included not only incompetence or deceit in medical practice but also all activities that had been disapproved of by the AMA, such as participation in certain health insurance schemes and even fraternization with "cultists" (chiropractors, osteopaths, etc.).

Social pressure exerted by the small county society took the form of informal ostracism or formal exclusion from membership. That type of control was effective because many of the essential aspects of medical practice depended upon continued collegial support, such as patient referrals and consultations. The reputation, income, and practice of many doctors were likely to be affected by their standing with the local professional society.

Such control through social pressure by local societies was good to the extent that it helped to maintain a higher quality of medical care. However, its negative effect was to inhibit the member physicians from taking innovative and autonomous actions. Membership in local county medical societies is no longer as important as it once was and so no longer exerts as much influence on physician behavior (Mechanic, 1979).

Control Over Other Health Practitioners. From its inception, the AMA has advocated the laudable social goal of licensure, understanding that, functionally, licensure protects the consumers as well as the physicians against quackery. As a result, organized medicine has maintained a fairly solid front against nonmedical health practitioners.

Since it is the custodian of the accumulated knowledge of medicine, the AMA does not limit its use of power to destroying quackery. It has shown an equal vigor in attacking health practitioners who are widely considered legitimate and useful but who represent a competitive threat to the medical profession, such as the osteopath and chiropractor. Having labeled them "cultists," which means "irregular" practitioners, the AMA has used many tactics to uproot their power—opposing their recognition through license, barring them from membership in local medical societies, or denying them the right to practice in AMA-dominated hospitals.

However, the AMA is by no means free from powerful opposition. Other highly respected and important organizations in the field of health care have clashed with the AMA on many occasions. Such organizations include the American College of Surgeons, the Association of American Medical Colleges, the American Hospital Association, and the American Public Health Association.

Control Over Society. In addition to controlling its own members and other health care practitioners, the AMA has been successful in exerting control over society for its own benefit. Basically, its power stems from three sources: consumer ignorance, medical licensure, and political lobbying.

Medical knowledge and technology has grown so complex that the physician's knowledge concerning the necessity for or consequences of treatment far surpasses the consumer's level of comprehension. Nevertheless, professional power solely based on public ignorance will be endangered if the professional knowledge is shared by too many people. As the number of physicians increases in a society, their technology ceases to be a scarce commodity. Hence, they are able to generate less power than before.

By restricting the supply of physicians through medical licensure, the AMA influences the patterns of medical care for the benefit of the medical profession. The policies of the various state boards of medical examiners are practically identical with those of the AMA because the medical society in many states recommends the appointees to the state board, nominates the candidates for the office, or lets its members actually serve on the board (Hyde et al., 1954). In granting sole authority to the boards to issue licenses, society in effect has given considerable power to the AMA. With the rationale of quality control, the AMA has exercised pressure on medical schools to curtail enrollment. Medical school are approved by the AMA's Council on Medical Education and Hospitals, and to remain on the approved list, they must meet the standards set by the council.

Finally, and most important of all, there is the political source of the AMA's power. Since politicians try to avoid tackling any organized opposition, the first step for those who want to influence politicians is to organize (Harris, 1966). In politics, the symbolic interactionist framework is applicable in the sense that the appearance of power is often as useful as its utilization as long as no one challenges it. The legend of the invincibility of the AMA appeared in the 1930s, and it was built up over the years while its existence depended on the politicians' characteristic reluctance to get involved in any test of strength.

The AMA's apparent power came to be substantiated by resolute lobbying in recent years. Because it has large financial resources, the AMA could engage in costly propaganda campaigns, extensive political activity, and vigorous lobbying (Rayack, 1967). That political power is all the more awesome in view of the fact that the AMA has been the biggest spender among the Washington lobbies. Its expenditures are far in excess of those of the rest of the lobbyists, including the powerful National Association of Manufacturers and the AFL-CIO.

Malcolm Todd, a member of the American Medical Political Committee's National Board of Directors, stated the position of the AMA clearly: "This is the only way to bring about the election of candidates who, . . . are sympathetic toward conservative government, free enterprise, and private practice in medicine. . . . We intend to be medicine's permanent political arm" (Rayack, 1967).

By keeping in constant contact with the key administrative agencies of the government, especially those that design health legislation, the AMA has combated third-party interference in the form of federal aid to medical education, health insurance plans, and socialized medicine. Professional autonomy has been the slogan.

Decline of Power. For some time, however, the "sacred trust" (Harris, 1966) in the medical profession as guarded by the AMA has been under attack by various forces both external and internal to organized medicine (Rayack, 1967).

The scientific and technological revolution in medicine, along with the rapid rise in the demand for medical services have produced structural changes in the medical marketplace. Consumers have begun to demand health service as their natural right, they have organized themselves into labor unions that in turn have shown concern for the cost and even the quality of medical care, and they have been successful in arranging health insurance to meet the cost of illness.

There have also been changes on the part of those who provide medical care. Institutional modifications include the growth of hospitals as centers of medical care, the increase in specialization in medical practice, and the appearance of a host of paramedical and other health professionals.

Above all, society is witnessing the growing role of the government at all levels in financing, providing, and regulating health services.

Collectively, these events have contributed to the lowering of the status and power of the physicians in private practice, those who are in the majority at the AMA. Using Rayack's (1967) expression, they have been "dispossessed," which implies a weakening of the AMA.

MEDICAL PRACTICE

Perhaps the most critical aspect of the medical profession is control over its own work, specifically, control over the evaluation of the technical knowledge used in the work (Friedson, 1970). In the preceding sections of this chapter, professional autonomy was examined in relation to the formal characteristics of the medical profession: (1) how formal medical training inculcates professional values in future physicians, and (2) how formal organized medicine has attempted to protect the profession.

Given the autonomy of the profession at large, how is that autonomy maintained by the individual physician in everyday work settings? Varied contexts for practice, whether viewed as social systems or processes, affect the physician's inclination to conform to professional values. Perhaps of primary importance is the amount of collegial interaction, which is influenced by the type of practice. Certainly there are different sources of control over a physician's performance, depending on whether the work setting is a solo practice or a group practice (Coleman et al., 1966).

Solo Practice

Some of the characteristics of solo practice are as follows: (1) a private enterprise—a physician works alone in an office that is equipped by his or her own capital; (2) a free market competition—a patient makes a free choice based on the quality of treatment and the price; and (3) a fee for service—a patient makes payments directly to the physician for services rendered.

Solo practice has been the prototype for medical practice in the United States. It has been cherished as a "sacred cow" by the medical profession for more than a century (Evang, 1960). Its rationale lies in the functionalist claim that only the solo practitioner who has internalized professional values can be autonomous in fulfilling societal functions.

Even when the functionalist assumption of internalization of professional values is not met, solo practice still has the romantic touch of classical capitalism with a minimum of centralized regulation and control. In such a model, conflict among solo practitioners is viewed as a healthy mechanism that will ensure high-quality performance.

However, a truly autonomous fee-for-service arrangement is inherently unstable except perhaps back in the nineteenth-century small community where there was but one physician. The balance of power among solo practitioners is a precarious one and is likely to tip toward the control of either patients or colleagues (Freidson, 1975b, 1979).

With a system of free enterprise and competition, colleagues can become rivals seeking one another's patients. In order to retain one's patients, a solo practitioner must cater to their demands. The doctors' performance is subject to the evaluation of patients who, as lay persons, utilize nonprofessional standards.

The positive aspect, on the other hand, of client control over solo practitioners is that physicians are compelled to treat patients as persons rather than as disease entities, which will improve doctor–patient communication. Yet there is a danger that physicians who are dictated to by clients may deviate from professional regimen in favor of clients' demands.

Collegial control upon solo practitioners is sometimes found in informal networks such as the fraternity type described by Hall (1946, 1948, 1949). It is a well-integrated system formed by established doctors with relatively loyal clienteles. The newcomer must start at the bottom of the hierarchy in order to be sponsored by senior members. This informal organization affects the careers of solo practitioners in many ways, such as the number of patient referrals received, the opportunity for hospital appointments, and the speed of promotions.

While Hall stressed the power of the inner fraternity upon individual physicians, Freidson (1970, 1975b) postulated a heuristic free market in which solo practitioners are free to choose the colleagues or the fraternity they associate with. Moreover, these networks tend to be independent of one another. Thus, someone who is excluded from one circle will find another circle of colleagues. Such patterns of collegial relations are likely to exist in areas that have a variety of hospitals and other hierarchically ordered medical institutions. Winick (1961) suggested that in larger cities a physician's behavior is more individualistic and diffuse, free from collegial controls.

However, unlike the practitioners of olden days who enjoyed a monopoly of patients in their respective communities, the twentieth-century solo practitioners in the United States are likely to be specialists who conduct a large part of their practice in hospitals. By definition, a specialist cannot operate alone but needs to be integrated into a collegial referral system.

The physician referral process has been investigated by Shortell (1972, 1973, 1974a; Shortell & Anderson, 1971; Shortell & Vahovich, 1975) using an exchange theory perspective. Among various costs and rewards to the interacting physicians, status was identified as an important reward factor. Enhancement or maintenance of status serves as a reward and loss of status as a cost. Also, one's status influences how one perceives all other rewards and costs associated with professional activities.

Studying private-practice internists, Shortell (1973) found that high status internists tended to refer primarily to high status physicians, while lower status internists referred more often to higher status physicians. It was interpreted that by choosing each other as referral partners, high status physicians validate their own status and the status structure of the group. In contrast, for lower status internists, referral to higher status consultants is rewarding because it enhances their professional image. At the same time it is less costly than referring to lower status practitioners, who might steal their patients.

This crossover among status groups is somewhat contrary to Freidson's (1970) early postulate that physician networks tend to be independent of one another. However, the norm of reciprocity between status groups does not apply here in that high status physicians do not send their patients to lower status colleagues.

Cooperative Practice

After World War II the modes of practice shifted from solo to cooperative patterns. Between 1946 and 1969, the number of medical groups increased by 1,576 percent together with the rise of 697 percent in the number of physicians practicing in multispecialty groups (American Medical Association, 1978; Bennet, 1976; Stevens, 1971).

Cooperative work settings can be divided into three types. First, there is the partnership, which is an arrangement whereby physicians share profits from fees as well as overhead expenses of maintaining common facilities and personnel. Second, in an association physicians have their own patients from whom they collect fees but they share expenses. Third, a group practice is a form of association that includes more than two people. It is a practice in which three or more full-time physicians are formally organized to provide comprehensive medical care through the joint utilization of equipment and personnel. These members of the group decide in advance upon the method by which the income from the joint medical practice will be distributed (Balfe & McNamara, 1968).

A group practice occasionally involves a third party who assumes responsibility for the welfare of the population. For example, various agencies such as the government, health insurance groups, or large business corporations, have organized and staffed bureaucratic group practices to serve a particular clientele or to provide for large-scale financing in the form of health insurance.

The origins of cooperative practice can be traced to the functionalist premise of efficiency that (1) a collaborating group is an integrated system; (2) each member plays a positive and complementary role in the attainment of commonly shared goals; and therefore (3) cooperative practice is more functional and efficient than solo practice.

What must be pointed out is that group members have more free time and far more flexible schedules than do solo practitioners. The former can take time off without the fear of losing their patients. Second, a pool of resources is expected to render higher technical quality, economic efficiency, and continuity. Specialists can consult and supplement one another. They can also operate on a larger scale, providing more diagnostic equipment and therapeutic facilities.

Furthermore, in cooperative practice where interaction with colleagues and their approval are necessary for work, the physician's performance is more likely to be controlled by professional standards maintained by other physicians than by the nonprofessional expectations of patients (Hoffman, 1958; Peterson et al., 1956; Payne & Lyons, 1972; Ross & Duff, 1978). From the functionalist's vantage point the third-party control in group practice is viewed as a force offsetting an imbalance between client and physician controls. The third party has the client's welfare in mind, yet that party is objective enough to use professional guidelines in order to advance the health of the population at large (Schwartz, 1968).

Examination of cooperative systems, however, have not always validated these functional arguments.

In fact, it must be pointed out, that in conformity with the conflict perspective, stress and strife are endemic in pluralistic practice. In partnerships, the division of pooled fees is a constant source of dispute, since the practices of the partners are not identical, especially among specialists. The addition of a third party into group practice only complicates the process of the power contest. A third party may act as an administrator whose goal of operational efficiency does not coincide either with professional values or with the client's needs. A detailed discussion on this subject will be deferred until Chapter 10.

Based on research findings, Graham (1972) concluded that the evidence is equivocal, that is, cooperative practice is not significantly better nor worse than solo practice on all the points listed above.

Freidson (1979), on the other hand, summarized the pros and cons of different arrangements of medical practice in relation to the quality of care, patient satisfaction, and physician satisfaction. He found that group practice has the advantage of (1) easy access to modern diagnostic and therapeutic facilities, (2) collegial consultation, (3) coordination of specialists, and (4) collegial supervision, all of which contribute to the improvement of the "science" of medicine (Mechanic, 1979).

While suffering from deficiencies on the above counts, the solo practice is likely to provide a better "art" of medicine. Compared with group practice, solo practitioners are more immediately responsive to patients' needs, showing personal interests and making themselves more accessible to patients.

Physicians' work gratification derives from various sources, such as autonomy, professional prestige, personal contact with patients, scientific accomplishment, and the like. On the whole, it is expected that the greatest satisfaction would be obtained by a doctor-owned, fee-for-service partnership or group practice, which lies between the two extremes—solo and bureaucratic arrangements.

Hospital Practice

Finally, there are physicians who have hospital staff appointments; these include specialists, medical school teachers, and doctors-in-training. Details of hospital practice will be presented in Chapter 7. Briefly, given the complexity of the division of labor in the hospital and the multiplicity of the sources of support and control, a physician in the hospital setting is under a great many pressures. Nevertheless, the dual authority system of the medical professional versus the bureaucratic administrator in hospitals has left the control of individual physicians largely up to their professional colleagues. This is primarily based on the premise that professional expertise cannot be evaluated by the lay personnel. Furthermore, a physician's status as a guest at the hospital is likely to shield him or her from administrative influence.

By virtue of collegial proximity in the work setting, hospital practice is thought to facilitate social control over physicians by making their performance more visible to peers, hence more responsive to critical evaluation. However, collegial evaluation and sanction have been more implicit than systematic or binding for individual physicians. Based on a study of a large medical group of over 50 doctors, Freidson (1975b) argues that effective peer review is extremely difficult.

To begin with, autonomy has been a cardinal tenet in the profession and is a disincentive for physicians to monitor the performance of their peers. They share the value that the individual physician should be trusted.

Second, uncertainty in medical work makes it difficult to adopt standardized rules by which to judge errors. Such ambiguity fosters the notion that certain mistakes are inevitable in medicine and hence the criteria for evaluation are permissive.

Third, much of the actual performance of physicians is not observable. With the limited opportunity to work directly with other physicians in the medical group, many physicians suspend their judgment about their colleagues, claiming that hearsay of patients and physicians is unreliable.

It may be anticipated that hospital settings are more conducive to the exercise of control than ambulatory settings such as the group-practice clinic of Freidson's study. Several investigators (Flood & Scott, 1978; Neuhauser, 1971; Rhee, 1977; Roemer & Freidman, 1971; Shortall et al., 1976) have given evidence that the greater the power the medical-surgical staff exercises over its own members, the higher the quality of care delivered. For instance, in a sample of short-term acute care hospitals, Flood and Scott (1978) found that the more stringent the regulations (e.g., requirements governing admission to the staff and the awarding of surgical privileges) imposed upon individual surgeons by the surgical staff, the better the quality of surgical care (e.g., the post-patient health status of patients).

On the other hand, there are other reports indicating the leniency of collegial control. In hospitals there exists among physicians a "rule of etiquette" that advises overlooking each other's mistakes to hide errors and incompetence from the patients and the public. Millman (1976) described how social control fails to operate even in a situation specifically developed for the purpose of such control. The monthly mortality review conference in his study of hospitals is officially intended to audit the physician's performance in cases where patients have died or suffered from complications. Millman observed how errors are justified and responsibility for the mistake is neutralized so that no doctor is made to appear guilty.

The Miofsky Case. A most devastating example of a hospital's failure in disciplining physicians is the recent Miofsky case. William E. Miofsky, the anesthesiologist at Sutter Community Hospitals in Sacramento, California, was arrested and charged with forced oral copulation on unconscious female patients in the operating room. This is the most sensational medical scandal in Sacramento history, but what makes the charges extraordinary is that these alleged incidents occurred over a period of nearly two years.

> On February 11, 1977, circulating nurse Sandra Doll Neri caught Miofsky engaging in oral sex with an unconscious 52-year-old female patient. Neri, unable to accept what she saw, brought in another nurse, . . . , who also said she witnessed Miofsky having sex with the patient. Neri . . . told head operating nurse. . . .
>
> The three nurses discussed the episode with . . . [the surgeon on duty] who refused to believe the allegations but urged . . . to report any further suspicious activity. . . .
>
> Sutter Community Hospitals administrator William Schaeffer . . . learned of the allegations in February 1977. Miofsky was . . . advised of the allegations, but . . . he denied them. . . .
>
> In June 1977, Neri went to the second-in-command operating room nurse . . . told [her] she believed Miofsky was continuing his questionable behavior.
>
> [The latter] notified nursing director [who met with Neri and personnel director]. . . .

> [The nursing director and the personnel director] advised Neri that she should monitor Miofsky's activities but not discuss the serious allegations with other staff members . . . they believed her because they had heard Miofsky's suspicious conduct from other nurses . . . ("Miofsky . . . ," 1979).

> During the first nine months of 1978, the nurses monitored Miofsky's activities . . . and after Neri reported a resumption in [them in] later 1978, the nurses decided to act. . . .
>
> Based on the new developments, . . . [head operating nurse] wrote a . . . letter to Schaeffer which he received on January 11.
>
> After nothing was done, the outraged nurses decided to go to the Sacramento County Medical Society January 15. ("Sutter nurses . . . ," 1979).

As a result, the Sutter Hospitals have been stripped of their accreditation status and may lose their licensure. Sutter's executive director, Schaeffer, has been indefinitely suspended, and the chairman of the Board of Trustees, E. William Rector, M.D., has been forced to resign. Both of them admitted they had knowledge of the Miofsky case at least for a year while they made no effort to check the allegations because they thought the nurses' allegations to be unbelievable and unestablished ("Sutter stripped . . . ," 1979).

The Miofsky case was interpreted as a hospital's breach of public trust in its ability to protect patients from an unethical doctor. There were no effective means of dealing with accusations against hospital employees and doctors in a timely and orderly manner.

The roots of the Sutter Hospitals' problems have been traced to their structure and operation. According to the report prepared, independent of the Miofsky incident, by a hospital consulting firm (Williams, 1978), Sutter Hospitals were doctor-dominated facilities with widespread administrative and personnel problems. As compared with California's other non-profit hospitals, Sutter's board was unique in physician dominance (i.e., nine of fifteen members were physicians).

Later, in the investigation of the Miofsky affair, the hospital called upon Gordon D. Schaber of McGeorge School of Law, and former Superior Court Judge, Elvin F. Sheehy, to co-chair its own investigation (Sheehy & Schaber, 1979). They identified three major sources for the failure of the hospitals' procedures in handling the Miofsky case:

> (A) The failure of Hospital administration to properly instruct Hospital personnel on the purpose and use of the incident reports and unusual occurrence reports . . .
>
> (B) Division of authority within the governing structure of a hospital as represented by the independent medical staff with its organization and a separate but independent administration of the non-medical staff personnel. . . . At no time was the Miofsky affair ever reported to the Executive Committee [of the medical staff] by the representatives of Hospital administration or vice versa. . . .
>
> (C) The institutional tradition that mandates that one professional does not publicly speak critically of a fellow professional (Sheehy & Schaber, 1979, pp. 8–10).

Schaeffer, the hospital administrator, claimed that when doctors wanted new equipment, more space, or almost anything else related to the medical staff that required administrative action, they would circumvent the administration and go to another physician, usually one of the trustees ("Suspended . . . ," 1979). Sutter Hospitals have less administrative control of doctors than some other area hospitals. For instance, the Sutter administrator cannot summarily suspend a doctor, even if he or she thinks charges have been made that are grave enough to warrant the action.

Situations where physician trustees vote on the quality of medical care and physician evaluation have been described in such unflattering terms as "putting the fox in charge of the chicken coop" ("Sutter stripped . . . ," 1979). Doctors' tolerance of alleged imcompetence of their colleagues results partly from a fear of retaliation. Responding also to the recent general distrust in professional autonomy, doctors have become increasingly secretive about personal and job-related problems. They will not betray the professional subculture by exposing the incompetent to the public. This is why doctors were so reluctant to believe accounts by several nurses ("Sutter nurses . . . ," 1979).

Further, unlike at other hospitals, an individual at Sutter cannot take an allegation directly to the administrator, the chief of staff, or the chief of a department. Instead, an allegation must be made to a chairperson of the staff or the department, who would channel it through the department, the executive committee, and finally to the governing board.

Thus, at Sutter, nurses cannot bring a charge into the disciplinary channels. They must have a doctor to do it for them. When the nurse reported what she saw, while Miofsky denying it, officials in the hospital chose to believe the doctor, not the nurse. The nurses were accused of having a personal vendetta against the anesthesiologist. Doctors warned the nurses about what would happen if they were wrong about the allegations. Even after they obtained evidence, the nurses were forced to turn to outside help from the Medical Society, since the hospital continued to drag its feet. At Sutter, nurses said that they could be transferred or forced out of the hospital if they complained too loud ("Sutter nurses . . . ," 1979).

The Miofsky case has attracted wide publicity not only because of the sensationalism of sex crimes but because of the seriousness of the inadequacy of hospital and physician services. It alerted the public to the need for increased concern with and surveillance over their health care. The imprisonment of Miofsky, and dismissals of Schaeffer and Rector alone will not solve basic problems inherent in the Sutter and other hospitals. Structural changes such as the reduction of physicians on the board and a more even balance of power between the medical and administrative staffs will be more effective in avoiding other, less sensational but nevertheless serious, problems in the health delivery system.

Professional Standards Review Organizations. Only recently has this method of quality control began to attract attention, not so much because of the increase in malpractice suits but because of the rising cost of medical care. The federal government, which has become a major buyer of health services, has begun to show keen interest in promoting procedures to evaluate medical practice, particularly its cost.

In 1972, legislation called for the establishment of Professional Standards Review Organizations (PSROs) under Medicare and Medicaid. The PSROs were to be composed of community groups who would conduct evaluations of the performance of various aspects of the medical delivery system. Physician organizations were provided with the first chance to create PSROs, but if they did not avail themselves of the option, the opportunity was to be passed to other community groups.

Functions of the PSROs include (1) the development of standards for medical practice in a given geographic region, (2) the delimitation of acceptable practices, (3) the review of the performances of providers in the area, and (4) the exercise of appropriate sanctions for noncompliance (Anderson, 1976; Decker & Bonner, 1973; Goran et al., 1975; Kavet & Luft, 1974).

The degree of success of the PSROs has not been very encouraging. Available data indicate that peer review, which is the principal component of quality control, has not been effective in hospitals, clinics, or private offices (Derbyshire, 1974; Stroman, 1976). Moreover, the initial goals of PSROs were inherently self-contradictory, aiming simultaneously at the improvement of the quality of care and the reduction of cost. If the standard of medical care is set high, its operation is likely to cost more.

It is too early to determine the fate of mandated peer review through PSROs. Its success or failure will be affected by several issues such as (1) the nature of the norms concerning the quality of care and cost of health services, (2) the type of decision making on the review board, (3) the extent of depersonalization of the review process to avoid personal involvement, and (4) the development of realistic sanctions.

Physicians' Strikes. The changing characteristics of their profession are reflected not only in the increasing loss of profession automony by physicians but by their attitudes toward strikes.

Traditionally, physicians did not join unions or engage in strikes. Physicians' strikes were once extremely rare in the United States and conjured up frightening images to lay persons—that of physicians abandoning patients. Now, strikes are becoming more common. In 1975, strikes occurred in the three largest American cities—New York, Chicago, and Los Angeles.

This is partly a result of the Congressional Act of 1974 in granting some 2-million hospital workers the right to organize, bargain, and strike under federal labor law. Until August 1974 only about a dozen states accorded hospital workers these rights ("Doctors hit the street . . . ," 1975).

In the first major strike ever undertaken by American doctors, about 2,000 interns and residents picketed for four days to protest their working conditions ("Doctors on strike," *Time,* 1975). The strike was called by the Committee of Interns and Residents (CIR), a union representing 3,000 physicians-in-training who work at private and municipal hospitals under a contract with the League of Voluntary Hospitals.

The strikers objected to:

> a hallowed hospital tradition: occasional work weeks of 100 hours or more, including tours of continuous duty that last for 36 hours or longer with only brief breaks for catnaps. As a result, they said, exhausted interns and residents sometimes make mistakes that could otherwise be avoided. Some of the striking interns and residents told horror stories of falling asleep on their feet during operations; one admitted that he had pulled out several stitches after dozing off while holding an incision open with retractors. ("Doctors on strike," *Time,* 1975, p. 81)

To reduce the chances of hospital accidents, the CIR demanded a cut in the average workweek to 80 hours, with no more than 15 hours to be worked daily. They also asked not to perform duties that are considered more appropriate for nurses, technicians, and other hospital employees.

> Most objectionable, for many of the striking doctors, is the so-called scut work they are forced to do. "Eighty percent of my job," said . . . a striking surgeon . . . , "should really be done by someone else. There are patients who die because you can't get to them." ("Doctors on strike," *Newsweek,* 1975, p. 71)

Hospital officials and many older doctors who had gone through equally grudging initiations into medicine for much less money insisted that long hours and menial chores are part of the necessary preparation for a medical career. However, the AMA lent support to the CIR's position, stating that "when a physician has to work 50 hours straight or 100 hours in a week, [it is] a threat to the quality of care a patient is receiving." ("Doctors on strike," *Newsweek,* 1975, p. 71)

Finally, the strikers and the League of Voluntary Hospitals compromised and reached a settlement stipulating that, except in emergencies, no doctor will work more than one night in three, that duty schedules are to be agreed upon by individual hospitals and that grievance procedures will be established.

The strike had little effect on patient care. Only 13 percent of the doctors walked out at Metropolitan Hospital; most New York University Hospital interns and residents refused to join the strike. Many of the struck hospitals were able to maintain their normal capacity by pressing senior physicians into service. Also, given adequate notice, the hospitals had moved patients to other institutions, closing down some clinics or rearranging clinic schedules ("Doctors on strike," *Time,* 1975).

Systematic studies of striking interns and residents are not available. Hence little is known about the feelings and actions of striking house staff members—their fear, guilt, and risk-taking.

Among few is the interview study of striking physicians by Kotz and Rosenblatt (1978). They observed that the goal of the doctors' strike is not to shut down the hospital completely, which may turn the public against doctors. Rather, its major function is symbolic and informational to let the public know that physicians are willing to strike. Many physicians felt ambivalent about joining the strike as they viewed it as a violation of the Hippocratic Oath. This ambivalence was resolved largely by the rationalization that the strike is in the best interests of patient care. Also feelings of cohesion and solidarity of the House staff helped overcome any initial feelings of guilt about striking.

Finally, Kotz and Rosenblatt added a remark which relates to the larger organizational structure of medical practice. According to them, house staff members are willing to strike at this stage in their medical career, while they are employees of a bureaucratic organization. Later, when they enter private group practice or become hospital administrators, they are less likely to strike against their patients.

SUMMARY

Physicians attained professional status because, in functionalist terms, they acquired the technology to perform an important function in society, that of saving lives. From the conflict perspective, however, the status and power of physicians had to be fought for.

Before the Middle Ages there was no clear identity attached to physicians even as an occupational group, not to mention as a profession. It was only after the appearance of the germ theory in the nineteenth century that physicians came to demonstrate techniques superior to those of other healers.

Since the mid-nineteenth century physicians have grown increasingly concerned with establishing scientific standards to set themselves apart from quacks. The AMA became active and effective in this endeavor after the turn of the century. During the early period, the AMA focused its efforts upon improving the quality of training at medical schools. Standardization of medical education served as a weapon to monopolize medical knowledge and to exclude others from practicing medicine.

The germ theory, which brought about advances in medical science, also dictated the goal of medical education. The school goal of scientific performance shaped the type of students admitted, the nature of their medical education, and the outcome of education as manifested in the characteristics of physicians. Medical schools from 1910 to 1960 had an elitist bias in recruiting students predominantly from the white middle class or upper middle class male population and also produced physicians who were oriented more toward the science than the art of medicine.

Having reached an elitist position, organized medicine had to be sure that it would not be eroded internally or externally. Through informal social control of local societies as well as by other measures, the AMA has succeeded in suppressing dissent and producing a united front. In combating outside pressures the AMA has engaged in extensive political lobbying and campaign activities to avoid third-party interference.

Victories by the AMA in political and other arenas firmly consolidated their elevated position as a medical profession. Consequently, physicians enjoy autonomy in their work without being subject to external evaluation. As a profession of experts, the medical profession has a monopoly on anything that can be considered to be illness (Freidson, 1970). Moreover, advances in medical science have expanded medicine's jurisdiction even to the domain of deviant behavior. In a sense the medical institution has come to play a role as an agent of social control.

As inviolate as it may appear, however, the status of the medical profession has been subject to a series of challenges since the middle of this century.

Through the upsurge of civil rights movements in the 1960s, demands were made for more sexual equality, and low-cost community health clinics. Thus, major changes in the medical school were required.

After about half a century of dominance, the AMA has begun to lose ground because of both internal and external forces, such as diversification of interests within the profession, the rising power of the clients, and the increasing governmental role in determining the quality and cost of medical care. Coupled with other changes in the field of medicine, the validity of professional autonomy has undergone reassessment. Systematic rather than informal peer review as a mechanism for quality control is currently being advocated and implemented.

In sum, both the status and power connected with the medical profession, which took centuries to build, are undergoing major structural changes. The special mystique of the medical profession no longer protects physicians as unassailable. The once tightly knit, closed system of the profession is finally being forced to open its doors to social forces. Thus, medicine is losing unique characteristics of a profession—work autonomy, elitist status, monopoly of knowledge, authority over clients, freedom from third-party interference, and so on. This trend has been identified by some (Haug, 1972, 1975, 1976; Toren, 1975) as "deprofessionalization."

There are several phenomena that account for this reversal of professionalization. First of all, there is the trend of bureaucratic invasion of the field of medicine. As knowledge becomes more specialized, more standardized, and more complete, the ability to codify tasks in a routine manner increases. Within the routinization of jobs, the mystery of the work (intellectual challenge and fascination), which has been claimed to be the essence of the profession, will be lost (Engel, 1969).

The fundamental blow, however, to the medical profession came from the changing values in our society. Only recently, medical care, health, life, and survival have come to be regarded as the inalienable rights of every American citizen. People have begun to demand ready access to medical care regardless of their ability to pay. In order to implement these new values, third-party involvement began to increase and to undermine professional autonomy.

In the midst of this turbulence at the crossroad of medicalization and deprofessionalization, how do professionals find satisfaction from work? Sarason (1977) delved into the aspects of professional life that are hidden in the private struggles of individual professionals.

The highly educated medical professionals came to their careers with great expectations that their lives would be filled with a vibrant sense of challenge, growth, and achievement. At the same time, placed on society's pedestal, physicians are seen by the public as masters of their fate in addition to being savers of lives. Sarason observed that these expectations make professionals especially vulnerable to the depressing effects of realizing that their professional dreams have become unrealistic. There comes a time when their careers are perceived by medical professionals as a boring and confining trap instead of a glamorous personal growth.

This dilemma may cause some to lose the desire to climb the ladder of the medical profession. Also, these internal struggles and conflicts may suggest that the mystique of the profession no longer exists.

CHAPTER 7
Hospital Organization

> "Where in the world am I?" said Alice. She opened her eyes to a strange surrealist landcape that looked a good deal like the inside of a modern hospital, only more so. To one side, as far as her eyes could see, stretched row upon row of little cubicles with seemingly thousands of people lying in bed and thousands of others rushing in and out doing things for and to those in bed. The center of activity was a huge operating room, brilliantly lit, with many tables, all kinds of elaborate equipment, and long queues of waiting people, some lying on stretchers, others hovering over them, all dressed—or undressed—in white or green.
>
> On the other side was a great mishmash of stores and booths and mail-order houses, selling pills, potions, and drugs of all shapes and colors, eyeglasses, crutches, false teeth, hearing aids, bandages, aphrodisiacs, anything and everything that people could be persuaded to buy in the pursuit of health.
>
> In between the beds and the stores were throngs of people sitting and waiting, some in little clusters as in a doctor's office, and others in huge lobbies as big as railway stations. In the background Alice could see long rows of people sitting at desks like in an insurance company, taking in and giving out checks (Somers, 1972b, p. 849).

> The American hospital is large, impersonal, and dominated by elaborate technology. The American hospital is small, inefficient, underequipped, and understaffed. The American hospital exists to serve the community. The American hospital is crowded to the point of inefficiency and even danger, and serious delays are encountered in obtaining admission. The American hospital is often half-empty, and many of its patients should be at home or in extended care facilities. The American hospital is a business run to show a profit for its owners.
>
> Will the "real" American hospital please stand up? Which of these many contradictory characterizations of United States hospitals is correct? To some extent, all of them are. No other country has such a heterogeneous collection of institutions comprising its hospital "system." In no other country is it as difficult to generalize about hospitals or to analyze their strengths and shortcomings (Fuchs, 1974, p. 79).

The above excerpts illustrate two major issues concerning contemporary American hospitals: (1) American hospitals are large, complex organizations with many functions to perform; and (2) they are heterogeneous in terms of ownership, size, complexity, structure, goal, efficiency, and quality of care delivered.

Types of Hospital. There are over 7,000 hospitals in the United States. According to ownership, they can be divided into three general categories: voluntary, government, and proprietary. Voluntary hospitals are operated and controlled by nonprofit corporations. A significant amount of their support comes from charitable contributions and subsidies. Government hospitals are owned and operated by some unit of the government. At the federal level are the military, Veterans' Administration, and Public Service hospitals. At the state level are the county and municipal hospitals. Proprietary hospitals are owned by private corporations or partnerships and are operated on a profit-making basis (American Hospital Association, 1968).

With respect to types of service, general hospitals provide a full range of both general and special services. Specialty hospitals, on the other hand, limit their services to certain areas, such as specific types of illness (tuberculosis sanatoriums and psychiatric clinics), certain age groups (pediatric and geriatric hospitals), and occupational groups (veterans', merchants', and seamen's hospitals).

Hospital services also vary from long-term care (mental hospital or tuberculosis sanatorium) to short-term care (childbirth and minor accidents). A short-term hospital is defined as a medical facility where over 50 percent of the patients stay less than 30 days. The term *community hospital* refers to a general or special type of institution that is short-term and nonfederal, and there are over 6,000 of them in the United States today.

Good statistical data are now available on most American hospitals, but such was not the case prior to World War II (Corwin, 1946). The American Medical Association collected data annually from hospitals until 1946, when the American Hospital Association began to register hospitals using a different criteria. To be accepted for registration by the American Hospital Association, an institution must meet the following standards: (1) more than six beds for an average stay of over 24 hours per admission; (2) safe and sanitary construction and equipment; (3) an organized medical staff, registered-nurse supervision, and nursing care for round-the-clock patient care; (4) maintenance of clinical records; (5) minimal surgical and obstetrical facilities or relatively complete diagnostic and treatment facilities; and (6) a diagnostic X-ray and clinical laboratory. In short, by AHA standards, a hospital was and is required to offer more intensive services than merely room, board, personal services, and general nursing care (U.S. Dept. of Commerce, 1975).

Based on the earlier statistical data that are available on medical institutions, there was a 41 percent leap in the number of hospitals between 1909 and 1920. This was in response to the increased number of patients who began to show confidence in medical science and who sought treatment in hospitals. When the initial impact of medical discoveries wore off, the rate of increase in the number of hospitals diminished to a 4.9 percent increment from 1920 to 1930, and again from 1950 to 1970 (see Table 7.1).

The proportion of short-term hospitals, however, has increased over the years from 64 percent in 1930 to 82 percent in 1970, while the proportion of

Table 7.1:
Number of Hospitals, by Ownership and Control

		Governmental			*Nonprofit*		*Proprietary*
Year	*Total*	*Federal*	*State*	*Local*	*Church*	*Others*	
1970[4]	7,123	408	577	1,680	([1])	3,600	850
1960[4]	6,876	435	556	1,324	1,241	2,338	982
1950[4]	6,788	414	([2])	1,654	([1])	3,250	1,470
1950[5]	6,430	355	552	1,005	1,097	2,072	1,349
1940[5]	6,291	336	521	910	998	1,903	1,623
1930[5]	6,719	288	581	943	1,017	3,890	([3])
1923[5]	6,830	220	601	915	893	2,439	1,762
1918[5]	5,323	110	303	–	–	–	–
1909[5]	4,359	71	232	–	–	–	–

Notes: [1] *Church-operated and affiliated hospitals included with "others."*
[2] *State hospitals included with "local."*
[3] *Proprietary hospitals included with "other nonprofit."*
[4] *1950–1970: American Hospital Association data.*
[5] *1909–1950: American Medical Association data.*

Source: U.S. Department of Commerce, *Historical Statistics of the United States* (Washington, D.C.: U.S. Government Printing Office, 1975), p. 79.

long-term facilities has decreased. The increase in long-term hospitals is due partly to the decline in tuberculosis sanatoriums after an effective cure was found for that disease. The decrease is also attributable to the growth of nursing homes, which care for chronically ill patients. Further, many chronically ill patients are cared for at special long-term care units established in general, short-term hospitals.

There were 7,123 hospitals in the United States in 1970. Of those, 5.7 percent were federal facilities, 8.1 percent were state controlled, 23.6 percent were supported by local governments, 11.9 percent were proprietary hospitals, and the dominant remainder (about 50 percent) were in the nonprofit category. In sum, the most typical medical institution is the general voluntary hospital dealing with short-term cases.

CONCEPTUAL FRAMEWORKS AND VARIABLES

Max Weber's Theory of Bureaucracy

In studies of the hospital as a large, complex organization, Max Weber's model of bureaucracy has served as a frame of reference for many researchers. Weber brought the model into being near the turn of the century as a reaction against the nepotism, capricious judgment, and personal subjugation that prevailed in management practices during the early days of the Industrial Revolution. Weber described bureaucracy as a "social machine" that operates by rules, reasons, and law. This definition is broad enough to include the bureaucracy of the hospital, and many studies have been made of hospitals from the perspective of this standard model of large, complex organizations.

According to Weber (Gerth & Mills, 1958), a bureaucracy has the following characteristics: (1) it has a division of labor that is based on functional specialization, which in turn promotes expertise among the staff members and enables the organization to hire employees on the basis of technical competence; (2) it has a well-defined hierarchy of authority, which serves to check arbitrary power and insures the disciplined behavior of everyone; (3) it has a system of rules and procedures covering the rights and duties of employees and work situations, which provides for a uniformity of operation and, together with the authority structure, enables effective coordination; (4) it has an impersonality of interactions, which prevents strictly personal judgment; and (5) promotion and selection are based on technical competence, which maximizes rational decision-making.

In short, disciplined performance that is governed by technical competence, rational judgment, abstract rules, and is coordinated by the authority hierarchy, serves the organization most efficiently in the pursuit of its goals.

When applied to the hospital, however, Weber's model of bureaucracy presents some difficulties. There are widespread criticisms of the model, which will now be analyzed from the functionalist, conflict, and interactionist perspectives.

Functionalist Critique of Weber's Model

One of the basic objections raised by functionalists concerns the "line" structure of Weber's model. Weber's bureaucracy is characterized as a one-dimensional, one-way communication channel in which commands are transmitted from the top to the bottom of a hierarchy.

Functionalists view organization as a system consisting of mutually dependent parts. They are concerned with the links of interdependence among parts rather than monocratic authority relations. As outlined in Chapter 2, Parsons (1960) envisions organization as a social system functioning with and related to a total society. A large, bureaucratic organization must be studied in relation to modern, complex society because it came into existence as an aspect of functional differentiation of society. It did not exist in primitive societies.

Having rejected Weber's monocratic model as inappropriate for professionals, Parsons sees a hospital as a "company of equals" with minimum hierarchical differentiation.

In addition to Parsons, there are others who used the systemic approach. For example, Georgopoulos and Matejko (1967) examined the interaction among the following variables: goal attainment, availability and allocation of organizational resources, coordination, integration, conflict resolution, and adaptation. They found that the basic question was not whether a hospital met its specified minimum requirements but rather how well it functioned as a unified social system. In sports terms, this implies that teamwork is more important than isolated individual successes.

Heydebrand (1973) went even further by identifying the levels of the individual factors that influence the patterns of hospital organization. He concluded that the hierarchy of variables begins with the most general level, dealing with the organizational interaction with the external environment. Included at this level are (1) the size and structure of the surrounding community, (2) the interests and power of the medical and other health professions, and (3) the authority and policies of governmental and legal agencies. This basic stratum is followed by the second level of variables, which consists of the complexity of the task structure and the degree of organizational autonomy. The third level contains technology and functional specialization. Finally, at the fourth level is found a nonbureaucratic mode of coordination (professionalization). This hierarchy of variables is a causal model in which the direction of causality is inferred from the lower level up through the higher bureaucratic levels. In addition, all of these levels of variables are considered to be determinants of organizational effectiveness.

Conflictive Critique of Weber's Model

While Weber posits no major conflict in his rational and efficient model of bureaucracy, others see contradictions in his logic, which destroy or at least modify his basis of bureaucracy. On the one hand, Weber described bureaucracy as reliant on expert technical judgment. On the other hand, it expects a disciplined compliance with the directives of superiors. Weber apparently saw no contradiction between these two principles; he assumed that the superior's judgment is always the best one in terms of technical expertise. This is not realistic, according to some (Gouldner, 1954), who contend that conflict generally arises between disciplined compliance with administrative procedures and adherance to professional standards.

Many investigators (Burling et al., 1956; Henry, 1954) have seen built-in conflict (Smith, 1955) in a hospital organization characterized by a two-line authority. The professional orientation held by the medical staff and the bureaucratic orientation of the administration are incompatible, and many personnel, particularly nurses, are caught between the two. Also, the power of lower-level participants in the organizations such as hospitals is an important facet of conflict. Cohen (1965) suggested that impossible work demands on lower-level bureaucrats lead to many situations where they can threaten to withdraw needed services.

Professional versus Bureaucratic Orientations. There are some similarities between professional and bureaucratic orientations such as (1) universalistic rather than particularistic standards applied to decision-making, (2) a specialized body of knowledge gained from specialized training, (3) specificity of expertise rather than generalized wisdom, (4) affective neutrality in relation to clients, and (5) achieved rather than ascribed status of a professional or bureaucratic person.

The major difference between the two orientations lies in control structure (Blau & Scott, 1964, p. 60; Freidson, 1975a, p. 172). Distinct from the hierarchical control exercised in bureaucratic organizations, professionals use self-control and collegial surveillance. As a result of long training, a professional is expected to have acquired and internalized a code of ethics governing professional conduct. Self-control is supplemented by the surveillance of performance by peers, who are in a position to observe his or her work, who have the technical competence to evaluate this work, and who are motivated to maintain professional integrity for the sake of the reputation of the profession.

To deepen the gulf between physicians and administration, there are structural sources of conflict. Doctors are "staff" members who have acquired professional skill from outside the organization, but they are also members of the "line" since they actually work on the raw materials. Hence, they are subjected to administrative power.

Despite built-in conflict, hospitals as organizations rarely dissolve. Litwak (1961) suggested the importance of studying ways in which the contradictory forms of organizational structure can exist side by side without ruinous friction. In line with the functional conflict theory, he proposed a model of bureaucracy that permits conflict as an integral part of the system.

According to Litwak (1961), there are three types of bureaucracy: Weberian, human-relational, and professional. Weberian bureaucracy is most efficient when the organization deals primarily with uniform events and with traditional areas of knowledge. The human relations model is effective in the areas in which events are not uniform and where social skills are needed. Professional bureaucracy is a combination of the first two. In this dual-model situation, certain mechanisms transmit the two conflicting forces so that they can be "harnessed to organizational goals." For example, activities can be separated physically and functionally so that different people performing different tasks conform to separate models of evaluation.

In a similar vein, Goss (1963) suggested dual control of authority and advisory relations within a single hierarchy. Structured authority relationships prevail in the area of administration and rest on the predictability of behavior that is essential for coordination. In contrast, the advisory relationship is found in the realm of professional work, leaving each physician's individual authority intact. Goss calls the latter an advisory bureaucracy: subordinates are obliged to take advice under critical review, but they are not necessarily obliged to follow it in making their decisions.

Along with functional conflict perspectives, Litwak, Goss, and others (Gouldner, 1954) have accounted for the fact that hospitals continue to exist despite built-in conflicts since they possess mechanisms to resolve conflicts.

Interactionist Critique of Weber's Model

Weber's preoccupation with the formally instituted aspects of bureaucracy and his neglect of the informal relations and unofficial pattern that develop in formal organizations have been criticized by interactionists. They claim that the formal relationship is only one aspect of the real social structure, and that the organizational members interact casually outside the realm of formal roles. Blau (1963) in his *Dynamics of Bureaucracy,* noted the many ways in which informal relationships in bureaucratic settings are necessary to make the organization really function. Strauss and his group (1963) described the hospital as an institution where negotiation and compromise are constant preludes to the informal agreements. Many other studies demonstrate that friendship patterns, unofficial exchange systems, and natural leadership arise to modify the formal arrangements (Mechanic, 1962c; Page, 1946; Turner, 1947). Labeling theory (which was introduced in Chapter 2) delineates the processes of informal interaction and the consequences of such transactions upon the individuals involved. This theory has been applied by many researchers to mental hospitals, which will be discussed later in this chapter.

Another variant of the interactionist perspective, exchange theory, has been useful in studying the interactions among various components of the hospital organization (Burling et al., 1956) and between the hospital and the external environment (Levine & White, 1961). Unlike Weber's unilateral chain of command, exchange theorists postulate a give-and-take between the parties concerned. For instance, the hospital receives community inputs in the form of patients, funds, and support. In return, the hospital must satisfy the community expectation for quality as well as efficiency of care.

Organizational Process Model

In this chapter, hospital organization will be examined as an open system (Georgopoulos, 1972a, Gross, 1967; Katz & Kahn, 1966; Thompson, 1967), whose boundaries are relatively elastic rather than fixed. In the process of mutual stimulation and response, the hospital is affected by the environment and in turn influences it. Through this continuous exchange with external forces, the hospital maintains its own identity and integrity as a system (Steeg & Croog, 1979).

The organizational process is cast in the "input–transformation–output" cycle (Georgopoulos, 1972a; Newhauser & Anderson, 1972). The hospital (1) receives input from a variety of personnel, resources, and patients from the community; (2) transforms some of these inputs through the organizational processes; and then (3) returns finished outputs to the environment, which in turn have a bearing on the hospital.

Figure 7.1: Organizational Process Model

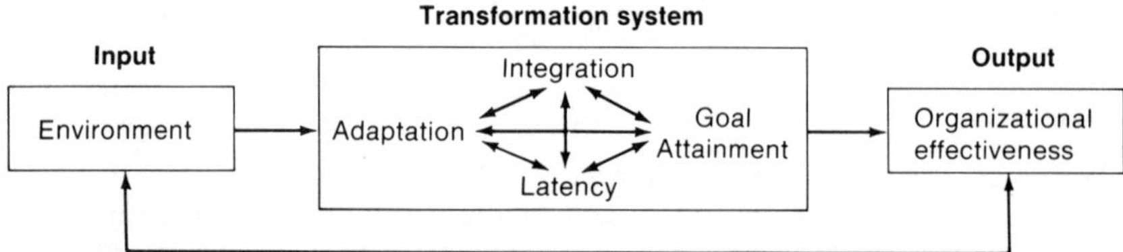

Environment. The hospital is directly dependent upon the environment for its inputs—patients, physicians, other personnel, facilities, supplies, and capital (Georgopoulos, 1975; Heydebrand, 1973). The hospital is also linked to other health service agencies such as the Department of Health, the pharmaceutical industry, insurance companies, and voluntary health care and research organizations. Of particular importance in recent years is the role played by the federal government as a purchaser and a deliverer of medical services. Increasingly, the hospital is forced to interact with third parties such as the Social Security Administation, planning agencies, state rate-review board, and Professional Standards Review Organizations (Shortell, 1976).

Less directly, the hospital is shaped by values, characteristics, and the needs of the community such as demographic composition, morbidity pattern, socioeconomic characteristics, the political power structure, and general attitudes toward health.

Another important component of the environment is technology (Comstock, 1975; Harvey, 1968; Perrow, 1967; Thompson, 1967), which influences the structure and process within the hospital organization. Historically, two of the major events leading to the hospital revolution were the technological ability to control surgical infection through antisepsis and the diagnostic developments surrounding radiology (Georgopoulos, 1972a). More recently, the relative value and geographic distribution of coronary care units, renal dialysis, and related life-saving technology have become serious issues of hospital operation.

The effect of technology upon the hospital may be indirect. An introduction of new medical technology affects values, attitudes, and knowledge of people toward the health delivery system, and results in a change in the structure and process of the hospital system.

System Variables. Structural variables of the hospital organization include size, complexity, and stratification. The size of the hospital has been chosen by many researchers as the most salient feature of the organization (Lena, 1975; Starkweather, 1970). This dimension is generally measured in terms of capacity—the number of beds and/or patient days.

The complexity of the organization may be narrowly defined as the degree of specialization of organization members, that is, the extent to which separate functions, goals, or tasks are assigned to different organization subunits (Hage, 1965). On the other hand, a broader definition covers the extent of goal proliferation, the number of divisions of labor, the levels of hierarchy, and the geographic dispersion (Hall, Hass, & Johnson, 1967).

Some researchers consider the above definition of complexity to be too inclusive and have focused their attention upon one dimension, namely, a vertical one in the form of stratification. Stratification refers to the manner in which various occupational groups are rank-ordered in the hospital. The researchers of hospital stratification have been concerned with (1) determining how many hierarchical levels exist in the hospital, (2) examining the characteristics of people at each level, and (3) measuring the social distance and power differentiation perceived among these levels.

The analysis of functional variables of the hospital in this chapter will primarily follow the Parsonian model of functional prerequisites. The most immediate requirement of an organization in its relation to the environment is its ability to adapt to external forces and carry on an effective interchange with it. This includes adaptation prerequisites: (1) securing resources and personnel from outside; (2) maintaining advantageous relationships with the community; and (3) responding properly to changes in the outside world.

The hospital must be able to cultivate the sociopsychological commitment of individual members to the organization. Development of common organizational values and shared norms is important to socialize and bind the members securely into the system. The organization must also provide mechanisms by which strains and tensions can be managed. These are latency prerequisites.

The task of organization involves the following integration prerequisites: (1) coordinating many diverse roles and interdependent activities of different staffs and members, and (2) integrating all parts of the system so that the hospital can attain its goal most efficiently.

Finally, the ultimate goal (or the goal-attainment prerequisite) of the hospital is to provide high-quality output to the community (e.g., patient care or health service) in terms of quantity, quality, cost, and acceptability. This involves the ability to maximize the efficient and reliable performance of every component of the organization.

The outcome of the organizational processes then will be evaluated by the community. The degree of community satisfaction or dissatisfaction with the hospital's performance will affect the community's future support of the hospital.

The volume of hospital research has been growing rapidly in recent decades and comprehensive reviews have been conducted (Georgopoulos, 1972a,

1975; Shortell, 1976). However, with few exceptions (Georgopoulos & Mann, 1962; Glaser, 1970), the majority of the studies do not attempt to examine all of the salient variables of organization research. They lack an integrative framework for the comprehensive study of health care organizations such as the general hospital, the mental hospital, and the nursing home.

THE GENERAL HOSPITAL

Historical Development

The general hospital as a social system has gone through a sequence of structural changes since its inception. Prevailing values of society are likely to define the priority of functions to be performed by the hospital. The importance of a particular task area (e.g., custody of the sick) is determined by the social values of the time (e.g., charity) (Sigerist, 1960).

Within an organization, the conditions under which certain members come to possess power was specified by Perrow (1963, 1969). Perrow hypothesized that an organization, as a goal-oriented system, will be controlled by those who can fulfill the most important assignments. Those who have the skill to perform these tasks will have the power to determine major operating policies and organizational goals.

Perrow further differentiated between the official and the operative goals of an organization. While official goals of an organization may be formulated by societal values, operative goals are needed to provide the specific content of official policies. These operative goals are likely to be shaped and implemented by the most powerful group to suit its vested interests.

Greek and Roman Hospitals

Greek temples, such as those dedicated to the cult of Asclepius (Rosen, 1963), were probably the earliest separate institutions concerned with the care of the sick. They were operated by the principle, technology, and personnel of religious medicine.

During the time of the Roman Empire, separate medical institutions for the care and shelter of the sick did appear, but they were primarily intended for the military. These hospitals were only an expedient result of the expansion of the empire, since great distances made it impossible for the Roman army to send sick soldiers home for treatment (Major, 1954).

The Medieval Hospital: Religious Domination

Christian values and the Church totally dominated medieval society. Charity was the basic Christian value that motivated the rise of medieval hospitals (Rosen, 1963); all Christians had a duty to the sick and the destitute. This charity motive was reinforced by another Christian value, namely, that grace and salvation might be achieved by giving alms. Not only was caring for the sick a Christian duty, but it was considered to be beneficial for the salvation of the soul.

The hospital as a concept and as an institution developed through another close link with the Church—medieval monasticism. The manner in which the monks cared for their own sick became a model for the laity.

> The strict rules of conduct and the equally severe regulations for the care of the soul made a medieval hospital almost like a monastry. Staff and patients all had to take part in religious services daily—matins, primé, tierce, mass, sext . . . all had to be observed. . . .
>
> It seems that as much—if not more—attention was paid to the spiritual well-being of a sick person as to the treatment of his ailments. Physicians were few and medical knowledge was limited (Dainton, 1961, p. 27).
>
> Treatment was a medley of pseudo-science and old wives' remedies. A traditional knowledge of herbs enabled the medical doctor to concoct useful medicine and ointment, but added to the herbs were nauseous ingredients of doubtful value, and their administration was controlled by astrological calculations (McInnes, 1963, p. 18).

As the medieval hospital developed, it was not only a center for medical care, but it became a philanthropic and spiritual institution as well. It not only cared for the sick, but it also harbored others that were in need, such as the poor, the indigent, the infirm, travelers, and pilgrims. In that spirit, hospitals also became places of refuge.

The early facilities were usually rough stone buildings with straw on the floor, badly lighted, and filthy. Sometimes several patients were put into a single bed with no regard to their diseases. In those days, there was no knowledge of bacteria or of the infectious nature of disease (Sigerist, 1960, p. 138). The level of medical technology was so low that the hospital was considered more a place to come to die than to be cured. The status of physicians was insignificant due in part to their ineffectiveness in curing patients, but that status was also the result of the hospital being dominated by religion.

Along with that domination, the concept of charity as a means to salvation tended to emphasize the role of the donor. In addition, the founder, sponsor, or patron of a medieval hospital had certain rights that were established by law. Such a patron could (1) decide what types of patient would be admitted, and therefore, excluded; (2) appoint administrators (warden, master, and keeper); (3) make visitations to inspect the hospital; and (4) set the rules of behavior.

This individualistic and private nature of charitable institutions also allowed for various abuses. Hospital funds were misappropriated and sometimes even provided an income for a cleric. Ecclesiastical authorities became aware of various abuses that grew notorious, and they eventually decreed that all hospital administrators had to swear to the ecclesiastic authorities honestly and to prepare an annual statement of hospital accounts for their bishop (Dainton, 1961; McInnes, 1963; Talbot, 1967).

Secularization of the Hospital

From the thirteenth century on, the hospital gradually came under secular jurisdiction. The Renaissance orientation toward life—the positive valuation of this world and an independence from clerical domination—was manifested in the changing attitudes toward disease and the goals of the hospital.

With the destruction of monasticism in England, many hospitals were temporarily closed. These closures were primarily a reaction to the abuses practiced by the patrons (Dainton, 1961). The shutting down of the hospitals drove the shelterless sick and poor out into the streets. Then, as the bourgeoisie grew wealthy and powerful, municipal and national authorities began to take over the health service activities of the church.

Concurrently, a feeling of citizenship developed in the place of religious ideas among the people of London, and it was collectively felt that action should be taken to help the poor. This concept was recognized officially, taking the form of the English Poor Law of 1601, which held each parish responsible for the care and feeding of its own poor.

That duty of social welfare was grudgingly accepted by the state and communities (Dainton, 1961), and it was extended to the establishment of hospitals that were supported by the "poor" tax and by certain voluntary contributions. Administratively, the municipal authorities were responsible for the hospital facilities. The overall administration was in the hands of a board of governors, which consisted of commoners (non-aristocrats), citizens (non-aliens), and free people (non-slaves, non-serfs, etc.) of the city, headed by a magistrate.

The essential function of the parish hospital was to help maintain social order by ameliorating suffering, by diminishing the effects of poverty, and by eradicating the practice of begging. Its goal continued to be a combination of the care of the sick and the needy, and the position of the physicians also remained unchanged.

The status of the doctors in these hospitals was low because medical care was not the primary goal of the hospital, the doctors were not able to cure the patients, and they were guests of the hospital. Actually, the physicians practiced outside of the hospital for fees, and they worked at the hospital gratis in return for the privilege of receiving instruction such as the monitoring of medically interesting cases.

From the Eighteenth to the Early Nineteenth Centuries

The growth in the number of hospitals during the eighteenth century and the early nineteenth century reflected the sociopolitical and medico-scientific climate of those times. The scientific revolution of the sixteenth and the seventeenth centuries laid the foundation for the establishment of institutions wherein scientific knowledge could be applied to medical care.

The early stages of the Industrial Revolution were accompanied by new social problems as well as by a different view toward the ill health of the poor. Not only did poverty and sickness become commercial problems, but there was a growing social conscience coupled with humanitarianism that led to a belief in the practical virtue of medical efficiency. The ideas of earlier centuries, such as mercantilism and social economy, became a motivating value for the eighteenth-century hospital movement. It was held that providing efficient medical care for patients at the hospital was cheaper for society in the long run than it was to leave them unattended (Abel-Smith, 1964; Abel-Smith & Gales, 1964).

Hospitals established (or reopened) in London during this period were chiefly the result of private initiative and contributions, along with some government assistance in the form of legislative action. The dearth of municipal support was partially due to the lack of training of the parish officers as well as to their reluctance to assume additional responsibilities (Rosen, 1963).

The United States followed the general pattern set by Mother England, but there was a considerable time lag. The first American general hospital was established by a group of Quakers in Philadelphia in 1751. The therapeutic and organizational situation in American hospitals between 1751 and 1859 corresponded with the condition of European hospitals during the Middle Ages. Improvements in American hospitals during the next fifty to sixty years correspond to those realized during the Renaissance in Europe (Duffy, 1968; Rothstein, 1972).

But then, much like the English hospitals during the eighteenth and the early nineteenth century, the ones in America were not governmental undertakings. They too were the outcome of voluntary efforts by private citizens, financed by subscription and bequest. The primary purpose of these voluntary hospitals, as it was in England, was social rather than medical. They were intended to serve the sick and poor whose home conditions were deficient and totally lacking in medical care.

The social rather than medical nature of the hospital goals as well as the low level of medical technology generated the policy of not admitting patients with chronic, incurable, or terminal illnesses. These patients were sent to the almshouse or to the workhouse. Even so, the death rate in the American hospital was very high. For example, the fatality rate in a major American hospital was 17 percent in 1847 and declined to 10 percent by 1850 (Duffy, 1968).

Trustee Domination. In short, until the early nineteenth century, the major goal of the hospital was social or religious rather than medical. Physicians lacked sufficient medical technique to fulfill the goal attainment function, and therefore, their status was deemed to be low.

The hospital was legitimized by the commonly held social values of the times, such as the Christian ideals of charity and salvation in the medieval period, and by social philanthropy during the thirteenth through the early nineteenth centuries. The hospital was loosely supervised by the Church or the local government lest it should violate those societal values.

The internal coordination function was performed by an administration whose structure was quite small and simple. Administrative performance was also directly supervised by the Church or the local government.

The most important task for the hospital until the early nineteenth century was the procurement of resources because most hospitals were totally dependent on private contributions. Since institutional survival depended on this vital function, the donors or their community representatives (trustees) exerted great power. Trustee domination was also due to the technological weakness of the other personnel. Physicians and administrators, for example, could not provide precise indicators of efficiency or goal achievement (Perrow, 1963, 1969).

Both physicians and hospital administrators maintained their status by seeing to it that the organization operated in conformity with societal values and that funds were not misused.

In the voluntary hospitals during this period, the trustees officially had the ultimate authority. Since they had access to the donors, the trustees could exercise not only financial control but also could control the appointments and the promotions of medical and nonmedical personnel. In comparison, the administration had little power, prestige, or responsibility.

Operative goals of the hospitals were set by the trustees, whose only responsibility was to the sponsoring community. They tended to favor conservative financial policies and to oppose high expenses for equipment, research, and education, thereby curtailing the authority of the medical staff. Trustees also frequently represented certain social groups in the community, and it was in their own best interest to promote the selfish interests of these groups.

The Hospital in the Twentieth Century

Medical Domination. Whether viewed as developmental stages of organization or as a dialectic conflict process, several drastic shifts of power can be observed within the hospital during this period. First, with the success of the germ theory, the trustees' domination was replaced by medical domination, and that was followed by administrative domination as a result of the growth, complexity, and political maneuvering in many hospitals in the twentieth century (Perrow, 1963, 1969).

It was also during the twentieth century that medical technology made extraordinary advances, such as the establishment of physiology and bacteriology and the development of antisepsis and anesthesis. This put medicine on a firm scientific basis. Since doctors monopolized the skills to utilize these technical advances, their status escalated.

Then, as the effectiveness of treatment improved, public attitudes toward hospitals also changed. For a long time, the rich received medical care including surgery at home, and the poor feared admission to the hospital as a death sentence. As advances in medical technology lowered the death rate in hospitals, the public realized that various illnesses could be treated more effectively in the hospital than at home. As a result, by the beginning of the twentieth century, hospitals were admitting increasing numbers of patients from various socioeconomic strata (Packard, 1963).

At the same time, the value of the hospital as an educational institution for physicians, students, and nurses was increasingly recognized. In the meanwhile, doctors began to organize themselves as a profession, thereby gaining control over standards of medical care and increased authority in their demands for resources.

All of these factors helped increase the power of the doctors in the authority structure of the hospital. Societal values of the twentieth century place a premium on good health instead of spiritual salvation, and so they defined the goal of the hospital as one of curing disease rather than simply caring for the needy. Doctors monopolized the technology to attain this goal, hence, they are in a position to command power.

The operative goals of a physician-dominated hospital were defined in strict medical terms: achievement of high technical standards, promotion of exemplary research, and provision of a good medical education. Just as the trustees once emphasized the selfish interests of the donors, there could be a danger that resources might be curtailed in areas which did not directly promote selfish medical goals.

When doctors fully exercised their potential power, the legal power of trustees became nominal. The latter were only consulted during a crisis situation. The administrative function also became that of "housekeeper." The administrative viewpoints on operative goals, policy matters, and personnel selection were neglected. All of these issues were dictatorially defined as medical in nature by the doctors. Hence, neither the trustees nor the administrators were considered qualified to voice their opinions.

Administrative Domination. Then, as hospitals became large and complex, the necessity to coordinate the multitude of nonroutinizable functions arose. Doctors could no longer direct an increasing number of personnel. The concern of the trustees, doctors, and patients with the economic operation of the hospital gave the administration its power (Perrow, 1963, 1969). Also, health services in general became so interdependent that the coordination of the hospital and other institutions in the community was important. For example, to facilitate hospital use, health insurance plans were inaugurated during the depression of the 1930s (Somers & Somers 1961) when hospitals were suffering from a reduction in donor contributions. Such needs for a specialized function of coordinating and administering gave rise to administrative dominance in the mid-twentieth century. The administrators were equipped to handle such matters because of their specialized training.

The operative orientation of the administrators tended to be toward financial solvency, careful budget control, efficiency, and the minimal development of services. Just as there are disadvantages to trustee and physician domination, so there are with administrators, who tend to discourage more expensive, long-term investments, such as for preventive medicine, research, and training.

Multiple Domination. As the hospital organization reached its current complexity and maturity, every component of the system tended to fulfill vital functions. Because of functional indispensability and interdependence, it is difficult for any single component to monopolize power in our large voluntary hospitals. More and more contemporary hospitals are viewed as multiple dominance models where medical, administrative, and community power structures are intricately interwoven.

In sum, the environmental influences upon the hospital have been most manifest in the areas of social values and technology. Commonly held societal values, such as religious and scientific values, molded the goals of the hospital. When religious value was predominant and scientific technology low, the hospital's goals were defined in terms of charitable custody of the helpless. Later, the ascendancy of medical technology through the advent of germ theory designated the hospital goal to be the curing of disease without much concern for caring about the patients.

Modern General Hospital

Adaptation

The hospital as an open social system is inextricably bound to the conditions of its environment. It must obtain support from the community both in the form of resources and in social legitimacy. Also a constant adjustment is necessary since the environment, especially its technological aspect, is rapidly changing.

The efficacy of a hospital depends upon the extent to which its organizational operation is appropriately matched with the nature of the environment (Thompson, 1967). Blankenship and Elling (1962) ascertained the extent to which hospitals closely aligned with the community power structure would fare better in obtaining community support, particularly funding. Schumaker's (1965) study also indicated a positive association between hospital prestige and administrators' participation in community affairs. Studying a 300-bed voluntary hospital, Perrow (1961) showed that the hospital's claim to prestige was based on indirect indexes of quality of care—reputation of staff and amount of free care. There are few occasions when the goals of a hospital may be properly evaluated by consumers, but emphasis on such external referents tend to subvert the quality of care.

In recent years, external control of the hospital has become more explicit than before. Third-party payers (the federal and state governments) and the public have been increasingly concerned about the enormous rise in hospital costs. Pressures have mounted to check these cost hikes. Since the enactment of the Medicare and Medicaid bills, various programs (preadmission testing, extended-stay review, and discharge planning) have been implemented to stabilize costs of hospital care (Somers & Somers, 1977).

For instance, in order to reduce the number of admissions, a preadmission certificate (PAT) has been required by some third-party payers (Israel, 1973). This certification process is intended to ensure that only those patients that require hospitalization are admitted. However, as initial results became available, abuse and ineffectiveness of PAT were discovered (Mebs & Brewer, 1971).

Based on the data of 60 Massachusetts hospitals, Dambaugh and Neuhauser (1976) confirmed that PAT has a negligible effect on the length of hospitalization. The result was attributed to (1) the lack of financial incentive to shorten length of stay through PAT because the hospital is reimbursed fully for patients who stay overnight; (2) administrative inefficiency in scheduling different admission flows for patients with and without PAT; and (3) the medical staff's reluctance to admit patients shortly before surgery.

Ideally, a PAT program will not only decrease length of stay but also enhance efficiency by redistributing workloads in the admissions and diagnostic departments. However, in order to attain the maximum benefits of a new program, such as PAT, installed in response to external pressures, the structure and functions of the hospital have to be rearranged. Shortell (1976) suggests that there is a greater need for internal flexibility when the hospital is operating in a highly complex, diverse, unstable, and uncertain environment.

Type of Hospital. It has been observed that the operational goals of the hospital vary according to its relationship to the environment. Roos, Shermerhorn, and Roos (1974) proposed an exchange model, which postulates that society exchanges resources with health services. In other words, hospital goals and structure will be shaped by the proportion of the organization's need for resources from outside.

The proprietary hospital is ineligible for government funds, neither does it attract philanthropic supporters. This, however, insulates the hospital from external pressures upon its operational decisions. The operational goal of the proprietary hospitals reflects their need to solicit paying patients and community doctors in the face of the general scarcity of capital. Thus, privately owned proprietary hospitals are likely to pursue the goal of efficiency in order to make a profit.

In contrast, community-sponsored voluntary (nonprofit) hospitals are unencumbered by the profit motive. They are exempt from federal income tax and local property tax, and receive community and government funds. These financial arrangements provide little incentive for efficiency. Instead, voluntary hospitals can concentrate on delivery of high-quality care. Traditionally, voluntary hospitals have been characterized as the "physician's workshop" where the physician comes to administer care to individual patients. Thus the community hospitals are closely bound to the demands and needs of their medical staffs, whose first loyalty is to the medical profession. Also, the suppliers of the funds (governmental and philanthropic) as well as the middle class and upper class patients to whom these hospitals cater expect high-quality medical care.

State and local government hospitals, on the other hand, must provide access to all members of the community, regardless of their ability to pay. Access is an important goal. Yet, being funded by government resources, these hospitals are highly susceptible to fiscal considerations. In order to meet staffing needs, the government hospitals rely heavily upon interns and residents. This affiliation with the medical school allows the medical school to exert pressure for quality care.

In short, the exchange model (Roos, Shermerhorn, & Roos, 1974) stresses the network of interdependence binding an organization to essential resource suppliers in its environment.

Board of Trustees. The board of trustees holds the hospital in trust for the community (Burling et al., 1956), and it is the responsibility of the board to ensure that the hospital fulfills the conditions of that trust. In this sense, the trustees constitute the ultimate source of hospital authority.

Board members are usually chosen from the residents of the immediate community and are prominent community members who have attained high status in business or in the professions. A potential board member's strategic position in the community is given first consideration and is chiefly a function of abilities to influence the press, the city government, the private donors, and public opinion for the benefit of the hospital. By and large, the composition of a board reflects the characteristics and social relations of the surrounding community, and the trustees act as a bridge between the hospital and the local community (Pfeffer, 1973). However, there are many studies indicating that the board members are recruited from elite groups and do not share the views on health policy generally held by consumers (Riska & Taylor, 1978).

Some social scientists claim that the board controls the organization in name only, while others maintain that the organization is controlled by the board. Still others (Pfeffer, 1973) identified two functions of the board—the links to the community and to the administration—and examined the power of the board in connection with the hospital's dependence upon its environment.

Support from the community is essential for hospitals that rely heavily on private donations for capital expenditures (i.e., private nonprofit hospitals). To the extent that large capital expenditure is needed for expansion, the success of such a hospital is reported by some (Blankenship & Elling, 1962; Holloway et al., 1963) to rest upon how well the board represents the economic powers in the community. However, as community life becomes more bureaucratized, the economic elite appears to withdraw from the more formal and visible statuses of power such as public offices. Instead, they manage to exert influence through less conspicuous channels such as secondary-level committee work (Form & Miller, 1960; Holloway et al., 1963).

On the other hand, in the government-sponsored hospitals the organization is not as immediately and directly linked to the support of the local environment. In these hospitals, administrative and technical expertise are emphasized (Pfeffer, 1973). According to Zald's (1969) study, the board's knowledge of hospital administration is directly related to the proportion of the budget supplied by the federal government and inversely related to the size of the budget.

Thus, the organization's relationship to the environment affects the adaptive function of the hospital board, which in turn influence other functions of the hospital.

Latency

The hospital as a social system with its distinct identity must be able to cultivate and maintain staff members' identification with organizational goals. However, staff consensus in beliefs, sentiments, and goals cannot be assumed but must be empirically verified (Kurtz et al., 1962).

For example, in his study of Yankee hospital, Wessen (1972) discerned five hospital goals: patient care, community service, education, instrumental aims, and research. Education refers to the training of personnel through formal programs, while community service provides health care valuable to all residents of the area whether they be sick or well. Instrumental aims pertain to the hospital's goal of self-preservation by maintaining the esteem of the community, by keeping patients and employees satisfied, and by remaining solvent. Wessen found that strikingly few of the above goals of a hospital could be verbalized by his interviewees. Although the primary aim of patient care was recognized quite universally by doctors, nurses, and other employees, the doctors emphasized educational and community service purposes more heavily than others. The nonprofessionals were most insistent upon the importance of the hospital's instrumental aims. Obviously, status differences in the hospital are associated with differences in perception of the goals of the institution. Furthermore, commitment to hospital goals has frequently been associated with an individual member's perceived fulfillment of important work values (Larson & Palola, 1961; Palola & Larson, 1965).

The board of trustees is likely to view the hospital as a community resource that is to provide an optimal quality of care to the community residents. The trustees are prone to see themselves as advocates and surrogates for the community's interests. They expect the hospital to be managed efficiently and to be financially solvent. Although they are not technical experts with respect to hospital affairs in either a medical or administrative sense, their identification with the hospital as its governing body is strong. They frequently intervene when decisions and policies of the administrative and medical staffs influence the direction of the hospital, especially in the case of the distribution of its resources.

The administrators tend to consider the hospital as a complex managerial apparatus, dealing with the aggregate of patients and staff personnel. The administrators may regard themselves as the coordinators and managers of the process of production of health care and community services. The function of the administrator is not only to direct and oversee the various business-oriented activities associated with the hospital, but also to ensure that the institution operates economically. Even a nonprofit designation does not exonerate the voluntary hospital from the demands imposed by ownership upon the efficiency of the organization.

Within broad limits, physicians are inclined to perceive themselves as the central authoritative figures and the final arbiters in the making of clinical and related decisions. In their minds, the hospital is an instrument designed to serve them and their patients. All other personnel are facilitators of their work. The power of the physicians stems from their monopoly of technical expertise, which is vital to the attainment of hospital goals.

However, professional autonomy is no longer completely intact. Physicians' performances are slowly but increasingly coming under scrutiny by patients and those third parties who are concerned with the quality of care in the face of soaring medical cost.

In general, the above three groups—the board, the administrators, and the physicians—constitute the power structure of the hospital and are more likely than other lower-ranking workers to identify themselves with hospital goals, although they diverge in orientation. In contrast, nonphysician, ancillary health workers (nurses, physician's assistants, therapists, technicians, and pharmacists) may be more inclined to identify with their immediate medical supervisors than with the hospital (Pearlin, 1962). Legitimacy of their work must be validated by the physician's approval that their performance meets the standards set by the physician.

More and more, however, ancillary health practitioners are asserting their right to participate in the decision-making process. They expect the hospital to provide a legitimate opportunity for the expression of their professional interests as members of the health care team. Also, they consider themselves as advocates for the patients against physicians who tend to view patients as disease entities rather than as persons.

Finally, there are the nonprofessional, lower-ranking workers. As hospitals have grown in complexity, an increasing variety of occupational skills are needed to meet the expanding demands. A large number of unskilled and semiskilled, nonprofessional and semiprofessional workers are now employed; without them hospitals could not function. For instance, white-collar workers prepare and transmit a large part of the paper work and the messages that keep the hospitals functioning.

Some of the lower-ranking employees feel a strong identification with the aims of their organization and develop a loyalty to the administration. Others view their work in the hospital as a stepping stone to a better job and do not complain about their low-ranking position. However, there are a great many lower-ranking employees for whom the job means merely earning a living and does not provide any psychological reward. To make it worse, their salaries have traditionally been low (Boyer, Westerhaus, & Coggeshall, 1975).

In line with the functionalist assumption, those with less important functions are less well integrated into the system. There have been many studies indicating the sense of alienation of low-ranking workers (Georgopoulos, 1975). In recent years, however, unionization of low-ranking employees is raising their power in relation to administrators as well as physicians. The immediate result of unionization may be an increased labor–management conflict, but the improvement of the status and working conditions for these workers is likely to enhance their sense of integration and identification with the organization.

Integration

The organization shown in Figure 7.2 is typical of the structure of the general hospital. In order to coordinate the diverse activities of various components, the hospital must be concerned with the four major tasks of integration.

First of all, the hospital is based on the delicate balance of a triadic power relation among the board of trustees, the administrative staff, and the medical staffs. The balance is affected by both internal and external forces. Second, the dual lines of authority, characteristic of a hospital, must be well coordinated. One line of administrative control runs from the governing board through administrative personnel. The other line of control is the medical hierarchy,

Figure 7.2: Organization of a General Hospital

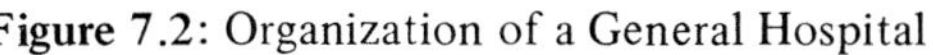

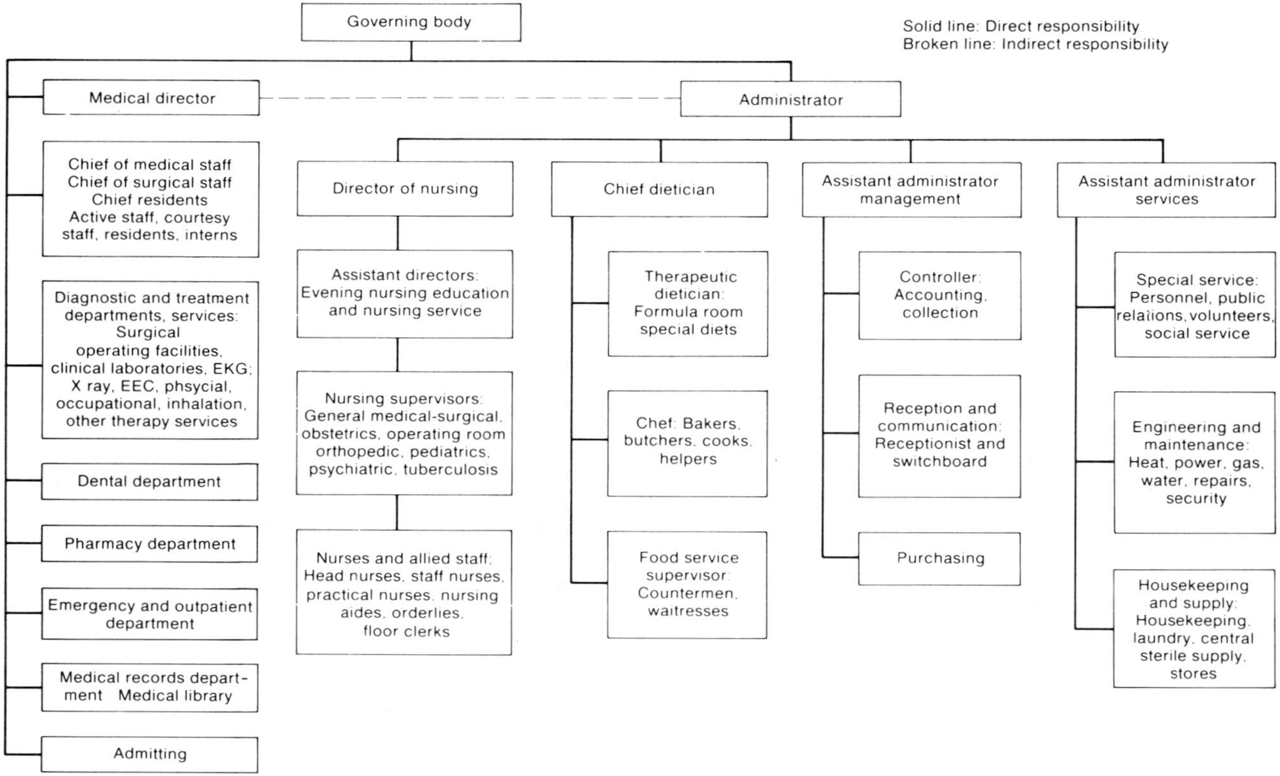

Source: U.S. Department of Labor, Manpower Administration, Office of Manpower Policy, Evaluation, and Research, *Technology and Manpower in the Health Service Industry* (Manpower Research Bulletin No. 14). May, 1967.

consisting of medical and paramedical staff members.

Third, the hospital must deal with the cleavage between upper- and lower-ranking personnel. In the upper brackets, medical staff members are likely to be committed to the medical profession, while administrative personnel tend to identify with the hospital organization. However, for those in the lower strata, whether they are orderlies or janitors, hospital employment may be nothing but a means for survival. The hospital must be able to integrate lower- as well as upper-ranking personnel into the system so as to motivate their work efficiency.

Finally, there is an important subunit in the hospital, the ward, which consists of regular members such as physicians and nurses, and of temporary ancillary personnel such as laboratory technicians, therapists, and social workers.The ward is also in close contact with other units in the hospital such as the medical chart room, pharmacy, laboratory, and the X-ray room.

Triad of Power Relations. Within the hospital, the board of trustees deals primarily with the administrative and medical staffs. The relations with both types of staffs are laden with the fundamental conflict of lay versus expert authority. The trustees are not technical experts with respect to hospital matters, yet they have prestige and power in the community that are usually at least as great as those of the physicians and the administrators.

Frequently, a number of the administrators are members or officers of the board of trustees, although the advisability of this mixture has been a relatively controversial issue among hospital officials (Rosenkrantz, 1967; Shortell et al., 1976). In comparison with the situation in a large industry, the hospital administrators are given much less discretionary power by the trustees and are tied much more closely to the board and its wishes. The trustees may intervene concerning the administrator's authority in such areas as long-range planning, capital financing, and selection and tenure of trustees.

The influence of the trustees on doctors is inclined to take indirect channels through liaison committees, or the administrators, or informal individual communications between a board member and a physician (Burling et al., 1956). The board has very little direct authority over doctors because the latter function on the basis of their professional self-regulation.

Dual Authority Lines. The hospital has been described by many investigators as a prototype organization, one that is under the conflicting imperatives of cost-saving efficiency and professionalism. Professional values encourage both the autonomy and the separation of managerial responsibilities from the medical staff. The norm of economic efficiency, on the other hand, imposes the requirement of close coordination and integration of the functional elements of the organization. This amorphous structure makes the hospital administrator's task difficult and even tenuous at times.

One of the greatest conflicts for the hospital administrator is found in the differential perception of authority that exists between the administrator and the doctors (Bates & Whites, 1961). Doctors exert power derived from their monopoly of technical expertise. Their ability to intervene in the hospital procedures on the basis of medical emergencies provides especially powerful leverage (Hall, 1954). It is actually possible for doctors to label an ambiguous event as an emergency (against the decision made by the administrative sector) merely to gain resources they believe they need.

A good example is provided by Taylor (1970). In the hospital he described, the normal procedure for patient admission requires that the request form be signed by a private physician and approved by the administrative personnel. When the latter finds the patient undesirable because of a previously unpaid hospital bill or a bad reputation as a credit risk, the patient would be refused admission. In such a situation, a physician might label the case as an emergency, which would override the administrative routine. Frequent use of emergency requests is viewed as illegitimate by administrators, resulting in conflict between the medical and administrative sectors.

Another source of power enjoyed by the doctors at the expense of the administrator is their socioeconomic independence from the hospital. A doctor who functions as a volunteer worker or who is a guest serving and being served by the hospital, is free from many bureaucratic obligations. However, the greater the physician's commitment to the hospital, the more inclined he or she is to use the regular channels of bureaucratic authority (Freidson, 1975b).

Usually, some agreement is reached as to who should have authority in what areas. Tasks involving everyday, routine hospital operations are left solely to the administrative staff even though those activities include the responsibility for the conduct of the medical staff. However, there are many grey areas, such as the purchase of medical equipment and employment of medical personnel, where both groups claim the legitimacy of their own power. When the hospital administrator decides to intervene in the use and payment of salaried medical specialists, to control the quality of surgery, or the use of proper techniques, his authority may be questioned by the medical staff. Thus, the administration tends to consider the medical staff irresponsible when it comes to spending money (Duff & Hollingshead, 1968), while physicians tend to judge administrators as being incapable of making decisions that involve medical services.

However, the antipathy between the administrator and the doctors may also be more ritualistic than real. Despite verbal distaste for administrative duties, a quarter of the doctors in a large hospital, according to a study by Goss (1962), did not rank administration as the least interesting among various other activities such as research, teaching, and community service. Also, the more time they spent in administration, the more they came to like it.

It has been suggested (Goss, 1962) that some doctors like administrative activities but feel compelled to express a ritual repugnation lest they should be judged as nonprofessional by their colleagues. In addition, physicians with experience and concern for the future may see the long-range policy implications of administrative activity upon professional areas and so may undertake administrative tasks willingly. Research findings indicate that the greater involvement and participation of medical staff members in hospital-wide decisions increases physician awareness, resulting in beneficial effects not only on control of hospital costs but on quality of care (Schultz, 1972; Shortell, 1974b; Shortell et al., 1976).

The Nurses. Nurses serve as an adjunct to both the medical and the administrative authorities, but their position carries a professional identity of its own. The functional quality of nurses is contingent upon their relation to physicians (Mauksch, 1965) in carrying out treatment and patient care. At the same time, nurses must manage an aggregate of cases in an administratively acceptable manner.

Functionalists view the nurses' role as marginal and stressful. In contrast, conflict perspectives emphasize the balance of power that the nurse holds in determining the outcome of any bargaining that may arise between a patient and the staff (Freidson, 1975b). Since they have the strategic advantage of being on the floor at all times, nurses have bargaining power with physicians, using their firsthand knowledge and professional evaluation of what is taking place with patients. Then, on the other side of the coin, they can negotiate for power with patients by utilizing their access to physicians. That two-edged position along with their possession of inside information makes nurses a key to patient comfort and recovery.

Within the formal structure of the hospital, the nurses' position is subordinate to a dual authority. Yet through the informal interactional process, they can exert power to the extent of changing the formal structure and of increasing efficiency. The amount of their power, however, is delimited by the rigidity of the social structure in the hospital, the degree of professional specialization, and the personal qualifications and personality of the nurses themselves.

Nonprofessional, Lower-Ranking Workers. In the past many lower-ranking hospital workers recognized that they had little or no formal authority. Also, the only kind of pressure they exerted was limited to informal and subtle manipulation of their superiors in relatively trivial matters that would not affect the basic structure of the hospital. For instance, a telephone operator could exert pressure on a doctor and bargain for cooperation by threatening to report him or her to the administration for not responding to paging.

Sources of such power were listed by Mechanic (1962c) as follows: (1) expertise—lower-ranking personnel with expert knowledge not available to higher-ranking personnel are likely to have power over them; (2) effort and interest—lower-ranking workers gain power when higher-ranking employees do not devote enough effort and interest to a task; (3) attractiveness—personality and appearance are universally related to a person's access to power; and (4) location and position—the closer a person is located to the center of an organization, the greater is his or her access to power.

In the long run, the accumulated influence exerted by low-authority groups could reach beyond everyday trivialities and affect the long-term organizational policies as well. Be that as it may, power of this type is an indirect force in comparison with the more direct approach taken by hospital workers' unions in recent years. In the past decade or two unionization has become the major tactic for low-authority workers to wrest control over their work from management.

A movement toward unionization was facilitated by several social factors in conjunction with dissatisfaction with low pay. During the 1960s the civil rights movement politicized blacks and women, who occupy the major portion of the low-ranking hospital positions. They were alerted to the powerless positions they held and began to organize themselves to bring about structural changes in the hospital. This movement of hospital employees is in conformity with the general trend toward unionization in contemporary society (Krause, 1977; Metzger & Pointer, 1972).

The immediate implication of the unionization drive for the hospital is an increased labor–management conflict. As workers establish themselves as collective bargaining agents, they are more likely to engage in strikes that are highly disruptive to organizational functioning. On the other hand, conflict may bring about needed change and improvement that would not occur in a system which is assumed to be integrated in the functionalist sense of the term. Whether or not the new structure born out of the dialectic change is more effective than the previous one in attaining hospital goals remains to be seen.

The Ward. The heart of the hospital is the patient ward, where the basic work of the hospital is performed. Various wards have been compared in terms of their stratification and integration since these characteristics are directly related to internal communications and to the activities of the personnel.

Status distinction is a direct result of stratification, and it is so pronounced in the hospital that the expected manner of deference is actually taught to student nurses as part of their professional adjustment course (Wessen, 1972). These status levels are reinforced symbolically by the distinctive uniforms worn by the various categories of personnel, by separate dining rooms, and even by separate seating arrangements.

Segregation through this caste-like arrangement puts strong limitations on informal interaction. Ward personnel tend to interact mostly with those of their own peer group. According to a study by Wessen (1972), while in the ward, doctors are three times more apt to speak to other doctors than to nurses, and they almost never talk with any of the other personnel. Likewise, the nurses are more than twice as likely to speak with other nurses than to other workers. These caste barriers to informal communications in the ward and in the hospital at large tend to foster disparate attitudes within the various strata and are dysfunctional to the system's integration.

Goal Attainment

The ultimate purpose of organizational research is to identify the determinants of organizational effectiveness: what are the variables that facilitate goal attainment? Thus, the effects of environmental factors, structural and functional variables of the hospital system, and their interlocking multivariate feedback effects on goal attainment need to be researched. However, there have been only a few studies that deal with the interrelations of all the variables as they relate to goal attainment (Georgopoulos, 1975). We will examine below some of the major issues discussed in the areas of hospital goal attainment.

Size–Complexity–Performance. There is a general correlation between hospital size and the distribution of most facilities and services. As hospital size increases, so does the likelihood that the hospital offers a particular facility or service. Those facilities or services that involve complex equipment, a large capital investment, more highly skilled personnel, and educational programs are more likely to be found in large rather than small hospitals (Heydebrand, 1973).

According to the survey by the American Hospital Association (1977), an emergency room and inhalation therapy are frequently offered in hospitals with more than 50 beds. The percentage of community hospitals with fewer than 50 beds that have an inhalation therapy department is markedly lower than the percentage that have an emergency facility. Among those services that are offered only in large hospitals are histopathology, electroencephalography, premature nursery, and therapeutic radioisotope facilities (see Figure 7.3).

Figure 7.3: Percent of Community Hospitals Reporting Selected Facilities and Services, by Bed-size Category, 1976

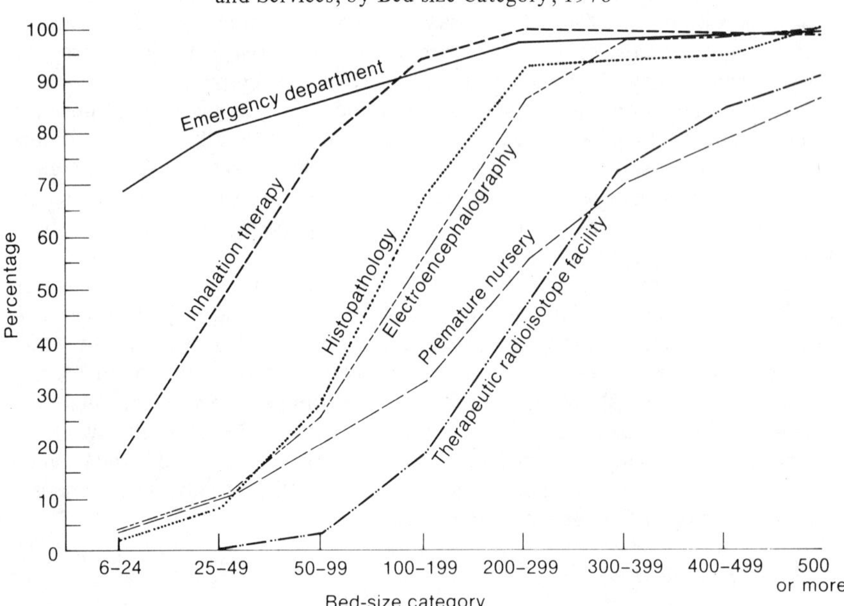

Source: Reprinted, with permission from *Hospital Statistics,* 1977 edition, published by the American Hospital Association, p. x, fig. 3.

This relationship between size and resources of organizations is also found in administrative spheres. Management qualifications, which strongly influence all organizations, tend to vary with the size of the hospital. It is not surprising that the administrations of the larger hospitals are better trained and more experienced than are their counterparts in the smaller institutions (Neuhauser, 1966). However, in terms of administrative intensity—that is, the proportion of organized resources allocated to administration—there is a tendency for the larger hospitals to be lower on this score (Anderson & Warkov, 1961;

Heydebrand, 1973). The smaller hospitals seem to place greater emphasis on bureaucratic procedures and to show a greater degree of intersector conflict, although this pattern varies with the type of organization and the operational definitions of size and administrative intensity.

Faced with inconsistent findings concerning the relationship between the size and resources with respect to goal attainment, some researchers have claimed that size is not in itself a critical characteristic of the organization. In fact, many investigators found that large size is not significantly related to better hospital performance (Scott, Forrest, & Brown, 1976; Starkweather, 1970).

Variables such as complexity, coordination, and centralization of decision-making have been identified as intervening in the relationship between size and organizational effectiveness (Georgopoulos, 1975). For instance, Thompson (1967) hypothesized that when the differentiation among hospital units is high, the greater the coordination of those units and the better the quality of care. Based on the data on surgical patients in 742 voluntary or community, nonprofit hospitals, Scott, Forrest, and Brown (1976) rejected, at the overall hospital or ward level, this hypothesis, that more highly differentiated hospitals provide better care only if they devote special attention to coordination. However, in the operating room, coordination was found to be important (Scott, Forrest, & Brown, 1976).

Stratification–Performance. As for vertical coordination (stratification), negative effects of stratification upon hospital goal attainment have been documented by many. These include the association found between rigid stratification and low performance of personnel, a sense of alienation, and job dissatisfaction.

The work of Seeman and Evans (1961) at a 600-bed university-affiliated general hospital serves as a good example. Stratification of the 14 wards was measured by nurses' descriptions of the attending physicians' behavior patterns—for example, requiring the nurses to follow the medical hierarchical dictates in reporting any marked change in the patient's condition, treating lightly suggestions made by those below them, or keeping professional distance from the other ward personnel. Performance was assessed by objective data based on medical records, reputational measures derived from superiors' ratings of the interns, and subjective reports of the interns on their own behavior.

Criteria of performance were developed in terms of hospital functions: selection (sorting patients to proper treatment categories), supply (distributing equipment, personnel, and supplies), service (such as providing medication to the patients), communication (channeling consultations among various physicians), control (guaranteeing required environmental conditions such as isolation of infectious diseases), discovery (advancing medical knowledge by way of research), and teaching (disseminating medical knowledge through nurses' training and instruction to patients).

Using the above method, Seeman and Evans found that ward stratification is related to performance. The highly stratified wards are characterized by (1) poor communication with and about patients, (2) poor teaching functions, (3) less adequate consultation (especially in psychiatric and social service areas), (4) a high turnover of nurses, and (5) lower-quality performance by interns. In short, a high degree of stratification appears to hamper the effective communication necessary for therapeutic teamwork.

Technology–Stratification–Efficiency. Having reanalyzed the data of Seeman and Evans (1961), Perrow (1969) demonstrated that the best performing units are the surgical wards, which are highly stratified, and the medical wards that are the least stratified (e.g., the emergency room). In other words, performance is a function of the combined effects of stratification and technology.

The importance of technology in determining the ward structure and functioning has been shown by many comparative studies. Different wards have distinctive assignments and use varied methods in performing these jobs. Technology available in the ward is likely to affect the social structure and the functioning of the ward (Burling et al., 1956; Perrow, 1969).

Coser's (1958) study illustrates the effects of technology upon ward structure and interpersonal relations. Comparing surgical and medical wards, Coser noted their basic differences in tasks and technology. In a surgical ward therapy is rapid, specific, and conclusive, and the surgeon's action-oriented, decisive decision-making is endorsed by strongly committed subordinates. In contrast, the tasks in the medical ward are frequently accompanied by ambiguous diagnoses, alternative therapies, tentative decision-making, and trial-and-error information processes.

Such variations in means and ends affect the communication and activities in the wards. The surgical ward is autocratic in that the attending surgeon, especially the chief resident, makes all of the decisions. On the next lower level of authority, however, a roughly equal status prevails between the assistant residents, interns, and nurses. This makes for a common bond between them. With so little authority delegated to them, the assistant residents and interns cannot hold a position that is consistently superior to that of the nurses. This equalitarianism under despotism encourages a collegial type of relationship between the nurses and the doctors. Hence, banter, joking, and informal interaction are seen in the surgical ward.

Actually, the position of the nurse in the surgical ward resembles what Jules Henry (1954) called the "oak tree" setup, a situation wherein orders come down to a particular person from many sources. This multiple subordination makes the nurse's role stressful, but it also gives him or her greater importance as well as a more active part in therapy.

In contrast, the medical ward is characterized by Henry's "pine tree" type, wherein authority is consistently delegated down the line. In that ward, nurses have few creative tasks in patient care, and they tend to perform routine jobs ritualistically. Interaction and communication in the medical ward are formal and polite and seldom are accompanied by joking or swearing. Unlike the surgical nurses, the medical nurses only talk to those immediately above them, and rarely communicate with the personnel at any higher level.

Another example of the effect of technology upon the ward structure is found in the study of the emergency room (Mannou, 1975). Here, the task is characterized by (1) uncertainty of workload, (2) inability to control the workload, and (3) urgency and decisiveness in decision-making (Roth, 1972). As a result, timing, the managing of patients, and decision-making are the paramount ingredients of technology required in creating an orderly environment with unpredictable patient problems. Because of the urgency of the decision-making and the open context in which the doctor's work is observed by ancillary personnel, decision-making tends to be shared and negotiated between the doctors and nurses.

The hospital ward dealing with the terminally ill has a special function to perform. The goal is not to cure but to respond to the psychological needs of dying patients. Technology adopted in this context is described by Strauss and Glaser (Glaser & Strauss, 1965, 1968; Strauss & Glaser, 1970) as a ritual of pretense. American physicians ordinarily do not inform the patient outright that death is imminent, since the news may be a fatal blow. The staff members as well as the patient carry on the pretense that death is not probable, or at least not imminent.

A persistent practice of such pretense affects the more permanent aspect of hospital organization. The personnel must organize themselves as a team to guard against disclosure. Another structural consequence is the increased nurse's burden, namely, the nurse's commitment to work relatively closely with and around dying patients. Teamwork and the functional importance of the nurse's role are likely to produce an equalitarian structure in the ward that deals with the terminally ill.

Control versus Performance. Traditionally, the hospital has been characterized by contradictory goals (quality versus efficiency) and incompatible structures (professional autonomy versus administrative bureaucracy). The assumption was made that the best medical care would be provided if professionals were free to exercise their judgment without external control. Recently, this position has been challenged by many organizational researchers, who claim that organizational performance will be improved to the extent that decision-makers can and do evaluate the consequences of their programs—in short, to the extent that "consequences are visible" (Becker & Gordon, 1966; Gordon, Tanon, & Morse, 1976). In other words, greater specification of procedures designed to increase the visibility of consequences is related to higher-level organizational performance, such as a better balance between centralized and decentralized coordination.

In order to test the above hypothesis, Shortell and others (1976) studied 42 of the 58 short-term, voluntary, nonteaching hospitals of 100 beds or more in Massachusetts. The degree of specification of work procedures is measured by the extent to which medical and nonmedical department heads and staff members are free to decide what, when, where, and how their work is done. Hospital efficiency is examined by direct costs per patient day in medical and nonmedical areas. Quality of care is assessed by the medical-surgical death rate and the postoperative complication rate (while controlling for the effect of severity of case).

Shortell and others (1976) found that the administrative visibility of consequences is related to hospital efficiency. Both medical and nonmedical costs are lower in those hospitals where administrators are able to compare the performance levels of their hospitals with those of other hospitals (Neuhauser, 1971).

In the medical sphere, Shortell's group also found a positive correlation between visibility of consequence and quality of medical care. In other words, the greater the degree of autonomy of doctors, the higher the death rates in the hospitals. Conversely, a more structured medical staff is associated with higher-quality care, which is in line with other research findings (Becker & Neuhauser, 1975; Rhee, 1977; Roemer & Friedman, 1971).

The relationship between control and quality of care has also been studied among surgeons. The data based on 8,000 patients treated by 500 surgeons in 15 short-term general hospitals (Flood & Scott, 1978; Scott, Forrest, & Brown, 1976) indicate a positive association between the quality of surgical care (i.e., mortality and morbidity rate adjusted to presurgical conditions) and surgical staff control (i.e., strictness of requirements for gaining admission to surgical staff membership).

Physicians on hospital medical staffs have in the past experienced much autonomy. Technical incompetence frequently went unobserved, uncommunicated, and unsanctioned, at least formally (Freidson & Rhea, 1963). The general tightening of professional standards and greater specification of medical staff activities in recent years seems to have resulted in a higher quality of care. However, the optimal balance between autonomy and control among medical staff members is yet to be reached.

The complexity of the relationship between control and performance is illustrated by Becker and Neuhauser's (1975) study comparing hospitals and other organizations. In the medical component of the hospital, where tasks are less routine and predictable than in the administrative section, general hierarchical specification of procedures (low physician participation and control) was *negatively* related to efficiency, while specification of procedures to increase visibility of consequences was *positively* related to efficiency.

As for the relationship between the administration and the medical staffs, Shortell and others (1976) reported that the increased administrative visibility of consequence had a positive impact on quality of medical care. Some of the mechanisms designed to increase visibility of consequences in administrative operations (e.g., determining the appropriateness of hospital admission or the numbers and types of tests and examination) is associated not only with cost control but with a higher quality of care. The more efficient hospitals (those with lower costs per case) deliver a higher quality of care as indicated by a lower death rate and lower postsurgical complications. Flood and Scott (1978) also reported that greater power by the hospital administration is strongly associated with better quality of medical care.

In order to interpret these findings some researchers have given credit to the administrative role in providing coherence and coordination in a medical work situation frought with fragmentation and overspecialization (Georgopoulos & Mann, 1962; Perrow, 1961). Shortell and others (1976), on the other hand, suggested that concern for efficiency may lead to more careful attention to patient care. In short, efficiency and quality of care are not contradictory. Furthermore, quality of care refers not only to a lower mortality rate but also to innovativeness. Gordon and others (1976) report that visibility of consequences permits a decentralized organizational structure to be effective, which in turn provides impetus for innovation (Morse, Gordon, & Moch, 1974).

Traditionally, professional autonomy has been considered an essential ingredient for high-quality medical practice. It has been assumed that professionals can perform best when they are left unencumbered by administrative bureaucratic regimentation. However, studies centering around the notion of visibility of consequences, such as those reviewed above, make this assumption suspect. In recent years the extent of specification of work procedures is increasing due to growing bureaucratization of medicine. Also, the attempt to increase visibility of consequences is more vigorously pursued by the third-party payers of medical expenses (Somers & Somers, 1977). And increased control over medical practice appears to be accompanied by better medical care, at least in some studies. However, in order to answer whether or not further control of medical practice will result in improved medical care, more systematic studies concerning the interrelations between the environmental and the organizational variables must be made.

THE MENTAL HOSPITAL

The "Total Institution" Model

The General Hospital versus the Mental Hospital

Both general and mental hospitals have the official goal of patient care and recovery. They each use the ward as the primary functional unit; the staff consists of the same major occupational groups; and they maintain a similar division of function. Their overall formal bureaucratic structures are also quite similar.

The major differences between the two organizations begin with their operative goals and the availability of technology to attain these goals (Perrow, 1969). In the general hospital, patients typically stay for a short period of time, during which recovery and healing through physical therapy is the primary goal. Staff–patient relationships remain limited in scope. In the case of mental patients, the hospital is their community in that it is where they receive treatment, engage in work, and acquire friends during their stay for an indefinite period. Thus, the operative goals of the mental hospital are custodial as well as therapeutic.

The technology available in dealing with these tasks varies between the two kinds of hospitals. Except for a few drugs and shock treatments, therapeutic success in psychiatry is much less definitive than is the case in the general hospital. This situation makes the role of the psychiatrist marginal (Holt & Luborsky, 1958; Sharaf & Levinson, 1964; Smith, 1957) and extends the role of the psychiatric aide (Belknap, 1956; Hyde, 1955; Schwartz & Shockley, 1956; von Mering & King, 1957).

These functional differences in operative procedures lead to structural differences in terms of the allocation of authority and the development of communication channels. In the mental hospital, many psychiatrists play administrative roles to the degree that custodial care is left in the hands of aides. Thus, the long-term impact of nurses and aides upon the patients becomes crucial to their recovery. In contrast, the general hospital is characterized by a clear division of labor between the medical, ancillary, and lay occupations.

There is also a sharp distinction between the short-term, acute disease and the long-term, chronic disease hospitals. The latter resemble the custodial mental hospital in their structure and processes (Apple, 1960; Coser, 1963; Freidson, 1970; Perrow, 1969).

Goffman's "Total Institution"

The mental hospital can be viewed as a bureaucracy (Appleby et al., 1967; Kahne, 1959), since it is an organization with a formally defined division of labor and is governed by a normatively defined code and authority pattern.

Some people have placed it in an analytically different rubric, as a community or small society (Caudill, 1958). For the patients, it is a relatively self-contained, tightly bounded world.

In an effort to combine the bureaucratic and the communal aspect of the mental hospital into a single model, Goffman (1961) developed the concept of the total institution. According to his concept, the total institution is identified by the following features: (1) it contains a large number of inmate-inhabitants whose lives are formally administered to and controlled by a small staff; (2) it is isolated from the wider society; and (3) it carries out a special goal, which influences the total personality of the inmates.

Total institutions are organizations built for the purpose of changing people and their identities, that is, for resocialization. To this end, the above mentioned characteristics of the total institution are deemed to be functional. The bringing together of co-participants to live in one place serves to break down the barriers separating different spheres of life. Isolation from outside influence and regimentation under one authority help organize different features of life within an overall plan. To the extent that inmates share the goals of the institutional administrators, the total institution has a positive effect upon them.

However, frequently the inmates of the mental hospital are not voluntarily committed. They are brought there against their will by the police, the courts, social workers, or family members. With the negative connotation imputed to mental illness, incarceration to the mental hospital distinctively stigmatizes the patient.

Furthermore, the bureaucratic management of inmates accompanied by a lack of financial and technical resources often results in generating adverse effects upon the patients. Being labeled as mentally ill and processed through the "rites of degradation" exercised by low-paid attendants, individuals are likely to become sicker as they stay longer in the total institution, Goffman claims. For details of the negative consequences of the labeling process in the total institution, readers are referred to Chapter 5.

Levinson and Gallagher (1961) criticized the image of the total institution as being too overgeneralized. They suggested that there exists considerable variation among total institutions, which range from a prison-like to a treatment-oriented center.

Functionalist Perspective. The functionalist perspective appears to be valid because the mental hospital as a total institution is a well-demarcated system to which the inmates are bound. Its operational goal is defined as custodial, that is, it protects the community from the patients (Appleby et al., 1967). The custodial task is mainly carried out by lower-ranking personnel such as nurses and aides in the relative absence of other personnel in the ward.

For a long time, this custodial goal had been endorsed by societal values that viewed mental illness as abnormal, irrational, and dangerous. The release of mental patients from the hospital was met with public criticism, and there were questions concerning the safety of the community from these people. The decision to release a patient from a mental hospital was influenced not only by a clinical evaluation of the patient but by the cooperativeness with authority figures during hospitalization as well as environmental factors such as the perceived threat to the community and the receptivity by family members to his or her return (Greenley, 1972).

The total institution may be considered well integrated to the extent that psychiatrists frequently play administrative roles, thereby minimizing value conflict between medical and administrative sectors. Although the system fans out to dual structures of medical and administrative personnel at the bottom, the organization converges again in the collaboration of attendants and business personnel who share the same negative views toward the patients.

Conflict Perspective. These functionalist assumptions of system integration have been challenged by empirical findings. The pioneer study by Stanton and Schwartz (1954), and later research by Smith (1966), Katz and Kahn (1966), March and Simon (1958), and Georgopoulos and Mann (1962), all suggest that the poor coordination that leads to organizational conflict naturally results from three different sources: poor communication, the vested interests of the occupational groups, and the lack of value consensus.

The barriers to adequate communication between echelons or departments are inherent in all large, complex organizations. In the mental hospital, staff departments, such as nursing or social work, may be completely estranged from contact with the treatment unit. Ward life may be a culture in itself that is connected with the upper stratum only by obscure written orders.

Poor coordination may stem simply from misunderstandings, but it may also result from differences in the vested interests of the subgroups. The nurses and aides may operate their wards following the principle of least effort by virtually ignoring the therapeutic goal of rehabilitating the patient. Consensus on values can never be attained in a mental hospital that subscribes to the official goal of therapy and the operative goal of custody.

In the light of these findings, the conflict perspective may be more useful than functionalism when analyzing social processes in the mental hospital. In particular, the framework of conflict functionalism, especially when dealing with functionality versus dysfunctionality of conflict within the system, may shed light and even validate hypotheses concerning incidents in the mental hospital. For instance, Stanton and Schwartz (1954) tested the hypothesis that the patients' collective disturbance is the result of staff conflict.

Interactionist Perspective. Because of the long stay of patients in the mental hospital and the all-encompassing nature of the total institution, staff–patient interaction has been of prime concern to many researchers. Beginning with the classic study by Stanton and Schwartz (1954), the interactionist perspective has been adopted by many. Numerous investigators have dealt with the patterning of everyday interactions between patients and staff in relation to the social structure and culture of the hospital.

Goffman's work in *Asylums* (1961) represents the first large-scale effort to examine the hospital from the viewpoint of the patient. Irrationality of staff behavior in dealing with patients is the key theme in his work. Perrow (1969) criticized this emphasis upon staff irrationality because it is counterposed by assumed sanity and manipulative ability of the patient.

Strauss and his associates (Strauss et al., 1963) have extended the interactive perspective from the staff–patient relation to that of the entire context of the hospital. To them, the hospital represents a series of negotiated settlements between staff members who hold different ideologies.

Historical Development

The history of the mental hospital has evolved around the rise and fall of the total institution. As a subsystem of a society, the interaction between the mental hospital and its environment has undergone vicissitudes along with changing social values.

Prior to Moral Treatment

In ancient times, the mentally disordered were viewed negatively (Rosen, 1968). Despite the occasional existence of legitimatized social roles for those who had visions or trances, psychoses per se did not lead to an exalted status. Under Roman law, the insane were deprived of civil rights such as the right to marry, to participate in elections, or to dispose of property, but there was no provision for treatment or confinement. The mentally afflicted of well-to-do families were likely to be cared for at home by a personal attendant. Those from the lower class or with no family ties became objects of ridicule, scorn, or abuse. Those who seemed to harm others were bound or placed in stocks.

Under the Christianity of the Middle Ages, mental illness was imputed to evil spirits or witchcraft more readily than under religions of antiquity. Exorcism became a widely used therapeutic technique (Mora, 1975).

By the fourteenth century, a few institutions appeared in different parts of Europe for the purpose of confining the mentally ill, often in abandoned monasteries or castles. These people lived on the periphery of society and were divorced from the world around them. The purpose of such custodial institutions was to protect the social order from the mentally disordered.

The Age of Enlightenment brought a new conception of mental disorder. The ferver for rational thought stigmatized the irrationality in the mentally disturbed, holding that it was due to a derangement of the mind. Lunatics who had been allowed to roam the streets were now beaten or confined. Foucault (1965) described the seventeenth and eighteenth centuries in Europe as the period of the "great confinement." In France, general hospitals were established, by royal edict, to provide a "reasonable regime" for those unable to govern their lives rationally.

By the early eighteenth century, the mentally ill were chained in jails and other institutions in much of Europe. At Bethlehem Hospital in London, the mental patients were even exhibited for amusement (Mora, 1975).

Moral Treatment

During the French Revolution the first great reforms in the treatment of the insane took place, based on an ideology of respect for the individual. These changing concepts were influenced by the belief in human perfectibility, which in turn suggested that insanity was not incurable. Liberal political philosophy contended that insanity was the result of the deprivation of the inflicted by a tyrannical church and government (Bockoven, 1957) and also the result of the abuse received after incarceration in the public asylums.

In the context of growing public sentiment in favor of individual rights and against oppression in all forms, the physician was favorably situated to institute a reform in the management of the institution. Mental illness was ascribed to a functional disorder of the brain that was induced by events external to the individual. It followed that treatment could be affected by arranging the environment so that the individual would be exposed only to those events which would restore inner harmony and the power of reason.

The insane were unchained and treated according to their moral rights as individuals (Bockoven, 1957). Complete humanization of the institution was advocated, and individual discourse with patients was found to be a more effective technique than medication. Consideration and a delicate feeling for the patient's state of mind were the keynotes of the moral treatment.

The superintendant-physician was in daily contact with all of the patients and saw them in a variety of situations provided by the institutional routine. The physician and attendants shared hospital living with the patients. The pattern of hospital life was not sharply different from the town or farm life of the period, when this society as a whole was not exceedingly stratified or differentiated.

The adoption of this moral treatment coincided with the ascendancy of a liberal theology and political democracy. In the United States, it was a cultural phenomenon of the nineteenth century (Foucault, 1965).

The State Mental Hospital

During the latter half of the nineteenth century, mental hospitals underwent extensive changes. With a rapid population growth, high immigration rates, increasing urbanization, dislocations due to the Civil War and to industrialization, and because of lax commitment procedures, the state mental institutions were filled rapidly. On the other hand, moral treatment was too expensive to be continued on a mass level.

From the middle of the nineteenth century, when statistics were first kept, until 1955, the number of patients incarcerated in mental hospitals increased each year, and by 1955 there were roughly 600,000 patient-residents in these hospitals.

In addition to the problem of sheer numbers, there were other, more basic reasons for the disappearance of moral treatment. In the first place many people never accepted the belief that the lunatic was curable. Second, and more important, mental illness came to be regarded as an example of nature's method of eliminating the unfit from among productive human beings (Bockoven, 1957). The idealistic philanthrophy of moral treatment was frowned upon as contrary to Darwinian evolutionism, which was taken as advocating the survival of the fittest.

The accounts that appeared in the 1940s and 1950s concerning state mental hospitals are quite similar. Large-scale sociological studies include those by Dunham and Weinberg (1960) and Belknap (1956). The state mental hospital was described in other words as a resource-deprived total institution, as later conceptualized by Goffman (1961), and it was treated more or less as a necessary evil by those responsible for its support (Perrow, 1969). The surrounding community that it served was generally ignorant of its problems, needs, and practices.

As the total institution emerged, the physician became an administrator. The superintendent of the state hospital was usually a doctor, often a psychiatrist, and the two incompatible hierarchies of administrative and medical staffs were under his or her direction. The two hierarchies merged at the bottom of the organization, where the business personnel and the attendants shared the view of the patients as incurable and disruptive.

On the medical side, the hierarchy consisted of a handful of doctors who had huge case loads but had to spend 60 percent of their time on administrative duties (Deutch, 1948). In many studies, doctors were criticized for failing to be good administrators, for being aloof from nurses and attendants, and above all, for being ineffective in treatment. But there was no appropriate treatment technology available for the public mental hospital. Electric shock treatment was performed simply to discipline the patients and to maintain order (Perrow, 1969).

Therefore, one reason why psychiatrists played administrative roles in mental hospitals was imputed by some to the fact that psychiatrists were not sure of their own role or of their technology and were fearful of incursions by others (Perrow, 1969). They wanted to hold administrative power as an extra buffer.

In the absence of therapeutic technology, the state mental hospitals adopted the goal of custodial care in place of therapy. The aim of technological treatment was of symbolic value only, and the operative goal was custody, control, and minimum care.

Using this frame of reference, Perrow (1969) described the dominance by the attendants as functional for the hospital's goal. Hospital budgets were very low due to legislators with social Darwinian beliefs who considered the level of care less important than the level of custody. Custody was in the hands of attendants who were prohibited from participating in the therapeutic role. Attendants were engaged in the most urgent and difficult task in the institution, that of controlling patients who engaged in destructive and disorderly behavior. Power most often goes to those who fulfill the most crucial assignment of any organization. Attendants, in effect, ran the wards, and thus, in many respects, the hospital.

The dominance of the business staff with its profit orientation was another consequence of the lack of any treatment technology. Budget considerations led to the replacement of the services of psychiatrists by those of less expensive personnel—nurses, social workers, and aides. Because of the symbolic importance of the psychiatrists' legitimatizing role, psychiatrists were placed in administrative positions to save the money that would normally be used to pay for professional administrators.

The Rise of Milieu Therapy and Outpatient Clinics

Ideology. A modern counterpart of the concept of moral treatment made an appearance around 1938 in the form of the "therapeutic community." There was a growing acceptance of mental illness as a disorder of the total personality that was due to and caused by the individual's interpersonal relations and life stresses. Efforts were made in mental hospitals to develop a social milieu that augmented the interpersonal and group interaction. This approach utilized all of the personnel therapeutically and tended to counter regressive tendencies (Howells, 1975).

Milieu therapy consists of (1) the development of the therapeutic potential of staff members through the cultivation in them of feelings of importance to the patients; (2) the removal of restrictive and punitive barriers between staff and patients; (3) the participation of patients in the therapeutic process; (4) the cultivation of the social environment as a therapeutic force by offering social activities; and (5) the merging of the therapeutic and larger communities (Greenblatt, 1957).

According to milieu therapy, rehabilitation of the mentally disturbed is considered more effective if the patient can remain a member of the community. The institution is desirable only for those who are dangerous to themselves or to others, or who are almost totally unable to function by themselves. President Kennedy supported the shift from inpatient to outpatient care when he signed the Community Mental Health Centers Act in 1963. That bill authorized $150 million for the construction of community mental health centers. The basic objective of that legislation was to provide mental health services for those with emotional disturbances that were too minor for hospitalization.

Inpatient service decreased drastically from 77.4 percent in 1955 to 32 percent in 1973 and has been replaced by outpatient services such as those given at community mental health centers. Even more dramatic, the 48.9

percent of psychiatric services furnished by state mental hospitals in 1955 was reduced to only 12.4 percent by 1973. Within the realm of inpatient services, those given by the state mental hospital declined from 63 percent in 1955 to 19 percent in 1973 (Dodge & Rodgers, 1976), and more and more people are using psychiatric services offered at general hospitals (Holden, 1973).

The community mental health movement was facilitated by the appearance of new therapeutic technology and new value orientations.

The adoption of certain drug therapies has reduced the number of patient-residents in the public mental hospitals. Tranquilizing drugs are considered to improve certain types of schizophrenics to a manageable state so that they can be treated outside the institution (Clausen & Huffine, 1975).

Another reason for the decline of hospitalization is found in the growing trend, during the past couple of decades, of emphasizing the harmful effects of institutionalization of the mentally ill. Moreover, the 1960s witnessed vigorous attacks on the concept of mental illness itself. Some activists attributed the etiology of mental illness to the social structure rather than to the individual psyche and advocated a therapy within the environment of ordinary community living instead of isolated hospitals (Cohen, Skhel, & Berger, 1977; Mechanic, 1978).

Implementation. The ideology behind the community mental health center movement has been well accepted in principle by psychiatrists, politicians, and the public. However, its implementation has met with many difficulties. Frequently, patients are returned to a community that provides them with few resources. The same disabilities associated with institutionalization develop in the community context in that the patients are socially isolated, unemployed, and receive little care. The mentally disabled are released to roam the streets, as they were 500 years ago.

> Five hundred years ago, boats were cruising the waterways of Europe with cargoes of unwanted madmen, castaways shoved from port to port in ships of fools.
>
> An enforced ocean voyage was an easy way to cleanse a town of strange and disturbing figures. Some were herded on pilgrimage ships taking the demented to shrines. Some were pushed off at the next harbor. Some were abandoned to the sea.
>
> In today's enlightened age of science and social conscience, thousands of mentally disabled persons are still voyagers, a fragile cargo released from state hospitals and cast adrift in contemporary ships of fools.
>
> They journey from hospital, from hospital to community—there to follow a circuit of halfway houses, flophouses and emergency rooms. Many return to the hospital (Graham, 1977, p. A6).

Because of this plight in the community there are some who want to go back to hospitals (Snider, 1973).

> A middle-aged woman kept returning like a homing pigeon to New York's Bronx State Hospital. She couldn't cope with a troubled daughter, late welfare checks and the East Bronx where she was robbed five times. She began to hear voices.
>
> Often, she would be found curled up asleep in the lobby of the hospital. Once re-admitted, she improved. "It's a jungle in the East Bronx," she says. "I'm afraid to

leave the apartment. That's slow death in itself. The hospital is better for me" (Graham, 1977, p. A6).

The lack of success of the community health movement is due to several factors: value orientation and the lack of financial and technical resources. In the first place, there is a gap between enunciation and implementation of the goal of community health service. The ideology was endorsed by President Kennedy and accepted by the public, but it was not accompanied by stable governmental funding or by a neighborhood endorsement of community mental-care facilities. Community residents subscribed to the idea so long as it was going to be practiced in other people's communities (Williams, 1977). Faced with massive resistance, mental health officials have tended to locate patients in already deteriorated areas, which is the least objectionable locale to middle class residents. The degree of community acceptance of the board-and-care facility has been shown to be the best predictor of whether or not the patient will become integrated into the community (Segal & Aviram, 1977).

Part of the difficulty with the community health movement resides in its meager financial resources. While communities were relatively quick in responding to the new administrative policy to reduce hospitalization, thereby lessening their financial burden, they have been slow in investing resources to meet the needs of patients in the community (Chu & Trotter, 1974). In an attempt to protect their budget, various agencies shift the responsibilities to others, leaving needy patients to nursing and boarding houses, substandard facilities run for profit, or even to migrant labor camps and prostitution (Graham, 1977). Privately owned facilities are operated mainly for monetary gain. Since these facilities are few in number and the demand is great, they never lack for clients awaiting placement and therefore are not motivated to provide more than elementary services at a minimum cost to themselves.

In addition to deficiencies in financial resources, community mental-care technologies are still underdeveloped. There are some excellent arrangements that improve the quality of the patient's life, but many facilities provide physical and social care not much better than, if not inferior to, that of public mental hospitals (Segal & Aviram, 1977; Stotsky, 1970).

The organization of effective community care distinct from traditional hospital programs requires a major shift from conventional bureaucratic and hierarchical perspectives (Morris, 1976). The decentralization process from the custodial to the therapeutic orientation is a complex and idiosyncratic one (Levy & Rowtiz, 1975). It is still tentative and no classifiable stages of development are clear. One of the major problems is a cleavage in the control structure. A large, centrally administered hospital has been broken up into small, autonomous divisions with decentralized staffs. Units are thus supposed to be autonomous, yet staff members are aware of many levels of control, such as institutional, managerial, and technical, by virtue of their residing in a broader organizational context (Costonis, 1966). It is a gross oversimplification to assert that democratic decision-making alone will result in greater therapeutic success. Different types of decision-making are needed to correspond to the goal emphasis of each institution and the contextual constraints (Ullman, 1967).

There has been considerable innovation in staff roles in many of these institutions. The professional psychiatrist must serve as facilitator, coordinator, and integrator as well as therapist by being sensitive to the community environment—community acceptance, the employment market, housing availability, the integrity of the welfare service system, and the like. Goals are thus diversified, varied, and intangible. Technologies available are not specified and are uncertain (Mechanic, 1978). The traditional model of bureaucratic organization cannot furnish guidelines for professional behavior in these new community settings, and new organizational norms have yet to be developed (Robin & Wagenfeld, 1977).

THE NURSING HOME

Before closing this chapter on hospitals, mention should be made of nursing homes, which are alternative, long-term health care facilities that have drastically increased in number in recent years.

In earlier days, long-term care was linked to concern for paupers. Through the almshouses or poorhouses the public assumed responsibility for the aged as well as the disabled, the unemployed, and the unprotected (orphans). The twentieth century witnessed a specialization of various types of institutions and segregation of different groups of residents, which resulted in the emergence of nursing homes as residential institutions providing nursing and personal care services.

The utilization of nursing homes by those who were not indigent appeared later than the parallel development in hospital care for middle class patients. However, the historical concept of charity is tenacious in that there still seems to be an expectation that the recipient of care should be grateful and submissive.

Expansion of the Nursing Home Industry. Nursing homes have increased rapidly during the past quarter-century. Bed facilities have more than doubled between 1963 and 1973 (U.S. DHEW, 1976). In 1977 the national expenditure for nursing home care was $12.6 billion, which was 7.7 percent of the total medical expenditure (Gibson & Fisher, 1978).

The growth of this long-term institution is largely due to the impetus coming from the external environment. The proportion of the elderly who require maintenance care has increased because of the extended life span accompanied by the decline of family care. Medicare and Medicaid (see Chapter 10) helped remove the financial barrier to the use of these facilities by many aged citizens. Federal funding stimulated the proprietary nursing home industry, which has mushroomed since 1966.

According to the 1970 census, a million people aged 65 or over, about 5 percent of the total elderly population, resided in institutions of various types. This figure underestimates the real exposure of the elderly to nursing homes since it was derived from cross-sectional rather than longitudinal population data. Kastenbaum and Candy's (1973) study suggests that there is at least a 20 percent chance of any aged individual entering a nursing home at some time in his or her life.

Extended-care facilities vary enormously in their label, objective, ownership, administration, bed capacity, service, quality, and cost of care. According to the national survey of nursing homes during 1973–1974 by the U.S. National Center for Health Statistics (1977a,b,c,d,e), approximately 70 percent of the 15,700 homes studied were proprietary and another 70 percent had a bed capacity of 50–200. The majority (71 percent) of all nursing home residents were attended to by their own physicians. About half of the homes provided physical therapy (53 percent) and counseling (52 percent); less than one third offered recreational (31 percent) or speech and hearing (29 percent) therapies; and a quarter had occupational therapy (23 percent). Of all full-time equivalent employees (i.e., two half-time employees are counted as one full-time equivalent worker), over half were members of a nursing staff, and nurse's aides comprised 46 percent.

As for the characteristics of the residents, the median ages were 78 for males and 82 for females. Although more than half of the residents (59 percent) were transferred from other types of institutions, the largest *single* category of residents lived in private accomodations prior to admission. The primary reason for admission was reported to be physical (80.6 percent)—illness or need for treatment. Over half (58.3 percent) of the respondents were reported to suffer from senility (broadly defined as decline in intellect, memory, judgment, loss of orientation, difficulty in speaking, or feebleness); one third indicated arthritis or rheumatism (34.3 percent), and heart trouble (33.5 percent). Many respondents exhibited behavioral problems such as confusion (57 percent), agitation or nervousness (42.3 percent), or depression (38.9 percent).

Abuses of the Nursing Home Industry. Nursing homes have, in general, improved greatly in recent years due to increased professionalism, licensure, accreditation, and certification. Licensing laws have began to incorporate standards for nursing and other care and to require certain minimum qualifications for personnel. To participate as a Medicare provider, a home must be certified as an extended care facility with 24-hour nursing service and at least one registered professional nurse employed full time. Participation in the Medicaid program requires a home to be certified as a skilled nursing home and/or as an intermediate care facility.

Despite these regulations, fraudulant practices within the nursing home industry have drawn much attention. Mendelson and Hapgood (1974) described the methods by which the government is swindled as its money passes through nursing home accounts. For instance, if a flat rate per patient per day is paid by the government, profit is made by the nursing home operator by cutting daily costs to the minimum. This can be done by providing the cheapest food in the smallest possible amounts, hiring a lower-paid practical nurse rather than a registered nurse, or paying the lowest rate for aides by hiring people who cannot hold a job anywhere else.

In those cases where the government reimburses the nursing home, the operators can increase their profit by padding their bills. The operators choose their suppliers, such as pharmacists, and decide how much they are to deliver; hence they can demand kickbacks (Apple, 1970). The operators and physicians can also report to the government goods and services that the patients do not need and have not received.

Nursing home operators can engage in these transactions because there is little risk of being caught or punished. Even if caught, all that is required generally is to return the money under the pretense of clerical error without criminal charges (Mendelson & Hapgood, 1974).

At a higher level of fraud, there is the manipulation of the ownership and mortgaging of nursing homes that receive guaranteed government income. Owners and operators of nursing homes can maneuver so as to extract the most revenue and pay back the least in income tax, all within the confines of the law.

According to the assessment by Mendelson and Hapgood (1974), the problem is not the absence of regulations but failure in their enforcement. Nursing home lobbying is influential at the state level where the Medicaid reimbursement rate is set and nursing home inspection is conducted. The federal government has failed to collect basic information about the industry, and it refuses to reveal its reports on nursing home inspections. Ultimately, however, blame is placed on the general public, which is indifferent to or ineffective in exerting pressure on state and federal government for reform.

Integration of Health and Social Services. Medicare, which is the federal funding arm for health care for people aged 65 and over, provides short-term, skilled nursing and active, rehabilitation-oriented care for old people following discharge from the hospital. Thus, Medicare legislation ties residence in nursing homes to sojourns in hospitals and appears to bridge a gap between the health and social services required by the elderly.

In reality, however, Medicare serves to separate the community in which the elderly live and their health delivery services because Medicare allows medical services only to those who are hospital-bound. The physicians must regularly certify not only that his or her patient is sick enough to need medical attention but that the condition requires only "part-time intermittent care." The program is not intended to subsidize long-term maintenance of the aged (Meyers, 1970).

This is attributable to the traditional disease orientation of medical practice (Brody, 1973). Historically, medicine has been concerned with the understanding and management of disease rather than the health maintenance and optimum functioning of the individual. The hospital, with its emphasis on acute, episodic treatment, has consumed the major share of fiscal, personnel, and facility resources. Health professionals in general are oriented toward acute illness and have limited experience in the management of long-term conditions, to which they give low priority.

However, for the elderly population physical disability is intermixed with mental impairment, immobility, and environmental hazards. The lower income status of the elderly results in their occupying inadequate housing in overcrowded areas with limited transportation services. There is a frequently quoted question: if a 75-year-old woman lives on the second floor of an apartment without an elevator, would she manifest a cardiac or a housing problem (Clark, 1971; Pollack, 1969)? The elderly are imprisoned in their homes due to lack of information concerning services that may be organized too complexly, physically dispersed, inadequately advertised, or so loaded with eligibility requirements as to be inaccessible.

Certainly acute medical care is vital for the aged; what is equally needed is a continuum of health and social services for the chronically disabled that will enable them to function optimally. The ideal of providing for "complete, physical, mental, and social well-being and not merely the absence of disease" (World Health Organization, 1946) is attained only by coordinating subsystems of the general environment such as the family, public and private organizations of income maintenance, housing, communication, and transportation as well as health delivery services (Brody, 1973; Shanas & Maddox, 1977).

The implication of the Medicare failure to assume a continuum of health and social services is seen in its effect upon new, so-called "comprehensive care" alternatives. Most of the current national health insurance proposals (see Chapter 10) are extensions of the Medicare principle characterized by the disease orientation. They tend to equate health coverage with medical and inpatient care for catastrophic illnesses and to exclude nonemergency services. The health delivery system needs a major restructuring to meet the needs of the elderly (Brody, 1973).

Nursing homes developed in response to external demands (aging population) and stimuli (federal funding). As a result, their operation is closely linked with the external environment. Power is concentrated in owners and operators who serve as a liaison with the outside world, consisting of the government, physicians, pharmacists, and so on. Nursing home managers can manipulate these outsiders to their advantage. Since maintenance care in nursing homes does not require a high level of medical technology, the role of the professional workers is under the control of the operators. The operators can decide the extent to which medical and other services are needed, what should be expended, and what should be reimbursed by the government to maximize their profit. Such an operation will survive so long as the public ignores the problem.

SUMMARY

In this chapter the hospital has been examined as a social system interacting with the environment. The hospital receives inputs from the outside world in the form of (1) patients, physicians, other personnel, resources, and capital; (2) technology; and (3) social values. These external influences help formulate the operative goals of the hospital, which in turn affect the structure and process of medical practice. The effectiveness of a large, complex organization is determined by the interlocking influences of the internal variables (structural variables, performance of functions, and technology available) and external variables (technology, funds, values).

Environment. The relationship between the general hospital and the environment can be viewed as one of exchange. The type and extent of financial support that the hospital receives from the outside are likely to affect the operative goal of the hospital—quality, efficiency, or access. Proprietary hospitals without government or philanthropic funding must strive for efficiency, while voluntary hospitals, unencumbered by financial considerations, can concentrate on medical quality. Government hospitals, on the other hand, are concerned with making their service accessible to everyone.

As compared to general hospitals, most mental hospitals are state owned. As such, demand for accessibility in the face of limited financing contributes to the poor quality of care delivered. The shortage of trained personnel and the low salary scale in the state mental hospital are partially responsible for inducing the hospital to concentrate on custodial rather than therapeutic goals. Because of this inadequacy of therapeutic effect in the hospital, the task of treating mental patients has historically been shifted back and forth between the community and the hospital—that is, from moral treatment to total institution and back to milieu therapy.

The link of the nursing home to the environment is primarily financial. The reimbursement by the federal government for the proprietary homes has generated a profit incentive in nursing home owners and operators.

Technology. In addition to financing, technology is another important component of the environment. Until the early nineteenth century medical technology was so primitive that the hospital was considered as a place where the poor came to die. The goal of the hospital was more social or religious than medical. During the twentieth century medical technology made extraordinary advances that elevated the position of the medical staff in the hospital. At the same time hospitals grew larger and more complex, which required the integrative role to be specialized by the administration.

Technology, or the relative absence of it, has played an important role in the history of mental health services. When insanity was considered incurable, the mentally ill were chained, beaten, or cast away. After a brief attempt at moral treatment, public mental hospitals with the characteristics of a total institution became the prevailing facilities. Because of the low level of therapeutic technology, the mental hospital adopted a custodian goal, which was carried out by nurses and attendants. The modern counterpart of moral treatment appeared in the form of milieu therapy, designed to avoid the negative effects of institutionalization. The ideology of the community mental health movement (milieu therapy) has been well received by society, but its implementation suffers from the underdevelopment of community therapeutic technology.

Stratification. Throughout the foregoing discussion it has been assumed that hospitals, as goal-oriented organizations, develop structures that reflect their goals and attempt to attain them by maximally utilizing available technology. In order to assess whether a particular structural arrangement will facilitate goal achievement or not, Max Weber's model of bureaucracy has been used by many researchers as a point of departure. To Weber, bureaucracy serves the organization most efficiently because it performs with discipline and coordination and is governed by technical competence, rational judgment, and standardized rules.

The applicability of this model to the hospital has been subject to much criticism. Objecting to the monocratic authority structure of Weber's model, functionalists envision the organization as a system consisting of mutually interdependent parts. The typical structure of the modern general hospital is characterized by a horizontal rather than a vertical emphasis at the top of the organization, where control is shared by the governing board, the administrator, and the doctors. Further, dual lines of authority extend from top to bottom in the administrative and medical staffs.

While Weber does not posit any major conflict in his rational and efficient model, others consider a conflict perspective more tenable because of the perpetual and basic dissension between the administrative and medical sectors. While the administrative sector of the hospital endorses the goal of efficiency and develops the bureaucratic structure to attain that goal, the medical staff adheres to the norm of professional autonomy, which is antithetical to Weber's concept of bureaucracy. Physicians believe that the ultimate goal of the hospital is to deliver high-quality care and that this goal will be realized most expediently if physicians are able to exercise autonomy.

This dichotomy in the definition of hospital goals—quality versus efficiency—has been accepted by many investigators as an inherent characteristic of the hospital organization. In recent years, however, a different approach has been adopted by some organization researchers to examine the relationship between control and performance. It has been reported by them that specification of work procedures designed to increase visibility of consequences (e.g., performance levels of staff members and hospitals) is positively associated with not only efficiency (e.g., cost control) but also with the quality of medical care (e.g., lower mortality and morbidity rates, therapeutic innovativeness). It is suggested that a certain amount of regulation serves better than complete professional autonomy to improve the quality of care.

At this point we do not have enough empirical evidence to ascertain the optimal amount of control needed for the maximum level of goal attainment. However, hospitals are faced with the trend toward an increasing degree of control exercised by nonprofessionals. One aspect of this is seen in the growing bureaucratization of the medical practice wherein physicians are subject to more and more specifications of work procedures. Another source of external control of hospitals is the third-party payer of medical costs (the government), which is establishing various evaluation measures of medical practice.

Thus, the hospital as a subsystem of society may be undergoing a major structural transformation and re-evaluation of goals. The increasing volume of hospital research is encouraging as it will shed light on the future direction of hospital development. However, there is a great need for more comprehensive research than that available today. Such studies should be based on an integrative framework that will deal with the interaction between the external environment and the internal structure of the hospital.

CHAPTER 8

Other Health Practitioners

In previous chapters, particularly in Chapter 6, attention was focused upon physicians as medical professionals. A profession in pure form is based on abstract, theoretical knowledge that is transmitted by formal and lengthy training; access to the profession is controlled through the licensure system. Because of the functional importance of such a body of knowledge and due to the limited number of people who are capable and willing to acquire the particular skill, professionals are likely to be accorded high social status. Technical expertise alone, however, does not warrant the professionals' high status. They generally form an organization that enhances in-group solidarity and fights against external pressures.

A corollary is that a profession enjoys autonomy in determining its membership and in deciding the manner of its practice, since the lay public cannot evaluate or control the performance of professionals. However, in order to protect the lay clientele, professionals are expected to be oriented to service rather than profit.

Outside the domain of the physician, there are many other health practitioners who aspire to the status of the professional. However, these other health occupations have not yet attained the full-fledged status profession.

There are health occupations, such as dentistry and clinical psychology, which have become professions in the last generation, but they have not yet attained the eminence enjoyed by medicine. There are also semiprofessions such as social work that may achieve professional status over the next generation. Some writers (Goode, 1969) have speculated that certain occupations, for example, osteopathy, nursing, chiropractic, pediatry, and pharmacy, will not become professions in the foreseeable future.

Classification of Semiprofessions. The semiprofessions have been classified and rank-ordered by various categories. Wardwell (1979) divided them into three groups: limited, marginal, and quasi. *Limited profession* refers to a health occupation whose service is usually confined to particular parts of the human body, for example, dentistry, podiatry, optometry, and psychology. *Marginal* practitioners are those whose approach to health and disease is in conflict with that of orthodox medicine, such as osteopaths and chiropractors. The *quasi-*practitioners utilize pseudoscientific methods, and they include spiritual healers, quacks, and the like.

Wardwell (1979) further compared health practitioners according to other criteria such as the rank of their occupational prestige, the quality of training required before practice, and their historical background. Medicine requires the longest period for training and enjoys the highest occupational prestige. Dentistry follows medicine in occupational prestige, while among the lowest in rank, as measured by various standards, are osteopathy, chiropractic, and Christian Science. The status of pharmacy, optometry, and clinical psychology lies in the middle.

Professional associations representing all of the above occupations act individually as political pressure groups to affect the formulation and administration of laws that will determine the status of their occupations. The founding of a new professional organization is frequently for the express purpose of promoting occupational legislation that will prevent other, already established professions from regulating the new group (Akers, 1968). Medicine was the first to organize at the national level (1847) and to achieve licensing in all states (1915). It was followed by pharmacy (first organized in 1852, and licensed in all states by 1955) and dentistry (first organized in 1859 and licensed in all states by 1935). Organizations for optometry and chiropractic appeared much later.

Akers and Quinney (1968) compared the organizational strength of various professional associations in terms of resources (size, wealth, and level of education) and structural integration (membership comprehensiveness, commitment, stability, and intragroup cleavage). The AMA is the largest and the wealthiest association. The American Dental Association (ADA) is also large and wealthy, but standard dental training does not match medical training in its rigor or comprehensiveness. The ADA, however, is more tightly organized and shows greater professional unity than the AMA.

Optometry and pharmacy have fewer resources and a weaker structural integration than medicine and dentistry. However, optometry and pharmacy duplicate the dental–medical contrast at a lower level, that is, pharmacy has greater personnel and financial resources but is less united as a group than is optometry. Finally, the chiropractic organization is weaker in every respect: underdeveloped in resources and insufficiently unified as an occupational unit. Historically, the degree of organization in conjunction with the levels of technology appear to have decisive effects upon the status of the profession.

Selected Semiprofessions. In this chapter three types of semiprofessions are selected for detailed analysis. The first is what Wardwell (1979) calls the limited professional (dentists and pharmacists), whose technology is accepted by the AMA as legitimate but not complete since it is limited to particular parts of the human body. The second type will be called the ancillary professional (physician's assistants and nurses), whose service is dependent upon and subordinate to the physician's discretion. The third group combines Wardwell's marginal and quasi-professionals (chiropractors and Christian Scientists), whose practices are largely unapproved of by the AMA as lacking in scientific validation.

Each health occupation is described in terms of the functionalist perspective as a social system whose goal is professionalization. However, the process of goal attainment is analyzed from the conflict perspective in that various health occupations are in constant struggle with other aspiring or emerging as well as established professions. The interactionist perspective will also be utilized in examining the public image of the practitioners and its impact upon the practitioner–patient relationship

Each occupation will be examined in four areas: (1) historical development toward a profession; (2) recruitment and socialization of its members; (3) characteristics of its practices; and (4) professional organization.

PROFESSIONALIZATION

The process of professionalization is examined below from the functionalist and conflict perspectives.

Functionalist Perspective. The functionalist's postulate of system integration makes the study of social change difficult. However, there is at least one type of social change that can be described within the functionalist framework, namely, the process of differentiation. This means that a unit or system that has a single, relatively well-defined place in society can be divided into subunits or subsystems which have different structures and functions (Parsons, 1966). For example, at some time in history, the physician dispensed medicine and ran a drugstore. Later, the preparation of medicine became the specialized function of the pharmacist, who did not have the same level of training as the physician.

In order to subsume the process of differentiation into the functionalist framework, additional assumptions need to be made. First, if differentiation is to yield a balanced and more evolved system, each newly differentiated substructure must have a greater adaptive capacity for performing its function than the previous undifferentiated system. Second, the operations of two or more new units must be coordinated within the broader system.

Within this framework, an industrializing society has been viewed as a professionalizing society (Goode, 1960a, 1969) in that (1) the percentage of the labor force that is professional and technical has increased over the years; (2) more and more occupations try to acquire the symbols of professional status; and (3) ultimately most occupations will become professions by developing and monopolizing a body of abstract knowledge dedicated to service.

The process of differentiating a profession out of an occupation has been analyzed by placing occupation and profession at the opposite ends of a continuum, where each possesses unique attributes. In order for an occupation to become a profession, it must acquire two fundamental features: (1) a prolonged, specialized training in a body of abstract knowledge and (2) a collectivity of service orientations.

From these two characteristics, many other traits of the profession have been derived: (1) Autonomy: Since lay people cannot evaluate professional knowledge, the profession has autonomy in determining its own standards of training and practice and in evaluating and sanctioning the behavior of the practitioners. (2) Socialization: The profession provides a more far-reaching socialization and training experience than other occupations. One method that can be used to determine whether an occupation has a sufficient knowledge basis to be accepted as a profession is to measure the amount of learning required to enter the occupation. (3) Professional organization: Members are more strongly identified with their profession than members of other occupations are with theirs. Professional organization serves not only to control the conduct of its members but also to protect their profession through legal and political mechanisms (Denzin & Mettlin, 1968; Goode, 1968; Pavalko, 1972).

This type of approach assumes the importance of internal change within an occupation, the maintenance of equilibrium within the process, and the profession's acquisition of a better adaptive capacity.

Conflict Perspective. The major difficulty in the functionalist approach to professionalization lies in its failure to study the external forces operating upon occupations, such as industrialization and bureaucratization, and the conflicting nature of interaction among various units, such as occupational, political, and legal institutions.

From the conflict perspective, all societies are systems of competition among component units such as individuals and occupational groups. Whether members of an occupation are united as in a labor union or remain merely a social aggregate, their total collective success or failure in the societal power struggle determines the rise or fall of the occupation.

Occupations that seek recognition as professions must win the contest in all three arenas: prestige, power, and income; and the most important of these is prestige. The attaining of professional rank is not a zero-sum game: the rise of some occupations will not necessarily cause the decline of others. The professional eminence of a certain occupation is likely to be earned independently, and it is not likely to have been stolen from another profession. Nevertheless, no occupation becomes a profession without a struggle and without generating antagonism among the established professions. Each time-honored profession tends to treat newcomers as either charlatans (not properly trained) or encroachers (illegal competitors) (Goode, 1960a).

In addition to the competition among occupations, other external forces must be specified with respect to how they hinder the process of professionalization. As E. C. Hughes (1958) put it, the fundamental task is to determine the circumstances in which people in an occupation attempt to turn it into a profession.

Having examined the context in which professionalization takes place, Taylor (1968) identified such counterforces as bureaucratization, commercialization, and unionization. In the 1970s a few sociologists even proposed deprofessionalization or antielitism as a plausible, alternative trend for the future of our society. Deprofessionalization implies the equalitarian expropriation of the unique qualities of a profession, particularly its monopoly over knowledge and work autonomy (Haug, 1972, 1976). Using a different label—proletarianization, Oppenheimer (1972) argued that a white-collar proletarian type of worker is now replacing the self-regulated, professional type of worker.

Viewed in this way, an occupation aspiring to reach a professional status may never attain it. Any occupation can deliberately extend the period of its training, but whether it can attain the autonomy and power needed is doubtful in the midst of this social trend toward deprofessionalization.

LIMITED PRACTITIONERS: DENTISTS

Historical Development of Professionalism

The history of dentistry involves the transformation from a craft to a profession. Like surgery and obstetrics, dentistry has suffered from the stigmatization attached to work with the hands.

Dentistry as a craft dates back to antiquity. Ancient Egyptians were familiar with dental surgery because loose teeth held in place by gold wires have been found in excavated skulls (Venzmer, 1968). Historical documents also indicate that ancient Egyptians knew how to expel an abscess of the gum or to treat an ulcerated gum with an application of cinnamon, gum, honey, and oil (Bremner, 1959).

The development of dentistry in Europe, however, was slow. During the sixteenth century, dental treatment was given by barber-surgeons, bathhouse keepers, peddlers, old women, and the like. Dentistry in their hands was merely the pulling of an aching tooth with a primitive instrument. In order to cover the gap made by a missing tooth, an artificial tooth carved from bone or ivory or a sound tooth from someone willing to sell was wired in place. Such repairs lasted for several years. No one in those days thought much about infection of the teeth or its consequences (Haggard, 1934).

During the Revolutionary period, some European dentists came to the United States, and in that unrestricted environment, dentistry made more rapid advances than it had abroad. In 1840, the first dental school, the Baltimore College of Dental Surgery, was founded.

It should be noted that this dental school was established partly because the medical profession in Baltimore refused to incorporate dental subjects into the curriculum of the medical school (Young & Cohen, 1979). The American Dental Association, on the other hand, appears to interpret the situation more as a reflection of the sentiment among the dentists as a whole, who wished to maintain an autonomous identity (McCluggage, 1959). At any rate, this event was one of the crucial factors that led dentistry to take a separate road from that of medicine. As dentistry matured and gained in technology, it grew increasingly protective of its own destiny (Bremner, 1959).

During their early days, dental schools not only had to struggle against the opposition of practicing dentists, who believed in apprenticeship but also against physicians, who were inclined to regard dentistry with low esteem. However, dental schools were saved from these obstacles when they, together with the proprietary medical schools, were recognized as a source of profit by the entrepreneurs of the period. This profit motive made possible the quick growth of an infant profession (Young & Cohen, 1979).

Twenty years after the Flexner Report, a survey of dental education was financed by the Carnegie Foundation. The results guided the American Dental Association in the 1920s to upgrade the standards of its professional education. Now that it is fully recognized as a profession, dentistry is the second best established of the group of independent health practitioners in terms of standards of professional training and requirements for license. Dental schools, without exception, are all affiliated with universities. The present course of training in dentistry requires at least two years of professional college work, followed by four years in dental schools before the degrees of Doctor of Dental Surgery or Doctor of Dental Medicine are awarded (American Dental Association, 1976).

Dentistry is the only health care occupation that has achieved a professional standing without being taken over by medicine. Ancillary medical techniques, such as anesthesiology and radiology, were absorbed into the jurisdiction of medicine. They became medical specializations before their knowledge base was sufficiently large to justify their recognition as independent professions.

In terms of its current position in the occupational prestige structure, dentistry is called the "second profession," a ranking just below that of medicine. However, the label of second profession is not necessarily intended invidiously. First of all, dentistry has attained a professional level of technology. Second, unlike physicians and lawyers, who are increasingly absorbed in a bureaucracy, the dentist maintains an independent practice in most cases. Another strength of dentistry lies in its professional organization, which is more cohesive than the AMA.

However, the public sees dentistry as something of a parvenu vocation and also as intrinsically less interesting, dignified, pleasant, and "clean." Unlike the other professions, which are romanticized in mass media, the dentist is rarely portrayed charismatically. But this negative image is accompanied by high income and professional autonomy, which collectively give the dentist an amorphous status (Sherlock & Morris, 1971).

Professional Training

Recruitment to the Dental Profession

From the symbolic interactionist viewpoint, it is hypothesized that the invidious label of the second profession leads dentistry to recruit different types of students than do the medical schools, specifically, those who failed to attain entry into a more preferred profession (Sherlock & Morris, 1971).

Socioeconomic Origin. Relative to medicine, the dental profession does not have a high rate of occupational inheritance. Only a small proportion of the fathers of dental students are dentists themselves (Fusillo & Metz, 1971; Heist, 1962; Lawson, 1976; Mann & Parkin, 1960; Quarantelli, 1961a; Sherlock &

Morris, 1971; "The 1968 survey . . . ," 1969). This is partly due to the fact that dentistry has grown at such a fast rate in the United States that it has not been possible for dentistry to replenish its ranks from within. In addition, as the second profession, dentistry is not in a position to recruit physician's children into dentistry since they are probably influenced to follow parental footsteps.

Recruitment to dentistry is more a matter of intergenerational status mobility than it is the inheritance of a specific occupation (Dick, 1960). Dental students are likely to have upwardly mobile parents who had made the historical exodus from a primary occupation, such as farming, ranching, and mining, into high-income positions, including professional, managerial, proprietary, skilled, and semiskilled occupations. This suggests that economic resources are more crucial than occupational status per se for sending an offspring to dental school, which is quite expensive (American Dental Association, 1969; Silversin & Drolette, 1977). An upwardly mobile parent can provide not only the financial resources but also encourage the mobility aspiration of the offspring toward a higher status, that is, some type of professional career.

Career Decision. The hypothesis of dental students being "frustrated medical students" has been rejected by many studies (Lawson, 1976). D. M. More (More, 1959, 1961a; More & Kahn, 1960) found that the top dental school applicants have credentials worthy of acceptance in most medical schools. For the majority of dental students, the commitment to their career was formed during the latter years of high school, and it grew throughout their college years (Sherlock & Morris, 1971). However, Sherlock and Morris (1971) indicated that at the age of ten, medicine was a much more frequent first choice than dentistry. They interpreted this finding to mean that the fantasy for medicine was replaced by a more realistic inclination toward dentistry when high school grades fell below the mark students assumed to be necessary for entry into medical school.

Wittemann and others (1975) have reported that ability, interest, and personality are major factors in directing students to a career in the health sciences. Dental students are likely to possess sociability, artistic interest, business management propensity, mechanical-technical skill, and quantitative, technical, and scientific aptitude composites. Unlike medical students, dental students show low physical science interest. Wittemann and Currier (1976) have pointed out an entrepreneurial orientation (freedom to carry out one's ideas or to develop one's full potential) among dental students.

However, the students' perception of the practitioner's motives is skewed toward pragmatism, for example, earning a good salary and building a professional reputation in the community (Wittemann & Currier, 1976). Other studies show a more utilitarian orientation among dental students, who tend to regard the dental profession as a realization of middle class aspirations for success and independence (Heist, 1962). The self-employment status of dentistry is an attractive feature in comparison to a bureaucratized medical practice (More & Kahn, 1960). Earning income from fees rather than from a salary and setting one's own working conditions are considered more important than prestige.

Pragmatism is best expressed by Sherlock and Morris (1971) as a "minimax" choice pattern adopted by dental students, that is, minimizing the difficulty for obtaining maximum rewards. Relative to medicine, dentistry is perceived as providing an easier entry into a profession, with easier admission and shorter training. At the same time, dentistry is seen as promising many practical advantages, such as independent practice, high income, flexible working schedule, and less responsibility.

Socialization

Unlike the study of medical students by Becker and others, which noted a change from humanitarianism to a cynical orientation, More (1960, 1961b) indicated that dental students maintained humanistic concern throughout their education. The reason for this has been sought in the marked difference in the educational experiences of medical and dental students. While medical students have almost no contact with patients during their basic training, most dental students have some patient contact at an early stage.

However, more recent studies contradict earlier findings. Rosen and others (1977) found that first-year students are more likely to identify with upper class students as professional models than with dental practitioners. These neophyte dental students also envision themselves in closer touch with patients than they perceive practicing dentists to be with patients.

In a similar vein, Sherlock and Morris (1971) noted an increase in cynicism and a decline in ethics over the course of dental education (Fusillo & Metz, 1971). The initial moderate degree of commitment to dentistry increased slightly during the early stages, but by the final year, it dropped to a level below that of the first year. In terms of the occupational identity cycle, the students adopted the self-image of dentists, but then increasingly thought of themselves as business people rather than as researchers, crafts workers, or administrators. They became more concerned with "good income" than "solving oral health problems," with "superior working conditions" than "opportunity to cure sickness," and with "community prestige" rather than the "relief of pain."

A review of studies of medical education shows that the lack of significant changes in medical students can be attributed to the development of an autonomous student subculture that is resistant to faculty influences. These studies indicate that the students' original values are of crucial importance. The values most first-year dental students hold reflect their social class origins and their aspirations. They value autonomy, prestige, social mobility, and income rather than professional service, altruism, or even technical competence. During their years of training, dental students realize that there is a similarity of values and lifestyles among themselves, and they band together. The students' original values are reinforced as the result of interaction with peers (Sherlock & Morris, 1971).

Dental Practice

Public Apathy. The nature of dental disease has had an important impact on dental practices and on dentist–patient relationships in that it has generated discrepant attitudes toward treatment between patients and dentists (Davis, 1976). While dentists emphasize preventive care, patients are likely to wait until the disease has progressed enough to give them intolerable pain. Despite the growing dental education of the general public, apathy remains the dominant feature of the lay attitudes toward dental disease. While the yearly average number of visits to physicians was 5.1 per person, the number of visits to dentists was only 1.6 in 1975 (Biro et al., 1976; U.S. Dept. of Commerce, 1977; U.S. Public Health Service, 1960). Comparing objective and subjective dental health statuses, Barenthin (1977) found that dental conditions, as judged by the dentists, made little difference in whether or not individuals were satisfied with their general dental condition. People tend to get used to bad teeth unless there is a sudden deterioration or discomfort. This explains why it is so difficult to entice people to take better care of their teeth (Keegeles, 1961).

This low utilization of dental care is partly due to the reluctance of a patient to experience the pain that generally accompanies dental treatment and also to the optimistic notion that death seldom accompanies dental disease (Biro et al., 1976). However, once under way, the courses of dental diseases are irreversible and are compounded when they are neglected by the patient. Thus, dental treatment in any population consists of continued prophylaxis for the disease and treatment of damage that has accumulated through neglect (Young & Cohen, 1979).

Work Settings. The majority (96 percent) of the dentists surveyed by the ADA in 1975 were independent workers. The term *independent dentists* includes those who are part owners of a practice, who practice alone and are the sole owners of a practice, or who practice alone but have an expense-sharing arrangement with other dentists. Those employed in an incorporated practice as shareowners of the practice are also considered independent dentists. Self-employed dentists, one type of independent dentist, constituted 77.5 percent of the sample. About 4 percent of the dentists in the sample were salaried dentists who are employed by another practitioner, have a partnership, or work in a corporation (American Dental Association, 1977).

As for auxiliary personnel, the majority (92.5 percent) of the sampled dentists employ at least one dental assistant, but more than half (58.7 percent) hire no hygienists and over a third (35.8 percent) do not use a secretarial staff (American Dental Association, 1977).

Traditionally, dentistry has been based on solo practice. The dentist's office used to be completely self-contained and depended on almost no outside resources, either from other practitioners or from the community. The practice could be isolated and insulated by that office, and not subject to review. The merit, however, of self-evaluation and peer review has been acknowledged by a significant segment of the profession (Schonfeld, 1969, 1970), even though norms are unknown and systematic mechanisms to assure quality are absent. For example, research results (Milgrom et al., 1978a,b) suggest a generally high level of care provided by practitioners who volunteered for evaluative projects and a significantly more critical self-assessment than peer appraisal.

In recent years, even solo dental practitioners are coming under some periodic review through the development of open-panel prepaid programs (Friedman, 1966). In the open-panel practice, beneficiaries are provided diagnosis or treatment planning at designated facilities and then referred for treatment to dentists in the community. This is in contrast to the closed-panel system in which a limited number of dentists are preselected to provide care for a group of patients. In these few instances of prepaid programs, dentists appointed by the local dental society or employed by a welfare agency are subject to financial review (e.g., the correctness of the fees charged and the ascertainment of the treatment performed) and occasionally to performance evaluation. Furthermore, in 1974 a new component was added to the peer review. The ADA modified its traditional principle of ethics based on autonomy in such a way that a dentist now is obliged to report instances of gross and continued malpractice of another dentist to an appropriate agency. However, dental practitioners are still reluctant to participate in peer review (Waldman & Schlissel, 1977).

With the increasing need for consultation with and referral to specialists and the growing hospital-centered medical therapy, the independent, solo practice is slowly declining. In addition, the professional tasks of the dentists are being supplemented by the dental auxiliaries, such as dental hygienists and dental laboratory technicians (Howard et al., 1976). Furthermore, the importance of teamwork between dentists and physicians has been increasingly emphasized, although its implementation is extremely limited as yet (Dunning, 1976; Odenheimer et al., 1977; Thompson, 1975).

Dentist–Patient Relationship. The dentist–patient relationship has been studied by many researchers from the symbolic interactionist perpsective (Davis, 1976; Linn, 1967; Quarantelli & Cooper, 1966). That approach was taken because the dental office of a solo practitioner is a milieu in which the dentist treats the patient literally on a face-to-face basis in a dyadic relation (Baseheart, 1975).

Value orientations and self-perceptions of both the dentist and the patient are brought into this system of face-to-face interaction. Much of their behavior can only be understood by taking into account how each defines the situation. The dentist acts on the basis of his or her self-image, which is unfavorable. This negative self-concept has been reported and interpreted by some (Cussler & Gordon, 1968; Quarantelli, 1961b) as reflecting a dentist's own definition of the situation rather than as an objective rating. For instance, in 1963, the North-Hatt replication study of occupational ranks (Hodge et al., 1964) indicated a rise in the public estimate of the dentist's status. Nevertheless, the self-image of many dentists has not improved significantly because they compare themselves with physicians.

A source of that negative self-image was identified by Quarantelli (1961b) when he examined the clinical work role of dental students. It was the students' belief that patients considered dentists to be "individuals who hurt people while doing mechanical work for which they charge too much." While recognizing the negative views of others, practicing dentists have learned to interpret these attitudes in ways that will soften the blow to their egos.

Dentists sidestep the charge that they inflict pain on others (Firestein, 1976; Hengst & Roghmann, 1978; Seeman et al., 1976) by (1) denying that pain is seriously involved in most of their work; (2) blaming the patient for ignoring a dental condition and allowing it to deteriorate so badly that any dental work will hurt; or (3) by asserting that pain is an unavoidable part of the treatment.

The image that the dentists possess "only a mechanical skill" has a serious effect on them because it is perceived as a rejection of the professional status of dentistry (Leatherman, 1978). The typical reaction to the "mechanic" label is a flat denial of its validity. However, dentistry as a skill-demanding job does provide many dentists with professional role satisfaction (Klein, 1978; Murray et al., 1975).

The accusation of high fees is handled by (1) a blanket denial that fees are high for the service rendered; (2) an acceptance of the blame in a limited context; or (3) a justification for expensive fees when necessary. For example, they claim that the cost of operating a dental practice rose 132.5 percent as compared with a rise of 61.9 percent in charges for dental care between 1967 and 1975 (Phillips, 1977).

If dentists perceive that patients have negative attitudes toward them, dentists are likely to feel the necessity to establish their authority early in the relationship (Cussler & Gordon, 1968). Toward this goal, they try to manipulate the impression they make upon patients (Cheney, 1977) by turning away those who are late for appointments, by directing rather than asking patients to go to specialists for particular problems, by taking X-rays even when patients are reluctant, by explaining authoritatively what needs to be done, and so on (Linn, 1967). Above all, dentists can always shut up obnoxious patients by making them keep their mouths open.

However, since dental care is a lifelong process, it is more important for dentists than for, say, medical specialists to cultivate patient loyalty. Therefore, in order to have patients come back to their offices, dentists must negotiate and bargain with patients rather than order them around (Albrecht, 1977; Fishman & Ortiz, 1977).

Based on his observational study in training clinics at dental schools and private dental clinics, Linn (1967) identified two major areas around which symbolic bargaining between dentists and patients are centered: authority relationship and pain management.

In order to gain control over social interaction, dentists assess the characteristics of their patients in terms of age, sex, social class, personality, and the like, and modify their approaches to the patients accordingly (Cheney, 1977). Dentists can control the amount and subject matter of conversation strategically by simply approaching a patient's mouth with some instrument in hand. While doing so, however, they try to make patients feel as if they had a choice of action, by such tactics as requests couched in polite language—for example, Would you like to rinse out your mouth?

Patients, on the other hand, are expected to be compliant (Davis, 1976) because of their awkward position in dental chairs and of the anticipated pain. There are various subtle ways of defying the dentists' authority. For example, some patients use delaying tactics by asking many questions, gagging, coughing, tightening the jaws, or not opening their mouths wide enough. Others assume an anesthetized social involvement, ignoring the existence of the dentist as a social being—for example, not talking beyond the bare minimum, closing their eyes, stretching or letting their hands hang loose as if socially unaware of the dentist (Linn, 1967).

As for the management of pain, dentists warn patients that pain or discomfort might be expected and that it is natural or normal. Patients usually do not openly express pain or discomfort but show indirect evidence of it by a grimace or body movements. They are embarrassed to reveal their weakness since they are culturally conditioned to be stoic.

When some mishap occurs—for example, an instrument is dropped, a drilling machine stops working, or the work does not progress as fast or as easily as anticipated—a dentist stays calm lest the incidence undermine the professional image. No sign of impatience or embarrassment is shown by the dentist. The patient in turn is also likely to pretend that nothing happened because it would not be advantageous to disrupt the therapeutic equilibrium at the moment, even though the patient may never come back to the office again.

Professional Organization

Membership. The American Dental Association was founded by 26 dentists in 1859, and its membership is now over 111,000 (Rothstein, 1970).

Its top legislative and policy-making level is the House of Delegates, which is composed of representatives of the constituent (state and territorial) dental societies. The constituent societies in turn are made up of component (district and local) dental societies. Except for dentists in the federal services, a dentist applies to a local society for membership, and when accepted, is automatically entitled to membership in the ADA. In general, membership requirements include graduation from an accredited dental school, licensure for dental practice, and a record free of professionally unethical conduct. However, as we have discussed in connection with AMA membership, the ultimate judgment about acceptance has sometimes reflected local biases with regard to race, ethnicity, and sex (Young & Cohen, 1979).

Functions. The professional organization serves and protects its members in various ways. Apart from offering individual fringe benefits such as group insurance plans, the primary function of the ADA is to enhance the status of the dental profession. This can be accomplished, first of all, by maintaining increasingly higher professional standards for its members. For this purpose, the ADA provides a mechanism for information transfer and exchange through professional conferences and journals. Also, it is the role of the professional association to establish standards for training and practice by means of the accreditation of dental schools, the licensure system, and the inspection of drugs and products related to oral health (American Dental Association, 1975; McCluggage, 1959; Young & Cohen, 1979).

Second, in order to elevate the status of the profession, the ADA develops unity and consensus among practitioners on important social issues, and it transmits their joint opinion to governmental and social agencies (Goldberg et al., 1976). The ADA is well aware of the fact that to be effective in influencing policies, legislations, and public opinion, a profession must present a united front.

As mentioned earlier, the organizational cohesion of the ADA is the strongest among health professions, including medicine (Akers & Quinney, 1968). The ADA has the most stable and comprehensive membership, a high membership commitment equal to that of the AMA, the second (to the chiropractors) highest participation in national meetings, and it shows the least amount of intragroup conflict. It should be noted of course that the current cohesion and comprehensiveness of membership are the products of a long history of endeavor toward unity (McCluggage, 1959). In terms of organizational resources, the ADA is the second strongest, following the AMA. Combining the factors of resources and structural cohesion, the ADA has an organizational power as strong as the AMA, and that equates directly with the political power manifested by these organizations (Young & Cohen, 1979). In sum, as measured by the standards of professional technique and by organizational power, dentistry has acquired professional status (Merrison, 1976; Nelson, 1977).

From the conflict viewpoint, dentistry has succeeded in winning the battle against medicine by establishing a separate and almost equal status in terms of economic (high income), political (the power of the ADA), and technical (dental science) spheres. Viewed from the functionalist perspective, however, dentistry has yet to gain public recognition of its functional importance. Except in educated circles, the public is still inclined to regard dental care as less important than medical therapy.

In the interactionist perspective, a negative label attached to dentistry affects the self-concept of the dentist, which in turn influences the dentist–patient relationship. Furthermore, the labeling process proceeds interactively between the labeler and the labeled. To the extent that dentists define the situation negatively by accepting the public image of dentistry as a second-class profession, they try to rationalize their selection of a dental career by a minimax theory, namely, that they have given up the higher prestige of the first profession for easier access to the second profession. By so doing, they attempt to maximize the practical rewards of dentistry, such as high income and autonomy at the expense of the service orientation, which is another necessary ingredient of the profession, and those practical rewards in turn reinforce the invidious image of the second profession.

LIMITED PRACTITIONERS: PHARMACISTS

Historical Development of Pharmacy

The first written reference to pharmacy as distinct from medicine appears in the records of the early charity institutions that engaged in caring for the sick and the indigent. Ordinances have been found from the twelfth century that specify the roles of physicians and pharmacists. These rules state that the physician is obliged to observe the compounding, or at least to be present until all individual ingredients are collected, by the pharmacist, thus forbidding the pharmacist to counterprescribe and the physician to dispense (Durgin et al., 1972; Kremers & Urdang, 1963; Sprowbs, 1970; Wootton, 1971). At some time during the fourteenth century, specialization in the two professions began to appear in England. After the plague of that century, the differentiation of pharmacy from medicine became an established fact, and hospitals of that era are reported to have had well-equipped pharmaceutical services.

Generally speaking, however, the right of the physicians to dispense has been retained in Anglo-Saxon countries. Unlike in other European countries, a profession based entirely on the art of pharmacy did not exist before the eighteenth or nineteenth century.

American Pharmacy. In the United States, John Morgan in 1765 proposed that pharmacy and medicine be distinguished. Morgan's prime object was to improve the entire field of health care by cultivating each department separately.

The gradual weaning of pharmacy from the medical profession appeared in the late eighteenth century when drugstores began to replace the physicians' drug selling activities. During the 1810s some state legislatures passed acts obliging an apothecary to take an examination for licensure. The Philadelphia College of Apothecaries was established in 1821 and represented the first obvious manifestation of a pharmaceutical profession in America.

The rapid industrialization after the Civil War helped pharmacy to continue to develop its own trade. Gradually, attempts by wholesale druggists to imitate English patent medicine evolved into large-scale, independent enterprises that had only incidental concern for professionalism.

However, since the wholesale druggists who provided physicians with imported or indigenous drugs were held responsible for their effects, they became interested in attaining a better knowledge of the chemicals. Some wholesalers began manufacturing chemicals, making the beginning of the large American chemical and pharmaceutical industries. People working as apprentices in these establishments gradually developed professional pride and aims.

With the turn of the century, the American pharmacy started to show progress in several fields, such as in education, industry, and supportive legislation. However, while pharmacists were gaining more knowledge and competence through higher education, they were also progressively losing their vital function of compounding medicine as a result of the growth of the drug industry and bureaucratization. Although 80 percent of the prescriptions still required the knowledge of compounding on the part of the pharmacist in 1920, that percentage dropped to 75 percent by 1930, 26 percent by 1950, and it was down to 4 percent by 1960 (Kremers & Urdang, 1963). Today, the percentage has decreased to about one percent, and the pharmacist's functions have been reduced to counting and labeling (Schumaker, 1977).

The period from the turn of the century to the mid-1950s is called the period of confusion (Bean, 1977). There was little consensus as to the roles to be played by these overtrained pharmacists.

However, by the 1960s, we can observe an effort among some pharmacists to redefine their role into a more positive one in a rapidly changing society (Bean, 1977). In both the community and hospital pharmacy, the new role of the pharmacist includes providing drug information and monitoring drug therapy in a clinical pharmacy (Millis, 1975; Silverman & Lee, 1976; Tyler, 1968). This new awareness of a pharmacist's therapeutic responsibility is due to various other factors in the health field. For one thing, there is a critical shortage of physicians, most of whom are overworked and unable to become drug experts and who need trained specialists to serve as drug information experts. Second, the public, who have been growing more educated and concerned about their health, now utilize more drugs and demand more information about them. Thus, in the 1970s, we see a new hope for professionalizing the role of the pharmacist.

Professional Socialization

Development of the Pharmaceutical Education System

Until the early part of the ninteenth century, pharmacy in the United States had been considered, by most pharmacists and physicians, as an art that did not require theoretical knowledge but rather could best be learned by practice (Kremers & Urdang, 1963). Prior to the founding of the Philadelphia College of Apothecaries in 1821, only a few ineffectual attempts were made to provide formal instruction for pharmacists. The era of pioneer pharmacy schools, which were established by the early pharmaceutical association (the College of Apothecaries), ended with the Civil War. From that time on, pharmacy schools were founded to promote the business interests of the pharmacists who created them.

In the midst of these conflicting currents, a revolutionary attempt was made in 1868 by the University of Michigan to establish the academic study of pharmacy as a full-time occupation. That bold innovation included extensive labortory instructions coupled with basic science, and the school refused to accept apprenticeship as a prerequisite to graduation. This program was started without the cooperation of the pharmaceutical practitioners, who in fact were opposed to the idea. However, the trend toward professionalism was irreversible. In 1892, the first four-year curriculum in pharmacy appeared in the United States, and that placed pharmaceutical instruction on a par with other academic disciplines.

The movement for higher and more uniform educational standards began at the turn of the century, and it was stimulated by increasing advances in scientific medicine. Since 1932, a four-year curriculum beyond high school is required for a pharmacy licence by all states. In 1950, the University of Southern California began the first six-year program, including two university years of prepharmacy for a Doctor of Pharmacy degree. These programs projected a model of the pharmacist as a disinterested scientist who understands the scientific principles behind pharmaceutical activities (Wardwell, 1979).

Recruitment and Socialization

Unlike the well-established medical profession, pharmacy as a semiprofession appears to appeal to lower income groups and to upwardly mobile urban families. According to McCormack's (1956) study, two-thirds of the sampled pharmacy students came from the small business or white collar classes, one-third from manual worker families, and none came from the high status professional group. The trend for schools of pharmacy to be attached to state universities or to other tax-supported institutions now makes that training accessible to lower income people.

As for the reasons for selecting pharmacy, importance was attached by McCormack's respondents to personal aptitude and economic security rather than to the social function of pharmacy, such as the desire to contribute to social welfare (Harvey, 1966; McCormack, 1956). When asked to describe the most important characteristics of a successful pharmacist, 56 percent of the respondents mentioned personality traits, particularly aptitude as a business person.

Their self-image reflected a small-business tradition, as owners of a retail drugstore (85 percent), located in medium-sized cities or a small town (73 percent), and carrying out their practices in residential rather than business districts (80 percent).

Occupational inheritance was relatively low in that only 17 percent of the sampled students were children of pharmacists and only 11 percent had some near relative who was a pharmacist. However, the majority of them (90 percent) had worked in drugstores, particularly in independent stores (79 percent), prior to their enrollment.

The role conflict between business and professional orientation, which historically has been present in the occupational structure of pharmacy, becomes manifest in the socialization process at pharmacy schools. While pharmacy colleges are primarily engaged in teaching scientific principles of pharmacy, the trend in the 1960s to expand their program from four to five years reflected a response to retail pharmacists' pressure to teach more business management. Thus, educational institutions themselves have incorporated a business orientation (Braucher & Evanson, 1963; Grosicki, 1963).

According to McCormack's (1956) study, pharmacy students, who tended to avoid thinking about the business–professional conflict, nevertheless acknowledged the conflict. Weinlein (1943) found that as students approached graduation, they were increasingly reluctant to enter retail pharmacy. A possible explanation is provided by the findings of other studies (Buerki, 1965; Knapp & Knapp, 1968), which indicated a process of realistic disenchantment and a development of cynicism as the students progressed through pharmacy school.

This attitude is not entirely the fault of the students since we must conclude from these earlier studies that the pharmaceutical education did not recruit professionally motivated students nor did it socialize them toward the altruistic goal of the profession. In addition, pharmacy schools have adopted an ethic of "noninvolvement" in the patient's medical problems. Rodowskas (1977) recalls that he and his graduating class of pharmacists in 1961 were instructed to function solely in a support role and to keep quiet.

With the emergence of the new role of the clinical pharmacist, recent graduates are reported to be more professionally motivated. They are looking forward to becoming active members of the health team and to serving as drug information specialists (Bean, 1977; Silverman & Lee, 1976).

Practice of Pharmacy

In the practice of pharmacy, the first dilemma for the pharmacist is found in the conflicting roles of a profession and a business. Second, within the sphere of the profession, the pharmacist must struggle against the deep-rooted power of medicine.

Professional versus Business Role Conflict

The sociological study of pharmacy began with Thorner (1942), who set the pattern of viewing the occupation as a unique combination of business and professional elements. He defined the societal function of the pharmacist as the preparation and the distribution of drugs. The conflicting nature of the pharmacist's role is apparent in that the preparation of drugs involves a professionally skilled service, while distribution represents a commercial activity.

The business versus profession dichotomy is traced back to Tawny (1920), who distinguished the business role as being inherently acquisitive and having a speculative profit-making goal. E. C. Hughes (1958) differentiated between business, where *caveat emptor* (let the consumer beward) prevails, and profession, where *credat emptor* (let the consumer trust) is dominant.

McCormack (1956) described the marginal role of the pharmacist in both functionalist and interactionist aspects. On the one hand, the marginality of the pharmacist matches the definition of the occupational function. As Thorner elaborated, marginality appears where the service objective of pharmacists is at odds with their pecuniary goals.

On the other hand, from the interactionist perspective, marginality can be seen as a discrepancy between the self-perception and the perception by others concerning the status of the occupation in question. McCormack found that pharmacy students tend to view their own prestige as being much higher than does the general population. This imaginary prestige is acquired by manipulating social reality, that is, by viewing themselves as part of the established medico-scientific profession. These students have similarly upgraded the ranking of the chemist and the dentist above the levels accorded by the general public.

Quinney (1963, 1964) compared the objective, structurally induced role conflict and the subjective perception of the situation. He found that while 94 percent of the retail pharmacists acknowledged the existence of a role conflict objectively, only a quarter of the business-oriented pharmacists were subjectively affected by the conflict. The business-oriented were more likely than the profession-oriented to have violated drug dispensing laws, presumably by attempting to maximize their financial self-interests. It was the professional pharmacist who was most likely to suffer from the role strain, yet he or she also indicated career satisfaction.

An alternative to the method of description by dichotomy is to describe the profession and the business from separate multi-dimensional perspectives rather than in terms of a single continuum of acquisitiveness versus altruism (Caplow, 1954). Following this method, Denzin and Mettlin (1968) viewed pharmacy as a case of incomplete professionalization. Although pharmacy has acquired certain features of a profession, for example, educational training, it does not have all of them, such as autonomy and prestige.

A second method is to reject the contrasting difference between profession and business. Parsons (1949) stated that both a business and a profession pursue similar goals of achievement and recognition. The only difference lies in the institutionalized patterns by which they realize these goals. Kronous (1975) found that both altruistic and pecuniary values are similarly important to pharmacists, whether they are profession or business oriented. Then, when the working environment was considered, altruism prevailed in the business-oriented setting, and prestige and income were deemed least important. Kronous concluded that an ideology of service is not the exclusive domain of a profession—it is a commonly professed value. The public spirit concerning that ideology has become a common advertising theme.

Finally, a third critique of the professional versus business role conflict is pursued from the perspective of contextual analysis, which focuses its attention upon the external circumstances in which pharmacists operate. For example, Bean (1977) stressed the importance of studying the behavior of pharmacists as the function not only of pharmaceutical group norms but also of global trends such as bureaucratization. Such a societal force tends to direct pharmacy as well as other occupations toward deprofessionalization, despite the intent of the individual occupation to do otherwise, that is, to professionalize itself.

Hierarchical Conflict of Pharmacy versus Medicine

Between medicine and pharmacy there exist some generic equivalents, such as (1) the performance of relatively specific, socially necessary functions; (2) the acquisition of a body of knowledge, a special technique, and competence, mastery of which requires theoretical study; and (3) the adherance to a generally accepted professional ethics of service.

However, pharmacy has been viewed as containing two conflicting roles, that is, the preparation and the distribution of drugs (Thorner, 1942). The former involves decisions as to who needs what medication. This requires specialized training to acquire scientific knowledge and skill. The distribution of drugs, in contrast, pertains to the business management of drugs, demanding sales talent.

The inherent strain in the relationship between medicine and pharmacy stems from the fact that medicine has tried to monopolize the function of the preparation of drugs. The prescription of drugs belongs to the domain of medicine, and not the province of pharmacy. Thus, pharmacy is an adjunct to medicine in functionalist terms.

The pharmaceutical professional code directs the pharmacist to follow faithfully instructions from the physician, and it condemns any substitution in a prescription. For the pharmacist, this functional limitation of judgment and initiative results in a paradoxical code of ethics, minimizing the exercise of initiative and judgment. Technical proficiency is the only pharmaceutical ideal, and there is nothing a pharmacist can do about a prescription when in doubt except to communicate with the doctor.

However, the relationship between pharmacy and medicine is not integrated by a hierarchical order alone, and it should be viewed as an interactive process with strain and conflict.

First of all, from the professional role perspective, blind adherance to directions does not constitute the pharmacist's whole duty. If a doctor makes an error on a prescription, it is the responsibility of the pharmacist to detect it. Should he or she fail to do so, the pharmacist as well as the doctor may be penalized. This position of professional responsibility gives leverage to the pharmacist, who evaluates the physician by the type of prescription given. As a result, the pharmacist looks down upon and considers incompetent those doctors who habitually call for patent medicine.

When doctors are legitimately too busy to keep up with the proliferation of new drugs, they may even consult with pharmacists from time to time. In the case of a hospital practice, the role of the pharmacist is being redefined as that of a working member of a coordinated group of health professionals (Cain & Kahn, 1971). Bean (1977) found that this new type, the clinical pharmacist, is patient-oriented and actively participates in patient care through drug therapy.

However, according to a study by Lambert and others (1977), other health workers feel that the pharmacist's clinical role should, but in reality is less likely to, include (1) reviewing drug utilization, (2) documenting professional activities, (3) directing patient involvement, (4) dispensing and administering drugs, and (5) prescribing drugs, in that descending order. Among retail pharmacists, those who show a tendency to recommend products to clients are business-oriented people (Linn & Davis, 1973). This suggests that their clinical orientation is derived from entrepreneurship rather than professionalism.

Thus, a second type of medico-pharmaceutical interaction involves the pharmacist's entrepreneurial role. The pharmacist's frequent contact with the public puts him or her in a position of power in relation to the physician (Hull, 1955). The pharmacist can refer patients to a particular physician or reward those physicians who send patients to him or her by providing rent-free office or other "business" considerations.

Under Medicare and Medicaid, kickbacks on pharmaceutical products have been criticized (Apple, 1970). According to these programs, financed by the third-party payment, the pharmacists' reimbursement is funneled through other facilities such as hospitals, nursing homes, and extended-care facilities. Since small hospitals and nursing homes do not maintain their own on-site pharmacies, they look to community pharmacists to provide such service on a contract basis. In most situations there is competition among the pharmacists to obtain such a contract. Consequently, they are often solicited for "under-the-table kickbacks," that is, granting illegitimate discounts to nursing homes and aiding the latter in submitting false statements to the federal government. The most bitter complaints, however, come not from the public but rather from pharmacists who have been seduced into this unfair, competitive practice.

Professional Organization

Local Organization. The history of the development of the professional pharmaceutical organization reflects the process of dialectic conflict rather than an evolutionary growth of professionalism through functional integration with other institutions of society.

First of all, we can identify the laissez faire state of pharmaceutical practice during its early period. Thanks to the American ideology of liberty and individualism, the quality control needed to raise pharmacy to the status of a profession was left to the initiative of individual pharmacists. They did not want any restrictions by a special group that thought itself superior to others, by their own associations, or even by law. Standardization and regulations were understandably objected to by the uneducated merchant druggists who could not meet any standards and who did not want to lose their unscrupulous business.

The conflicting pressure came from an external group—the medical profession. Medical science, which was flourishing in Philadelphia at the time, began to take some control of the drug trade in 1820. It was then that a suggestion was made by the medical faculty to grant an honorary degree to apothecaries who had shown their mastery of pharmacy by passing an examination.

Resentment toward such an action led Philadelphia druggists to hold their first meeting to propose counteraction. They acknowledged the necessity to raise the standards of their trade in order to place their business on the respectable footing of a branch of the science of medicine. To that end, they established the College of Apothecaries (1821), which later changed its name to the College of Pharmacy. Since the college was founded as an association of practicing pharmacists, its activity was not limited to the establishment and management of its school. Its power extended to the inspection of drugs, the settlement of disputes, and the like. The leaders of the college published the first *American Pharmaceutical Journal* in 1825.

National Organizations. Like the development of the local association, a central, nationwide organization did not originate through a growing understanding of the necessity of professional solidarity, but rather developed as a response to pressure from the outside. In this case, it arose from bad conditions in the drug trade.

The external challenge came from British manufacturers who exported pharmaceutical preparations that were substituted for, adulterated, or even weakened in strength. A petition to Congress, signed by pharmacists as well as physicians all over the country, resulted in the passage of a law that required the observance of standards (1848). The need to set up standards for drug inspection and to establish a national organization led to the emergence of the American Pharmaceutical Association in 1852. Gradually, those who became dissatisfied with the limited status and sphere of activities provided by this organization formed other associations such as the National Association of

Retail Druggists (1898) and the American Society of Hospital Pharmacists (1942).

Thus, the rise of local and national associations was an accommodative response to external forces more than to the professional enthusiasm of member druggists. However, in accordance with the dialectic conflict viewpoint, any movement carries within itself the seed of its own destruction. Organizations that were established to avoid legal restrictions in the practice of pharmacy, became the initiators and guardians of American pharmaceutical legislation. A series of pharmacy laws transferred the responsibility of drug control from the hands of pharmacists to those of law enforcement agencies.

For instance, the Food and Drug administration was given the power to classify every new drug into categories of "by prescription only" or "over-the-counter" (OTC), or to classify certain drugs as unsafe except under the supervision of a physician. That external power thereby reduced the frequency of OTC prescribing, and hence the responsibility of the pharmacist.

Organizational Strength. Although pharmacy has its several national, state, and local societies, these organizations have been ineffective in representing and controlling the whole profession. Due to the proliferation of subspecialization, pharmacy fails to hold together in a cohesive organization. Some pharmacists have moved in opposite directions without strict censure from the pharmaceutical societies. For instance, the pharmacy societies have made little attempt to take a definite stand in two movements: (1) the proliferation of small apothecary shops and (2) the development of the large, chain, discount drugstores.

The weakness of structural cohesiveness is also found in the absence of a clear-cut organizational bond between the national and state levels in many areas. Except in a few states, membership in the national association is not contingent or automatic upon membership in state societies (Akers & Quinney, 1968).

Such organizational weakness has resulted in incomplete professionalization of pharmacy in that it has failed to insure its control over the social object around which its activities are organized, namely, the service of preparing drugs (Denzin & Mettlin, 1968). For example, retail drugstores tend to engage in selling nondrug items. Also, pharmacists have lost to the drug manufacturing industry their function of compounding ingredients.

ANCILLARY PRACTITIONERS: PHYSICIAN'S ASSISTANTS

The Emergence of the Physician's Assistant

The concept of a physician's assistant and the delegation of the physician's tasks are not new. For years physicians have entrusted a wide variety of duties to nurses and medical assistants (i.e., the title for the nonprofessional office helper with clerical or technical capacity). What is new since the mid-1960s is the desire to formalize the training for a new category of personnel who perform services delegated by physicians.

According to the AMA, the physician's assistant is defined as a skilled person qualified by academic and practical training to provide patient care under the supervision and direction of a licensed physician, who is responsible for the performance of that assistant (Todd & Foy, 1972).

The emergence of this new occupational classification is due to several factors. The most immediate is the health workforce shortage and maldistribution, particularly in the supply of physicians (Carnegie Commission, 1970; Petersdorf, 1975). The scarcity of physicians is partly due to the restrictive policy adopted by the AMA in training physicians (which was discussed in Chapter 6). There is also the increasing utilization of medical care facilities by people who have come to believe that health care is a right. Since many of a physician's functions are routine and repetitious, specially trained personnel such as the physician's assistant can assume these tasks (Lewis et al., 1969; Yankauer et al., 1970).

The first physician's assistant training program was begun at Duke University in 1965. Personnel in the health field were too few in number and inadequately trained to meet the demands placed on the medical profession, which generated the need to create a new career program for physician's assistants (Stead, 1966).

The following years witnessed a mushrooming of diverse curricula. For instance, the University of Washington began the Medex program in 1969 for the military corpsmen and corpswomen returning from Vietnam, who possessed extensive medical training and work experience in remote sites without physicians' supervision. While specialty programs such as the orthopedic assistant and urologic assistant programs required fairly intensive training, there also appeared a four-month health assistant program (1970), which required only the attainment of age 18 for admission.

By 1970, the Department of Health, Education, and Welfare reported 80 physician's assistant training programs in various stages of development in addition to 50 programs to extend nursing roles (U.S. DHEW, 1972), although less than 200 physician's assistants had graduated ("Survey . . . ," 1971). In the torrent of diversity, some efforts toward consensus were being made.

In 1970 the Board of Medicine of the National Academy of Sciences classified physician's assistants into three categories according to the degree of specialization and level of judgment exercised (Estes, 1970). Type-A physician's assistants are qualified to act as the primary patient contact, collect historical and physical data, and analyze and report the data so that physicians can grasp the problems and determine the next appropriate steps. They can also perform diagnostic and therapeutic duties specified by physicians. In limited settings they function without direct supervision of physicians (Barkin, 1974).

The job description and training of Type-B assistants are concentrated and narrow, but in their special areas their skill may exceed those of average general practitioners. Finally, the formal training of Type-C assistants is limited both in the depth and breadth of theoretical base. They are expected to work under the close and direct supervision of the physician.

Interest in training physician's assistants has been primarily stimulated by educators, congressional representatives, and government officials. Although organized medicine did not originate the concept, it has taken upon itself the responsibility for developing this new occupation so that it will become a formal adjunct to medical care.

In 1977 the AMA reported 53 accredited educational programs ("Allied health . . . ," 1977, p. 2813). Two institutions sponsor accredited programs for surgeon's assistants. There are a small number of new, as yet unaccredited, educational programs for radiology, pathology, and anesthesiology assistants.

Despite the fact that these programs have been in existence for over a decade, the variation in training and the failure to impose any standard evaluation makes it difficult to reach an overall conclusion about their impact on access to primary care. The evidence available indicates that physician's assistants have made additional primary care services available to specific population groups such as children and those in certain urban areas (Fisher & Horowitz, 1977; Lave & Leinhardt, 1975; Schonfeld, Heston, & Fals, 1972). Those physician's assistants placed in community health centers or located with family practitioners in rural areas have had a significant bearing on access (Raba, 1979). Some studies indicate that more than 42 percent of the graduates are located in nonmetropolitan counties with populations between 10,000 to 50,000. However, no conclusive statement can be made because of the fluidity of employment and the variations in state legislation (Fisher & Horowitz, 1977). Also, to the extent that physician's assistants remain tied to physicians as their employees, supervisors, and source of reimbursement, physician's assistants will be maldistributed in the same pattern as physicians.

From a financial viewpoint, provision of some of the physician's services by nonphysicians should reduce medical expenditure in terms of the cost of medical education and the medical fees that consumers must pay. Furthermore, personnel resources for physician's assistants are readily available among those who are partially trained but fall short of becoming physicians, such as returning military corpsmen and corpswomen (Smith, Richard, 1969).

Any effect on financial efficiency should be seen in a reduction of the cost of services billed directly to patients served by physician's assistants. There are no national data to allow generalizations yet. In some cases it is reported that patients are billed at 50 to 75 percent of the prevailing fee schedule for the same services when provided by physician's assistants (O'Hara-Devereaux et al., 1977; Seigel, Jensen, & Coffee, 1977). However, in many instances no significant differences seem to have been made (Lewis, Fein, & Mechanic, 1976).

In the context of medical practice, the physician's assistant contributes to the quality of medical care by alleviating the burden on overworked physicians (Stead, 1967). Also, the assistant can offer services for primary, preventive, and emergency needs. With growing specialization, many physicians are educated beyond primary and general practice functions and are likely to prefer to practice in specialized areas. Thus, physicians and physician's assistants can be complementary.

Furthermore, it was hoped that physician's assistants would be able to reduce the social distance between patients and physicians. Physician's assistants are expected to approach patients through different styles of interaction to eliminate a patient's psychological barriers to the medical establishment. However, available data suggest that many physician's assistants adopt traditional modes of interaction (Lewis, Fein, & Mechanic, 1976). In sum, whether or not the physician's assistants remain marginal additives to scarce physicians or play a strategic role in improving medical practice remains to be seen.

Physician's Assistant Training

Recruitment. Only a limited number of students may be enrolled each year. Consequently, the physician's assistant selection process is highly competitive (Fisher & Horowitz, 1977). There are several avenues of recruitment for physician's assistant programs. First of all, there are those who chose the physician's career but failed. In 1970, 24,987 people applied to American medical schools, which had space for only 11,348 (Dube et al., 1971). According to the Association of American Medical Colleges, as many as one half of the remaining 13,639 were fully qualified to become physicians. Many of those people may be eager and able to deliver primary care as physician's assistants.

Second, the physician's assistantship offers an opportunity to enter medicine without the lengthy training required for an M.D. degree. Many college graduates are interested in the health care field but do not wish to go through medical school. Third, there are highly intelligent, motivated individuals who are interested in direct patient care. For them, primary care is where the action is in the health field. Fourth, being a physician's assistant can be a way out for some registered nurses, pharmacists, inhalation therapists, and laboratory technicians who feel that they are in a dead-end career. Finally, the physician's assistant is a useful civilian health occupation for military medical technician who otherwise find it difficult to fit into the traditional medical practice system.

An interview with a class of 40 students in the physician's assistant program at Duke University in 1972 revealed that the average age was 28 and nearly all (33 out of 40) were married ("A glimpse . . . ," 1972). However, all the students had begun their careers in health-related fields long before entering this program. One entrance requirement for the Duke program is at least 2,000 hours of direct patient contact. The interviewed stduents had an average of five years of experience as military medical technicians, X-ray operators, nurses, medical technicians, inhalation therapists, or similar specialty.

As for their motivation for enrolling in the program, the legal consultant to the program observed: "They're not frustrated docs'—they see themselves as valued members of the health care team." Students tended to speak in more pragmatic terms—upward mobility. The starting salary of $14,300 in 1975 (Fisher & Horowitz, 1977) may not be a great step upward for veterans with many years of experience, but they expected to climb quickly once they built up experience. In addition, upward mobility to them meant more than a raise in pay; it meant an elevation from the position of mere technician to that of a health-team member. They viewed the physician's assistant program as a chance to upgrade skills either by broadening their experience or by learning medical specialties. Most of the students viewed the physician's assistant occupation as a career, not a stepping-stone to some other profession, which is in conformity with the original purpose of the Duke program (Association of PA Programs, 1976; Estes & Howard, 1970; Stead, 1966).

Socialization. There have been three types of training identified: the Medex program (three-month didactic work followed by nine to twelve months of preceptorship); the two-year university medical center-based program; and the two-year college or university program in a nonmedical setting. All these programs begin with intensive didactic work in basic and clinical sciences, followed by a preceptorship with practicing physicians in various clinical settings such as fee-for-service sites, solo and group practices, university medical centers, Health Maintenance Organizations or other prepaid group plans, public health departments, prisons, specialty hospitals, and military installations. This is to provide a broad experience that orients the students toward primary, ambulatory care.

Physician's assistants are trained to be interdependent practitioners under physician supervision. For this purpose, curricula are intended to develop the ability to elicit a comprehensive health history, to perform a comprehensive physical examination, to make simple diagnostic laboratory determinations, to provide basic treatment for common illnesses, to make an appropriate clinical response to commonly encountered emergencies, and to be concerned with preventive medicine (Fisher & Horowitz, 1977).

Because of the short history of the program, few systematic studies of student culture and socialization processes are available. However, from available reports ("A glimpse . . . ," 1972) and the structural arrangement of the training program, a certain amount of conflict is anticipated.

First of all, the physician's assistant program operates under the direction of a physician who is chairperson of the admission committee, who organizes the course materials, and recommends certification by the medical center (Stead, 1966). Not only are the physician's assistant trainees under the physician-teacher's authority, but also they are frequently placed side by side with medical students, who enjoy higher academic status. Many programs (Kempe, 1968; McCally et al., 1977; Stead, 1966) are conducted in close association with medical schools in order to give future physicians an early appreciation for and understanding of the value of the physician's assistant. This will place students for physician's assistantship at the bottom of the totem pole, except that in the clinical setting they have nurses below them. The students for physician's assistantship tend to think that their training is more rigorous than most nursing programs and that they can outperform the nurses clinically ("A glimpse . . . ," 1972).

Physician's Assistants in Operation

A recent study of 1,250 physician's assistants who graduated prior to 1975 indicated that 67 percent of them were employed in primary care: 23 percent in family practice, 22 percent in general medicine, 15 percent in internal medicine,

5 percent in pediatrics, and 2 percent in obstetrics/gynecology (Fisher & Horowitz, 1977). However, there is a danger for physician's assistants to be "swallowed whole by the whale that is our present entrepreneurial, subspecialty medical practice system" (Sadler et al., 1975, p. 28). The attraction of specializing is partly financial, since the physician's assistant without specialization may not earn much more than nurses (Sadler et al., 1975). In the interview of 40 students at Duke University, 14 reported their expectation to specialize in surgery, and 18, in medicine ("A glimpse . . . ," 1972). Many training programs are seeking to prevent such cooption. For instance, primary care in rural areas is emphasized at the stage of clinical rotation in many programs (Godkins et al., 1974).

Physician's Assistant versus Physician. Once in a practice setting, the position of the physician's assistant is ambivalent in relation to the physician and the patient. Practicing physicians in Wisconsin were surveyed by Coye and Hansen in 1969 to determine their attitudes toward the concept of the physician's assistant and the roles to be filled in practice. Of the respondents, 61 percent believed that they would use physician's assistants in their own practice. Physicians in the survey sample saw the physician's assistant almost exclusively as a technician rather than as an independent health professional. The majority of them thought the following areas inappropriate for physician's assistants: routine anesthetics, uncomplicated deliveries, portions of physical examinations, and many emergency room procedures. What were considered as more "disposable" jobs included taking a medical history and discussing illnesses with the patients (Ford, 1975).

The American Society of Internal Medicine found that its members believed that many tasks of their practice could and should be delegated to an allied health worker, such as history taking (60 percent), home visit (65 percent), patient instruction (70 percent), nursing home visit (43 percent), and pap smear (34 percent) (Riddick et al., 1971). The American Academy of Pediatrics also reported that over 70 percent of surveyed pediatricians favored delegation of such activities as recording of history and counseling on child care (Yankauer et al., 1970).

In the above studies as well as in others (Hellman et al., 1970), a discrepancy is found between what the physicians believe they could and should delegate and what they would delegate in reality. Many studies revealed that while about 60 percent accept the physician's assistant concept in principle, only 30 percent would be inclined to delegate many of their responsibilities. However, there are other studies indicating that the physician's assistants have achieved "negotiated autonomy" in relation to physicians (Duttera & Harlan, 1975).

To some extent, the physician's task delegation to paramedical personnel varies according to the work setting. Breslau, Wolf, and Novack (1978) found that physicians in large, complex organizations on the average delegated more than did small, independent practitioners. The large organizations are expected to avail themselves of greater paramedical resources. However, physicians in the modern, presumably rational, health service organizations are more likely than traditional solo practitioners to utilize physician's assistants only in routinized, technical duties but not in patient care tasks. In short, irrespective of the work setting, the transfer of medical tasks to nonphysicians has been very limited.

The relationship between the physician's assistant and others on the health team depends on his or her position in the organization. Sadler and others (1975) classified three types of organizational alternatives: (1) a vertical or authoritarian structure in which the physician's assistant is dependent on the physician; (2) a horizontal or egalitarian setting in which the physician's assistant is independent; and (3) a circular arrangement whereby everyone, including the physician's assistant, is interdependent upon one another. If the health team is to become a workable entity, the circular model is desirable. Yet, this model seems to be more widely talked about than implemented (Breytspraak & Pondy, 1969). Also, there is a great variation from state to state in the degree of autonomy enjoyed by physician's assistants. In some states physician's assistants function independently even to the extent of prescribing and dispensing drugs, while in other states such as in California they work under the supervision of physicians (Raba, 1979).

Physician's Assistants versus Patients. The public perception of the physician's assistant was surveyed by Litman (1972) in rural Iowa and Minnesota. Although respondents were generally supportive (65 percent), a substantial portion of them (31 percent) showed lack of confidence in the training, experience, and competence of the physician's assistants. Frequently, public acceptance of physician's assistants required the personal endorsements of local family physicians. Particularly strong objection was raised against allowing former military corpsmen to provide maternity services such as prenatal care and routine delivery.

A systematic study was done to evaluate the Medex trainees in primary care in upper New England (Nelson et al., 1974). The vast majority of patients in the sample who had been cared for by Medexes reported that they were "very competent" (89 percent), "very sure of themselves" (83 percent), "very professional in their manner" (86 percent), "respectful" (100 percent), and "courteous" (96 percent). Furthermore, 83 percent of the patients definitely would want the Medex to participate in their care again.

Patients were very favorably disposed toward allowing a Medex to perform routine technical procedures, such as giving injections (93 percent) and recording vital signs (98 percent), but there was considerable opposition to their performing normal deliveries (36 percent) or running a prenatal and well-baby clinic (58 percent).

In terms of background characteristics of patients, more positive attitudes toward Medex were elicited from (1) younger patients, (2) women, (3) lower socioeconomic class patients, and (4) patients in remote rural areas, who suffer from a physician shortage. It should be noted that the above findings concerning the socioeconomic status of patients differ from those by Breytspraak and Pondy (1969), who reported that both the lowest and highest income groups were less likely to accept the physician's assistants than were middle class people.

There are many other contradictions among the available research findings. Part of the problem is that few systematic comparisons have been made because of the newness of the programs. Another source of discrepancy is the instability of the patient's receptivity to the physician's assistant. Nelson and others (1974) found that as the degree of interaction with Medex increases, so does the patient's acceptance of Medex.

Quality of Care. Many studies have been conducted to assess objectively the quality of care provided by physician's assistants. Having reviewed much of the literature, Celentano (1978) concluded that within the officially defined tasks for which physician's assistants are trained, the levels of quality are equally high when compared to physicians.

However, Celentano raised questions regarding the applicability of generalizing from these research findings. First of all, the quality of care is multidimensional (Cohen et al., 1974). Measures used include (1) the degree of concurrance between physicians and assistants concerning diagnosis and chart- and record-reading; (2) comparative rates for complication, disability, hospitalization, and mortality of patients treated by physicians and assistants; and (3) patients' utilization of hospital emergency service versus physician's assistant services. Most of these indexes used as measures of quality have extremely questionable reliability and validity. They are unstandardized and lack comparability.

Second, samples are generally small and biased. Many studies were conducted upon newly graduated physician's assistants. They may be better trained and more highly motivated to maintain high standards than those who got the degree earlier and have been practicing several years.

Third, few studies have given attention to structural variables such as practice setting and geographical areas. As is true with physicians (Rhee, 1977; Ross & Duff, 1978), the quality of care is likely to vary significantly depending on the organizational context in which physician's assistants practice.

Thus, despite a rapidly increasing literature on the quality of care by physician's assistants, there still exist numerous issues to be resolved. A more sophisticated analytic design is called for before generalizations can be made.

Organizational Control by the AMA

Physician's assistants are subsumed under several national organizations—the American Academy of Physician's Assistants (AAPA), the Association of PA Programs (APAP), and the National Commission for Certification of Physicians' Assistants (NCCPA). These physician's assistant organizations remain closely linked with the AMA and the Association of American Medical Colleges (AAMC) (Glazer, 1977).

The status of a profession, as characterized by autonomy, is difficult to conceive of for the physician's assistant. By definition, physician's assistants are dependent on physicians. They are selected, trained, and supervised by physicians, and administratively they report directly to physicians. There is no distinct body of knowledge monopolized by the physician's assistants, since virtually all of their activities are ones delegated by the physicians.

It was exactly this fear of losing whatever professional autonomy gained by nurses that caused the nursing organizations to reject the AMA's invitation for them to become physician's assistants. In 1969 the AMA announced a plan to make 100,000 nurses physician's assistants. The responses from the nursing organizations were immediate and wrathful. They objected to the AMA's unilateral decision to meet the physician shortage by compounding the scarcity of nurses. Later, disagreement appeared among nurses, some of whom viewed the physician's assistantship as the only opportunity for nurses to extend their functions (Sadler et al., 1975). Nurses are trying to establish their professional independence by raising their educational level. In contrast, physician's assistants enjoy more medical responsibility and higher income than nurses by assuming a legally dependent position.

The pressures to raise the standards of training and practice for physician's assistants came from the AMA rather than from physician's assistants, who had not yet established a single national organization with resources and power (Todd, 1972). The primary concern of the AMA is that services rendered by allied health workers be consistent with standards acceptable to the AMA.

With regard to licensure, a basic question is whether physician's assistants should be licensed at all, or whether the sanction for their performances should be considered as an extension of the legal authorization conferred upon the physicians (Carlson & Athelstan, 1970; Kissam, 1977). Currently, many of the state legislature proposals are of two basic types (Todd, 1972): (1) an exception to the medical practice act to codify the physician's legally required right to delegate tasks to competent allied health personnel; or (2) a broadening of the power given to the state board of medical examiners so that the board may approve training programs or certify graduates of approved programs.

The original intent of licensure was to place very specific restrictions and standards on the license as a means of clearly assigning liability. If physician's assistants are not licensed, their negligent acts become liabilities of their supervising physicians. This will inhibit physicians from delegating tasks to their assistants.

On the other hand, a rigid licensure code could severly restrict the range of the physician's assistant's activities. Also, proliferation of licensing laws for specific categories of allied health care tends to fractionalize the provision of health services and inhibit the flexible utilization of the allied health workforce at a time when innovation is needed (Raba, 1979).

Furthermore, the general philosophy governing licensure has been challenged in recent years (Forgotson & Cook, 1967). Traditionally, the ability of a licensee is determined by the satisfaction of educational training requirements (input) rather than by performance after graduation (output). Hence the licensure system leads to the arbitrary escalation of educational requirements with little attention given to the product.

Thus, instead of customary licensure, certification is being proposed. In 1971 the AMA adopted a proposal to assume a leadership role in the developing and sponsoring of a national program for the certification of the physician's assistant who functions at the highest level of responsibility (Type-A, mentioned earlier). This certification process is to include two components: (1) proficiency tests to assess an individual's knowledge and skills related to the actual demands of an occupational specialty or a specific job; and (2) equivalence tests to sanction learning gained outside of formal training programs.

ANCILLARY PRACTITIONERS: NURSES

History of Nursing

Medieval Nursing. Two great influences during the Middle Ages—religion and the military—shaped the nursing practice into a distinct occupation. One of the most astonishing undertakings of the feudal system was the Crusades, which necessitated the establishment of hospitals staffed by physicians and nurses.

Formal groups or orders of nursing were developed and sponsored by the Church. The assumption of worldly responsibility by the Church led to care for the poor and the sick, and devout Christian women became devoted to nursing. Absolute devotion to the sick without selfish motives made the nursing order acceptable to all, and it was thus able to survive for many centuries.

Nursing in the Middle Ages was technologically primitive; an important duty of the nurses was to minister to the spiritual needs of the patient. The nursing order was not yet firmly associated with the medical profession because nursing was dominated by the Church, and medicine had not advanced enough to exert its leadership over nursing. Since it was attached to the Church, nursing had to share in its vicissitudes (Bullough & Bullough, 1969; Dock & Stewart, 1938; Griffin & Griffin, 1973).

From the Late Seventeenth Century to the Midnineteenth Century. The period from the end of the seventeenth century to the middle of the nineteenth century witnessed remarkable advances in medical sciences. However, as was described in Chapter 6, there was a large gap between medical discoveries and the adoption of the new knowledge into medical practice. Since medical practice at that time was based on superstition and assumed knowledge, it could not possibly stimulate the evolution of nursing as a profession.

Nursing sank to its lowest level in those countries where Catholic organizations were upset by the Reformation. The state closed churches, monastries, and hospitals. As a result, nursing lost the dignity of the Church. Nurses were recruited from the lower classes and were without organization and social standing. Before nursing could be fully accepted as a worthy occupation, the importance of secular nurses had to be recognized. This was difficult because of the position of women in society. The reform of nursing was made possible only by a series of social revolutions during the eighteenth and nineteenth centuries that led to the emancipation of women in general.

Within this social setting, the Crimean War broke out in 1854. Medical care for the wounded became a great public issue, and public pressure was brought to bear to improve the status of nursing and medical care. Florence Nightingale returned from the war a heroine because her nursing administration was effective in reducing the death rate (Dock & Stewart, 1938).

The Nightingale Fund and the Nightingale School of Nursing were established. Nightingale emphasized the importance of training nurses and was successful in refuting the commonly held notion by physicians that nursing could be done by instinct. Thus, nursing was elevated from a lowly craft supervised by an order of the Church to a respected, formal occupation. None of these developments were received with enthusiasm by physicians, but the changes were accepted so long as control over nurses remained in physicians' hands (Bullough, 1976; Glaser, 1966a).

American Nursing. During the early days, American nursing resembled that of the Reformation period in Europe in that nurses were ill-paid individuals from the lower classes. Hospitals were for the poor, while middle class patients were taken care of at home and were nursed by family members.

In the same year, 1873, three important schools were founded. They were Bellevue Hospital School of Nursing in New York City, the Connecticut Training School in New Haven, and Boston Training School of Massachusetts General Hospital. Each tried to gain independence from the hospital administration for its nursing education by establishing two principles: (1) the school must be considered an educational institution and not a source of cheap labor for the hospital; and (2) the school of nursing must be administratively independent from the hospital. In 1894 and 1896 forerunners of the American Nursing Association (ANA) and the National League for Nursing (NLN) were established. They were able to gain control over the profession and to stem the growth of substandard nursing schools by means of the state licensure system (Dietz, 1963; Goodnow, 1930; Nutting & Dock, 1912).

Between the two World Wars, a reform movement succeeded in instituting university-based nursing education and the accreditation system (Davis, 1966; Fenwick, 1901). By the 1950s nurses were well educated, but their role did not include diagnostic and therapeutic functions. It has only been since 1971 that many states have began to enact amendments to their nurse practice acts to facilitate the assumption of diagnostic and treatment functions by nurses (Brown, Swift, & Oberman, 1974; Reeder & Mauksch, 1979).

The history of nursing is viewed by some (Ehrenreich & English, 1973; Twaddle & Hessler, 1977) as a process of conflict among healing practitioners, or rather, as the process by which female healers and nurses were defeated by male physicians.

Early healers, whether male or female, had no more scientific knowledge than that of herbal remedies. Nonetheless, it was only the women healers who were persecuted and murdered during the witch hunts by the church and the state. During the early 1800s in the United States, physicians who called themselves "regular practitioners" had no better knowledge than did the "irregulars." However, the former succeeded in consolidating their status by associating with the elite and powerful members of society and by fostering favorable legislation. The consequent decline of the irregular practitioners forced women healers to join forces with regular physicians, on a subservient basis, and to accept nursing as the only option open to women as health careerists.

Such a perspective of sexual and social class conflict tends to de-emphasize the role of technology. While physicians were acquiring knowledge and techniques that were distinct from those of the irregular practitioners, nurses did not establish a base of knowledge that was the exclusive property of the nursing domain. If nurses are able to develop a unique "art" of medicine that is competitive in healing power with the physicians' "science" of medicine, job recruitment into nursing and medicine may be based more on an individual's work orientation than on sexual status.

Nursing Education

At present, students can become registered nurses in three programs: a three-year hospital-based diploma program, a two-year associate degree program at a junior (community) college, or a four-year baccalaureate program at a university or college (Rowland, 1978).

In 1965 the ANA presented a position paper that advocated granting the baccalaureate degree for professional nursing and the associate degree for technical nursing, although it was not accepted by the majority of its membership (Walters et al., 1972). The *professional nurse* was defined as one who: (1) has at her command a theoretical as well as an empirical body of knowledge; (2) shares the responsibility for total patient welfare and progress, coordinating medical and other services; and (3) has the freedom to think and act independently, consulting with but not being supervised by physicians. The *technical nurse,* on the other hand, (1) exercises judgment within clearly defined limits, dealing with common and concrete nursing problems; (2) works under the supervision of a physician or a professional nurse; and (3) renders direct technical assistance to the professional nurse engaged in research and practice innovation (Fagin, 1976; Reeder & Mauksch, 1979).

Interest in developing and implementing a doctoral program in nursing has accelerated during the past 15 years. Several major university schools of nursing have, since the early 1960s, initiated programs to stimulate nurses to gain research skills and theoretical insight and to broaden their general scholarship (Leininger, 1976).

Recruitment and Socialization

Recruitment. In view of the fact that the three-year hospital based diploma students constituted 81 percent of the total nursing student body in 1959 and 53 percent as late as 1968, it is understandable that most of the earlier research on nursing students was conducted in the diploma schools.

While baccalaureate programs tend to attract middle and upper class students (Knopf, 1972; McPartland, 1957), other programs tend to recruit students from the lower middle class and from the upwardly mobile group (Mauksch, 1972). Upwardly mobile students from working or middle class families with the economic means for their education view nursing as a road to greater social mobility. More recent studies, however, indicate some changes in the social background of the nursing students, i.e., higher-income families

(Reeder & Mauksch, 1979).

The decision to enter nursing is reported to occur quite early, long before high school age (Fox et al., 1961; Martin & Simpson, 1959; Williams et al., 1960). However, the two-year associate-degree students tend to be older and to have had prior health care experience (Knopf, 1972; Wren, 1971).

Motivations for entering nursing are reported by the diploma school students as the desire to serve patients, to serve physicians (Reeder & Mauksch, 1979), to be needed, and to work closely with others. Many studies (Ginsberg et al., 1951) indicate that nursing combines functional pleasure (i.e., helping patients) and symbolic status (i.e., being needed), and it gratifies needs for affiliative and nurturant relationships. As a corollary, these same nursing students tend to avoid individual risks or blame-producing situations, and they are not characterized by assertiveness or radicalism. In short, nurses in the hospital-controlled diploma schools are not the type who would rebel against medical domination in order to gain professional autonomy.

Baccalaureate students, on the other hand, express as their reasons for selecting nursing that it is a means for achieving personal advancement as well as for helping people (Wren, 1971). Students in the associate degree program tend to be tied to a vocational rather than a professional motivation.

Socialization. The nurse's role in diploma schools is defined as being subordinate to the physician's. This is closely linked with the traditional female role in which a woman is expected to support and protect the dominant male, since nurses are still predominantly females (Schulman, 1972).

Socialization of students into this submissive role is done by designating compliance as a component of "professional" behavior. For instance, if a nurse goes to the nursing office and complains about a patient, she is simply told that she has not behaved professionally, which in this case implies not acting with dignity, deference, and distance (Mauksch, 1963). This early and forceful emphasis on professional behavior is important because a role failure reflects more on the nursing occupation rather than on the individual (Reeder & Mauksch, 1979).

In contrast, baccalaureate students are reported to be socialized to a nursing role that values individualized patient care, rational knowledge, and innovation, and to view themselves as autonomous, professional persons (Brown, Swift, & Oberman, 1974; Kramer, 1970). Nevertheless, compared with the general college population of females, nursing students attach greater importance to altruistic and philanthrophic service and less importance to personal influence and the dominance of others (O'Neil, 1973).

The sources of their disillusionment also appear to be different for the diploma and baccalaureate students. Since the diploma school emphasizes practical training, those students begin their systematic contacts with patients at an early stage, which tends to disillusion them sooner. Patients are often rude and ungrateful. For diploma student nurses, patients present a challenge to rather than a gratification of their desire for nurturant relationships. They gradually learn that nursing is just a job to be done (Ingmire, 1952; Meyer, 1960).

In contrast, baccalaureate students are prone to experience major disappointment much later—not until they find that the professional autonomy taught at school is dysfunctional in the bureaucratic work setting of the real world (Kramer, 1974; Wren, 1971).

In sum, one of the difficulties faced by nursing in establishing itself as a profession is the seeming absence of a distinct knowledge base. Despite doctorate programs and higher education, it is not easy to claim that the domain of nursing knowledge is independent of that of the physicians' domain.

Nursing Practice

Professionalism and Role Conflict. Is nursing a profession? There is a disagreement even among nurses, and many take a negative or neutral position. From their leaders, nurses are under pressure to become professionals, while physicians and nurses themselves are apt to doubt their qualifications as professionals. The physician's concept of the perfect nurse has traditionally been couched in the following aphorism: "She must feel like a girl, act like a lady, think like a man, and work like a dog" (Pratt, 1965).

The marginality of the nursing profession is due to its relative absence of a functional autonomy and to its subordinate position in work settings. Nurses are hampered by being expert in the delivery of services that are substantially controlled by others who do not wish to be expert in such areas of health care. Here, the assumption is made that a nurse's care of a patient is different from the physician's treatment of a patient.

The degree of autonomy varies with the type of nursing, and that, in turn, ranges from uncomplicated activities such as those dealing with personal hygiene to complex ones demanding expert skill, judgment, and technical experience. Among those who enjoy a relative autonomy are the nurse practitioner, clinical specialist, anesthetist, industrial nurse, public health nurse, school nurse, and the like. For instance, nurse practitioners provide direct care to individuals, families, and groups; they engage in independent decision-making about the needs of clients; they collaborate with other health professionals; and they may even plan and institute health care programs as members of the health care team (Bliss & Cohen, 1977; Kinlun, 1972; Ostrea & Schumar, 1976; Raba, 1979). According to Wright's (1976) study, registered nurses are strongly supportive of the new role of family nurse clinicians, especially in the delivery of primary health care ("Role of the nurse . . . ," 1977).

However, two-thirds of all employed registered nurses work in hospitals. This means that most of them are in a highly bureaucratic setting (Reeder & Mauksch, 1979). The role conflict of nurses who are caught in the dual authority systems of the hospital—physicians and administrators—has already been discussed in Chapter 7. To recapitulate, the professional autonomy of hospital nurses is hampered by three factors. First of all, because of the caste system of physicians and nurses, nurses occupy a subordinate position (Bullough & Bullough, 1975; Kramer, 1974). Even if nurses make diagnostic decisions, they protect themselves by engaging in an elaborate game that keeps the physician in a superior decision-making role (Bullough & Bullough, 1975; Stein, 1967). The aim of this doctor–nurse game is to avoid open disagreement between the players. Thus, the nurse makes significant recommendations to the doctor in a manner that appears passive and totally supportive of the "superior" physician.

Second, unlike physicians, nurses are directly under administrative authority, whose orientations are different from those of the medical professionals. Third, as employees of large, bureaucratic hospital organizations, nurses have little opportunity to exercise any initiative.

Role conflict is particularly severe for baccalaureate nurses, who have cultivated a professional role concept while at school (Corwin, 1961; Hogstel, 1977). Many studies (Kramer, 1967) have reported that rather than adhering to their professional role, they either increased their loyalty to bureaucratic values or dropped out of nursing (Kramer, 1974).

Instead of making a generalization to fit all nurses, Habenstein and Christ (1963) distinguished three types of nurses: the professionalizer, the traditionalizer, and the utilizer. The professionalizers, who are likely to have baccalaureate degrees, believe in the utility of formal, rational knowledge. They strive toward the future attainment of a professional status for nursing. The traditionalizers are oriented toward informal and nonscientific knowledge about tender, loving bedside care. Finally, the utilizers' primary concern is the technical and organizational details of work in exchange for wages.

Changing Roles. The mother surrogate role of nurses (Schulman, 1972) has been undergoing changes during the past 15 years (Reeder & Mauksch, 1972). The public image of the subordinate and self-sacrificial nurse was altered when in 1964 over 3,500 nurses in the New York City Department of Hospitals demanded higher salaries with a threat of mass resignation (Griffin & Griffin, 1973). In the first six months of 1966, 140 threatened strikes were reported all over the country. For the first time in history, nurses banded together to act as a cohesive social force in a battle to win improved working conditions and increased economic security. Public support went to the nurses when it was learned that the resignations and strikes were due not only to low salaries but to inadequate hospital conditions and poor patient care.

Such assertiveness by nurses was and is well justified in view of the fact that many of them are well trained and are performing highly technical duties. During the 1970s the nurse's role has been extended to include prescriptive and therapeutic tasks, which has raised their traditionally subordinate position (Bullough, 1976; Reeder & Mauksch, 1979).

There are several forces facilitating the changes in nursing roles (Brown, 1970; Pratt, 1965). First of all, there is the change in the nature of disease from acute, short-term illness to chronic sickness, and that trend is coupled with the larger cohort of elderly population with chronic health problems. While a physician's treatment is decisive for an acute illness, a nurse's care is very important in chronic cases.

Second, the gap between the increasing consumer demand for medical service and the shortage in the health work force creates a need for nurses to perform technical services. Also, the increasing specialization in medical care, such as in a breathing clinic, requires specially trained nurses. Third, the growing specialization and complexity within the organization of medical practice has produced the work pattern of the medical team, a pattern in which the nurse can be an active team member.

However, changes in nursing practice have been slow in coming. External barriers to change include the reluctance of physicians (O'Dell, 1974) and administrators to accept new roles for nurses. Physicians are willing to delegate responsibilities to physician's assistants but not to nurses (Hessler & Griffard, 1976). Then, due to the trend toward institutionalized licensure, hospital administrators tend to exert legal control over the functions of nurses and to limit those functions accordingly (Hershey, 1969). Even the distinction in training background does not seem to impress many employers. Based on survey data, Hogstel (1977) reported that nurses with associate degrees and those with baccalaureate degrees are not differentiated in relation to position, function, and salary.

Part of the problem resides in the psychology of nurses themselves. Many of them are not equipped with such value orientations as power, influence, and dominance that are necessary to achieve functional autonomy. Even many of the skilled nurses do not try to extend their role beyond that of physician's assistant. They seek attention, encouragement, and praise from physicians for performing skilled techniques well rather than seek to be autonomously in charge of the psychological care of patients (Brown, 1970).

Let us examine, finally, whether or not nurses could mobilize enough organizational power to affect professional autonomy.

Professional Organization

Numerically, the nursing profession has the largest number of members among the health service occupations. With regard to the organizational membership, the American Nurses Association (ANA) is also the largest in size among the professional organizations in the nation. However, only 40 percent of the nation's registered nurses are members of the ANA, and no more than one-third of all active nurses subscribe to the *American Journal of Nursing* (American Nurses Association, 1974; Kelly, 1975).

Until recently, the majority of nurses trained at the hospital-based diploma schools were accustomed to a subordinate position, and they preferred to use their organization for conservative and affiliative relations rather than for assertive fights against dominant groups (Brown, 1970). Another source of organizational weakness stems from the diversity of nursing training and practice. The goals of the professionalizers, traditionalizers, utilizers, and the hospital administrators are very different, and that makes it difficult for nurses to form any united front. Furthermore, the dual organizational system of the American Nurses Association and the National League for Nursing disperses power to too many segments of the nursing profession. While the membership of the ANA is limited to nurses, the NLN includes lay members who are concerned with nursing, as well as nurses (Reeder & Mauksch, 1979).

To date, the major contributions by the nursing organizations have been focused upon self-improvement (i.e., raising the educational standards), although there have been some attempts made to establish collegial roles of nurses in relation to physicians. For example, the National Joint Practice Commission was established in 1972, sponsored by the AMA and the ANA. It provides an arena in which physicians and nurses can discuss their congruent roles and make recommendations for optimal working relations ("The changing status," 1978).

There is speculation that nurses may direct their efforts to unionization rather than to professionalization. Unions seem to offer a more direct threat to management and so may provide nurses with greater control over their working conditions ("AFT will organize . . . ," 1979; Denton, 1976).

Notwithstanding its subordinate position to medicine, however, nurses are members of the Council on Allied Medical Services, together with hospital administrators, and dentistry and pharmacy workers (Akers, 1968). This alliance does not include chiropractors or optometrists. In fact, one of the reasons the council was organized some years ago was specifically to combat chiropractors and optometrists. In this sense, nursing is under a big protective umbrella.

MARGINAL PRACTITIONERS: CHIROPRACTORS

So far, we have dealt with occupations approved by the AMA. Now we move on to those that have been largely rejected by the AMA as nonscientific.

Historical Development of Chiropractic

Origin of Chiropractic. Prior to the late nineteenth century, the majority of doctors in America had no formal medical education, and they practiced the healing art together with others such as ministers, innkeepers, magistrates, or the local barber. It was during this period that Daniel David Palmer, a self-educated man, performed his unique experiments with spinal manipulation, and he is said to have discovered chiropractic in 1895. He claimed it to be a great leap forward in manipulative therapy and in the understanding of the disease process. The word *chiropractic* is derived from the Greek words *kheir* (hand) and *praktikos* (effective) (Cowie & Roebuck, 1975; Dintenfass, 1970; Smith, Ralph, 1969; Wilk, 1973).

In 1897, D. D. Palmer and his son, B. J. Palmer, who was more entrepreneurial than his father, founded the Palmer Infirmary and Chiropractic Institute. B. J. Palmer frankly admitted that their school was operated as a business and not on a professional basis, and he widely advertised for students by emphasizing the absence of prerequisites. The school had one pupil in 1898, three pupils in 1899, twelve pupils in 1903, 800 pupils in 1915, and by 1918 the student body had expanded to 1,862. By 1910 the school had acquired an X-ray machine, and its curriculum required 12 months of full-time attendance. Stimulated by this success, other schools were established, and most of them had moderate success.

Chiropractic versus Medicine. From the beginning, chiropractic was developed completely outside the field of medicine. D. D. Palmer stated that chiropractic was a separate, distinct, and independent science, art, and philosophy of life, one that holds nothing in common with any other system of health care. He claimed that otherwise there would be no excuse for its existence (Cooley, 1949; Wardwell, 1978).

Organized medicine stated its disapproval of chiropractic almost as emphatically. It claimed that there was no pathological basis for the theory of chiropractic and that it was presumptuous to allude to it as a science (Reed, 1932). Due to the Medical Practice Acts (1880)—which established the monopoly of the healing arts by physicians and prohibited nonmedical persons from engaging in any form of healing, chiropractic developed very slowly during the first two decades of its existence.

The long and bitter struggle for legal recognition and for a broader scope of practice began in 1909. Leaders in this occupation began a concerted effort in various states to gain what they considered minimal legislation and freedom to practice. In California, which currently contains the largest number of chiropractors, the conflict between chiropractic and medicine was the most intense, according to one historian (Turner, 1931). In 1909 a group of exponents of various healing arts including chiropractic organized themselves into the Naturopathic Association of California; they advocated a method of treating disease, using food, exercise, heat, and the like to assist the natural healing processes. They won an amendment to the medical law granting license to practice to the members of the Naturopathic Association. Although this law was repealed two years later, many drugless practitioners had managed to be licensed by then.

Following the repeal of this law, chiropractors renewed their efforts through a new organization of their own to obtain a licensing system under a state board of chiropractors. In the meanwhile, many chiropractors were arrested and jailed for practicing medicine without licenses. After a long period or organizing, fund-raising, and public relations activity, the California chiropractors succeeded in 1922 in getting licensing laws passed (Turner, 1931). During the decade of the 1920s numerous states enacted licensing laws.

In addition to such active mobilization of chiropractors, the survival of chiropractic in the face of opposition by organized medicine was facilitated by historical events as well as social conditions at the turn of the century. Shatin (1977) speculates that the demands for extra health care services were intensified by a series of incidents in the early part of the century—wounded World War I veterans returning home, relief-seekers in need of an immediate cure to replace the opiate of alcohol during the era of Prohibition (1917–1933), and the unemployed in search of psychological solace and less expensive therapy during the depression years. Chiropractors could fill the vacuum created by the undersupply of physician care in meeting all these demands.

By this time, however, chiropractors had begun to focus on special areas of therapy instead of claiming to provide cures for everything (Weiant, 1973). This was in line with the increasing division of labor and specialization of occupations. Chiropractors provided health care for such cases as hypochondria and other psychosomatic, or incurable (e.g., arthritis) ailments (Schwartz, 1973). Cases like these were likely to be neglected by disease-oriented physicians, but the chiropractors' holistic approach gave psychological satisfaction to patients suffering from psychosomatic illnesses (Rushmore, 1922).

As chiropractic achieved higher educational standards, greater clinical success, and public recognition, it also gained legislative acceptance. The Social Security Act of 1950 provided that expenses incurred for chiropractic treatment may be paid out of federal and state funds. Chiropractic is now licensed in all the states and is officially classified by the U.S. Bureau of the Budget as one of the four major healing professions, together with medicine, dentistry, and osteopathy. The U.S. Office of Education has attested to the validity of the academic degree of doctor of chiropractic and has began accrediting chiropractic colleges. Medicare, Medicaid, and most private insurance companies also recognize the service of chiropractic. During the 1970s, in the battle to win federal legislation such as Medicare and Medicaid, chiropractic gained support from varied interest groups such as senior citizen's associations, organized labor, and veterans' groups (Shatin, 1977; Wardwell, 1979).

While the AMA continues to attack chiropractic as a pseudoscience, in recent years medicine has begun to infringe upon the chiropractic domain by adopting spinal manipulative methods (Savage, 1971). In 1968, a group of prominent medical physicians formed the North American Academy of Manual Medicine. In that same year, the formation and a meeting of the First Congress of the International Federation of Manual Medicine took place. An increasing number of physicians are using spinal manipulative procedures under the banner of physiology, manipulative medicine, manual medicine, and the like. Propositions have even been made by physicians to hire chiropractors as physical therapists.

At present, this trend toward cooperative coexistence has split both medicine and chiropractic into two camps. One supports it as a healthy collaboration, and the other rejects it as a medical encroachment upon the chiropractic. In any event, starting in 1975 there have been many conferences to bring together representatives of both chiropractic and medicine (Wardwell, 1978).

Chiropractic Training

Chiropractors have been growing more and more self-conscious about upgrading the quality of their training (Dubbs, 1970; Haynes, 1967; Kimmel, 1964; Leis, 1971; U.S. DHEW, 1968). By 1970, all state licensing laws required at least a high school diploma, and two or more years of college was required in most states as a prerequisite to a four-year chiropractic curriculum. Furthermore, many states now require that chiropractors pass the Basic Science Examination of the National Board of Medical Examiners (U.S. DHEW, 1968).

Recruitment and Socialization. Given the marginal status of the occupation and the relatively lengthy period of preparation, who become chiropractors and for what reasons?

Most studies indicate that prior to entering chiropractic there exists a role model through exposure to a chiropractor, either as a patient or as a friend. Many of the chiropractors surveyed (Lin, 1972; Stanford Research Institute, 1960; White & Skipper, 1971) were involved in a serious illness or injury either to themselves or to someone close that was not treated successfully by a medical doctor, but was by a chiropractor.

According to White and Skipper's study, such seemingly miraculous incidents generally took place early in an individual's life and prompted the decision to enter chiropractic in the early days of high school. In contrast, however, half of the chiropractors studied by others (Lin, 1972; Stanford Research Institute, 1960; Wild, 1978) made the career decision after the age of 25, and most chiropractic students had considered or had actually worked in other health or health-related fields before enrolling in a chiropractic program (Wild, 1978).

As for career motivation, many chiropractic students report such altruistic reasons for entering the occupation as the opportunity to help people (Stanford Research Institute, 1960; Wardwell, 1952; Wild, 1978). White and Skipper (1971) interpret this as the influence upon the students exerted by the chiropractors who served as role models. Unlike medical doctors, who are trained to be affectively neutral to patients, chiropractors are encouraged to overtly display concern and interest in people. The personal interest manifested by the chiropractors whom students emulate is likely to help mold the latter's humanitarian orientation.

On the other hand, aspiring to move up a social class or two has been noted by many researchers as a motivation for entering chiropractic. Students are likely to come from working or lower class family backgrounds, and a career in chiropractic offers them a much higher social or economic status than that of their parents (Lin, 1972; Stanford Research Institute, 1960; White & Skipper, 1971; Wild, 1978; Wrestler, 1974).

The development of the occupational identification of chiropractors as marginal professionals was studied by Wrestler (1974) through the symbolic interactionist approach. Based on participant observation and interviews, Wrestler reported that chiropractic students perceive their healing technique as significantly different from, but equivalent with or superior to those of medical doctors. As students advance in school years, they come to show a greater appreciation of chiropractic as a distinct role.

However, chiropractic students see the image of the chiropractor, as perceived by society, as inferior to that of the medical doctor (Wild, 1978). If entering students are unaware of this negative label, the faculty and administration soon make them cognizant of what their future status is likely to be. The faculty members try to prepare students for the low esteem they will receive later, attributing the blame to the medical establishment, which does not want competition.

When chiropractic students come in contact with the outside world, they are further reminded of their marginal role. Many students who work in hospitals as orderlies or laboratory technicians to earn their tuition are harrassed by doctors, interns, or nurses if they are open about their healing philosophy. From friends and acquaintances, too, they hear such remarks as "Oh, you are going to be a bone snapper" (Wrestler, 1974).

In chiropractic, the development of the students' identification with their profession depends on the mixed reactions of significant others: (1) the faculty, who attempt to transmit specific views of chiropractic; (2) patients, who convey the public image of the chiropractor; (3) relatives and close friends, who are either ego boosters or ego deflators; and (4) fellow students, who are reflections of their own image.

Chiropractic Practice

Chiropractic Principles. Chiropractic is based on the following premises: (1) the relationship between the musculoskeletal structure and the functions of the body is a significant health factor; (2) in particular, the relationship between the spinal column and the nervous system is of the greatest importance; (3) the normal transmission and expression of nerve energy are essential to the restoration and maintenance of health; and (4) the human body has an inherent recuperative power (Bourdillon, 1973; Levine, 1973; Wilk, 1973).

Although chiropractic has a codified body of knowledge, in a narrow sense, the AMA has rejected the classification of chiropractic as a profession by claiming that most of the chiropractic principles have not been scientifically demonstrated as accurate. The AMA also argues that chiropractic is based on a single-cause theory that ignores such proven health theories as the pathogeny of bacteria.

Against these charges, chiropractors argue (Wilk, 1973) that they do not adhere to a monolithic doctrine but rather a two-factor theory of disease, one that is constituted of "exciting" and "predisposing" factors. While the microorganism is the exciting factor that causes disease, lowered tissue resistance is a predisposing condition. Chiropractic does not treat the disease, but it deals with the patient in an attempt to help return the body to a normal state of function, thereby letting the body overcome its ailments.

Although chiropractors agree on these basic principles, they are divided into two types of practice: "straight" and "mixers." While straight therapists depend on spinal adjustment, mixers supplement that with other methods such as physical and nutritional therapies.

Straight therapists tend to practice alone with little office assistance, and they maintain a separation from medicine. In contrast, the mixers are likely to hire more office assistants and to make referrals to physicians, with the view that chiropractic will eventually become part of the team of health professionals.

Chiropractic Clinic. Although chiropractic is now legal (licensed), it continues to endure a deviant status in American society. Roebuck and Hunter (1970) identified five formal, rule-making bodies that have labeled the chiropractor as a deviant: the AMA, federal agencies, the scientific establishment, commercial associations, and state agencies.

From the symbolic interactionist perspective, the chiropractic clinic presents a stage where actors (patients and staff) behave according to their definitions of the situation. Patients bring to the clinic the societal label of the chiropractor as a deviant (Wardwell, 1955). Nearly four out of ten chiropractors surveyed in California are "not very satisfied" with the recognition they are afforded in their communities. They attribute this low esteem to public ignorance about chiropractic (43 percent), the lack of group solidarity among chiropractors (19 percent), and suppression by the AMA (14 percent). However, more than seven out of ten chiropractors reported that they would definitely or probably enter chiropractic if they had to do it all over again (Stanford Research Institute, 1969).

Despite this negative evaluation, a large number of people visit chiropractors every year, at a rate of frequency greater than that for visits to such medical specialists as psychiatrists, dermatologists, podiatrists, and orthopedists (Schmitt, 1978; U.S. DHEW, 1966). These patients have special expectations about chiropractors: "curing" illnesses that medicine has failed to and "caring" about patients that physicians have neglected. Chiropractic appeals to an emerging cultural need for a less technocratic and bureaucratic medical system with an emphasis on holistic natural therapies and interpersonal psychological support (Denton, 1978).

This factor is particularly important because patients not only enjoy personal attention but are apt to see it as an indication of technical competence (Koos, 1954; McCorkle, 1961; Wardwell, 1955). On the part of chiropractors, personal relations with patients are considered as important as technical competence. They spend on the average more time with each patient than medical doctors do (Stanford Research Institute, 1960).

There is some evidence that chiropractic attracts patients with rural (McCorkle, 1961; Shatin, 1977) or lower class background (Koos, 1954; Stanford Research Institute, 1960), and women more than men (U.S. DHEW, 1968). It has been suggested that chiropractic offers a commonsense, single-cause theory of disease that appeals to the above types of people (McCorkle, 1961). They prefer chiropractors' specific statements about the cause of illness and the concrete treatment of the condition (e.g., the adjustment of the backbone) as compared to the more diffuse explanations offered by medical doctors (Koos, 1954; McCorkle, 1961).

However, other studies (Parker et al., 1976) indicate that chiropractic patients are not significantly different from the normal population in terms of socioeconomic status, personality, and psychological symptomatology. The majority of these people have received medical treatments without success and visit chiropractors as a last resort (White & Skipper, 1971). When a physician cannot find anything organically wrong using available diagnostic procedures, the physician is likely to dismiss the case with "Nothing wrong" or "It's just in the nerves." Physicians are frustrated by patients with functional or psychosomatic disorders and may label them "crooks"—trouble-making patients who waste their precious time (Coombs, 1978). In contrast, chiropractors validate the patient's belief that some definable organic pathology exists by empathizing with the patient and assuring him or her of a cure (Firman et al., 1975).

Whether the cure is really effective or not, at least the psychological needs of the patient are better met by chiropractors than by physicians (Jorgenson, 1978; Woodley & Kane, 1977). Furthermore, chiropractors serve the medical establishment by providing an outlet for many potentially time-consuming and troublesome patients. At the same time, by labeling chiropractors as irregular practitioners, physicians can maintain their own professional prerogatives. Thus, from the functionalist perspective, the social utility of chiropractors as a marginal group can be seen as a boundary-defining mechanism for the dominant medical profession (Firman et al., 1975).

Another predominant reason for seeking chiropractic help is familiarity with chiropractic culture due to prior exposure. Many patients had been acquainted with chiropractors or were referred to them through friends who had received manipulative therapy (Jorgenson, 1978).

In sum, having reviewed past studies and theories, Schmitt (1978) concludes that more research is needed to clarify utilization patterns of chiropractic. In particular, in their current form, theories about chiropractic use do not specifically incorporate the relationship between traditional medicine and chiropractic as an alternative.

Most patients come to chiropractic clinics for musculoskeletal problems, seeking relief from pain. The effectiveness of the treatment is difficult to assess even though some researchers report that more than half of the patients expressed unqualified recognition of a successful cure (Parker et al., 1976).

> "I feel as if my body were breathing in places it never breathed before," my friend Dick told me after his first visit to a chiropractor (Kruger, 1974, p. 136).

More systematic research is needed to determine whether an illness was self-limiting and healed naturally, or was cured because of chiropractic principles and therapy, or because of a placebo effect ("Chiropractors . . . ," 1977).

Faced with patient demand and the socially imposed marginal status, chiropractors must create and maintain a rationalization for their conduct. Of special importance is the initial encounter. When patients come into a chiropractor's office for the first time, they expect something strange or different from that of the physician's office. Thus, the first task for the chiropractic staff is to orient the patients so that they come to share the chiropractic definition of the situation and to understand the ground rules of conduct.

In an ethnographic study of the chiropractic clinic, Cowie and Roebuck (1975) underlined the strategic function of the physical setting and the preliminary interaction in the waiting room. The waiting room walls were heavily decorated with pictures, signs, and posters that communicate the chiropractic message with an air of professionalism. While the patient waits, the chiropractic assistant tries to engage the patient in casual conversation endeavoring to provide credence to the effectiveness of chiropractic. The chiropractic assistant thereby meets an implicit demand from the patient for a satisfactory definition of the deviant situation.

Upon entering the treatment room, the patient is welcomed by the practitioner with easy warmth. However, from the outset, the practitioner assumes control of the interactional situation by initiating, directing, and sustaining the conversation.

According to the study, the chiropractor defines his own role in terms of the nature, purpose, and philosophy of chiropractic by admitting that "I give him the works right off the bat. . . . spell it out for him in black and white. If he is going to buy it, I've got to find out right away." (Cowie & Roebuck, 1975, p. 82). Through that approach and during the early stages of the interaction, the practitioner can divide patients into three classes: (1) the one-timer who remains passive and nonaccepting of the chiropractor and will never come back again; (2) the problem patient whose attendance is irregular and whose overt behavior is unpredictable; and (3) the regular patient who is supportive of chiropractic.

Thus, the chiropractor is viewed by Cowie and Roebuck not as a passive recipient of a deviant label, but as a practitioner with a considerable degree of power within the practice setting.

Chiropractic Organization

Historical Development. In 1906, the Universal Chiropractic Association (UCA) was founded. Gradually the mixers began deviating from the group and branched out in 1922 to form the American Chiropractic Association (ACA). In order to "clean house," the straights expelled the mixers and founded a caucus within the UCA, which later became the International Chiropractic Association (ICA).

While critics have attempted to exaggerate the differences between these two national organizations, the ICA and the ACA, chiropractors claim that the diversity among themselves is no greater than the differentiation that is typical of all professional groups, especially medicine.

In 1969, a comprehensive report prepared by the U.S. Public Health Service for Congress recommended that the Social Security Act not be amended so as to permit chiropractors to participate in Medicare (U.S. DHEW, 1968). The ACA and the ICA responded by jointly issuing a White Paper, which asserted that chiropractic services were already authorized in 17 states under the Medicaid program of the Social Security Act, that all departments of the federal government accepted statements from chiropractors for employee sick leaves, and that worker's compensation claims for chiropractic services were paid in 48 states and the District of Columbia (U.S. DHEW, 1968). Congress realized that there was a significiant public demand for chiropractic and voted to include it in Medicare in 1973.

While one segment of medicine castigates chiropractic as a worthless cult, another admits its value and is negotiating with chiropractors to obtain their manipulative skills. Recent issues of medical journals have suggested that chiropractors might find a place in the M.D.'s office as physical therapists. The ACA has objected to this idea. As a physician's assistant, they claim that the chiropractor, like the nurse, will be reduced to being a servant to the medical profession and will cease to exist as an independent healing professional.

Organizational Strength. The ACA has the third largest budget within the health field, next to the AMA and the ADA, partly because of its large menbership dues. But since these dues have been in effect since 1963, the average assets of the ACA is not large compared to those of the AOA (American Optometrist Association) and APHA (American Pharmaceutical Association) (Akers & Quinney, 1968).

Due to the lack of federal financial support until recently, chiropractors had to depend solely on their own organizational resources for the improvement of their educational training. The ACA spent 40 percent of its total membership dues for educational and research purposes and established a department of research and statistics in 1959.

In contrast, expenditures for legislative activities have been relatively small. The ICA spends about 9.5 percent of its annual budget on research and about 4 percent for legislative activities. The ACA spends about 4 percent of its budget, amounting to $35,000, while the AMA spent $155,935 in 1965 alone to defeat the Medicare bill (Wilk, 1973).

The ACA is weak in terms of personnel resources and has low membership stability. However, it has a high participation rate as measured by attendance at its professional meetings (Akers & Quinney, 1968).

Another weakness of the ACA is that it is solely a national organization. There are no formal organizational representatives on the local level because of the intraoccupational cleavage into mixers and straights. In spite of the division, chiropractors have united to fight for self-protection, legal recognition, and public acceptance, but they do not have a mandate that would enable them to prescribe the health goals to which the public should aspire ("The AMA antitrust suit . . . ," 1978; Nofz, 1978).

The Future Direction. The future outlook for chiropractic has changed from the negative to the neutral to the positive. In 1960 the Stanford Research Institute suggested the general continued decline of chiropractic as a marginal profession. Based on a survey of California chiropractors, the institute denied other possibilities such as the emergence of the straight practitioner as a specialist like a dentist or a psychiatrist, or the transformation of the mixer practitioner into a medical professional like an osteopath. This prediction was based on survey data that indicated a declining number of chiropractic practitioners and students, a small number of clients, inadequate financial resources, and ingroup dissension.

In reviewing medical sociology textbooks, Skipper (1978) noted that chiropractic is not mentioned at all or discussed briefly and rather negatively. Gold (1977) interprets the situation as a manifestation of medical bias shown by medical sociologists. Given the fact that organized medicine does not consider chiropractic as legitimate, medical sociologists have paid little attention to it as a worthwhile research subject.

A less negative view is expressed by Firman and others (Firman et al., 1975; Shatin, 1977), who predict that chiropractors will thrive in their marginal role without being either upgraded to becoming professional competitors with medicine or being downgraded to the role of paramedic. According to their observations, the marginal and deviant qualities of chiropractic have stablized to the point where chiropractors serve positive functions to their patients and even to organized medicine. As mentioned above, there is always a small but steady number of clients who are attracted to chiropractic. With such a devoted and congenial group of clients and with their increasing participation in health-payment programs, chiropractors are not ready to relinquish their unique identity and be absorbed into medicine. Physicians also find it beneficial to keep chiropractors in a marginal role rather than denouncing them or absorbing them completely.

In contrast to these views, there are others who have taken a much more positive stance, stating that chiropractic is not a marginal profession at all, but rather is an attractive alternative to medicine for a sizable number of health care consumers (Denton, 1978; Nofz, 1978; Wild, 1978). They claim that the notion of marginality is outdated in view of growing public acceptance (U.S. Dept. of Labor, 1976). Thus the marginality of chiropractors is seen to exist only in the political arena, but not in the social or sociopsychological domains.

> Chiropractors are members of a major, if not the major, type of alternative medicine. They also constitute one of the most organized groups among those that present alternatives to mainstream medicine (Denton, 1978, p. 122).

> Chiropractic is not only alive and well but is prospering. Applicants, who now are required to have at least two years of preprofessional college work, have increased several-fold. All thirteen colleges in the United States have either added new buildings or have purchased the campuses of defunct Catholic schools (Wardwell, 1978, p. 14).

MARGINAL PRACTITIONERS: CHRISTIAN SCIENTISTS

The last group of healers to be discussed in this chapter are the Christian Scientists, who also are disapproved of by medicine as being unscientific. However, unlike laws concerning chiropractic, laws pertaining to medical practice ordinarily exempt religious practitioners from their purview probably because such healers are regarded as filling some other primary function, that is, a religious role (Wardwell, 1965, 1972). Christian Scientists are not subject to the expense of business licensing for operating as drugless healing practitioners because the Constitution protects their freedom to practice religion.

The History of Christian Science

Christian Science was born in the midst of the divided house of healing in nineteenth-century America. The healing world embraced not only conventional practitioners, but also homeopaths, eclectics, and many other cults. During that period, the AMA made its first feeble attempt to get started in 1846, the American School of Osteopathy was established in 1892, and Daniel D. Palmer founded the chiropractic movement in 1895. In with the rest of them, the cult of Christian Science was launched with the revelation experienced by

Mary Baker Eddy in 1866 and with the publication of her book, *Science and Health,* in 1875 (Peel, 1971).

Prior to 1866, Eddy was preoccupied with sickness, healing, and religion. She sought knowledge from different schools—allopathy, homeopathy, hydropathy, eclecticism, and from various other methods. During this period of search, her most significant influence came from a P. P. Quimby, who believed that the healing process was purely mental and was to be achieved by inculcating particular attitudes of mind in the patient (Wilson, 1961).

Briefly, Christian Science teaches that the power of the Divine Mind can manifest itself at the behest of believers by curing their illnesses, harmonizing their interpersonal relationships, and by providing for their material needs. The Christian Science practitioner explains to the patient that since humans reflect God, they cannot be sick. Therefore, the causation of disease is in the mind, which controls the body.

In 1879, the Christian Science Association resolved to found a church, the First Church of Christ, Scientist, in Boston. Eddy was its first pastor and the movement experienced rapid growth. Christian Science reflected the dominant values of nineteenth-century America—its optimism, belief in progress, pragmatism, and subjective idealism. The stern tenets of Calvinism had broken down, and the new faith, while supporting spiritual values, emphasized the growing belief in expansion, progress, and success. By 1890, the *Christian Science Journal,* first published in 1883 under a different name, listed 250 healers, 20 incorporated churches, 90 societies, and 53 academies.

Then, in 1889, Eddy decided to close all of the existing organizations of Christian Science that has grown up so haphazardly—the Massachusetts Metaphysical College, the Boston College, and the National Christian Science Association. She declared that there was too much reliance on material organization, and she cleared the way for the establishment of a highly centralized and unified organization.

During the last twenty years of her life, Eddy built an entirely impersonal system of control, except for her own charismatic leadership. Pastors were replaced by readers who read from prepared texts, the Bible, and *Science and Health.* All churches became branches of the Mother Church. They were governed by the Board of Directors, which was appointed and dismissed by Eddy during her lifetime. After her death, this board became self-perpetuating, allowing the transition from charisma to bureaucracy (Gottschalk, 1973).

Christian Science continuously increased its membership until 1936, when it began to decline (Braden, 1958). There are several reasons for this. To begin with, the movement had not fulfilled its earlier promises in its healing practice, and by then, medicine had gained public confidence. Second, Eddy's mental therapy had been relaced by various theories concerning psychosomatic illness. Third, social values had changed from those of the time of Eddy, and also the movement ceased to be a novelty.

The Education of Christian Science

In 1881, Eddy's Massachusetts Metaphysical College was established to offer a primary course, a normal course, and a course in metaphysical obstetrics. The college charter granted power to confer degrees. Those who studied there became healers and teachers who eventually set up their own practices.

In her day, Eddy appears to have accepted, enrolled, and taught anyone who came to her. Today, teachers are counseled to carefully select those who have good past records and who show promising proclivities toward Christian Science. Those who seek primary instructions are usually persons with considerable knowledge of the religious beliefs and of the therapeutic system of Christian Science.

In the primary course, instructions are given purely from one chapter of *Science and Health,* "Recapitulation," which consists of 24 questions and answers on the theology of Christian Science. Teachers are also required to teach pupils to defend themselves against malpractice. Primary instruction lasts about two weeks. Although class instruction is not mandatory to be officially listed in the *Christian Science Journal,* such a listing after completion of the primary course serves as the equivalent of certification as a qualified practitioner.

After three years of full-time successful practice of healing, practitioners may apply for the normal course to the Board of Education, which is given only once every three years to a limited number of pupils. The normal class lasts six days, and earns one the degree of C.S.B. (Bachelor of Christian Science). A graduate of the normal class is certified as a teacher and may give primary class instruction to not more than 30 pupils each year. Subsequently, teachers call their pupils together once a year for an associate meeting where further instruction is given.

In principle, any Christian Scientist can become self-educated solely through the study of the Bible, *Science and Health,* and other documents. Yet, class instructions are surrounded by an aura of secrecy. For example, note-taking in class is either forbidden or severely restricted (Wilson, 1961).

The bond between teacher and pupil is considered to be very close. If a teacher falls out of favor with the church authorities and becomes disqualified, all of the pupils who were trained by that instructor are also disqualified, and they remain so until they are reinstructed by another teacher.

Although Christian Science has no clergy, it has its own professional body of those whose livelihood comes entirely from the religion: the teachers and the practitioners. Below them is the laity, which can be divided into the ordinary members and the class-instructed members. Teachers and practitioners do not perform any special function in the services or worship of Christian Science churches or in the organization. However, they informally command considerable prestige, and they frequently play a commanding role in the business life of the church.

Christian Science Healing Practice

The elements of emotional ecstasy through group ceremonies that accompany most faith healing are not used in the healing practice of Christian Science. The function of the practitioner is minimized to the extent that his or her physical presence is not always necessary. The patients are encouraged to attain the correct belief through their own prayer and mental concentration along with the reading of the Bible and *Science and Health.*

When a practitioner is present, the first step is to allay the fear of the patient. God's "all-ness" and goodness are reaffirmed, and it is argued that harmony (and health) is the fact. It is repeatedly explained to the patient that sickness is a belief, or a fear manifested on the body, and it must be annihilated by the Divine Mind (Eddy, 1934, p. 493).

This is a ritualistic denial of reality, which is a tenuous psychodynamic reinforcement. Without the emotional ecstasy characteristic of faith healing, the Christian Scientist teaches a psychological mechanism through abstract and impersonal metaphysics (Wardwell, 1972).

The patients of Christian Science practitioners are drawn from a relatively narrow range: the converted or the desperate. Apart from the Christian Scientists, there are patients who call in practitioners for a variety of reasons: (1) they have heard of Christian Science from relatives and friends; (2) they have lost hope and faith in medicine; or (3) they have been given up and declared incurable by doctors.

The Christian Science practitioner demonstrates knowledge of the doctrines of that faith, a knowledge that transcends that of clients and of the lay public. However, that knowledge, which cannot be validated scientifically, may mean little to the person who does not share the belief of this religious group. The essential benefit that the patients receive is psychological, although it is not conceptualized as such by the practitioner.

Psychotherapy is an unintended product of the spiritual therapy. The Christian Science method does not coexist with medical treatment because it is based on different theories of disease. While Christian Science views disease as a mental and moral issue, medicine treats disease on a physical and chemical basis. The occasional use of medical treatment by Christian Scientists is justified according to circumstances: (1) special cases such as the setting of a bone, which is a mechanical adjustment without drug therapy; (2) the person does not have strong enough faith; or (3) the patient is under family pressure.

Mechanic and Volkart's (1961) study indicated that with the increase in severity of illness, Christian Scientists rely on medicine as well as on Christian Science principles. Nudelman and Nudelman (1972) further differentiated two types of Christian Scientists: devout and unreligious ones. The unreligious Scientists turn to medicine as well as to religion in cases of severe illness. When the illness is mild, unreligious Scientists are likely to ignore either medical or religious therapies because turning to religion requires diligent study of the Science. Devout Scientists, on the other hand, rely on Christian Science healing whether the symptoms are mild or severe.

Confidence in the efficacy of their therapy, compared to other healing arts, is evidenced by Eddy's suggestion in 1909 that Christian Science practitioners should make their charges for treatment equal to those by reputable physicians in their respective localities. Today, a practitioner charges a fee at his or her own discretion. The Church has little to say about healing practice except that a practitioner shall not sue to recover from patients and that he or she shall reduce the fees in chronic cases or in cases where the therapy fails.

It is doubtful whether many practitioners earn enough in practice alone to maintain themselves because of the limited source and types of patients. And yet there is a large pool of class-instructed Scientists from whom practitioners may be recruited, particularly after their retirement from another vocation. There is no restriction on the entry into the occupation to protect the interests of the already established practitioners. Their competitive financial situation seems to be eased by the fact that the majority of the practitioners, 77 percent in 1953, are married women who do not have to rely on the income from their practice for subsistence (Wilson, 1961).

The Organization of the Christian Science Movement

In the first edition of the book, *Science and Health,* Eddy described Christian Science as not needing a church organization. She obviously had no idea as to the extent of the organization that was to emerge from the students of that textbook.

The first organization developed by the movement was the Christian Science Association in 1876. In 1879 a charter was obtained for the Church of Christ, Scientist, and in 1881 Eddy received a further charter for the Massachusetts Metaphysical College.

Then, after the reorganization of 1889–1890, the resulting streamlined organization provided one central church, its branches, and the centralization of authority vested in the Directors of the Mother Church. Members of the movement had no vote or control in the central direction of the organization. The bureaucratization of the movement was thus begun early and at Eddy's own command. Her foresight in providing a stable organization in her own lifetime prevented a major disruption after her death (Peel, 1971).

The new organization, under the Mother Church, is unique in that it resembles a business corporation. Today, it is typically bureaucratic: fixed official jurisdiction in accordance with the law of the larger society; authority delimited by rules; formal appointments; an impersonal examination system; a full-time specialist administrative class; salaries, and fixed fees.

The policy of the movement—the control of its publications, censorship of its lectures, the appointment of teachers, and the disciplining of its members—are all vested in the Board of Directors. They are a self-perpetuating body of five.

Since the organization consists of only one church with many branches, each branch follows the identical order of service as conducted in the Mother Church. The branch churches do not confer with each other except when the churches within one state need to meet to promote their status in that state, or to unite for action with regard to the laws of the state. The business of each branch church is virtually restricted to its own maintenance.

The dual membership system meets the needs of a modern, mobile civilization. Membership in the Mother Church and in the branch churches are distinct and separate processes, and they entail different obligations. A Christian Scientist normally becomes a member of the Mother Church at the age of 12. In order to be accepted as a member of the Mother Church, a candidate must believe in Christian Science free from other denominations and accept the Bible, *Science and Health,* and the other works of Eddy as the only textbooks for teaching and practicing metaphysical healing. One can join a branch church only when one leaves Sunday School at the age of 20, and only if permanently settled in the district.

While most Christian Scientists are church members, the church is an association for the perpetuation of the cult rather than a prerequisite to special redemption or salvation. The Christian Science church is an impersonal institution and does not provide a guiding pastor, a spiritual confessor, or an opportunity for emotional release. The Sunday church ritual is less important than the private study and practice of the belief (Eddy, 1936).

Because of such impersonality, the associational nature of the church, and the sophisticated metaphysics of the belief system, Christian Science attracts members from the urban-suburban middle class rather than from manual workers, factory workers, the poor, and the uneducated. Another reason for its appeal to the middle class is that Christian Science demands a willingness to attribute poverty to the wrong set of mental attitudes. Naturally, poor people are not drawn to such a doctrine. Finally, another unique feature of the membership is the preponderance of women, probably due to the charismatic feminine leadership of the founder.

The most effective defense for Christian Science practice has been the use of the constitutional right of religious freedom. Christian Scientists argue that discrimination by law between healing methods would create a state healing monopolized by physicians and, in effect, establish a state religion, depriving the people of the right to choose (*Christian Science and legislation,* 1905, p. 41). In 1911, shortly after Eddy's death, a case brought against Christian Science practice was ruled in favor of it, with one judge commenting: "I deny the power of the Legislation to make it a crime to treat disease by prayer" (Braden, 1958, p. 254).

However, Christian Science opposition to medical aid has led to serious legal conflicts, particularly when it involves a third party ("Compulsory medical treatment . . . ," 1975). In 1957 the California Supreme Court ruled that "freedom to *believe* is absolute but freedom to *act* remains subject to regulations for the protection of society" (Braden, 1958, p. 257). Public and legal intolerance is especially intense in the areas of communicable diseases and sanitary matters. In 1957 a Superior Court judge in Chicago ordered a Christian Science mother to allow a physician to give her child polio shots if he felt it necessary. In California law all cases of venereal disease must be reported and controlled. The question arises, however, as to how the Christian Science practitioner is able to determine whether the disease is contagious or not, since for them any disease is unreal and only a mental construct.

At first, judges and juries denied Christian Scientists compensation in accident and other damage suits. Their premise was that the Scientists could not at the same time pronounce their injuries unreal and then also claim damages under the law. The climate has gradually changed. Now practitioners are authorized by statute to sign certificates for sick leave and for disability claims. Some insurance companies recognize the services of Christian Scientists in their health, accident, and hospitalization policies. Medicare and other welfare programs take care of the expense incurred by Christian Science practitioners and nursing homes. They are also exempt from the health examinations that are usually necessary for marriage, summer camps, school entrance, employment, and the like.

In order to reach and retain this status, Christian Scientists have maintained a surveillance over state legislation and mass media. Their lobbyists carefully study all bills related to health practice. They examine mass media constantly. If they find anything harmful to their status, they publicly denounce it and try to correct the situation (Akers, 1968).

FOLK MEDICINE

In addition to marginal health practitioners such as chiropractors and Christian Scientists, there are many less organized healers. For instance, there are practitioners of folk medicine, which is a mixture of natural, magical, and religious elements. Illnesses are divided into two types: those caused by natural forces (environmental hazards) and unnatural forces (divine punishment for wrongdoing or witchcraft). In this age of medical technology, why do some people seek care from nonscientific practitioners?

Folk medicine tends to be widely practiced among people who are isolated by geographical distance, cultural difference, poverty, or other factors from the mainstream of society (Coe, 1978). Compared with urbanites, rural people tend to be less secularized and their lifestyle, whether in agriculture or in medicine, is pervasively religious. Further, due to the lack of exposure to technological and scientific development, their control over their environment is limited; hence they seek supernatural explanations (Twaddle & Hessler, 1977).

Then, there are people who are marginal in the social and economic sense. Being unable to achieve middle class status, marginal people fall back on a cultural system where religion and magic allow them to deal with the hostile world. After reviewing the studies on low-income blacks, Southern whites, Puerto Ricans, and Mexican Americans, Snow (1974) observed that illness ascribed to witchcraft reflects distrust and lack of ease in social interactions. Witchcraft involves the magical expression of the fear that strangers, friends, or relatives may wish you harm. This is based on a mistrusting world view that society is a hostile and dangerous thing and that the individual had better look out for himself or herself. Snow claims that so long as there are socially and economically marginal people, folk medicine will have a clientele.

SUMMARY

To summarize, compare the different degrees of professionalization of the six occupations discussed in this chapter in terms of knowledge base, style of practice, group organization, and relationship to the medical profession.

Knowledge Base. To begin with, a profession must be founded on an abstract, theoretical knowledge base, one that is transmitted by formal and lengthy training and is monopolized by the profession through the licensure system.

The limited professions—dentistry and pharmacy—are built on two types of knowledge base. First, there is medical knowledge, which is given full credit by the medical profession for its scientific validity but is considered part of the domain of the medical profession. The second knowledge base—dental or pharmaceutical technology—is distinct and independent of medicine and historically has been looked down upon by medicine as being limited in scope and being a craft rather than a theory. Consequently, medicine did not allow dentistry or pharmacy to be incorporated into the medical profession as a specialty field. Both dentists and pharmacists have suffered from being labeled as limited or secondary professionals despite the fact that they have attained a high level of skill through long training.

The knowledge base possessed by the ancillary practitioners—physician's assistants and nurses—is almost entirely subsumed under medicine. Although some physician's assistants and nurses claim to use a method of patient care that physicians neglect or are incapable of, this method has not been systematized into an abstract body of knowledge. Furthermore, the educational levels for physician's assistants and nurses are much lower than those required for dentists and pharmacists, with the exception of specially trained people.

In case of the marginal practitioners—chiropractors and Christian Scientists—their claim of unique methods of healing is denounced by organized medicine as scientifically unverifiable. Yet, there have been some attempts at a merger with medicine—physical therapy and chiropractic, or psychotherapy and Christian Science. To a large extent chiropractors and Christian Scientists have chosen to suffer from the negative label of irregular practitioner rather than accept the merger.

In short, successful establishment of a professional status in healing practice seems to require the acquisition of a knowledge base that meets three conditions: it must be (1) scientifically verifiable, unlike in the marginal occupations; (2) distinct from and independent of medicine, unlike in the ancillary occupations; and (3) a comprehensive system, unlike in the limited professions.

Style of Practice. Monopoly of technical expertise by the professionals leads to two styles of practice: autonomy and service orientation. Since the lay clientele is unable to appraise professional performance, the professionals are granted self-disciplined autonomy over the manner of their practice, and in return they are expected to work with a service, instead of a profit, orientation.

However, inherent in the limited profession is the potential for the minimax career choice strategy. That is to say, many dental and pharmacist students are aware of their second-class status but are attracted by the financial reward and professional type of work, accompanied by a shorter training period than at medical school. Such utilitarian motivation tends to persist through dental and pharmaceutical practice, resulting in a role conflict of profession versus business. The business aspect is intensified by the predominantly fee-for-service type of practice. Many dentists are solo practitioners competing for clients, and retail pharmacists are generally paid directly by the clients since third-party payment frequently excludes drugs. In addition, as an adjunct to medicine, the role of the pharmacist excludes diagnosis and prescription, which curtails professional autonomy.

In the case of the ancillary occupations, a service spirit appears to have arisen, at least partially, from the lack of autonomy. While physicians are busy "curing" diseases, nurses and physician's assistants are expected to "care" for patients. Dating back to Florence Nightingale, service is of primary importance to nursing, and it has sometimes been considered more crucial than technical competence. Physician's assistants are also expected to show interest in the patient as a person, while specialty physicians tend to view the patient as a disease entity.

Having been stigmatized as irregular practitioners, the marginal practitioners —chiropractors and Christian Scientists—have fought against organized medicine to have their practice legitimized and at the same time not be absorbed into the territory of medicine.

Marginal practice requires technical expertise as well as business sense because it must engage itself more in attracting clients than does medicine (Coe, 1978). However, apart from possible pecuniary motivation, many of these marginal practitioners take a holistic approach to health care, viewing a patient as a whole person rather than as a germ-carrying organism. They are more expressive of their humanitarian concern and the service spirit than disease-oriented physicians.

Without being recognized as full-fledged professionals, the limited professionals seem to have developed a business orientation to compensate for the missing reward of the full profession. Being subordinate to the physicians, the ancillary workers have been forced to adopt a service orientation. The marginal practitioners use the service orientation partly as a challenge to the mechanistic approach of physicians. In short, aspiring occupations that are partially or totally rejected by organized medicine seem to cope with the difficulty by emphasizing utilitarian or service orientations.

Group Organization. Organizations are established when the members of an occupational group come to recognize common interests; when they desire to distinguish themselves from others who do not have the qualifications; and above all, when they attempt to gain and maintain power over other competing occupational and social groups (Vollmer & Mills, 1966).

In the process of professionalization, or even in an attempt at simple survival, the role of occupational associations as political pressure groups is important especially as they affect the formulation and administration of the law (Akers, 1968). While many alternative healing practices die out as fads, others survive because of their effective organizations. The latter are able to confront physicians in state legislatures where laws affecting the relative power of various groups are debated and voted on.

The strength of organizations can be measured by their resources (financial and personnel) and membership cohesion (Akers & Quinney, 1968). The American Dental Association is a cohesive and wealthy organization, whose political power is comparable to that of the AMA. The American Pharmaceutical Association suffers from internal conflicts and has not been effective in gaining absolute control over drugs against third-party interference. Generally speaking, organized medicine has established cooperative working agreements with the limited professions so long as the latter have accepted a limited status.

The ancillary occupations tend to have difficulties in developing a coalition against organized medicine because their occupational tasks are dependent upon medicine. The nurses' organizations are handicapped by their internal differences and the low level of participation by nurses, who are usually oriented toward traditional, subordinate roles rather than professional and assertive roles. As for physician's assistants, their organizational links are still weak due to the newness of the occupation, diversity in training and activities,and their dependency upon physicians.

Occupations that refuse to accept a limited or subordinate status to medicine (e.g., chiropractic, osteopathy, naturopathy, Christian Science) are still officially regarded as cults and are largely excluded from participation in medical activities and installations. Chiropractors are split into two organizations with different perspectives toward medicine and are not able to present a united front except for emergency cases. Christian Scientists are well organized as a religious group rather than as a health practitioners' organization. They have attained legal recognition to practice, but their clients are limited.

In sum, part of the organizational weakness of aspiring professions seems to be generated by their indeterminancy about their relations vis-à-vis physicians: merger versus independence.

Relationship with the Medical Profession. A common dilemma shared by emerging or aspiring health professions is how to establish an equal but distinct status in relation to the medical profession. Because of the monopoly of health practice by physicians, it has been extremely difficult for others to develop a separate profession. Organized medicine has tried either to absorb or denounce any such attempt. The relative status and power of the limited professionals (dentistry, podiatry, optometry, pharmacy) and medical specialists (ophthalmology, radiology, anesthesiology, etc.) vary depending on historical, technological, and political factors. If an occupation remains within the territory of medicine, it can borrow the prestige of medicine, but may never become an autonomous profession.

This quandary is more critical in the case of ancillary health occupations because their role is defined in terms of assistance to physicians and their knowledge base is subsumed under that of the medical profession. However, in recent years the shortage of physicians, particularly in primary care, accompanied by rising health care utilization, has given impetus to developing allied health workers not as subordinates but as extenders of physicians. The roles of physician's assistants and nurse practitioners are being redefined as being members of a health team instead of servants to physicians. These teams should be built upon the unique strength and expertise of each member, which are maximally utilized in an atmosphere of collegiality and mutual respect. Whether these middle-level practitioners will grow into full-fledged professionals remains to be seen, but their appearance can bring some changes to the existing medical delivery system.

Another blow to traditional medical practice is coming from alternative health care offered by marginal practitioners. Recent attacks on traditional medicine in the name of iatrogenesis—high medical cost, ineffective cure, harmful medical therapy—have caused public attention to be directed to alternative health care, be it chiropractic, acupuncture, health food, or physical fitness programs (Kruger, 1974). Health is too important to be left exclusively to doctors, and the American lay public with its tradition of individualism has always engaged in do-it-yourself medicine, resorting to irregulars and cultists (Duffy, 1976). In order to meet such public needs, marginal occupations must maintain their uniqueness and cannot merge with medicine even at the expense of a higher social status.

PART 3

Medicine Within the Social System

CHAPTER 9

Community Health Care

In Part 2, medical care services were viewed as social systems with internal conflicts. Chapters 5 through 8 described how physicians have elevated their status, organized themselves into a system, and established the medical profession; how hospitals have grown into complex bureaucratic systems; how other health practitioners are subordinate to the established medical profession and hospital organizations; and how the physician–patient relationship is dominated by the power of organized medicine.

This medical domination has caused many problems: (1) the alienation of the profession from the community; (2) a shift from primary care to specialization; (3) an impersonal patient care; (4) the maldistribution and shortage of physicians; (5) the abuse of power by organized medicine; and (6) the escalation of medical expenditures.

In recent years these problems have led the public to question the legitimacy of traditional medical practice. Consumers have begun to test the strength of the ramparts of established medicine. One approach to the medical citadel has been through citizen participation in community health programs.

Much has been said recently of community health, community psychiatry, and community participation. One assumption behind these activities is that health has to be dealt with in relation to the whole community environment. This "holistic" approach to health is an open challenge to the disease model, which views a patient as only a disease entity.

In order to treat the patient as part of a community with socioeconomic problems, physicians must receive information from counselors, social workers, and community residents. For dealing with community health, the health care team is quite useful.

Community health programs have existed for centuries, but in the 1960s community groups began to demand better services and more control over policy decisions in health care delivery systems. Thus, two unique kinds of local health care services were developed. One was the neighborhood health centers, which were established in impoverished areas with federal funding. The other was the emergence of free clinics, which were initiated and operated by volunteer workers to serve the needs of adolescents, "hippies," and racial minorities.

This chapter will open with a description of the conceptual framework in which the health center is viewed as a subsystem within the social system of the community. Then, it will review the evolution of community health programs and the forerunners of today's neighborhood health centers. After examining the social structure and processes conducive to the decline of these earlier local health care programs and to the birth of new ones during the 1960s, the mode of operation in the federally sponsored neighborhood health centers and privately run free clinics will be compared.

CONCEPTUAL FRAMEWORK

The Community as a Parsonian Social System

Sociological interest in the community lies in the amount of common activities rather than the territorial demarcation (Anderson, C. L., 1973). In this sense, the community may be conceptualized as a social system (Nelson et al., 1960; Reiss, 1959; Sanders & Brownlee, 1979; Sutton & Kolaja, 1960). When defined as a social system, the community is viewed as the totality of the interactions between its members and its component institutions. For an analysis of the community system, functionalist postulates include patterned behavior, consensus of values, group integration, and group control of individual behavior.

Neighborhood health centers are bound to generate a great deal of resistance because they challenge the status quo in the traditional community. From the functionalist perspective, the development of these centers is the process of regaining equilibrium in a community where the establishment of the centers has disrupted the balance maintained by the medical monopoly.

Following the Parsonian model, repercussions to the disturbance will be examined in terms of four prerequisites that a social system must meet for its survival: latency, goal attainment, adaptation, and integration. These four functions are in turn analyzed in relation to the major components of the community: cultural values, the polity, the economy, and stratification, respectively.

Latency: Cultural Values. Latency contributes to system maintenance by means of the commonly held cultural values that motivate individual members to act toward the attainment of shared goals. Here the latency function will be discussed in relation to ideologies such as individualism and equalitarianism. It is in the name of individualism that physicians have chosen affluent areas for practice, leaving the poorer neighborhoods deprived of medical services.

Goal Attainment: The Polity. The function of attaining the collective goals of a community is attributed to the polity (Parsons & Smelser, 1956, p. 48). The polity has the authority to maximize the use of resources—wealth and personnel, and it has the power to mobilize people to achieve community goals.

Thus, the function of the polity includes the establishment of neighborhood health centers as a part of government antipoverty activities.

Figure 9.1: Parsonian Functional Subsystems of the Social System

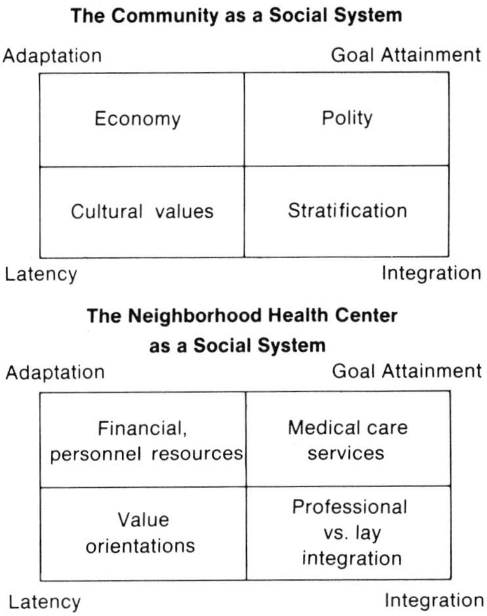

The Community as a Social System

Adaptation	Goal Attainment
Economy	Polity
Cultural values	Stratification
Latency	Integration

The Neighborhood Health Center as a Social System

Adaptation	Goal Attainment
Financial, personnel resources	Medical care services
Value orientations	Professional vs. lay integration
Latency	Integration

Adaptation: The Economy. The adaptive function deals with the problem of controlling the environment for the purpose of attaining the goals of the community. Parsons and Smelser (1956, p. 21) regard the economy as being specialized in this function because it produces facilities—wealth, goods, and services, for a community to use as it adapts to its limiting conditions. The neighborhood health center movement is not only a health program but is intended to have socioeconomic impact upon the poor by breaking up the vicious cycle of poverty and illness.

Integration: Stratification. The integrative function of a community is to articulate a set of norms for the members as a whole and for various categories with differentiated status and roles so that the community can maintain unity and cohesiveness. The normative ordering of the community yields a stratification scale: the scale of the prestige and status of persons as community members. The stratified community must be coordinated with the universal norms that govern individuals. The emergence of neighborhood health centers can be analyzed in relation to the stratification system, since its main feature, the participation of the poor in the decision-making process at the neighborhood health centers, presents an open challenge to the traditional hierarchical system in the community.

Having identified the components of the community as a social system, we will evaluate the validity of the functionalist assumption of integration from the conflict perspective. To Coleman (1957), for example, the major issue of a community is the resolution of conflict. He claims that the study of conflict serves as a means of focusing attention on specific attributes of communities, such as the conditions leading to equilibrium or the mechanisms of decision-making.

The community can also be broken down into person-to-person interactional units (Anderson, C. L., 1973). The degree of face-to-face interaction varies according to the characteristics of the community, such as the number of participants, awareness of action, the goal of action, and the recipients of action (Sutton & Kolaja, 1960).

The Neighborhood Health Center as a Social Subsystem

The operations of the neighborhood health centers will first be described in terms of the activities contained within a more or less integrated social system. Parsonian functional prerequisites are identified as specific task areas in the health centers (see Figure 9.1).

First, value orientations supporting the neighborhood health center will be examined in terms of the degree of value consensus held by various workers at the center and by the consumers' attitudes toward the program as measured by the rate of their utilization of the services.

Second, the level of the attainment of goals of the neighborhood health centers will be measured by the general quality of medical care, the effectiveness of the health care team, and the utilization of paraprofessional workers.

Third, the focal issue of the extent of integration in the center will be determined according to the degree to which consumers and professionals are coordinated. Finally, a measure of the adaptation of the health care system to the external environment will be determined on the basis of financial and personnel resources obtained.

The neighborhood health center will also be examined from the conflict perspective. When viewed as a political power struggle, disharmony in the center is not so unusual or threatening (Gordon, 1969). The neighborhood center operations proceed according to the normal progression of disequilibrium, arbitration, and compromise.

In that perspective, Coser's (1966) theory of functional conflict is useful since intergroup conflict is sometimes functional to enhancing the ingroup cohesion. Also, conflicts stimulate new rules, norms, and institutions, and they save society from stagnation. In short, conflict theories assume that an innovative program such as the neighborhood health center is likely to be in constant disequilibrium.

HISTORY OF COMMUNITY HEALTH PROGRAMS

Prior to 1850

There was little interest in community health in colonial America. Community health action was taken only during epidemics and consisted essentially of isolation and quarantine.

Despite the rapid industrial expansion and the growth of cities during the early part of the nineteenth century, organized health measures were slow in coming. The modern era of public health only dates back to 1850 when a health report was drawn up that served as a guide for community health for the next century (Anderson, C. L., 1973).

From 1850 to 1920

One of the two most important developments affecting community health in this period was the control of communicable disease by virtue of the discovery of the germ theory. The other was the development of neighborhood health centers in the immigrant settlements.

"Miasma Phase" (1850–1880). C. L. Anderson (1973) called the years between 1850 and 1880 the "miasma" (noxious air or vapor) period. During this period, disease was believed to be caused by noxious air, vapor, dirt, or a general lack of cleanliness. Public health consisted of promoting general cleanliness and quarantine. Medicine in these days was not significantly more effective than quackery for controlling disease.

Disease Control Phase (1880–1920). The period between 1880 and 1920 was labeled by C. L. Anderson (1973) as the disease control phase. It was during this period that the germ theory of disease came into being and was able to answer the pertinent questions of causation and prevention of communicable diseases. Public health efforts were concentrated on controlling communicable disease by inoculation and environmental manipulation (Mountin, 1940; Mustard, 1945; Viseltear, 1973).

The boundary between the professional and administrative domains of public health and medical care was less sharply delineated before about 1920 than it was later (Shonick & Price, 1977). While sanitation and the control of communicable disease were the primary public health activities, physicians also addressed themselves to the other health needs of the public. They did this because their private practices were not nearly as prestigious or lucrative as they later came to be, after medicine had established itself as a science and a profession.

Immigrant Settlement Days (1860–1910). While medical science was progressing, social changes were also taking place. Urbanization and industrialization flooded the cities and factory towns with rural and foreign migrants. The majority of the immigrants from southern and eastern Europe during this period were unskilled workers who had to accept poorly paid jobs (Rosen, 1971).

An awareness of the widespread prevalence of disease among the poor and the inadequacy of the health care available to them motivated efforts to establish settlement houses, or welfare centers, among the poor immigrants in large cities. In 1893, a nursing settlement house was opened in New York City in order to bring the benefits of public health nursing to an entire neighborhood. In the same year, a public dispensary was organized at the immigrant settlement, or neighborhood, in Chicago. In addition, various studies and programs were undertaken to improve health conditions where the settlements were located. They offered programs such as the improvement of housing and garbage collections, the fight against cocaine addiction among minors, and the regulation of midwifery (Adams, 1910).

The settlement house workers understood the devastating health problems suffered by the oppressed, poor immigrants, and they also recognized the problems created by cultural alienation. So they knew that effective application of health programs required an approach to the people on their own terms and in their own neighborhoods (Hiscock, 1935). By locating a settlement house in the section of town where the immigrants lived, public health care workers avoided strangeness and distance as well as language barriers and waiting periods (Davis, 1921). These settlement houses were the forerunner of the health center movement that began around 1910.

Nevertheless, even such a localization of health and social services was not enough to help the indigent immigrants, who were confronted with a multiplicity of uncoordinated agencies. By 1910, the idea of the neighborhood health center was expanded to include a requirement that geographical localization must be accompanied by administrative coordination and by active participation of the population served (Philips, 1940).

The First Health Center Movement (1910–1919). In response to these expanded needs, an extensive neighborhood health center movement began around 1910. Rosen (1971) described the movement of this period as largely being a series of experimental demonstrations. The neighborhood health center was meant to be an experiment in applying democracy to the health field. The movement endeavored to develop a consciously self-governing local unit in the midst of a large city. As such, the neighborhood health center was an experiment in social organization intended to create a community in which members would work together rationally and intelligently for the common welfare.

Stoeckle and Candib (1969) identified four features of the early neighborhood health centers: district location, community participation, bureaucratic organization, and preventive care. Financed by local taxes and philanthrophy and organized by voluntary agencies or municipal health departments, the early centers were located within city neighborhoods or districts, and their work was confined to the immediate population. Neighborhood residents were enlisted as aides to recruit patients, to take household surveys, and to participate in the governing of the center. Despite this decentralization of power, a bureaucratic form of organization was adopted to provide efficiency and to coordinate the centers, which were scattered and under diverse management. Most health center supporters viewed the program as preventive and educational. They regarded the center as complementing the curative work of physicians in private practice rather than competing against them.

Health Promotion Period (1920–1960)

C. L. Anderson (1973) referred to the period from 1920 to 1960 as the health promotion phase. When communicable diseases had been controlled, other health hazards were recognized. Public health efforts shifted from disease control to the promotion of the highest possible level of health for each individual.

Voluntary health agencies, which had been established prior to 1920, played an increasingly important role. Health centers financed by foundations, voluntary health agencies, or other social welfare organizations, as well as by local governments, were established in many parts of the United States (Anderson et al., 1976). Nevertheless, the concept of a local health center, which had developed largely to accommodate the needs of the urban poor and immigrants, declined toward the end of the 1930s due to changing social circumstances.

To begin with, the end of immigration during the war years and the restrictive legislation of 1921 and 1924 reduced the number of new immigrants. In the meanwhile, as the foreign-born and their children became acculturated into the American way of life, they moved up economically and moved out of the city slums. They also began to use more and more private medical care rather than the local health centers, which could provide only limited services.

Another factor, the changing pattern of financing medical expenses, made it easier for more people to seek private medical care. The concept of social insurance won greater public support during the depression of the 1930s, while voluntary health insurance was made available through labor–management negotiations. The postwar economic affluence of the 1950s also helped people to obtain private health care (Somers & Somers, 1977).

The same period witnessed another factor that undermined the health center movement. The function of social agencies changed as the federal government began to take an active role during the depression, and as a result, social agencies withdrew from health centers and moved to other loci, such as psychoanalytic case works, where they could exercise more power. In addition, there was a general political resistance to the further development of health center programs, and that was augmented by administrative infighting within municipal health departments (Rosen, 1971).

Finally, from about 1920, the boundary between the domains of public health and medical care was widened through the efforts of organized medicine (Shonick & Price, 1977). With the rapid development of the biomedical sciences and the establishment of medicine as a profession, the medical fraternity was successful in precluding all other health workers from practicing medicine (Betten & Austin, 1977). The power to grant or withhold approval to persons or institutions was formally lodged with the local medical societies. Thus, organized medicine proscribed the provision of curative medical care under local public health agency auspices. The latter, in turn, became conditioned to avoid trespassing on the domain of private medicine, and that resulted in a drastic curtailing of the functions of local health centers.

Social Engineering Phase

By 1960, the medical monopoly by private-practice physicians began to concern other health practitioners, who saw that the advanced medical technology offered by private-practice physicians and in large-scale hospitals was not available to everybody. The poor were especially neglected and even left out completely from improved health care services. C. L. Anderson (1973) calls the years since the 1960s the social engineering phase because the social aspects of health care have been given a new priority. A quest for social equalization of opportunity and access to health care took various forms, such as federally sponsored Medicare and Medicaid bills (to be discussed in Chapter 10).

It should be noted that until the mid-1960s most of the political actions were taken at the national level. The experiences of the New Deal of the 1930s and the civil rights struggle during the late 1950s and early 1960s seemed to indicate that all major social issues including health and welfare would be resolved by Congress, the federal courts, or by the President (O'Brien, 1975).

It was during the latter half of the 1960s that the long neglected concept of community health programs re-emerged in the form of neighborhood-based centers and free clinic movements. In the following sections, we will concentrate on the development and operations of the contemporary neighborhood health centers.

THE EMERGENCE OF THE NEIGHBORHOOD HEALTH CENTER

The Political Climate

Before 1964, the poverty of disadvantaged groups had rarely been a special focus of the federal government. However, during the late 1950s and early 1960s, the social consequences of poverty were so overwhelming that the federal government had to pay attention (Plotnick & Skidmore, 1975). Also, by the mid-1960s the federal government was in a better position to influence the health care system, since medical domination had been weakened. Third-party financing, such as through Medicare and Medicaid, was becoming more common (Fox & Crawford, 1979).

Under these circumstances, in 1964 the War on Poverty program was launched. Also in 1964, the Economic Opportunity Act was passed, and it mobilized a group of dedicated people from diverse backgrounds. Health care was viewed as a way to break the vicious cycle of poverty. Furthermore, it was recognized that existing institutional arrangements for the poor were defective and that health care for the poor would not be improved without a change in the health delivery system (Mooney, 1977).

In order to effect this structural change, the Office of Economic Opportunity (OEO), and later the Department of Health, Education, and Welfare (DHEW), sponsored the establishment of neighborhood health centers through federal grants-in-aid programs. By emphasizing consumer participation and the localization of neighborhood health centers, these facilities served as government-sponsored demonstration projects (Hollister, 1974, p. 1) that worked to strike a balance between federalism and decentralization (Kaufman, 1969; Swanson, 1972).

The Economic Background

It is not easy to explain why the War on Poverty gained such immediate support. Although unemployment remained at about five percent, general prosperity prevailed. The problem of poverty had been largely ignored during the post-World War II years, and social welfare legislation had a low priority (Levitan, 1969).

Some (Hollister et al., 1974a) attributed the success of the program to the evolving popular definition of a "health crisis," that is, rising medical costs coupled with consumer backlash in the form of malpractice suits. Due to the increased utilization of medical facilities, laissez-faire medical marketplace practices, inflation, and a host of other factors related to economic prosperity, medical expenses had risen to the point where they were considered to constitute a crisis. The problem was particularly severe for the underprivileged.

Another interpretation has been given in terms of demographic changes. Post-World War II migration among regions of the country produced fiscal problems for some local governments. This was aggravated by federal policies that encouraged minority residents to press their demands for better local government services (Moynihan, 1969; Piven & Cloward, 1971). Gradually the federal government was induced to assume some of the financial burden, and it did so by providing grants-in-aid to local governments, which in turn provided improved medical care for the indigent (Shonick & Price, 1977).

Stratification

During the post-World War II prosperity of the 1950s, there appeared a myth to the effect that wealth as well as health resources were more evenly distributed among the people than before. It was true that the general prosperity had raised the living standards of the underprivileged minorities and the poor. However, that had by no means decreased the gap between the rich and the poor. Rather, it sharpened the sense of relative deprivation experienced by the disadvantaged, who were just beginning to develop a taste for a better life.

The civil rights movement in the 1960s succeeded in focusing the nation's attention on the poverty of minority groups and supplied political pressure for a program to aid the poor. Health was seen as a crucial link in the cycle of poverty. The inadequacy of health care facilities in poor areas was considered a primary cause for unemployment, poverty, crime, social inequality, and conflict. Physicians in private practice were seldom found in neighborhoods in which large numbers of the poor and nonwhites lived (Gibson, Bugbee, & Anderson, 1970; Reskin & Campbell, 1974).

Cultural Values

If American values are considered to reflect a dichotomy between individualism and equalitarianism, as will be discussed in Chapter 10, then these values usually maintain a precarious balance. To illustrate, in recent years the idea of health as a right (i.e., an equalitarian value) rather than a privilege has come to be generally accepted. On the other hand, socialized medicine or compulsory health insurance has been largely rejected as a threat to individualism. In this respect, the neighborhood health center may be at a happy medium between equalitarianism and voluntarism. The model of decentralized neighborhood centers and consumer decision-making is appealing not only to the poor but to those who are increasingly dissatisfied with the bureaucracy of our contemporary society (Hollister et al., 1974a,b).

Intergroup Conflict

To the extent that the neighborhood health center has the potential for changing established relations in society, it finds itself at the focal point of conflict. Neighborhood health care served as a superb vehicle for the OEO activists to outflank the defenders of the status quo.

Conflict Between the AMA and the Neighborhood Center. To begin with, the criteria upon which neighborhood health center proposals were based departed radically from the stance taken by organized medicine. The neighborhood center's comprehensive ambulatory health care at a local level goes against the AMA's traditional distinction between therapeutic medical care and preventative public health. Also, organized medicine's dominance is challenged by the neighborhood center's emphasis on consumer participation and group practice. Finally, and most important, federal subsidy of the centers violates the AMA's long-cherished principle of fee-for-service.

However, the AMA's position on neighborhood health centers has been described as "schizophrenic" (Levitan, 1969, p. 60) rather than antagonistic. A series of defeats in congressional fights against Medicare seems to have mellowed the AMA's attitude toward third-party intervention. Also, the AMA's frequent and excessive warnings for so many years against socialized medicine may have lost their effectiveness. The AMA's ability to persuade the public was possibly diluted by the time neighborhood health center proposals were introduced. In addition, the AMA has in the past been tolerant of legislation on behalf of the poor who could not pay the standard fees.

In sum, some sectors of the AMA endorsed the notion of the neighborhood centers, while others issued unsolicited warnings to the federal government to stop meddling in health affairs.

Conflict Between Institutions. Beyond the AMA and the neighborhood centers, there was an even broader context of conflict from the onset since the OEO itself evolved out of a conflict situation. In the beginning, the OEO was a compromise between the vested interests of various groups such as the Labor Department, the Council of Economic Advisors, and Congress (Feingold, 1970; Levitan, 1969; Plotnick & Skidmore, 1975). Workers in existing institutions and government programs were worried about losing their functions through the birth of a new executive department. The professionals who staffed the OEO showed their primary allegiance to political constituencies, while other workers in the OEO directed their efforts to help communities far removed from Washington, D.C. (Davis & Tranqueda, 1969). There was also an ideological conflict even among the proponents of the neighborhood centers. Some advocated the creation of prepaid group practices to provide neighborhood health centers with greater financial stability than would be the case if they depended exclusively on the OEO (Hollister et al., 1974a).

These struggles between special interest groups were never completely resolved during the early operations of the neighborhood health centers, and as a result, the existence of OEO-based health centers is still rather tenuous.

Symbolic Aspects of the Movement

While some (Hollister et al., 1974a) view neighborhood health centers as a social movement that emerged out of widespread ideological and social support from the general public, others (Rein, 1970a) regard them as a demonstration of an approach to reform by the federal government. In line with the labeling theory, they argue that the federally sponsored health centers were primarily intended to gain for the government a label of political liberalism by demonstrating a fashionable, politically attractive, and rationally appealing program.

As a demonstration program, the symbolic aspects of the movement were far reaching. In the first place, the neighborhood health center was meant to be an innovative alternative to the traditional medical delivery system. The neighborhood health centers were to demonstrate that comprehensive, high-quality care could be provided at a reasonable cost. Further, the impact of the movement was to extend beyond the health care field and to reach the community at large. The participation of community members in health care service and policy decision-making at the health centers symbolized the ideologies of equalitarianism and decentralization.

However, since it is only a demonstration program, the government is not bound to develop the centers on a regular and continuous basis but only to maximize the effectiveness of the political label given to the program. This is highlighted by Rein (1970a) when he identifies the classic scenario of a government-sponsored demonstration project. It begins with unrealistically high expectations and promises that are used to gather political support. These are followed by claims of immediate success with a minimum amount of evaluation, but soon the program begins to run into financial and technical difficulties. By this time the proud promises by the government are replaced by hard-nosed evaluations so as to justify government withdrawal from the project.

From whatever perspective the neighborhood health centers are viewed, the agony of the successful birth of a new health delivery system is readily apparent. In the following section, the operation of neighborhood health centers will be examined to determine the extent to which these initial problems were resolved or aggravated, and the unexpected difficulties will be identified.

THE OPERATION OF THE NEIGHBORHOOD HEALTH CENTER

At first the neighborhood health centers were located mostly in inner-city areas, although some were established in rural areas. For the most part these centers were sponsored by medical schools, departments of public health, hospitals, or other health care facilities that had received federal funds to establish and to manage the centers in cooperation with community representatives.

The centers provided primary and preventive health care, including laboratory work, X-ray examinations, and minor surgery all under the same roof. Further, dental care, mental health services, and social welfare services were offered in many centers. Originally the program attempted to furnish at least one physician per 1,500 residents. In addition to physicians, the centers were to have many paraprofessional staff members who practiced medicine as health teams. Clients were generally low-income whites, blacks, Native Americans, Spanish-speaking, and other ethnic and racial minorities.

The operation of the neighborhood health center will be examined with reference to the four functionalist prerequisites for a social system.

Value Orientations

The underlying value of the neighborhood health center can be described as equalitarianism. The War on Poverty was conceived of as a means to equalize the opportunities for health, wealth, and welfare.

More specifically, the neighborhood health center was built on the assumption that sickness and poverty reinforce each other and that this new program would interrupt the vicious cycle of poverty and disease. However, some (Davis & Tranqueda, 1969) attacked this exclusive linkage of health and poverty as a "cop out" on the part of the federal government, one that evades the more complex issues of poverty.

As a derivative of the vicious-cycle theory, the holistic approach to health care was adopted in that health services must deal with a patient as a part of a family and of a community, both of which are laden with social and economic problems. Such comprehensive care could only be delivered by a team of professionals and paraprofessionals, not by a solo practitioner. In other words, these values signaled a reform in the health care system.

Finally, an equalitarian orientation assumes that poverty is a result of social injustice rather than personal imcompetence. In order to remedy the situation, consumer participation in the decision-making was prescribed. Poverty, defined as the result of a lack of power, self-respect, and money, is expected to be mitigated by active and meaningful involvement in constructive programs.

Differential Perception of Values

Along with the high aspirations and the lofty goals of the program, a need was felt from the outset for joint decision-making among the participants of the program—the community, the university (medical school), and the Office of Economic Opportunity. The OEO and the universities were quite explicit about the necessity of involving the community poor in the development of health centers in order to obtain financial support. However, the functionalist premise of value consensus in the health center system was tenuous because the selection of an appropriate area for joint decision-making was in itself a source of conflict.

There was also no agreement regarding the order of priority of stated goals among the groups involved. For example, at the Watts Neighborhood Health Center (Davis & Tranqueda, 1969), the Community Health Council members represented the values of a black community in its quest for power, and particular agencies within the community as well as individuals struggling for daily subsistence. The medical school at the university was interested primarily in solving health problems rather than in the community self-help action programs. Then, as a political bureaucracy, the OEO was concerned with financial solvency and immediate success to secure further financial support (Geiger, 1967b; New & Hessler, 1972).

Davis and Tranqueda (1969) further noted that the functionalist assumption of system integration was not validated. Discrepancies in the perception of reality and a definition of the situation were not cemented by a free exchange of ideas to enhance group solidarity. Instead, conflict resolution was accomplished largely through an interactionist bargaining by players of the power game.

Consumers' Attitudes toward the Neighborhood Health Center

The neighborhood health centers were established to make health care services more accessible to the disadvantaged. However, the question is whether or not, and to what extent, the persons for whom the centers were intended did in fact use them. Robertson and others (1968) were pessimistic in their prognosis of the acceptance of the health centers by low-income families.

This pessimism was derived from the prevailing value orientations of the destitute. Along with the Marxian characterization of the proletariat in a capitalist society, the poor have been described as powerless (Binstock & Ely, 1971; Cohen & Hodges, 1963), apathetic, and present-oriented (O'Brien, 1975; Tumin, 1967). For the indigents, pressing issues are daily bread and a job rather than immunization for the prevention of a possible disease in the future. Also, the poor are isolated from the rest of society, particularly from the complexities of modern medicine in big institutions, which tend to be biased against low-income and racial minority clients (see Chapter 5).

One of the tasks of the War on Poverty was to change these value orientations of the powerless poor through their maximum feasible participation in the program (Kramer, 1969). The supposition was that the sense of insecurity and powerlessness would be reduced by forging a network of relationships among hitherto alienated but similarly circumstanced people who could provide one another with a sense of status, worth, and well-being (Cohen & Hodges, 1963).

Have neighborhood health centers facilitated access to health care? Positive answers are found in many studies. Bellin and Geiger (1970) reported that 71 percent of the target population was using the Columbia Point neighborhood health center in Boston two years after its establishment, and that the center was the main source of care for five out of six of the people in the community. The annual average number of encounters with health center physicians for users of that facility was 6.1. This compares favorably with the health care utilization rates of other low-income population and even with more affluent populations. For example, a national health survey revealed an annual average of 5.0 physician visits for the total population (U.S. DHEW, 1962).

Furthermore, the Columbia Point program demonstrated some change in attitudes and behavior toward health care and its utilization. A marked increase in the use of preventive medicine was noted, such as asymptomatic checkups, immunization, and a reduction in postponing needed care (Bellin & Geiger, 1972). Above all, users' responses to the center were favorable.

Columbia Point is a Boston community that is somewhat geographically isolated, and its experience may not be typical of neighborhood health centers. However, there are other studies (Strauss & Sparer, 1971) indicating a more frequent use of neighborhood health centers by their target population as compared with that of other people in a national sample. Wan and Gray (1978) reported that regular users of health centers had received the same number of immunizations and physical checkups as users of private physicians.

The study of 21 centers by the OEO (Langston et al., 1972) revealed that an average of 66 percent of all eligible individuals and 55 percent of the eligible families had used the centers. These users of health centers appeared to express greater satisfaction with the care they received than middle class people using other facilities. The former group of people were more likely to recommend the centers to someone else than the latter would recommend their physicians or hospitals to others. Also, the users of the centers tended to avail themselves of the services of preventive medicine.

Nevertheless, the validity of these favorable responses has to be analyzed more carefully. For instance, the above mentioned target population of 21 centers evaluated by the OEO reported that they used the centers for their "usual source of care." Yet, 20 to 30 percent of these same people mentioned that their last physician visit was to another facility (Langston et al., 1972).

In the same vein, Hillman and Charney (1972) recognized that comprehensive health care is accepted with enthusiasm by a large number of indigent patients, but a significant minority could not be weaned from their traditional medical care facilities. Part of the problem is that people expect too much. The users of neighborhood health centers are pleased with the services they receive but they want more, that is, a 24-hour facility that would completely replace the outpatient and emergency room of a hospital and yet remain a convenient local facility (Salber et al., 1972).

A look at emergency room use as a manifestation of the accessibility to neighborhood health centers was supported by some (Gold & Rosenberg, 1974), who showed a reduction of emergency room use with the appearance of the neighborhood health centers. However,other investigators (Moore et al., 1972) saw nonsignificant changes. On a broader scale, the Health Interview Survey conducted by the National Center for Health Statistics discerned a rise in the rates of medical facility utilization by the indigent population from 1963 to 1973. Yet, with all other contingencies uncontrolled, we cannot determine how much of these results are due to the operations of the neighborhood health centers.

Thus, the findings concerning the effectiveness of changing value orientations among the poor are inconclusive. Even favorable studies do not usually indicate changing value orientations, but simply show reduced barriers of supply, distance, and cost. All that can be said is that the neighborhood health centers are reaching out to those who need the assistance most. The registration rates for those centers have been highest in families with the lowest income: young families with a large number of young children, and in general, blacks (Langston et al., 1972; Reynolds, 1976; Salber et al., 1970, 1972).

Patterns of Medical Practice

The primary goal of the neighborhood health center as a health care institution was to provide the best possible comprehensive health care to the poor. From their inception, however, neighborhood health centers have had to contend with charges that they were delivering substandard health care.

The Quality of Medical Care

Extensive and systematic evaluations of the quality of medical care at neighborhood health centers are scarce because of the costliness of evaluative research, the difficulties in establishing evaluative criteria, and the heterogeneity of the centers.

Among the few studies available, positive results were reported by Morehead and others (1971), who made a systematic comparison of OEO-based health centers and other health care providers. They found that, with the exception of the few small, highly organized and richly staffed Children's Bureau programs, the neighborhood health center performance rating was generally equal to that of the medical school hospital outpatient departments and was superior to the performance in the few solo practitioners' offices studied.

Kessner and others (1974) studied medical care processes, such as screening, diagnosis, and follow-up management. Neighborhood health centers, as well as prepaid group practices, were found to do a better job than hospital outpatient departments in performing routine screening tests. However, a significant number of the abnormal symptoms discovered were not appropriately diagnosed or treated at neighborhood health centers.

In terms of the outcome of the service, Gordon (1973) compared the incidence of rheumatic fever for children in the populations who were served by health center programs and for those who were not eligible. He found that the incidence was one third lower among children who were eligible for the neighborhood health centers. He further compared two time periods: before and after the establishment of the centers. A reduction of incidence by 60 percent between the two time periods was noted among children receiving center services, while the incidence was unchanged among the other children. Studying blacks in southern counties that had neighborhood health centers, Anderson and Morgan (1973) also reported a decline in infant mortality after the appearance of the health centers.

On the negative side, Breyer (1977) mentioned that the centers failed to offer comprehensive services except for the most basic primary care, and that they did not provide physician continuity when patients were transferred from the centers to hospitals.

Most of these findings, however, are inconclusive mainly because other factors were not sufficiently controlled.

Innovative Health Care: The Health Team and New, Allied Health Workers

In order to achieve the goal of providing comprehensive medical care to the indigent population, neighborhood health centers adopted two innovative approaches: health team operations and the training and use of new, allied health workers.

The health care team deals not only with the physical problems but also the social problems of clients in an attempt to bridge the sociocultural gaps between medical professionals and low-income patients. However, due to the complexity of the tasks and the underdeveloped definitions of the roles of the participants, the health team is more aptly described from the conflict perspective rather than as a functionally integrated social system (Rubin & Beckhard, 1972).

Role strains in the team work are illustrated by the experience at Columbia Point, the first OEO-sponsored center, which opened in Boston in 1965. A typical team consisted of an internist, a pediatrician, two public health physicians, two social workers, and two nurses. The proposal to hire family health workers—indigent residents in the target neighborhood who are trained to work as health care assistants; their job will be described in the following section on community health workers—generated so much conflict that these workers were not incorporated into the team until later.

The interview study conducted by Banta and Fox (1972) at Columbia Point examined the perceptions of the physicians, public health physicians, nurses, and social workers. First of all, the physicians who took a leadership role failed to recognize the Center's formal allegiance to equalitarian, peer-type relations (New & Hessler, 1972; Rubin & Beckhard, 1972). The public health physicians, in turn, did not have much respect for the staff physicians. The nurses deferred to the physicians, but also complained about the physicians for not sharing information and not becoming involved with the community. Finally, the social workers viewed the physicians as authoritarian. In short, the physicians were not using the group efficiently.

Public health physicians who lacked a definite commitment to serve the poor were assigned to Columbia Point. They would have preferred to work in a hospital or with middle class clients. Other team members were sympathetic about this situation, but they criticized these doctors for their inexperience, laziness, arrogance, and uncooperativeness.

Between the public health nurses and the social workers, there was an overlap of job territories. Instead of referring problem families to social workers, public health nurses tended to become involved in the counseling. The social workers, being proud of their objectivity, regarded the nurses as too emotional and lacking in professional understanding of the issues.

In short, the dynamics of this early health team were characterized by diffuse definitions of roles, a complex role set, and diverse orientations of the participants as well as the unfamiliarity of the members with one another (Breyer, 1977).

The Community Health Worker. In Chapter 8, new, allied health workers such as nurse practitioners and physician's assistants were discussed. One of the more innovative uses of health personnel at neighborhood centers involved the employment of poor and uneducated residents as community health workers (Smith, 1973).

The community health workers at neighborhood health centers (1) receive training and employment as residents in their own low-income area; (2) furnish neighborhood health centers with trained medical services without the expense of specialized physicians; and (3) act as a link between the center and the community because of their familiarity with the community (Zahn, 1968).

Among the community health workers, the family health workers deserve special attention since they represent a major program innovation in health careers. Their training lasts for six months. The first eight weeks of the core curriculum covers basic health skills, a survey of health career and community resources, and remedial training in English and mathematics, as required. Of the remaining 18 weeks, two-thirds are spent learning health skills taught by the nurses, and one-third is spent on knowledge of community resources taught by a lawyer. Seminars are given by community organizers, health educators, anthropologists, internists, pediatricians, obstericians, psychiatrists, and physical therapists. Trainees receive modest remuneration during the training (Wise et al., 1968; Zahn, 1968).

In addition to the physical care of patients, much of the family health workers' time is spent making home visits and dealing with social and environmental problems. Their job also includes community work such as locating available community resources and helping people to negotiate with agencies. As indigenous members of the community, family health workers can readily identify with their clients' lifestyle and thus are able to act as client advocates (Meyer, 1969).

The family health workers' role as a liaison between the health care facility and the community places them in a marginal position. On one hand, their employment in the medical establishment attenuates their claim of loyalty to the community, and on the other hand, as subprofessionals they are alienated from the health care team. Furthermore, their medical task is defined as being supportive of the physician's work, and their lack of professional autonomy subjects them administratively to redundant chains of command (Holton et al., 1972; New & Hessler, 1972).

Despite this built-in structural strain, however, there is a positive view of marginality (Levinson & Schiller, 1966; Smith, 1973). In a national survey of new career health personnel programs quoted by Smith (1973), more than half of the trainees were inclined to perceive their role as one of bridging the gap between the agency and the community, a role that was viewed as innovative and leading to career advancement. Another example by Wise and others

(1968) demonstrated that a neighborhood resident, trained for six months and supervised by public health nurses, could effectively coordinate many of the functions traditionally assigned to public health nurses and social workers.

Professional–Lay Integration

The neighborhood health center was built on the idea that the fight against poverty is best accomplished by getting the poor to participate in the decision-making process, thus helping them to gain a sense of power and self-esteem. The OEO funds, therefore, were assigned to the sponsoring group (i.e., hospital, medical school, health department, etc.) on the condition that the indigent residents participate in the program in a significant way. On the other hand, the official sponsors, who were in large part traditionally trained professionals, felt that they should command the center since they would bear the responsibility of fiscal and professional management.

The major issue of integration, in functionalist terms, evolved around the coordination of the professional staff and the consumer representatives. Because of the built-in structural stress, conflict perspectives were adopted by many (Coser, 1956; Feingold, 1970; Gordon, 1969), who envisioned the center as an arena for political power struggle.

From the interactionist's angle, consumer participation is considered a game (Moffet, 1971). Yette (1971) postulates that the outcome of the game is indeterminant because even the power of the oppressor is limited by the resourcefulness and alertness of the oppressed. Thus the oppressors must be observant about the moves made by the oppressed. In this regard, while professional staff members advocate the slogan of maximum feasible *participation* by the poor, they may actually be using participation as a tactic to accomplish the maximum *pacification* of the poor (Arnstein, 1969; Thompson, 1974).

Since the neighborhood health center emerged as an innovative institution, it is more realistic to examine the process of its development rather than to categorize it. Several process models have been advanced, such as Gordon's (1969) life cycle, which consists of instant community, conflict-inducing insight, and disintegration or cooperation. Geiger (1967b) distinguished four phases: confrontation, conflict, compromise, and accommodation. For Twaddle and Hessler (1977), three stages were apparent: formative, charismatic, and routinization.

Whatever terminology is used, three basic stages can be identified: contact, conflict, and accomodation.

Contact Stage. In most cases, the plans for the neighborhood health center are worked out by university or professional organizations long before the center begins its operation and without the participation of community representatives. However, since community participation is one of the requirements of funding, the sponsor organizations go out to the community to recruit representatives.

Many of the medical professionals may sincerely believe in community participation as a vehicle to correct social inequality (Geiger, 1967a). Yet, other motivations and expectations exist, such as using the community as an extension of the medical school's laboratory facilities (Twaddle & Hessler, 1977), or trying to coopt the poor and to protect themselves from charges of ignoring the community. What the professionals often want is a "passive, window-dressing, grateful, powerless advisory committee" (Geiger, 1967a).

The community deputies can be self-selected, elected, or appointed (Twaddle & Hessler, 1977). Frequently, when the physicians and administrators begin to search the community, they tend to encounter a readily available group of indigenous people "who stand up and say 'Here I am' " (Gordon, 1969). They may be either the type of people who actively involve themselves in various service organizations, or they are grassroot consumers who take an interest in the health center. Whether such people are the community elite or populists (Twaddle & Hessler, 1977), they are ready to assume the leadership role in their community. They tend to be happy with the status gained by the association with the center sponsors, impressed by the wealth and power of the professionals, and are therefore content to become a passive board member.

Thus, during this formative stage, a symbiotic relation develops into what Gordon (1969) called an "instant community," and Geiger (1967a) called a "great honeymoon."

Conflict Stage. Latent discrepancies between providers and consumers during the formative stage gradually become manifest. For one thing, there are differences in the ways the participants conceive of their organizations and activities. The medical staff, who is responsible to the university and medical school, is committed to attaining a specific goal, a rational health care program. By comparison, the administrators and community employees, who are held accountable to the community, are concerned with the survival of the center. From the global perspective, they tend to make decisions to the advantage of the organization as a whole, which, in this case, involves social and economic as well as medical spheres (Brandon, 1977).

The second major conflict arises from the unequal distribution of power. As the two groups work together, they begin to probe for the locus of control at the center (Twaddle & Hessler, 1977). Typically, consumer participants realize that they have little power over the major decision-making mechanism. That built-in handicap is due to the fact that, in the beginning, the OEO normally did not allow poor people to constitute a majority on the board of directors.

In spite of that ground rule, the consumers begin to demand "control" rather than mere "participation." Medical professionals, in contrast, do not see consumers as capable of making professional decisions. Despite their good intentions of objectivity and neutrality, it is difficult for anyone on the staff or on the board to remain neutral. As a result, the center is likely to become polarized, and sometimes the conflict will be severe enough to close down the whole operation.

As Twaddle, Hessler, New, and others (New et al., 1973; Twaddle & Hessler, 1977) observed, charismatic leadership may emerge during this period. Since the neighborhood health center is an innovative agency without a traditional role model, it is likely that its survival rests upon the ability of a charismatic leader to coordinate the conflicting parties.

Accommodative Stage. Perpetual conflict is unpleasant and destructive for everyone concerned, and some compromises are likely to be made. Three types

Table 9.1:
Typology of Decision-Making Patterns

Theoretical orientation	*Functionalism*	*Interactionism*	*Conflict*
Conflict resolution	Debate	Game	Fight
Strategy	Problem solving	Persuasion bargaining	Pressure
Congruence of interests	Consensus	Difference	Dissensus
Concentration of power	Low	Medium	High
Coalition capacity	Low	Medium	High

Source: Modified from Ralph M. Kramer, *Participation of the Poor: Comparative Community Case Studies in the War on Poverty,* © 1969, pp. 182, 185. Reprinted by permission of Prentice-Hall, Inc., Englewood Cliffs, N. J.

of conflict resolution have been identified by Kramer (1969) in his comparative study of neighborhood health centers. They are debate, game, and fight (see Table 9.1), and these types are determined by the degrees of consensus, concentration of power, and capacity for coalition (i.e., the capacity to organize and mobilize minority members against the opposition).

Debate is an effort to persuade or convince others with an open, formal, parliamentary procedure. The strategy is a rational one of collaboration and constructive problem-solving. This is made possible where there is a high degree of agreement, a diffusion of power, and a slim chance for coalition. This resembles the functionalist model of a social system that is based on common values. However, group consensus is not necessarily functional to the system because it may be generated by apathy, low salience of the issue, or by deliberate selection of homogeneous board members.

On the opposite end of the continuum is the fight as a method of conflict resolution. When there is a dissensus of interests and no likely alternatives, a fight will take place in which coercive pressure is utilized. The extent to which power is concentrated and structured along partisan and racial lines will heighten the stakes of vested interest groups, and that increases the possibility of a fight.

Game playing can be viewed from the interactionist perspective; actors use strategies of persuasion, negotiation, and bargaining. Kramer (1969) placed the game in the middle range between the debate and the fight. It is likely to take place where there is a divergence of opinions but where an agreement is perceived as a possibility.

As a result of some kind of conflict resolution, homeostasis will be reached. This accommodation may simply mean a task-oriented working arrangement rather than a reflection of group integration (Gordon, 1969). On the other hand, a new form of equilibrium can be reached. In some health centers, decision-making cliques were created outside the existing institutional structures. This emergent interest group or pressure group consisted of upwardly mobile and assertive members of ethnic minorities. Although it was still formally allied with the traditional community elites, its role had shifted from mere participation in a coalition to that of control (Kramer, 1969). Furthermore, a change in the organizational structure was accomplished. The consumers became a governing board of directors, and they received the grant directly from the OEO without the intermediary of medical schools and other organizations (Brandon, 1977; Twaddle & Hessler, 1977).

The type of accomodation varies for the individual centers. Some become more inclined in favor of the consumers, and others, the reverse. When equilibrium is reached, that stage may be called "routinization" (Twaddle & Hessler, 1977, or maturity.

Financial and Work Force Adaptation

The organizational survival of the neighborhood health center rests upon its ability to adapt to the external environment. Since it was created as a novel program at variance with the established institutions, its task of adaptation is perilous, particularly in gaining financial and personal resources from the outside.

Financial Adaptation

Financing. Initially, the supporters of OEO grants for neighborhood health centers assumed that long-term financial aid would come largely from Medicare, Medicaid, and other financial sources. These expectations appeared reasonable in the mid-1960s when federal financing programs were being enacted (Roghmann et al., 1971). However, such optimism on the part of the health centers was soon frustrated by the fiscal difficulties and restrictive policies of Medicaid.

When confronted with its own budget constraints, the federal government began to seek ways of improving third-party reimbursement by encouraging, for example, the Health Maintenance Organization model (see Chapter 10) to provide a more stable income source.

The financial problems of the health centers are unique and arise from a unique administrative structure. Most of the centers were supported, at least in the beginning, on a yearly basis by the granting agencies, and the centers were subject to evaluation and revision. This uncertainty discouraged the formulation of long-range programs. Also, rigidity in the OEO budget system was not conducive to a flexible utilization of resources.

Cost. From the beginning, neighborhood health centers have been criticized for their high operational costs. On a practical basis, however, it seems natural that comprehensive health care for the destitute should cost more because the morbidity rate is higher than in more affluent communities.

A major difficulty in comparing service costs at neighborhood health centers with those at other facilities lies in the fact that the centers deliver a whole host of services that are beyond those available elsewhere. To illustrate, extensive social services, outreach training, health education, the provision of transportation, and other such activities are an integral part of the health care at the centers (Zwick, 1972, p. 84).

Based on a systematic comparative study, Sparer and others (Sparer & Anderson, 1972; Sparer et al., 1970) concluded that the costs of medical care at the centers were competitive with other institutional providers, including hospital outpatient departments and clinics and large, prepaid group practices. In the centers, about 55 percent of the costs were directed toward primary clinical care, while activities for the support of health services averaged 18 percent in urban areas and 24 percent in rural areas. Similar favorable findings are reported for child and youth projects (MCHS, 1971).

Conversely, Breyer (1977) found deficiencies with regard to efficiency and physician utilization. This was interpreted as a weakness of the government funding since it was devoid of a penalty for nonmaximization of resources. Reynolds (1976), in comparison, attributed the cost inefficiency to the size of the centers.

Facilities. The scarcity of physical facilities to house high-quality health services in poverty areas was one of the most serious obstacles. Wherever possible, neighborhood health centers took over available sites and used the funds to expand their services. They also intended to use indigent labor to remodel buildings but ran into difficulties for violating construction codes and the like (Levitan, 1969, p. 55).

Some new centers were built by loans made available through an extraordinary cooperation between federal agencies (OEO, DHEW, Department of Housing and Urban Development, and Office of Management and Budget) and private mortgage and insurance companies (Zwick, 1972, p. 73).

Staffing of the Center

Physicians. Uncertainties existed in the beginning about the capability of the neighborhood health centers to recruit physicians to meet the program standard of one physician for every 1,500 people (Levitan, 1969, p. 56). This anxiety was understandable in view of the widespread preference of professionals to avoid poverty neighborhoods (Reynolds, 1976) and the low regard shown for the program by the AMA.

According to Tilson's (1973) study, health center physicians are characterized as (1) young (under 40 years old); (2) female (twice as many women as men); (3) black (more than four times as many blacks as others); (4) primary care specialists, notably pediatricians; and (5) largely uncertified by specialty boards.

Salaries are usually set by the OEO at levels competitive with other institutional modes of practice (Zwick, 1972, p. 81). Nonetheless, the characteristics of the center physicians listed above—primary care, younger age, lower rate of certification—help to lower their income level.

The turnover rate appears to be relatively high. In Tilson's (1973) study, fewer than half of the physicians remained at centers for more than two years. Those who stayed were more often black, older, and board-certified, and they had faculty appointments at medical schools. Many younger physicians seem to have used the health centers as a stepping stone to a more traditional medical practice. Even so, Tilson's data rejected the hypothesis that the mass exodus of physicians from health centers was due to (1) the professional versus consumer conflict, (2) the use of paramedical personnel and team practices, and (3) the low salary. He postulated that the surviving physicians are influenced by a combination of idealism and intellectual interest in the experimental mode of health care delivery.

The motivations of physicians to work at neighborhood health centers vary significantly. For younger physicians with family responsibilities, health center careers may represent convenient, steady jobs with regular hours, or, as stated above, they may offer the opportunity to gain enough experience to move on to more established institutions (Tilson, 1973). Women, or racial-minority physicians, may have no place to work except at the neighborhood centers. On the other hand, there are many physicians who are dedicated to the objectives of the centers and are in rebellion against traditional medical practices and the power of organized medicine (Brandon, 1977).

The data are not sufficient to determine whether the variations in physicians' characteristics are attributable to the economic process of the medical marketplace or the structural and operational aspects of particular neighborhood health centers (e.g., flexibility versus rigidity).

Outlook for Neighborhood Health Centers

Along with the changing political climate, the neighborhood health centers have experienced vicissitudes.

The neighborhood health center movement, a creation of the federal government's War on Poverty in the mid-1960s, met with opposition from the Nixon administration beginning in 1968. Republicans viewed the centers as poorly managed, too expensive on a per-patient basis, insufficiently linked to mainstream medicine, and a duplicate of Medicaid.

Another reason for the stagnation of the program is attributed to the general discontent with the War on Poverty campaign. During the 1960s a number of reform ideas were linked, but these ideas were not knit into a logically tight model. The neighborhood health centers became a focus of various progressive ideas advocated by different groups of people, such as President Johnson, politicians, racial minorities, and civil rights activists.

With time, however, the loose alliance of national constituencies that supported neighborhood health centers has eroded. Various groups have come to perceive differences in their goals, values, and methods concerning community health care. Gradually, the original design of neighborhood centers has begun to be transformed. Some basic aspects of the centers—emphasis on team practice, environmental causes for poor health, and social services related to health care—have been phased out, while other functions are taken over by other ambulatory care models such as prepaid group practice, reorganized hospital outpatient departments, and Health Maintenance Organizations (HMOs).

One of the competitive models is the HMO (see Chapter 10) (Anderson et al., 1976), and there have been attempts to convert neighborhood health centers into HMOs. Like a neighborhood center, an HMO is supposed to provide comprehensive health services to the residents of a defined area. Unlike the neighborhood center, however, the HMO is financed by the prepayment of a flat rate by its members. HMOs serve a different income-level clientele, and there is no provision underwriting the cost of participation by the indigent. In order to convert neighborhood centers to HMOs, the former must expand the original target areas to include those with the ability to pay. While the HMO model stabilizes financial sources, it generates the fear that services to the poor may be diminished in order to provide services more attractive to middle class members of the HMOs.

Thus, the enthusiasm for neighborhood health centers is being replaced in the 1970s by an increasing scrutiny concerning the indispensability of the neighborhood centers in improving primary health care.

Between 1970 and 1973 the administration of the neighborhood health center was gradually transferred to the Department of Health, Education, and Welfare (DHEW), and the units are now called community health centers. As a result of changing politicial priorities and budgeting constraints, DHEW did not expand the program but concentrated on maintaining existing centers (Reynolds, 1976). In significant contrast to its predecessors, the Carter administration has decided to bolster community health centers. Carter's health budgets call for the creation of 131 new centers. DHEW estimates that the new funds will provide services to one million additional individuals, bringing the total number of people served to 5.6 million in 705 centers. Even with the budget increase, however, community health centers would serve only 11.4 percent of those living in areas defined as medically underserved (Iglehart, 1978; "Policy and issues guidebook . . . ," 1978).

A question constantly raised is, Can the goals of the community health centers be accomplished more efficiently and effectively by other service delivery models?

FREE CLINICS

While the federal government was planning neighborhood health centers, spending $100 million (OEO, 1969), and debating free care through national insurance, the completely separate free clinic movement was taking shape in 1967. Left out of the rigid government planning and only supported by volunteer workers and by donations, the community-based free clinics appeared sporadically but eventually spread throughout the country (Smith, D. E., 1969).

Since no-pay or charity medical care has been available for years, it is essential to define the concept of a "free clinic." Schwartz (1971b) distinguished several criteria for the free clinic: (1) direct delivery of medical, dental, psychological, or drug abuse care that is provided by a facility during specified hours of service; (2) presence of professional as well as nonprofessional volunteer workers on the staff; and (3) services available to everyone in need without eligibility restrictions and without direct charges. The basic difference between free clinics and the OEO neighborhood health centers is that the clinics began on a voluntary basis without public funding, and they provide free services to anyone without bureaucratic discrimination.

History and Types of Free Clinics

The first free clinic opened in the Haight-Ashbury district of San Francisco in 1967 (Schwartz, 1971b). A few farsighted and concerned physicians saw the acute need for "no deposit, no return" somatic medical-crisis intervention to be provided for the youthful drug abusers who had congregated in that district.

Then, a series of free clinics were established ad hoc in other large cities (Smith et al., 1971). Gradually, clinic organizers began to reach out to one another for advice and to exchange information, which led to the formation of the National Free Clinic Council. Its first symposium was held in San Francisco in 1970 (Smith & Luce, 1970; Smith et al., 1971).

From its start as a "bad trip" center and from the incidental offering of crisis intervention, the Haight-Ashbury Medical Clinic has grown into a conglomerate of medical and psychological sections that include nonpsychiatric counseling and encounter-group centers. While some clinics were short lived, there are many others that have survived despite the public prediction that the free clinic movement was a transient phenomenon.

Types of Clinics. Among a host of free clinics, at least three major types have been differentiated (Schwartz, 1971b; Smith et al., 1971): neighborhood, street (or hippie), and youth clinics.

The neighborhood free clinic was frequently founded by politically organized racial minority persons—for example, Black Panthers—for helping inner city ghetto dwellers or migrant workers. Most of them receive more government funds, but they operate with a governing board composed of neighborhood residents. The street (hippie) clinic offers drug abuse treatment, including psychological and physical therapy related to drugs. Since the community consists of transient youths, policies are often decided by the staff, the administrator, or the medical director. Some clinics, however, have functioning boards, made up of the staff, street people, students, and community residents.

Finally, the youth clinic was typically organized by adults, service clubs, or an official board to deal with drug use among high school students. Many were started with a small amount of community funding, and their policy boards consist of housewives, business people, city officials, and professionals.

Need for Free Clinics. During the 1960s, in addition to the OEO clinics (which received the most attention), there were many other federal health care programs being funded. Why then was it necessary for the free clinic movement to be initiated?

In the first place, most of the clients of the free clinics deviate from social norms. They are alienated from the mainstream of society, including traditional medical service. As Smith and others (1971) aptly stated, unconventional people with unconventional problems must seek unconventional help.

The second main factor for the birth of the free clinics is found in the shortcomings of all federally sponsored health projects. Since they have strict eligibility criteria, many indigent and sick people feel themselves outside the reach of such clinics. Furthermore, federal funding is likely to be accompanied by federal control, despite the slogan of consumer participation.

Hence, a social niche was available for the free clinic, which is operated voluntarily by private citizens and provides health care to anyone without social discrimination.

The Operation of Free Clinics

The operation of free clinics will be examined by using the four Parsonian functional prerequisites to describe task areas.

Value Orientations

A major problem for an organization that claims to represent a constituency is to convince society that it indeed is a legitimate spokesperson for that constituency (O'Brien, 1975). The legitimacy of free clinics was difficult to establish because their clients were from the so-called "hippie" movement or counterculture of the 1960s (Roszak, 1969). Their unconventional lifestyle—communal living, sexual freedom, drug use, and reluctance to work in a traditional occupation—and their rebellious attitudes against the establishment, whether government, school, industry, or medicine, antagonized the public. Several clinics met with bitter opposition from the police and legal authorities, city health departments, and conservative local groups (King, 1971; Kroll, 1970).

The agony of the birth of free clinics in the midst of animosity is revealed by their affirmation of their values. To them, the word *free clinic* means more than just expense-free medical care. It symbolizes freedom from conventional values. More specifically, free clinics do not exercise any traditional judgment upon patients or label them as deviant or immoral. To register at free clinics, clients need to give only their names, ages, and addresses.

Freedom from the establishment also takes the form of antibureaucracy and antiprofessionalism. Simplified administrative procedures and equalitarian relations among professionals, paraprofessionals, and nonprofessionals are valued in the free clinics.

Patients' Attitudes toward the Free Clinics. In spite of an open policy for everyone and a tolerance for nonconformity, deviance, and minority status, clinics do vary in selecting or being selected by patients.

Schatz and Ebraham (1972) compared patient attributes at three clinics—a street clinic, a health department youth clinic, and a student health center at a college. They found that the clients were very similar in their backgrounds and demographic characteristics, but that the patients differed markedly in their lifestyles and consequently chose the clinics that provided acceptable cultural contexts.

The rapport and trust that greet them upon entry appeals to the patients of the street and youth clinics. Besides, these clinics use special symbols to "turn on" their youthful clientele—psychodelic decor, posters of rock celebrities, background rock music, and an informal, casually dressed, long-haired staff (Stoeckle et al., 1971). However, such ideological complicity with patients can result in a loss of authenticity and professional role rather than gaining the acceptance of the street community. Some patients, after visiting free clinics, expressed their preference for "real doctors."

Medical Care Services

Services Provided. The most common diagnoses at the three types of facilities are as follows: street clinics primarily deal with venereal diseases, birth control, pregnancy, upper respiratory infections, urinary infections, drug problems, hepatitis, dermatitis, trauma, physical examinations, and miscellaneous infections.

At youth clinics, venereal diseases, infections, and skin problems of adolescents are prevalent.

In comparison, the neighborhood clinics have a wide range of patients, from babies to the aged. Their most common problems involve prenatal and child care, and the respiratory infections and urinary complaints of older people (Schwartz, 1971b).

Clinics that provide drug care generally have flexible hours plus hotline switchboards that are open 24 hours a day to handle crises. Medical care, on the other hand, is limited to the specific hours when the voluntary physicians are available. However, when the patient load is heavy, volunteer health workers tend to stay beyond closing hours.

Physicians. Schwartz (1971b) made a national survey of the free clinics that opened from 1967 to 1969. He reported that in 56 clinics physicians spent an average of 14.5 hours per week, primarily in the evenings, since it is difficult for regularly practicing physicians to offer voluntary help in the daytime. Over half of the clinics were open to provide medical care for from 8 to 17 hours a week.

Some of the clinics drew interns and residents from medical schools as well as physicians. Medical students frequently volunteered as part of their community medicine elective or as a preceptorship.

Because of the negative label given by "straight" society to the clinic and its street people, clinicians are likely to suffer from a sense of marginality. Bartel and Weisser (1971) observed that while functioning as helpers for the deviants, some clinicians sought acceptance in the straight society by denouncing their clients in public. It is also noteworthy that the interaction between the "straights" and the street people has been more symbolic than actual because neither party desires actual contact with the other.

Quality of Care. In the beginning, free clinics rejected the issue of quality control pressed upon them by the larger society and organized medicine. They maintained that without free clinics there had been no medical service for particular groups of people, and that within a tight budget, any service would be better than none. Also, they were afraid that prejudiced public authorities would use their evaluation procedures to close some of the clinics.

Nonetheless, the quality of care has always been a great concern of free clinics. In fact, they have tried to demonstrate that their innovative methods are better than those of fragmented and bureaucratized conventional medical practices (Gordon, 1976). Systematic studies are lacking, but it may be assumed that free clinics which have had time to mature and to gain some stable resources are able to provide quality care.

Integration

There are several reasons to believe that the free clinic is a well-integrated social system. It is a nonbureaucratic small group where conflict, if any, is easily identified and resolved through personal interaction. Also, the values of antiprofessionalism and the diffusion of power cultivates equalitarian relations among all of the participants at free clinics (Stoeckle et al., 1971).

One of the major difficulties that hinders integration at free clinics stems from the fact that many of the workers are part-time volunteers. Without sufficient funds, clinics can only have inexperienced coordinators to organize part-time and full-time physicians, medical students, nurses, technicians, pharmacists, and other miscellaneous personnel.

Peterson (1974) vividly illustrated the important role of the triage worker at a free clinic where approximately 30 staff members came together for four hours, four nights a week. The physician may be scheduled for as little as one night per month and is not expected to know all of the volunteer workers present that evening. It is the triage person's role to serve as a liaison among all of the workers. For instance, the triage person is generally responsible for overseeing the medical operation and deciding beforehand, with the aid of the medical director and the laboratory technician, which tests are to be run.

While community participation is required in the OEO health centers, it is not considered important at the free clinics because the power, money, and jobs there are too scarce to manipulate (Stoeckle et al., 1971).

According to Schwartz's (1971b) survey of free clinics, about 40 percent of them reported a weak consumer participation, while in some others, community control of the clinics is exercised by local board members.

For street clinics, the community is difficult to define because it consists of transient youthful runaways with drug problems. They normally do not want to take part in policy making.

All that may be said is that in free clinics, the cleavage between providers and consumers is not as large as at the OEO centers because in the free clinics the providers (the physicians) are there voluntarily, and they do not act as sponsors of federal funds.

Adaptation

Free clinics run mostly on a voluntary basis. A medical student serves a few hours here, and a nurse donates some time there. There is seldom a salary even for the regular staff because there is so little financial support. Working with volunteer professionals is tenuous because there is constant pressure to find and schedule a full range of professionals (Schwartz, 1971b). As a result, clinics are mostly operated by nonprofessionals without any official credentials.

Operating a clinic with an all-volunteer staff can only continue for a limited time, and in the long run, some type of financing is necessary for its survival. Various alternatives have been proposed (Schwartz, 1971a) and implemented, such as charging patients small fees; claiming reimbursement from Medicare and Medicaid where possible; affiliating themselves with existing community health programs such as OEO centers; raising funds from industries, voluntary associations, hospitals, and individuals; or by applying for grants. Free clinics may also transfer some of their functions to regular hospitals.

However, there is the problem of whether or not the free clinics can maintain their freedom once funding is secured and the staff is paid. Free clinics are regulated de facto through funds, and de jure through statuses and regulations. Clark (1974) warned that as medical schools and government co-opt free clinics, they will be less and less free unless they become nationally unified and establish a lobbying force.

On the other hand, a functionalist perspective is expressed by Stoeckle and others (1971), who stated that the free clinic movement is not a radical revolution because it is integrated into the American tradition of voluntarism. In that light, and despite their rhetoric of freedom and innovation, their operations do depend on the excess energies within local, established medical practices, such as the several hours an evening a month donated by an established physician.

The free clinics are not transient phenomena; they have shown the ability to survive. As their novelty has worn off, public attention has been drawn in other directions. There are an estimated 400 clinics around the country that take care of some two to three million outpatient visits a year (Gordon, 1976).

Some clinics have gone through their life cycle quickly and have disappeared; others have evolved into major neighborhood facilities with the assistance of government funding; but most of them persist with little change—a voluntary staff, much spirit, and meager resources (Gordon, 1976).

SUMMARY

With over 7,000 hospitals in this country that are equipped with outpatient departments, emergency rooms, and the like, why was it necessary for the neighborhood health centers and free clinics to emerge in the 1960s? Or, do they simply reflect the social climate of the 1960s, and are they destined to disappear in time? How do they operate differently from the hospitals? These are the issues with which this chapter is concerned.

Factors that necessitated the birth of neighborhood health centers are found in the institutional structure of the health care system and the sociopolitical climate of the 1960s.

With the growth of specialization in medicine, the number of general practitioners has declined, particularly in poor urban neighborhoods. Prior to the recent expansion of government insurance programs, purchasing power for medical care was relatively low in the low-income neighborhood; hence few physicians would locate there.

In addition to specialization, the practice of modern medicine is marked by bureaucracy, which makes hospital care complex and impersonal. The result is that greater consumer sophistication is now required to reach the appropriate source of care. This factor has a prohibiting effect upon low-income, educationally handicapped people in using hospital facilities. Furthermore, prejudice against lower class patients shown by medical institutions oriented to the middle class has further deterring effects upon the poor.

Thus, the indigent have been isolated from the medical care system both physically and psychologically. This was the pre-existing condition that led to the birth of such facilities as neighborhood health centers. These needs were accentuated during the mid-1960s when civil rights movements shaped the climate of public opinion. Equalitarianism and antiauthoritarianism were the values advocated in every sphere of society. Health was perceived as a human right to be enjoyed by the poor as well as by the rich. Also, a change in the traditional medical establishment was called for in order to improve primary care services. It was in this social climate that the government launched the neighborhood health center project and that voluntary free clinics emerged in the 1960s.

Neighborhood health centers were started with ambitious goals to bring about changes not only in medical practice but also in the broader social structure. Innovative features of the centers included (1) the health team practice involving physicians, paramedical personnel, and social service workers to replace the hierarchical system dominated by physicians; and (2) consumer participation in policy making to enhance the level of self-determination of the poor.

How effectively have these goals been carried out? Although the neighborhood health center concept has been extensively described and debated, the overall effectiveness of the program has been less well documented. Many centers are not able to provide comparable operating statistical data because of the expense of installing reporting systems. Particular areas of performance have been described for individual centers, but the findings have been largely inconsistent and inconclusive.

Many studies, including the evaluation of 21 centers commissioned by the OEO, indicate that neighborhood health centers have been quite effective in enhancing the supply of available services in their target areas. However, the increased utilization of health services does not necessarily mean a change in attitudes toward health among the indigent. Moreover, there are still a large number of people who are not weaned from the traditional type of medical service (Hurwitz, 1972).

The idea of creating a health team with paraprofessionals trained on the job seems to remain primarily a promise. Most centers report stresses and strains between traditional and new occupational roles. Part of the problem resides in the intractable resistence of the traditional medical profession to new ideas. Physicians are likely to consider a neighborhood center as an outpost of the medical school (New & Hessler, 1972). Medical students are sent to the centers, which serve them as a community laboratory to carry on traditional medical training. The guardians of old careers are unwilling to adapt themselves to working with new staff members.

As for community participation in policy making, the medical establishment has also exerted power. Its ability to enter into or leave the health center project at will is illustrated in the following statement by a medical school official:

> Citizen participation in an advisory sense is mandatory. . . . Citizens should not be involved in the operations of the health center. . . . I can't have an education program run by citizens. If it comes to that, . . . then I will pull the medical school out of the neighborhood health center (New & Hessler, 1972, p. 48).

The traditional medical institution is not the only one to blame for ineffectiveness in the health center operation. Although the government mandated the community representation, it neither promoted nor assessed the rationale for lay participation (Metsch & Veney, 1976). Furthermore, the government operated these centers as demonstration projects rather than as permanent activities. The difficulty with a demonstration program is that it does not have the power over the government to bind it to continuing support. The fragmentation of financial support and the subsequent lack of federal governmental leadership led to the internal war within communities over anti-poverty funds and local political controversies.

In case of free clinics, the lack of public support affects not only the financial but the psychological spheres. Dealing with youthful drug addicts, free clinics are subject to social discrimination and must rely upon voluntary services only. Unlike neighborhood health centers, the operation of free clinics is characterized by a lack of coordination among professionals, paraprofessionals, and clients rather than power conflicts among them.

By the middle of the 1970s, the novelty of neighborhood health centers and free clinics had worn off. Public attention has shifted to the health maintenance organizations (HMOs) and the issue of national health insurance, although community-based health care services are still very much in evidence. From the beginning the neighborhood health center was a vulnerable concept, based on a diffuse alliance of reformers with a number of important conflicts:

> When a professional development or trend is in "fashion," the name by which it is designated acquires an aura of approval, and is used to describe activities and enterprises that differ widely, so that they may share some of the aura. This was also the fate of the health center concept, and is in part responsible for its decline (Rosen, 1971, p. 1630).

When the aura of the label "War on Poverty" faded, various elements of the neighborhood health center concept began to be implemented in other medical service methods. However, there is nothing wrong with this phenomenon. The whole process can be viewed as a natural evolution (Hollister, 1974).

The future of neighborhood health centers is not certain because of their deficiency in performing their manifest functions such as providing quality care along with reasonable and predicted costs. Furthermore, the establishment of an innovative, health care program in the context of a substantially unchanged traditional medical delivery system carries the risk of the potential development of a dual system of medical care: the neighborhood health centers for the poor and hospitals for the rich (Lewis, Fein, & Mechanic, 1976).

Even so, the latent function of the neighborhood health centers as an agent of social change should be properly acknowledged (Elinson & Herr, 1970; Smith, 1973). Perhaps the very persistence of free clinics may be indicative of faulty operations in our present medical bureaucracy. Because of their presence in the community and their local publicity, the free clinics have served as advocates for changes in the medical delivery system, and, even more broadly, for changes in the distribution of power and resources in society.

CHAPTER 10

National Health Care: Forms of Social Insurance

> "National Health Insurance: An Idea Whose Time Has Come?" (Berki, 1972)
> "National Health Insurance—The Dream Whose Time Has Come?" (Margolis, 1977)

At the time of writing of this textbook, the question posed by the above article titles is one of the major issues discussed in Congress as well as on the street. Since first proposed by President Truman, national health insurance came closest to becoming a reality in 1974. However, passage of any form of national health insurance now seems unlikely before the 1980 elections because of the wide discrepancies among key proposals and the cumbersome legislative route health bills must pass through (Fogg, 1979). The primary argument for changing the existing health care system is the enormous and growing cost of medical care.

Cost of Medical Care. In 1977, the total national health care expenditure was \$162.6 billion; for the average person, that is \$737 (Gibson & Fisher, 1978). This national figure is close to four times the amount spent in 1965. It represents a yearly increase of 12 percent compounded continuously and a much larger percentage increase in terms of yearly compounding. Health care spending has climbed steeply when compared to the gross national product (GNP) since 1965. On a per capita basis, \$297 was spent for hospital care in 1977, more than ten times the amount spent in 1950. During this same period, expenditures per person for physician's services rose more than eightfold.

Back in 1929, more than 88 percent of personal health care expenditures were paid directly out of the patient's own pocket. Even in 1950 consumers were paying almost 70 percent of their health bills directly. Then, between 1950 and 1965, the private health insurance industry grew rapidly, and since 1965, around a quarter of all health expenses have been covered by private insurance (see Figure 10.1).

Table 10.1: Aggregate and Per Capita National Health Expenditures, 1929–1977

Fiscal year	Gross national product (in billions)	Aggregate health expenditure			Per capita health expenditure				
		Amount (in billions)	Percent of GNP	Percent public[2]	Total	Hospital care	Physician's service	Dentist's service	Drugs
1929	$ 101.3	$ 3.6	3.5	13.3	$ 29.16	$ 5.29	$ 8.08	$ 3.87	$ 4.88
1940	95.4	3.9	4.1	20.1	28.98	7.23	7.06	3.00	4.66
1950	264.8	12.0	4.5	25.5	78.35	24.09	17.52	6.12	10.70
1955	381.0	17.3	4.5	25.5	103.76	34.06	21.75	8.72	13.66
1960[1]	498.3	25.9	5.2	24.7	141.63	45.56	30.57	10.65	19.67
1965	658.0	38.9	5.9	24.5	197.75	66.87	42.74	13.87	23.63
1970	960.2	69.2	7.2	36.7	333.57	124.74	64.80	21.56	34.29
1975	1,454.5	123.7	8.5	42.3	571.21	223.36	110.07	36.34	47.82
1977	1,838.0	162.6	8.8	42.1	736.92	297.38	145.84	45.11	56.72

Notes: [1] *Prior to 1960, private expenditures exclude Alaska and Hawaii.*
[2] *Refers to the percentage of national medical expenditure that is financed by public funding against private payment.*

Sources: Robert M. Gibson and M. S. Mueller, "National Health Expenditures, Fiscal Year 1976," *Social Security Bulletin,* 40 (1977):3–22.

Robert M. Gibson and Charles R. Fisher, "National Health Expenditures, Fiscal Year 1977," *Social Security Bulletin,* 41 (1978):3–20.

The upward trend in federal subsidies began with the advent of Medicare and Medicaid programs in fiscal year 1967. In 1967, for the first time, third-party payments represented more than half of all personal health care expenditures. By 1977, almost 70 percent of personal health care was financed by third parties (see Figure 10.1). Nevertheless, the total personal expenditure for health care is still high because direct payment refers only to deductibles, coinsurance, and costs of care not covered by insurance, and it excludes health insurance premiums or the proportion of the individual's social security tax that goes into Medicare.

The portion of personal consumption expenditures spent for health care almost doubled between 1950 and 1975, while the percentage for housing remained relatively stable and the percentage spent on food and clothing went down during this period. In 1975, 8.9 percent of total personal health expenses went for health care, while 25 years earlier, only 4.6 percent was spent for health care (see Figure 10.2).

The Consumer Price Index (CPI) provides a convenient measure of price change. Taking 1967 prices as the indexing base, the CPI for all items more than doubled from 1950 to 1975, while the CPI for medical care tripled. The most outstanding escalation has been in hospital room rates, from 57.3 to 299.5 between 1960 and 1977. The CPI for physicians' fees rose from 77.0 to 206.0 during the same period (see Figure 10.3).

Thus, despite the public financing of health care costs and the increase in taxes needed to cover those programs, the direct burden upon individuals for health care alone is still quite heavy. It is primarily these disquieting statistics on the price of ill health that have stimulated the public to entertain the notion of national health insurance in recent years. The traditional ideologies of voluntarism and laissez faire have been severely criticized as factors contributing to the rising cost and maldistribution of health care resources. The need for a nationally regulated and coordinated health care system is now expressed by many sectors of our society.

The seed for social insurance can be sought in the European heritage that was brought to this country. In order to understand why it has taken such a long time for the United States, as compared with European countries, to contemplate national health insurance (NHI), this chapter will trace the development of the concept of social insurance. The gradual shift from the voluntaristic operation of an open medical marketplace centrally enforced equalitarian programs will be analyzed from the functionalist, conflict, and interactionist perspectives. Based on social insurance milestones, American history is divided into (1) pre-Social Security years (prior to 1934); (2) the birth of Social Security; (3) from Social Security to Medicare and Medicaid (1935–1965); and (4) from Medicare to national health insurance (1965–present). For each period, health care services will be examined in relation to the social structure and processes.

Conceptual Framework. Some people (Glasser, 1972; Reuther, 1972) have criticized health care in the United States by calling it a fragmented and disjointed "nonsystem." They make references to the inability of the poor to afford medical care; the inflated cost of hospitalization caused by private

Figure 10.1: Per Capita Amount and Percentage Distribution of Personal Health Care Expenditure by Sources of Funds

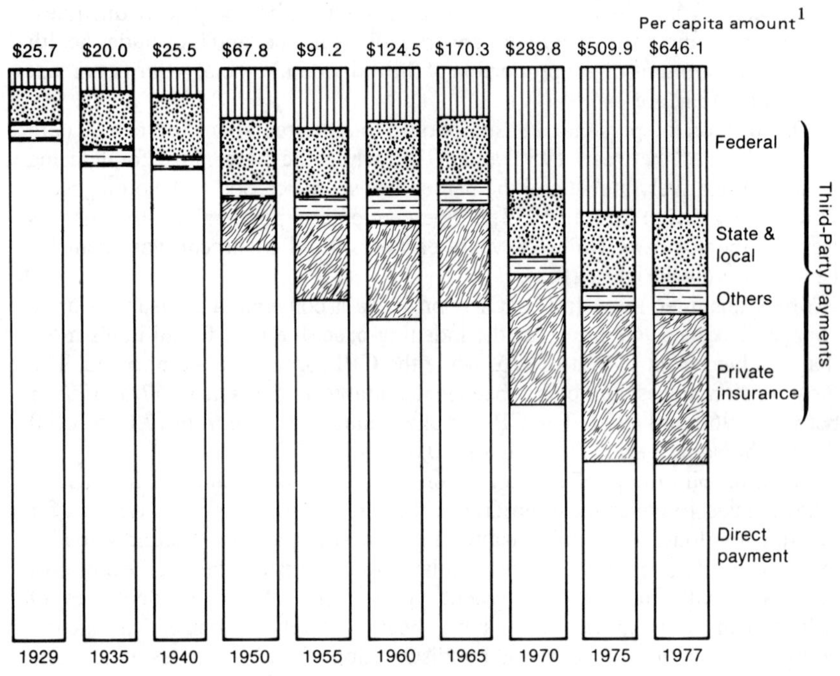

Note: [1] *Excludes expenses for prepayment and administration.*

Sources: Robert M. Gibson and M. S. Mueller, "National Health Expenditures, Fiscal Year 1976," *Social Security Bulletin,* 40 (1977):3–22.

Robert M. Gibson and Charles K. Fisher, "National Health Expenditures, Fiscal Year 1977," *Social Security Bulletin,* 41 (1978):3–20.

Figure 10.2: Percentage Distribution of Personal Consumption Expenditure, 1930 to 1974

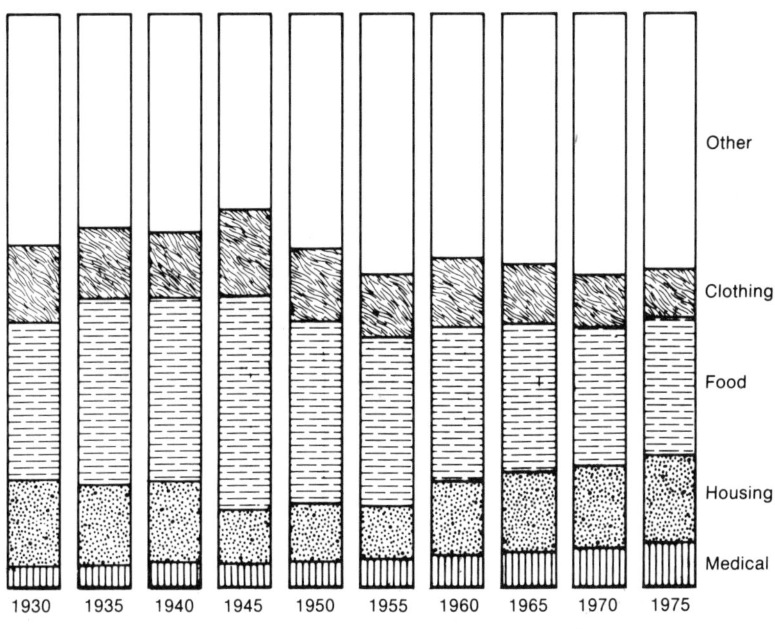

Sources: U.S. Department of Commerce, Bureau of Census, *Statistical Abstract of the United States* (Washington, D.C.: U.S. Government Printing Office, 1930-1975).

U.S. Department of Commerce, Bureau of Census, *Historical Statistics of the United States* (Washington, D.C.: U.S. Government Printing Office, 1975).

Figure 10.3. Index of Medical Care Prices, 1950 to 1977 (1967=100)

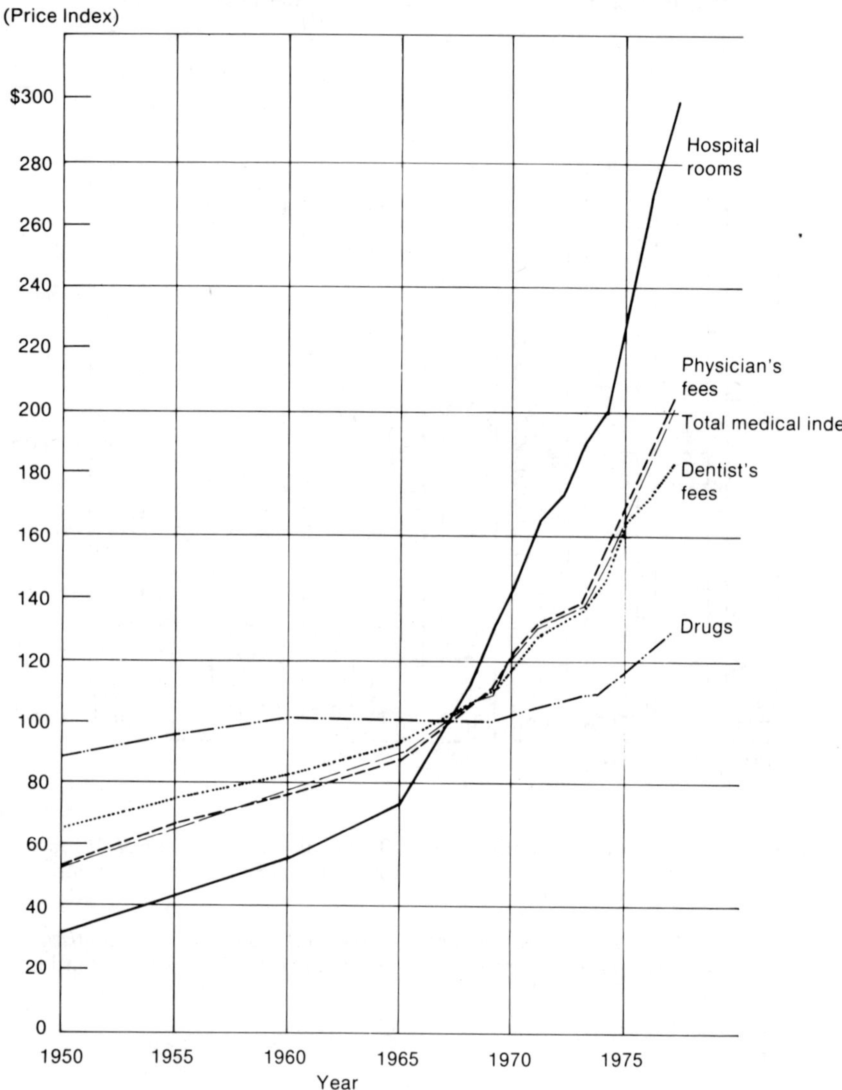

Notes: *Excludes Alaska and Hawaii prior to 1965.*
Base year: 1967=100.

Source: U.S. Department of Labor, Bureau of Labor Statistics, *Consumer Price Index* (Washington, D.C.: U.S. Government Printing Office, 1950–1977).

insurance mechanisms; and the absence of coordination among specialists. In short, they claim that inefficiency and higher costs are due to the absence of a national program of health insurance.

In contrast to this nonsystem perspective, others (Knowles, 1970) attribute the difficulties in bringing about any change in the medical delivery process to opposition from organized medicine. The notion of national health insurance dates back to the nineteenth century, but it has been continuously defeated through the efforts of the American Medical Association, which has maintained a relatively united front on this issue.

Thus, Twaddle and Hessler (1977) distinguish two viewpoints: from the consumer's standpoint, everything may appear to be chaotic and without system. On the other hand, medical care is a well-organized system as far as physicians are concerned, in that no one else has been able to break down the power of the AMA.

However, physicians and patients are not the only participants in the practice of medicine. Third-party intervention, whether by government or religious authority, is as old as the history of the healing arts (Somers & Somers, 1977). In this chapter, a societal perspective is adopted, which includes physicians (the first party), patients (the second party), and the government, insurance companies, and the like (the third party).

The interrelations between health care and other elements in American society will be analyzed in terms of the Parsonian model of a social system. For a detailed discussion of this analytical framework, see the first section in Chapter 9.

In order to examine how various components of society can be identified and how they are integrated into a more or less unified whole, this chapter begins with the functionalist assumption that there is a system. Then we will shift our analytical viewpoint to that of conflict theories in an attempt to determine if a system integration exists in spite of conflict, or if the conflicts serve as a source of equilibrium. Simultaneously, the interactionist approach will be utilized to assess whether or not the existence of a system is an artifact of the labeling processes. For instance, fear of socialism or communism, heightened by political propaganda, may lead Americans to assign the label of "democratic system" to the most disorganized state of affairs.

HISTORICAL DEVELOPMENT OF NATIONAL HEALTH CARE SERVICES

Pre-Social Security Period

Social Structure and Processes

Cultural Values. The cultural values of American society can be traced to the heritage of European tradition and to the revolutionary break with that tradition. As Lipset (1963) put it, from the interplay between the Puritan tradition and the revolutionary ethos, there emerged two major cultural themes: equality and achievement.

Equalitarianism is an expression of revolt against the traditions of the Old World: the Church, monarchy, hereditary aristocracy, and any other traditional institutions (McDonald, 1968, p. 2). In the domain of religion, equalitarianism is the outcome of the Protestant Reformation in Europe in the seventeenth and eighteenth centuries and the further rebellion of those various Protestant sects who moved to the New World in the seventeenth century. Equality of human beings is based on the ideal that individuals are created equal in the eyes of God and that they will determine religious truth without the influence of the authority of a clergy or the tradition of a church (Curti, 1943).

Another important ingredient of the Protestant ethic is the emphasis upon hard work and achievement (Weber, 1958). In addition to these religious factors, the establishment of a New World of free people on a vast and raw continent inspired individuals to maximize their abilities to achieve success in a land of opportunities (Greene, 1976; Williams, 1960).

Stratification. Immigrants to America did not transplant the feudal institutions or the aristocracy of the Old World because of their spirit of revolt and also the accessibility of land. Because there was an abundance of land, people could not be kept in a position to quasi-serfdom (Curti, 1943, p. 52). The ideal of equal opportunity regardless of one's social origin was institutionalized in an open society in which success was to be the goal of all. It was assumed that achievement determined one's position on the stratification ladder (Lipset, 1963).

Despite the equalitarian ideology, however, achievement could not be the only determinant of one's social status. The colonies varied from one another because of differences in soil, climate, and natural resources as well as because of their ethnic background. Ethnic stratification developed and passed through various stages, such as Anglo-conformity, melting pot, and cultural pluralism (Glazer, 1954; Gordon, 1964).

A greater gulf occurred between the whites and nonwhites. Racial groups resembled castes in that their socioeconomic achievement did not allow them to enter the higher, ascribed status of the whites. Blacks, Native Americans, Asians, and other nonwhites were excluded from the American creed of liberty and equality (Genovese, 1967).

The Economy. The Protestant work ethic leads to the sense of self-responsibility for economic welfare. It was assumed that diligence would bring success to anyone and that the poor deserved their lot because it was caused by their idleness. It was a disgrace to receive charity from private or public sources. In this framework, the notion of a welfare economy or public assistance had no place (Channing, 1917).

Economic individualism in the land of opportunity found a supportive rationale in the eighteenth century economist Adam Smith's laissez-faire principles (Smith, 1976). In line with conflict theories, Adam Smith claimed that (1) a maximum productivity could be achieved when economic competition was left completely free from third-party intervention; (2) natural forces ("an invisible hand") will reconcile the requirements of supply and demand as well as that of individuals and groups; and (3) the pursuit of one's own interest will result in promoting the welfare of society (Becker & Barnes, 1961, p. 523).

Until 1900 the United States grew rapidly in size and wealth despite occasional agricultural and industrial depressions. Corporations grew large and made large profits. It was generally believed that this concentration of economic power was an inevitable result of the modern capitalist and industrial process. The merger movement was justified as a step toward rationalization of economic organization—that is, corporate consolidation leads to industrial efficiency, avoiding the waste of small-scale production and the destructiveness of unregulated competition (Kolko,1963; Weinstein, 1968).

However, by the turn of this century big business was realizing that the merging of industries brought neither greater profit nor less competition. This was partly due to the fact that though industrial leaders had a limited knowledge of how their own corporations worked, they did not understand that operation in the larger economic context. The failure of the merger movement to establish stability and control within the economy led big businesses to seek federal regulation of the economy. Laissez faire was perceived as great in principle but intolerable in practice because it created economic instability. Thus, it was partly big business that prompted the so-called progressive period, 1900–1916, during which the central government exercised control over large industries.

The Polity. Out of the revolutionary independence from traditional European authority emerged the political liberalism of the United States (Channing, 1917; Commager, 1950; Hartz, 1955; Morison & Commager, 1950).

Many colonists came to America in order to escape from laws they disliked and from the power of the established institutions. In the "New Land," they frequently made their own local laws. In the beginning, a tendency toward local self-government was strong enough to hinder the development of a centralized government. Americans were suspicious of government power and, as a result, they favored democracy and abhorred socialism (Commager, 1950; Potter, 1954). The Declaration of Independence states that governments derive their just power from the consent of the governed, and that all people are born with equal rights to life, liberty,, and the pursuit of happiness.

Thus, the United States began more as a confederated league of separate and independent states. Later, federal control over that confederation was tested and won by the Civil War. There were other attempts to increase federal power from time to time during the nineteenth century, but the spirit of Jeffersonian antifederalism continued.

At the turn of the century, however, the nation entered what has commonly been called the progressive period. Progressivism was initially a movement wherein political regulations were used to attain stability, predictability, and security in the economy.

This was partly a response of the federal government to the desires of big businesses to attain economic stability. The progressive movement also served to pacify Populists, trade unionists, socialists, and other discontented groups who were becoming potential threats.

Theodore Roosevelt and other political leaders during this period consciously used government regulation of big business to save the capitalist system from (1) itself in its self-destructive competition; (2) from socialism, which was gaining support in Europe; and (3) from the masses, whom political leaders considered irresponsible. The injustices that Roosevelt attacked were not structural evils inherent in a capitalistic economy but were a few exceptional corporations that took advantage of other law-abiding corporations.

Thus, despite its radical appearance, the government remained conservative in that it preserved the basic social and economic relations essential to a capitalist society (Kolko, 1963; Weinstein, 1968).

Health Care Service

The Polity and Health Care. In 1880, Bismarck developed a governmental program of health insurance for the working classes in Germany in order to steer them away from the attractions of socialism and Marxism (Myers, 1970, p. 3). This stimulated some people in the United States to study the general movement toward governmental participation in health care services.

However, from the colonial years until 1935, welfare provisions were almost entirely the responsibility of individual localities and states. The federal role was limited to the provision of emergency services and socially necessary services to selected groups of people, such as members of the armed forces, merchant seamen, and veterans (Carter & Lee, 1972, p. 13). The U.S. Public Health Service, now part of the Department of Health, Education, and Welfare, was founded by the Marine Hospital Service Act (1798) as a protection of merchant seamen and thus, of trade.

Possibly the first national advocacy of governmental health insurance in the United States was a political stand taken by the Socialist Party in the early 1900s. Subsequently, when Theodore Roosevelt founded the Progressive Party before the 1912 elections,a plank supporting national health insurance was included in its platform (Faulkner, 1952, p. 35).

The Economy and Organized Medicine. Starting around the 1900s, a group of large, industrial concerns initiated medical programs to cover illness as well as occupational disability. As in Europe, worker's compensation had an appeal for both humanistic and economic reasons: the sooner a worker was cured, the sooner he or she could get back to work.

Another source of pressure toward such medical programs, called "welfare capitalism" in the 1920s, was the threat of unionism felt by the employers. Out of a similar fear of radicalism, a number of businesspeople effectively promoted legislation designed on behalf of the workers (McDonald, 1968, p. 50).

In the meanwhile, dissatisfied with the efforts of self-interested employers and laborers, other supporters of the progressive movement began to take active roles. The American Association for Labor Legislation (AALL) was founded in 1906 as an organization of trade unionists, social scientists, and social reformers (Myers, 1970, p. 4). Inspired by the United Kingdom's national health insurance legislation in 1911 and the domestic success of worker's compensation laws, the AALL turned its energies toward health insurance. It established the Committee on Social Insurance, which was largely composed of economists, statisticians, and physicians. In 1915, the committee produced a "Standard Bill," which was a compulsory health and disability law to be enacted by the states without the intermediation of the federal government.

During this period (1915–1919), the leaders of the American Medical Association supported the drive for social health insurance (Rayack, 1967, p. 137). The lead article in the January 30, 1915 issue of the AMA *Journal* was a pledge for social insurance. It stated that such insurance was the only way to solve both economic and ethical problems of medicine "without pauperizing the patient or degrading the physician" (Rubinow, 1915).

Then, the nation's attention was detracted from domestic to international affairs by World War I. Also, since health insurance ideas stemmed from Bismarck's welfare plan in Germany, opponents of health insurance attacked it as "German," hence "un-American" (Skidmore, 1970, p. 40).

By 1920, the official attitude of the AMA was reversed until it was in passionate opposition to social health insurance. This change is explained by Rayack (1967) in terms of the relative position of the medical profession in society.

Between 1900 and 1920, the AMA was trying to achieve professional autonomy by raising the standards of medical education and practice. The leaders of the AMA, as scientists and educators, were in tune with the progressivism that characterized the first two decades of this century. By 1920, however, the AMA had achieved its goal of educational reform, and its attention was directed toward increasing the power and prestige of the medical profession. The academic and scientific leadership of the AMA was replaced by a vocal minority of practicing physicians (Freymann, 1964) who were preoccupied with medical economics. It should be noted that medical care in those days was almost totally in the hands of solo practitioners on a fee-for-service basis.

During the 1920s, organized medicine was disturbed by changes in the patterns of medical care, such as the growth of group and contract practice, and the spread of group hospitalization plans. Influenced by these developments, the Committee on the Costs of Medical Care (CCMC) was self-constituted voluntarily in 1927 as a private organization by people from various disciplines concerned with public health and medical care. They were concerned with (1) the fractionalism of medical care services due to increasing specialization; (2) inadequacy of size of the health work force; (3) the rising cost of medical care; and (4) the need for better organization of services (Falk, 1973, p. 2).

The committee's studies were well received by many groups in the nation, but the committee itself suffered from a schism. The majority recommended a comprehensive group practice linked with prepayment; the minority espoused the continuance of solo practice and the fee-for-service payment method.

By endorsing the minority position, the leadership of the AMA committed the profession to "preservation of the inherited and then prevailing system of medical care . . . and to the continuing professional domination and control of the system," deaf to appeals from others (Falk, 1973, p. 4; Kessel, 1958). As functionalists might interpret it, the AMA managed to maintain its system equilibrium despite external and internal disturbances.

From the perspective of labeling theory, it is interesting to note that the AMA *Journal* denounced those in group practice as "medical Soviets" ("Editorial," 1932) and "unethical." What was involved in the label of unethical practice was really a question of medical economics (Rayack, 1967, p. 150).

The Depression and the New Deal

Social Structure and Processes

With the Great Depression and the New Deal, American society appeared to be undergoing major structural changes in the 1930s (Curti, 1943, p. 710).

Cultural Values. Amidst the economic dissolution and the dislocation of old values, new formulas for recovery and reconstruction were being sought. Marxism, which found an audience among intellectual circles and to some extent among the working class, argued that the depression presaged the inevitable collapse of capitalism. Marxism compelled Americans to evaluate class relations and the nature of capitalist economy.

Launching the New Deal program, Franklin Delano Roosevelt spoke of four types of freedom: freedom of speech, freedom of religion, freedom from want, and freedom from fear. The last two embraced the notion of security, constituting a departure from the traditional values of individualism and achievement. By introducing these new ideas as "freedoms," Roosevelt retained the vocabulary of traditional ideology (Skidmore, 1970). From the labeling theory perspective, the familiarity of the traditional label of freedom persuaded the public to readily adopt the New Deal.

The Polity. Through both the progressive period (1900–1916) and the depression of the 1930s, the American government was emancipated from the Jeffersonian ideal, which equated democracy with state or local autonomy, identified tyranny with centralized government, and made people suspicious of responsible official leadership (McDonald, 1968, p. 61). From 1933 on, the federal government took many actions that had hitherto been left to individual states. The problems caused by the depression were so complex and pervasive that separate states could not find solutions by acting alone (Morison & Commager, 1950).

The Constitution has always given Congress the power to provide for the general welfare, so the way was open for many new laws to be passed. In addition, government agencies were set up to help business, to control business, and to put the government itself into business. New agencies also provided direct help to individual citizens who had never been helped by the government before: farmers, the disabled, the retired, the unemployed, and even union members. Perhaps the most important product of the New Deal was the Social Security Act, which will be discussed in the next section. Critics of the New

Deal objected to all these procedures and lamented the creation of what they called the "welfare state."

The Economy. The depression made people realize that economic liberalism in itself was not sufficient to insure economic well-being for everyone in a complex society (Skidmore, 1970). The basic idea of the New Deal was to provide a balanced economy in which the government tried to maintain an equilibrium between producers, consumers, merchants, and workers within the framework of capitalism (Curti, 1943).

Being aware of the importance of big business to America, Roosevelt provided for a government that was favorable to big business and at the same time able to control it. With his slogan of checks and balances, he convinced voters that he was championing the "little fellow" (McDonald, 1968, p. 61).

The development of organized labor was facilitated by the passage of much prolabor legislation. The Wagner Act, for example, prohibited employers from punishing workers for belonging to a union, and it required all employers to deal with union leaders that were elected by the workers.

Confronted by vast unemployment, Congress set up agencies to lend money to state and local governments to create new jobs. The agencies relieved unemployment directly by funding federal activities such as the building of offices, dams, highways, and national parks, the writing of guidebooks, and even the painting of murals. These projects helped to maintain the Protestant ethic that one should earn one's income and not receive charity.

Stratification. Widespread poverty in the middle class due to the depression educated the public that people can be poor through no fault of their own (Stevens & Stevens, 1974). General redistribution of goods and services by the government came to be regarded as necessary in the face of the growing supremacy of liberalism heavily influenced by equalitarianism.

Commitment to equality brought some changes, though small, in racial stratification. In line with the general New Deal policy of promoting the well-being and happiness of the less privileged groups, the government modified its traditional policy of the Americanization of Indians toward that of cultural pluralism, and it began to stimulate the economic rehabilitation of tribal economy through federal assistance (Curti, 1943).

Health Care Service

Voluntary Health Insurance. A comprehensive prepaid health insurance plan had been defeated by the AMA prior to the depression. However, when the Great Depression left the nation's hospitals with empty beds and unpaid bills, hospitals began banding together and organized citywide rather than single-hospital insurance plans (Rayack, 1967, p. 156). The American Hospital Association (AHA) played a major role in establishing hospital service plans and in developing the Blue Cross Plan. In contrast to private insurance companies, Blue Cross had a public service philosophy. However, this did not mean that hospitals would allow Blue Cross to become a spokesperson for the public (Somers & Somers, 1977). Thus, the idea of voluntary health insurance came not from the insurance companies nor from medical societies, but actually from sporadic consumer and hospital efforts.

The AMA responded to those hospital activities negatively by emphasizing the defects and minimizing the virtues of voluntary health insurance plans (Burrow, 1963, pp. 179–180). Organized medicine was apprehensive about hospital prepayment plans because of the threat of competition, the loss of physician control of the medical marketplace to the third-party insurance, and the possible reduction of their income (Rayack, 1967, p. 159).

When the American College of Surgeons announced its approval of voluntary health insurance in 1934, the AMA was arrogant in rebuking the surgeons, stating that the latter did not represent the views of organized medicine. In short, the AMA was a powerful and passionate opponent of private health insurance during the early 1930s.

As the depression deepened, however, public interest in health insurance grew steadily, and federal and state legislatures began to consider seriously the enactment of compulsory health insurance laws. Also, a growing number of physicians within the AMA opposed its rigid stance. Due to fear of a possible government compulsory insurance plan, the AMA finally embraced the idea of voluntary health insurance, and called it "the American way" (American Medical Association, 1959, p. 315).

The Social Security Act (1935). In 1935, the initial legislation for what was eventually to become the Social Security Act was passed. The President's omission of compulsory health insurance from the Social Security Act reflected his fear that the entire program might have been jeopardized by provoking the AMA's opposition (Davis, 1955, p. 277). Instead, Roosevelt simply appointed a Medical Advisory Committee to study the field of health insurance and to make recommendations (Myers, 1970, p. 12).

In its original design, Social Security was a modest insurance scheme financed by compulsory employer and employee contributions to a trust fund that would provide wage-related benefits to retired workers. Many Americans viewed with suspicion the notion of a government old-age insurance program, and they feared that it would undermine Protestant virtues of work and thrift.

In 1940, a critical change in Social Security funding was made that was a recognition of the principle of social adequacy, or need. The benefit schedule was weighted in favor of low-income workers by providing them with greater benefits relative to their earnings and contributions.

The idea of incorporating two principles—social insurance (individual equity) and public assistance (social adequacy)—was appealing to Americans who cherished the traditional values of freedom and individualism (Skidmore, 1970, p. 47; Stevens & Stevens, 1974).

In line with the functionalist perspective, conservatives viewed the program as charity from the government rather than as the emergence of a new concept of government responsibility for those in need. By making the plan a form of insurance, conservatives felt, Social Security would not threaten the self-esteem of the recipient of the "charity" or the established social order. Liberals concurred with the functionalist view by deprecating social insurance as nothing more than a private enterprise operated by the government. From a different angle, that of labeling theory, Skidmore (1970, p. 29) laments the fact that a new concept of social welfare, which was germinating in the Social Security Act, was castrated because of the public's adherence to the traditional symbol of "freedom."

From Social Security to Medicare and Medicaid

Social Structure and Processes

Between the enactment of the Social Security Act (1935) and the passage of the Medicare and Medicaid bills (1965), the nation underwent World War II and enjoyed postwar prosperity.

The Economy. The first Social Security benefits were hardly paid before the United States had to gear up for a war. Drawing on the experience of World War I and the depression, the government undertook the task of raising American industrial and agricultural production (McDonald, 1968, p. 312). As a result of being organized on a vast scale by the government, the American economy reached a height of productivity that it had never known before.

Postwar economic readjustment and reconstruction was far less difficult than after World War I. The conversion from wartime to peacetime production was facilitated by economy forces (e.g., increased consumer purchasing power) as well as by government policies.

In the prosperous 1950s and 1960s, large-scale corporate businesses were considered to be legitimate once they labeled themselves as being more democratic and efficient than small enterprises. They claimed to be democratic because their corporate power was counterbalanced by the forces of labor unions, the government, and voluntary associations (Curti, 1943; Lipset, 1963). As business and industry grew, so did trade unionism, and in 1955 the AFL and the CIO merged into a single organization.

It is not as simple to generalize about the American economy of the 1950s and 1960s as the Republicans did with the motto of "peace and prosperity." Rapid social change—industrialization, urbanization, bureaucratization, unionization—was accompanied by many social problems: inflation, unemployment, shortage of facilities, and inequality in the distribution of wealth. However, with respect to health care services, the public utilization rate increased between 1935 and 1965 because of (1) increased buying power; (2) the growth of health insurance plans promoted by labor unionism; and (3) the technological advances facilitated by economic prosperity.

The Polity. The wartime mobilization and coordination of the work force and facilities implemented by the government gave an enormous stimulus to the growth of federal power. During the war federal government expenditures soared not only for military purposes but also for civilian activities (Morison & Commager, 1950).

After the war, federal spending continued to rise until it surpassed by far the level of expenditure during the years of the New Deal (McDonald, 1968, p. 322). The tremendous leap in the nation's productive capacity during the war implied that a certain amount of governmental intervention might cause the economy to grow at a rate never dreamed of. Thus, Truman's Fair Deal policy (1948–1953) was a derivative in name and in spirit of Roosevelt's New Deal. It extended the function of the government to include the regulation of the overall rates of economic growth and business cycles as well as the supervision of private business practices. The federal government's concern for the social well-being of its citizens was also emphasized in the Fair Deal by an extension of Social Security benefits and by an unsuccessful attempt to establish a prepaid medical insurance plan.

In the meanwhile, fear began to spread that the federal government had grown too powerful. Phrases such as "creeping socialism" began to appear in the Republican Party's literature (McDonald, 1968, p. 352). Eisenhower viewed the various domestic problems as resulting from excessive New Deal and Fair Deal programs. On every level possible, the Eisenhower administration tried to reverse Truman's policies.

As McDonald (1968, p. 322) noted, however, once government and the people grow used to the magnitude of federal government activity, there is little chance to diminish it. Extensive activities financed by the government through its enormous budget tended to condition people to look to Washington whenever they were in trouble. People gradually became accustomed to their "welfare state," particularly governmental participation in health and welfare fields.

Stratification. The development of large corporations and unions in postwar America made the class structure more complex. Even a multidimensional approach could not place many occupational groups within the simple dichotomous categories of the propertied or propertyless. For instance, small businesspeople were not only in conflict with big businesses, but they also had problems with trade unions. Yet, attached to the Protestant ethic, they were all opposed to welfare state legislations (Polsby et al., 1963, pp. 809–824).

In the domain of race relations, a more dramatic change than that of class stratification took place. In 1954, segregation in public schools on the basis of race or color was ruled unconstitutional. Commencing with this date, the courts began to strike down state and municipal segregation ordinances. During this same period (1954–1962), passive resistance to integration spread over the nation. Unfortunately, nonviolent civil disobedience was sometimes responded to with violence. Frustrated with the tediousness of progress, the civil rights movement underwent a rapid transformation from a nonviolent, integrationist approach to a violent, secessionist revolution during the period between 1963 and 1966 (Laue, 1965).

In both the domestic and international scenes, causes for the racial revolution have been identified as (1) the sense of relative deprivation experienced by upwardly mobile blacks who began to compare themselves with whites (Kurokawa, 1970); (2) the rising expectation of minorities frustrated by obstacles to achievement (Wilson, 1973); (3) the stimulation for independence by the emancipation of African nations (Baker, 1975); and (4) the Communists' criticism of racial injustice in a presumably democratic country (Baker, 1975).

The civil rights movement (1) cast doubt, for the first time in history, upon the traditional model of American democracy because of its exclusion of nonwhites; (2) encouraged a redistribution of resources and power more evenly in social strata; and (3) sensitized the public to the health and welfare needs of the poor and powerless.

Cultural Values. Many social scientists (Lipset, 1963; Whyte, 1956) portrayed America in the 1950s as being in an age of conformity. Americans had given up their traditional belief in self-reliance, individual salvation through work, thrift, and competitive entrepreneurship, and had come to accept the cult of belonging, security, accommodation, and congeniality to corporate structures.

Riesman (1950) posited a metamorphosis of the American character from an "inner direction," which is guided by a set of internalized values to an "other direction," which responds to the demands and pressures of other people. The Protestant ethic was replaced by the "social ethic," which is based on a belief in the group as the source of creativity.

The vogue of conformity has been attributed to the need of Americans to understand the major structural changes occurring in their society. Thus, it was explained that the anonymity of urban life eroded individuality; automation depersonalized the individual; mass media standardized everyone; bureaucratization killed individual initiative; and so on.

It should be remembered that there was considerable dissent from these views that Americans were conformists (Lipset, 1963). Nonetheless, the spirit of pastoral individualism and frontier entrepreneurship had been modified to suit a social climate that was governed by formal, large-scale organizations. In the field of health care, the needs of individuals were expressed more and more by organized interest groups such as the AMA, labor unions, and racial coalition groups. Yet, neither individuals nor groups appeared to be ready to give up their opposition to socialized medicine.

Health Care Service

Organized Medicine and the Economy. Since the late 1930s, the number of commercial companies, nonprofit organizations, and others that offered voluntary health insurance increased at a phenomenal rate. For the Blue Cross Plan alone, subscribers increased from 27 million in 1937 to 52 million in 1958 (Somers & Somers, 1977).

Among the many reasons for this rapid growth was the failure of the Social Security Act to provide medical care benefits, and this increased the reliance on private insurance companies. In addition, the wartime economy led the installment of private health insurance through employment contracts. Since employer expenditures for health insurance were accepted as tax-deductible business expenses, employers did not discourage this development.

As for the AMA, the fear of compulsory health insurance induced its members to endorse private insurance by advocating the "the voluntary way is the American way" (Rayack, 1967, p. 179). Besides, the private insurance schemes fitted the fiscal needs of hospitals and the traditional fee-for-service system of physicians (Falk, 1973, p. 14).

Medicine and Public Health. While comprehensive medical health insurance bills were being defeated, federally subsidized health programs were invading the field of public health—research projects in the Department of Public Health Service, the maternal and child health and welfare programs, crippled children projects, cancer and heart disease research, etc.

Nevertheless, the scope of these programs was limited; none threatened the overall medical dominance of research, education, and practice. The cleavage between the spheres of public health and the private system of medical care (Falk, 1973, p. 11) resulted in a differential federal fiscal commitment to each. This cleavage has been also identified as that between applied versus basic research. It was also demonstrated by the unresponsiveness of medical schools to public health personnel needs.

Historically, the American Public Health Association (APHA) had not included personal medical care within its purview (Falk, 1973, p. 11). Little by little, however, when sensitized by public needs, the APHA came to embrace personal health care and to support comprehensive health care programs in opposition to the AMA (Bellin, 1970).

Organized Medicine and the Polity. In 1935, the AMA did not make any serious objections to the principles of Social Security ("Proceedings of the Special Session . . . ," 1935) but did reaffirm its opposition to all forms of compulsory sickness insurance.

The years after the enactment of Social Security saw many proposals for medical care. In 1939, Roosevelt planned to submit to Congress his health program, which included compulsory health insurance. It had won widespread support from many sectors of society but not from organized medicine. The AMA began to show strong support for private voluntary insurance to prevent the enactment of compulsory health plan legislation (Falk, 1973, p. 6; Rayack, 1967, p. 176).

Compulsory health insurance drafts were introduced to Congress again and again. These proposals avoided a revolutionary leap to a centralized national plan, and they adhered to an evolutionary course by relying on modest federal grants-in-aid to several states for elective program developments. However, the milder the proposals, the stronger became the opposition by the AMA (Falk, 1973, p. 7).

Proposals for a compulsory national health insurance program that would cover everyone were made during the 1940s, but they met with little success. Thus, in the 1950s, tactics were redirected toward the realization of a plan limited to the aged and to disadvantaged people.

The elderly are likely to incur greater medical expenses yet are less likely to be covered by employment-based private health insurance than are young and middle-aged people. By 1960, health insurance for the aged had become a major political issue for both Republicans and Democrats. Furthermore, the aged as members of the voting population were becoming more numerous, and they were also politically articulate (Stevens & Stevens, 1974).

Additional support for the aged, the disabled, and the unemployed came from the labor unions. Organized labor shrewdly analyzed the situation and could see that the disadvantaged might turn into union enemies, so union lobbies assumed the burden of fighting for the underprivileged. Also, medical benefits for the retired, the disabled, and temporarily laid-off workers were a natural extension of collective bargaining gains (Somers & Somers, 1977).

Finallly, the improvement of health care for the disadvantaged became one of the major targets adopted by the civil rights movement in the 1960s (Fox & Crawford, 1979). By helping the aged and the poor, the movement championed the greater cause of remedying the maldistribution of health care facilities in this country (Reskin & Campbell, 1974).

Thus, the public was dichotomized on the issue of health insurance for the elderly. Proponents consisted of the AFL-CIO, organizations for the aged, APHA, nursing organizations, social workers, civil rights movement promoters, and consumers. Opponents, on the other hand, included the AMA, the AHA, business groups, and insurance companies (Rose, 1967; Vuori, 1968).

Faced with great opposition, organized medicine and the insurance industry began to worry that their position against medical care for the poor might backfire and generate support for proposals toward medical programs for everybody. That fear prompted them to assent to legislation for the aged and the indigent (Falk, 1973, p. 13).

Though the programs being discussed involve a trend toward rationalizing the health care system, they emerged as the result of political bargaining rather than rational planning. The conflict over health insurance for the aged mirrors the broader ideological polarization of "money-providing" versus "service-demanding" groups in society, of socialized medicine versus the voluntary "American way," and of private enterprise versus federal government control.

These two sides were represented by relevant executive, legislative, and pressure groups, which struggled with all the power at their disposal. Two leading pressure groups—the AFL-CIO and the AMA—derided the imagined (or real) power of their opponents to rally support for their own side. Some of the power of pressure groups, however, was a manifestation of congressional conflict. For example, the Democratic administration helped create an image of a powerful AMA to focus attention away from its own incapacity to manipulate Congress. The executive bureaucracy played an intermediary role between these opposing sides, tacitly incorporating compromises into legislative proposals (Feingold, 1966; Marmor, 1973).

Medicare and Medicaid. Finally, in 1965, the health care plans known as Medicare (for the aged) and Medicaid (for the indigent) were passed by Congress. They are a major legislative milestone in federal financing of health care. Nevertheless, the specifics of these plans indicate a compromise among various groups (Corning, 1969; Falk, 1973, p. 18; Feder, 1977). For example, the inclusion of a voluntary insurance scheme for physicians' services in

Medicare reflects (1) the legislators' fear that, otherwise, doctors would not cooperate in implementing Medicare, and (2) an opportunity for Republicans to reduce their losses in the face of a Democratic victory. To enlist the support of the medical profession, the law also avoided prescribing a fee schedule for physicians.

Medicare is a program for persons aged 65 and over and consists of two parts. Part A provides hospital insurance to all individuals covered by the Social Security system. It is financed through the Hospital Insurance Trust Fund, which is made up of Social Security taxation money. This part is compulsory health insurance in that those who pay Social Security contributions during their working lifetime cannot opt out of the health insurance payments.

Part B is a supplementary medical insurance that helps the elderly to pay doctor and other health care expenses. The fund is derived from the premiums paid by the elderly on a voluntary basis, and is matched by federal tax revenues.

Both parts inherited major features of private health insurance—deductible and copayment characteristics—that require some direct payment by the patient. For Medicare, before the benefits are available, the patients must pay a certain amount (deductible); and after that, they still must bear specified portions of the cost (copayment).

Medicaid, on the other hand, provides health care coverage for the poor, or rather, for those who fit into the categories of public assistance. In addition, this program covers the medically indigent whose incomes are not low enough for social welfare programs but who do incur high medical expenses.

There are important differences between Medicare and Medicaid in their legislative philosophies and in their administrative structures, although these differences are frequently blurred in practice (Newman, 1972).

A primary ideological distinction is that Medicare is viewed as social insurance and Medicaid as social welfare. Medicaid is built on the concept of income redistribution from the rich to the poor. The person covered by this program is viewed as a "recipient" of a benefit through the largesse of society. Except for the case of the medically indigent, Medicaid places no cost-sharing burden on its recipients. It is much more comprehensive in its scope and service than Medicare.

In contrast, Medicare fits into the social insurance model in that the participants are regarded as "beneficiaries." Participants are seen as deserving the services because they have paid for them through Social Security contributions. Furthermore, as insurance, Medicare contains deductible and copayment aspects, and it assumes that most of the population covered can afford to pay something for medical care and that the elderly would prefer being treated as independent persons rather than as objects of charity. Coverage is also limited since it is not meant to finance all necessary health care. However, there is no guarantee that workers presently contributing to the fund will receive benefits in the future. Program costs are so arranged that current contributions are needed to finance medical care for those already retired rather than being held for future needs.

Administratively, Medicare is a single federal program under the Social Security system. It establishes a federally defined, uniform package of medical care benefits for a defined group in the population, i.e., those aged 65 and over.

Medicaid, on the other hand, is a series of 52 separate and different programs within the jurisdiction of each state. The federal role is limited to setting general standards, issuing guidelines, and to overseeing the states' operations. Each state defines the level of income for eligibility and the scope and duration of the benefits. The income limits for a family of four, for example, range from a high of $6,000 in New York to $2,448 in Oklahoma (Spiegel & Podair, 1975). As a result, there are substantial regional variations in the degree of coverage of the low-income population. In the Northeast and the West a large proportion of the low-income population is covered, while the Southern states have the smallest proportion of low-income populations covered.

All programs offer basic required services (inpatient and outpatient services, other laboratory and X-ray services, nursing home services, and physicians' services), but the extent of coverage of optional services (e.g., dental, optometry, physical therapy, chiropractic services) varies considerably from state to state. One factor explaining this variation in medical benefits is the differential rate of federal matching in state Medicaid programs. Although a strong negative relation exists between state per capita income and the rate of matching—i.e., low-income states having high rates of matching funds—the largest proportion of the federal expenditure flow into a relatively small number of states such as New York (28 percent) and California (17 percent) (Lewis, Fein, & Mechanic, 1976).

The Medicaid legislation was designed to ensure that a minimum of benefits would be available to all those in need without interfering with the rights of the individual states. Consequently, however, the benefits are not equitably distributed among states.

Tenacious adherence to the "American way" is manifest in both programs. Medicare resembles voluntary, private insurance coverage in organization and administration. To avoid the label of socialized medicine, the law specifically requires no federal or employer control over the medical practice. Prevailing private facilities—hospitals, doctors, insurance carriers—are used to absorb federal funding. In fact, proponents of Medicare viewed it as a means to forestall socialism by helping the population to finance its health costs. Even Medicaid was applauded as an example of "creative federalism," that is, a state program made possible through federal funds (Stevens & Stevens, 1974, p. 77). Thus, instead of being presented as revolutionary changes toward compulsory health insurance, both programs are made to appear as "American" as possible

From Medicare and Medicaid to National Health Insurance

Social Structure and Processes

The Economy. Since the mid-1960s an increasing number of welfare acts have been passed. Legalization and nationalization of equality have ideologically shaped America into a welfare state, one in which the government protects minimum standards of income, nutrition, health, housing, and education as a political right.

However, instead of solving economic problems, welfare legislation seems to be producing the so-called welfare crisis. Welfare and health costs as well as taxes are soaring, while many of the unemployed recipients still fall below the poverty line.

At the same time, the taxpayers' rebellion against inflated government expenditures has been heightened by a new awareness of limited resources, which was brought about by the energy crisis of the 1970s (Horowitz, 1977). In contrast to the rising expectation and growth of the 1950s, the 1970s has been a decade of finite resources and prudent restraint. The public is critical of large welfare systems established by the government without recognition of the high cost factors involved.

Cultural Values. With this awareness that resources are limited and growth must be curtailed, progress itself becomes problematic. Instead of asking, "Can science remove the physical limits to growth?" this generation is wondering, "Do we want science to remove the physical limits?" (Horowitz, 1977). This constraint upon expansion and progress deviates significantly from the American frontier spirit of the preceding two centuries.

The decade after the enactment of Medicare and Medicaid has witnessed a transition to a new equilibrium between individualism and collectivism. During this period, equality has gained protection by the federal government instead of being left to the conscience and efforts of individuals. Such weight placed on equality has the tendency to countercheck individualism and freedom (Kelly & Miles, 1976). On the other hand, some people discern the persistence of basic values (Lipset, 1963), claiming that what appears to be conformity may actually be a step toward more genuine individuality (Kluckhorn, 1958).

Stratification. Along with the rise of equalitarianism, American society has become, according to Horowitz (1977), a place where the war of all against all, rather than Marxian class conflict, is conducted with ferocity. The gap between organized and unorganized working classes, and between proletariats (the poorest class of working people) and welfare recipients is itself a focus of struggle in the 1970s, coupled with inherited class and racial antagonisms.

Probably the most dramatic triumph of the racial minorities since 1965 is the implementation of affirmative action legislation (Kelly & Miles, 1976). The federal government has taken upon itself not only to prohibit segregation based on race, sex, and other categories, but also to remedy the consequences of past social inequality. Special quotas are established based on race, sex, and other criteria for school admission and employment so that minority groups who have been discriminated against in the past will receive preferential treatment. On the other hand, affirmative action has been challenged by the white male population as being reverse discrimination.

The class struggle is no longer limited to the conflict between capitalists and proletariats. The unemployed poor who are supported by government welfare programs have caused antagonism in the taxpayers and trade unionists. The economic interests of employed workers have been protected through collective bargaining by labor unionism.

According to Horowitz (1977), awareness of the limitations of resources and growth has intensified intergroup conflicts because every group is anxious to obtain a greater share of the pie before the whole society is frozen into a fixed-size pie.

The Polity. In response to various national crises of recent generations, for example, depression, war, undeclared war, and energy crunch, the power of the federal government has expanded since the New Deal (Kelly & Miles, 1976). Exercise of the executive authority of the President and the legislative power of Congress have been demonstrated in the enactments of Social Security, Medicare, Medicaid, and the like. The Social Security Act virtually confiscates money from employers and employees to support the elderly. The federal judiciary has also expanded. For instance, the federal government frequently came to the rescue of strikers and rioters who were penalized by state or local laws.

The ascendancy of federalism, however, has been attacked from both above and below. The capitalist elite and proletarian union workers have joined together in negating any effort on the part of the government to increase the welfare program. The task of the government has become that of allocating scarce resources in such a way as to prevent an explosive civil war (Walker, 1974).

In short, the period since the passage of Medicare and Medicaid can be described as a time of transition during which a search for a new equilibrium between individualism and collectivism and between local autonomy and federal intervention is taking place. It is in this context that national health insurance as federalization of a health service system has become a national issue.

Health Care Service

Aftermath of Medicare and Medicaid. The passage of Medicare and Medicaid was a source of pride for Congress because it was viewed as a legislative victory. However, this euphoria did not last long. To ensure the programs' survival in a hostile environment (e.g., opposition by organized medicine), the Social Security Administration made compromises that perpetuated inadequate health delivery institutions. Aversion to political risk made the Social Security Administration comfortable with the status quo and resistant to change (Feder, 1977). After several years of operation, many people concluded that the passage of Medicare and Medicaid was a "Phyrrhic victory" (Falk, 1973, p. 20).

As was expected and hoped for, consumer utilization of health services increased. For example, in 1963, 56 percent of low-income persons (less than $5,000 annual income) saw a physician as compared to 65 percent in 1970, while the use of physicians' services by other income groups did not change much during 1964–1969. By 1969, their use of ambulatory facilities surpassed that of middle income and upper income persons (Lewis, Fein, & Mechanic, 1976). However, when health status was controlled in the 1969 figure, the use of physicians' services increased with income.

Although Medicare and Medicaid were intended to provide uniform medical care to the elderly and the indigent regardless of income, race, or geographical location, differentials existed in the distribution of benefits. Examining Medicare patients, Davis (1975a) found that higher income elderly persons received more medical care and a more expensive kind. On the other hand, those elderly with the poorest health (i.e., the poor, blacks, southerners) were the lowest utilizers of medical resources. This was not so much because of the educational or motivational levels of patients, but rather the result of cost-sharing provisions in Medicare. For the indigent, the financial burden of deductible and coinsurance premiums were so heavy as to deter them from using health services.

Davis also found geographical variation in utilization, specifically, a lower utilization rate in the northcentral and southern states. This reflects regional differences in availability of medical facilities. Thus, the primary determinants of utilization of medical services under Medicare and Medicaid are the income level of the patients and availability and accessibility of physicians. Medicare and Medicaid exemplify the failure of an effort to ensure access to physicians without changing the structure of medical practice. The programs may have been successful in enrolling eligible persons, but they have not been able to improve the accessibility of care to the needy (Lewis, Fein, & Mechanic, 1976).

Overutilization of medical services has appeared not only among patients but also among physicians. Since the programs do not provide incentives to control costs or to reduce unnecessary utilization, they tend to encourage physicians and hospitals to be more extravagant than before (Stevens & Stevens, 1974). It is more convenient for physicians to attend patients in the hospital rather than as outpatients. So long as the government funds are available, physicians are inclined to encourage hospitalization, which turns out to be also advantageous to patients because the outpatient services are often not covered under standard policies (Newman, 1972).

In addition to overutilization (performing and charging for superfluous services without therapeutic or preventive justification), fraud—that is, charging for a service that is not performed—is reported in many studies (Bellin & Kavaler, 1970; Cons, 1973; Spiegel & Podair, 1975). In 1975 and 1976, New York City investigators disclosed that over $300 million a year had been paid to doctors for false claims (Makofsky, 1977). The development of utilization review mechanisms, peer review, and prior authorization have decreased some problems of unnecessary utilization, but more improvement is needed.

Although the volume of medical utilization has increased drastically (Coe, 1967), it is extremely difficult to demonstrate that the health status of the population covered has indeed improved significantly (Newman, 1972). Based on various measures of mortality and morbidity, there seems to be no evidence that the gap in health status between the poor and nonpoor narrowed in the decade of the 1960s, although the use of doctors and hospitals by the indigent increased (Edinson, 1977; Lerner & Stutz, 1977). In the 1960s mortality declined somewhat for low-income people, but there was an even greater decrease for the nonpoor, which resulted in the widening of the gap between the poor and nonpoor. Besides, some of the improvements in the utilization of health services by the poor over the past decade are part of a long-term trend, not necessarily the consequence of the government programs (Wilson & White, 1977).

With the absence of definitive conclusions, the results of many studies concerning physicians' performance and patients' utilization (Bellin & Kavaler, 1970; Bierman et al., 1968; Cashing, 1970; Cashman & Myers, 1967; Coe & Sigler, 1970; Colombotos, 1969b; U.S. DHEW, 1968, 1970) were likely to be used for political campaigns to promote or reject the program. For instance, examples of overutilization of health resources by patients and physicians are quoted by the opponents of compulsory health insurance (Feingold, 1966).

The increased utilization, whether necessary or not, of medical services and the enlarged administrative cost have steeply raised the government expenditure in health care. This affects the public by raising taxes. By the mid-1970s, it was painfully clear that comprehensive health services to the needy would not be attainable under Medicare and Medicaid without massive expenditures and without a powerful regulatory mechanism. The problem arose from the fact that the legislation provided no incentive to change the existing system of medical economics based on fee-for-service. Since no provision was made to encourage the formation of new health resources or the redistribution of existing resources (Mooney, 1977), the already inadequate facilities had to be extended to absorb the patient traffic created by these programs (Newman, 1972; U.S. Senate Committee on Finance, 1970).

Despite the soaring cost, it was rapidly becoming clear that the scope of these programs was too limited both in the benefits provided and in the population covered (Falk, 1973, p. 21). In 1970, Medicare paid only about 43 percent of the aged's total health bill (Cooper & McGee, 1971, p. 12).

Another major difficulty stems from the complexities of the programs, which led to widespread confusion and misunderstandings by the public as well as by the providers. Having one system of medical care for the aged, another for the poor and near-poor, and still another for everybody else contributed to strains in the administration of the programs.

Thus, by the late 1960s, the momentum of the health care crisis was building. A consensus was emerging that a comprehensive health program for the entire nation was needed. Various groups undertook to develop proposals, which have been in and out of Congress during the 1970s (Waldman, 1976).

Health Maintenance Organizations (HMOs). While these groups were playing out their medical service plans, the notion of a Health Maintenance Organization (HMO) was crystalized as a relatively uncontroversial, compromise scheme. HMOs are usually defined as "organizations of health care providers which operate in groups and are reimbursed for providing services to enrolled populations on a prepaid per capita basis instead of the traditional fee-for-service system of payment" (Bauman, 1976; Newman, 1972, p. 123).

An an alternative to Medicare and Medicaid, HMOs aim at increasing the group organization of physicians and the extent of prepaid group practice. The rationale for such goals is derived from the assumption that group practice and prepayment will (1) improve the practice of scientific medicine, (2) provide economies of scale in the use of medical technology and ancillary personnel, (3) result in a reduction in hospitalization and other expensive services because of the emphasis on preventive medicine, and (4) produce a model of a medical care system that is between laissez-faire capitalism and federalization of health care.

It is argued that group practice, as compared with solo practice, can offer better quality of medical care because it provides (1) better technical facilities due to economies of scale, (2) peer consultation, (3) regularized schedules and opportunity for continuing professional development for physicians, and (4) efficient use of paraprofessionals.

The prepayment method is expected to encourage early detection of illness, since enrollees, unhampered by immediate cost considerations, will seek care in the early stages, when physicians may still be able to avoid far more costly hospitalization. Furthermore, physicians have a direct financial interest in keeping the patient well, that is, the HMO financial structure encourages physicians to practice preventive medicine (Havighurst, 1970). HMOs reverse the profit incentive inherent in a fee-for-service practice, where services increase income and fees rise along with the increasing volume of services. HMOs also motivate physicians to seek cost efficiency because there is no third-party subsidization (Enos and Sultan, 1977).

As a prepaid group practice on a local level, the HMO serves as a bridge between laissez-faire solo practice and the federalization of medical care system. The HMO was intended to stimulate private physicians to participate in prepaid medical programs. This market-oriented and private sector approach of the HMO was appealing to both liberals and conservatives who had been disillusioned with the government's inability to realize access of medical service at a reasonable cost (Stevens & Stevens, 1974).

At the local level, the HMO operates in a series of competitive private health service organizations, each of which offers patients a health maintenance contract. Consumers buy contracts at the HMOs of their choice, and the HMOs compete among themselves for clients in a free medical marketplace. The HMO is presented as a direct antithesis to national health insurance, which is based on centralized authority and regulation. The assumption is that self-contained, local HMOs would stimulate the decentralization of government decision-making and serve as a model of "new federalism" or "creative federalism" (Stevens & Stevens, 1974, p. 129).

These were the political promises of the HMOs. There is a difference between what the HMOs were expected to achieve and what has really been accomplished. HMO performance in comparison with that of other modes of health care delivery has been reviewed by many, although most results are not conclusive yet (Lewis, Fein, & Mechanic, 1976; Roemer & Shonick, 1973).

With regard to enrollee access to health care services, most studies indicate that financial barriers appear to have been significantly reduced by the HMO prepayment method. Although initial premiums are higher under the HMO than those of other types of health insurance, out-of-pocket expenses and thus total cost for all services are consistently lower (Greenlick, 1972; Hetherington, Hopkins, & Roemer, 1975; Lewis, Fein, & Mechanic, 1976).

The utilization rate of physician services is higher in HMO plans compared with other nonHMO plans. However, contrary to general expectation, the comprehensive benefit packages of the HMOs have only a slight effect on low-income familys' visits to doctors. Barriers of access to physicians in HMOs are found in the financial burden of cost-sharing (higher premiums and deductibles) and in the bureaucratic operation of large group practice. Hetherington, Hopkins, and Roemer (1975) found that in group practice the utilization of HMOs for purposes of preventive medicine is higher among those who are highly educated, have higher income, and who are more sensitive to health care than among those who are physically vulnerable to illness—those over 40 years of age, women of childbearing age, or families reporting at least one chronic or acute illness.

Although there is often a broader range of services available to the HMO enrollees than those under other plans, this does not guarantee easier access to the services. Many studies (Lewis, Fein, & Mechanic, 1976; Mechanic & Tessler, 1973; Shortell et al., 1977) report the dissatisfaction of HMO members with difficulty in making appointments, lengthy waiting for appointments, and problems in reaching the facility or physicians by phone. In large HMOs especially, there seem to develop bureaucratic mechanisms to constrict utilization, such as the single, all-purpose, central appointments telephone, which is constantly busy. Demand tends to adjust itself to the services available as conditions become more inconvenient to patients (Mechanic, 1972b, 1976).

Hence, the HMO's claim for cost containment must be examined carefully. Lower operational expenses for HMOs as compared to other plans may not necessarily be due to their increased physician productivity or effective use of allied health personnel, but rather it may reflect the administrative control of the use of services. Also, since there is not financial reward for each service rendered, there is a potential danger that HMOs might provide as few services as possible. Although this allegation is not supported by hard evidence, an incentive to avoid expensive care could lead to dangerous medical practices.

The lower rate of hospitalization under HMOs, compared to fee-for-service patients with health insurance, has frequently been quoted as evidence of the successful practice of preventive medicine. However, no causal relationship has been established between decreased hospitalization and increased access to ambulatory care (Lewis, Fein, & Mechanic, 1976). The low rate of hospitalization may be at least a function of the low availability of hospital beds in some HMOs. Based on a comparative study, Luft (1978) concluded that the greater use of preventive services by HMO enrollees is attributable to their better financial coverage, not to the ideology of preventive care.

From available evidence, it is hard to conclude that HMOs can solve the problems of accessibility, cost containment, and comprehensive services. However, most studies to date are based only on a few HMOs, and any definitive generalizations should be withheld. Using a flexible formula, HMOs can take various forms and their efficiency and quality control remain to be proven (Enos & Sultan, 1977).

National Health Insurance Proposals

At the time of writing this book it is difficult not to predict the appearance of some form of national health insurance in the near future. It is the health crisis, perceived not only by receivers but also by providers of health care services, that prompts interest in national health insurance. The health crisis as felt by the users of medical services is the failure of the existing system to deliver adequate health care to everyone at a reasonable cost. Those who provide health care or, as third parties, pay for it face a different crisis—rising costs and deficiency of funds.

In a search of solutions, various plans for national health insurance have been proposed by various groups who have a stake in the health care system. A large amount of specific legislation has been introduced and reintroduced to Congress in the 1970s (Berki, 1972; "Controversy . . . ," 1977; Davis, 1975b; Eilers & Moyerman, 1971; Fain, 1977; Falk, 1977; Somers, 1971; Somers & Somers, 1972).

In this section, major trends in the proposals will be identified without going into details. Although all of the proposals appear under one label, "national health insurance," a polarization is apparent among them. One type reflects the functionalist view by proposing an evolutionary approach within the existing social system. Thus, national health insurance is seen to evolve out of a long history of private health insurance based on voluntarism and individualism. Supporters (Falk, 1977; Somers & Somers, 1972) of this approach warn the public, who are disenchanted with private insurance, that centralization of the medical delivery system can only bring rigidity, stagnation, and authoritarianism. They advocate pluralism, which would embrace both the private and public sectors.

In contrast, others (Navarro, 1973) call for the reorganization of the whole health care system. In line with the dialectic conflict theory, they claim that the prevailing health care system has within itself the seed for its own destruction, that is the private medical marketplace is malfunctioning. These conflict theorists contend that a total restructuring of the medical delivery system is imperative. And according to them, this revolutionary change must be acknowledged as such, instead of being disguised under the rhetorical label of the "American way" (Alford, 1975; Skidmore, 1970).

Partly because of analytical convenience, but also because national health insurance is supposed to represent a new "system," the various proposals will be examined in terms of the Parsonian functional prerequisites.

Values underlying national health insurance proposals can be categorized according to the presence or absence of the traditional American values of equalitarianism and individualism. Equalitarianism takes the form of universal coverage of the resident population without discrimination as to income or premium contributions. Equalitarian proposals contend that access to comprehensive medical care is a necessity and a human right, not a luxury. Individualism is reflected in the options allowed for individuals to select certain (or no) types of benefits at their own prepaid costs.

The adaptational function of the national health insurance system involves its economic solvency. Evolutionary proposals try to adhere to the classical free market principle, although tempering it to a regulated competition. Mechanisms to maximize the efficient and effective use of resources are the issues of the adaptive function.

The type of integration within the national health insurance system varies according to the proposals' administrative policies. The crux of the issue is private versus public administration, or rather, the extent of governmental intervention in financing and administering the health care system.

The ultimate goal of national health insurance is to provide the best available medical care to anyone who needs it. The different proposals address the issues of how and who will supervise the quality of medical care and how health care facilities will be distributed.

Three major categories of national health insurance proposals are summarized in Table 10.2.

Category 1: Voluntary Incentive Proposals. The first category includes proposals for taxes or other incentives to stimulate voluntary purchase of private health insurance. For example, a federal income tax deduction is allowed for an insurance premium, or federal grants are given to states to buy insurance for the poor. These plans have been endorsed by the AMA, the AHA, and private health insurance companies.

The major characteristic of this group of proposals is their voluntarism. However, voluntarism cannot guarantee equality. These plans are intended to protect everyone, but they are not universal in their coverage. For instance, the tax incentive is too low, and for moderate income taxpayers, it would be negligible.

Benefits are not comprehensive and are accompanied by deductibles and copayments.

Financially, a federal fund is used to support the private purchase of more private insurance. Cost control is gained by a restructuring of the private medical system such as by encouraging HMOs and other prepaid plans.

Administration of private plans will entail state advisory board approval of policies and the monitoring of financial operations. This board will prescribe regulations, establish standards, and develop programs to improve the quality of care. However, the quality control of medical delivery is predominantly left in the hands of the private sector (e.g., physicians, hospitals, and private insurance companies) with minimum federal control.

Category 2: Employer-Mandated Insurance. In the second category is the Nixon administration's employer-mandated insurance, which has been reintroduced to a subsequent Congress under a different title. This contains a compulsory feature imposed upon employers—mandatory purchase of private health insurance by employers for their employees. However, voluntarism prevails in that it is a private purchase of private insurance.

The value of equalitarianism is not realized in this plan either. To begin with, as an employment-based plan, it excludes migrant workers, part-time or casual workers, multiple-employer domestics, unemployed single persons, and so on.

Table 10.2: National Health Insurance Proposals

Functional prerequisite	*Category 1* Voluntary incentive proposals (AMA, AHA, insurance companys)	*Category 2* Employer-mandated insurance (Nixon Administration)	*Category 3* Public insurance (Senator Kennedy)
Latency			
Equalitarianism (universality)	Nonuniversal coverage	Nonuniversal coverage	Universal coverage
Individualism (voluntarism)	Voluntary insurance	Voluntary and compulsory	Compulsory insurance
Adaptation			
Finance	Tax credit for private insurance purchase	Mandates employer purchase of private insurance	Payroll tax and federal revenue
Cost control		Federal assistance plan	
Integration			
Administration	Private sector administration	Employer plan—state agencies	Federal administration
Goal Attainment			
Quality control of medical care	Primarily physicians' autonomy	Implicit standards, not specified and only for group practice	Health Security Board with centralized control

Also, for small employers, the cost burden is staggering. In fact, this proposal is a complex aggregate of separate programs for different income classes because high premiums, deductible aspects, and copayment features necessitate the continuation of a welfare program for the poor. Federal assistance would be provided for the nonemployed and self-employed.

Benefits are not comprehensive, and coverage of employees, nonemployed, and self-employed is on a voluntary basis. Quality control is to be exercised only by implicit, nonspecific standards.

Governmental administration of the program would be limited to prescribing regulations and federal standards for state insurance departments and to reviewing the effectiveness of the program. Basically, this plan retains our current medical care system.

Category 3: Public Insurance. In the third category is the Kennedy Health Security Act, which is a unitary, all-embracing federal program. This measure has received the endorsement of organized labor, which would like the federal government instead of private insurance companies to run the program. Unlike the other two types, this proposal attempts to reorganize the entire medical delivery system. The underlying philosophy is equalitarianism rather than voluntarism. The plan proposes compulsory coverage of all of the civilian population with broad and relatively comprehensive benefits.

The program would be financed by a combination of payroll taxes and general revenues, and it would be administered exclusively by the federal government without the use of private carriers. Funds would be allocated by Washington to each of ten regions on a per capita basis, and their use would be specifically itemized (e.g., institutional and physician's services). It would be the prerogative of the federal government to regulate costs, reallocate resources, and develop health resources.

Power would be centralized in a unitary, self-contained, five-member Health Security Board. The authority of the Board would extend beyond financial domains and would include the regulation of internal hospital practice, professional licensing standards, etc. In short, the professional autonomy of physicians would be replaced by third-party intervention. Physicians would have the freedom to choose among alternative compensation methods: payment on a capitation basis, salary, or fee-for-service. Whichever method is chosen, however, payment would be subject to a predetermined budget for physicians' services.

Carter's Proposal. The Carter administration's proposal should be mentioned because it sheds a different light on the whole issue of national health insurance. What distinguishes Carter's plan from others is its tight financial constraint. This reflects Carter's general restraint in the health budget, carefully charting priorities with limited dollars (Iglehart, 1978). This may mirror the social climate of the 1970s as a decade of restraint resulting from the energy crisis (Horowitz, 1977).

Carter's plan will involve no additional federal spending until the fiscal year 1983. Thereafter, the plan will be phased in gradually, taking into consideration such factors as the economic and administrative expenses under each phase. Carter keeps the option to delay a phase of the plan, should the country in a particular year be faced with serious unemployment or other economic hardships. Further, he proposes to have a self-destructive mechanism—that is, the program could be halted if it becomes too expensive. He claims that the national health insurance program should not be set in motion without regard for the cost or the general state of the economy.

Carter's plan is to be financed through multiple sources, including government funding and contributions from employers and employees. The plan also includes a significant role for the private insurance industry (*Congressional Quarterly,* 1977; Herrington, 1978).

The national health insurance proposals have been researched, investigated, compared, and debated in and out of Congress. Each of the proposals if enacted would generate significant additional expenditures for health services. For instance, estimated costs by 1980 are given as around $11 billion for the voluntary incentive proposals; $20 billion for the employer-mandated plans; $25 billion for the Kennedy Health Security Act (*Congressional Quarterly,* 1977, p. 17), and $25 to 40 billion for the Carter plan (Herrington, 1978). However, these figures, publicized by the proponents of the different plans, are usually substantial understatements of probable costs. Moreover, the advertised figures are rarely comparable, because they often use different definitions of costs and may relate to differing time periods. Whether improvements in efficiency of the delivery system will be sufficient to fully counterbalance the increased demand and prices remains to be seen.

The trouble with most of these proposals is that their sponsors deal with a limited aspect of the health crisis—financing of medical care. Few plans seriously confront other components of the crisis—the basic issues of the organization of a health delivery system, the relationship between the providers and recipients of care, and the power distribution in the health care system (Ehrenreich & Ehrenreich, 1971).

THE POLITICS OF HEALTH CARE

By tracing the origin and development of the concept of national health insurance, we have become aware of the politics of health care services in this country. Politics here is broadly defined as competition between interest groups for power. Power refers to the ability of one individual or group to compel another to do something.

Interest groups in American health politics include the government (federal, state, and local), medical groups (physicians and hospitals), corporations in the health business (drugs, medical supplies, and equipments), third-party payers (insurance companies and the government), the capitalist class, unions, and consumers (Fox & Crawford, 1979; Krause, 1977).

The power struggle among these groups has been carried out within the constraints of the American way: laissez-faire capitalism and decentralized government apparatus. Thus, until the depression of the 1930s, the role of the federal government in the health delivery system was minimal. Since the passage of the Social Security Act, however, the ascendance of federal power has accelerated. In the contemporary arena of health politics, the federal government plays a major role as a financier of health services.

Krause (1977) envisions the federal government as a "marriage broker" in the medical-industrial complex, since the government spends the citizens' money in a strategic area (health) through the relationship between government funders and private contractors. Each outside interest group (e.g., private corporations, the academic researchers) works with its internal counterpart interest group within HEW to develop a new law and push for the appropriation of funds.

In order to answer questions such as who is really in charge or who is responsible for the medical crisis (high cost, inefficiency, and inequality) there are several interpretations, such as professional dominance, industrialism with government control, or capitalist dominance.

Professional Dominance. The politics of health care has been examined by many from the perspective of professional dominance. The source of this power is derived from the fact that society grants to the medical profession the right and responsibility to control its own affairs largely because that requires an expertise which the public lacks. The qualities that are exclusive to the medical profession—technical expertise, precise and detailed scientific knowledge, useful function, and service orientation—have given the physicians more or less a self-regulating autonomy over quality control, the selection of specialties and geographical areas of practice, and the choice of financial arrangements (Friedson, 1970, 1975).

However, the medical profession acquired this elevated status not so much because of exclusive qualities but rather through a process of political negotiation and persuasion. The foundation of physicians' control over their work is political in nature, involving the aid of the state in legitimating the profession's pre-eminence through licensing laws that prohibits others from practicing medicine.

Further, the large income of the professionals enables organized medicine to engage in a wide variety of political lobbying and public relations activities. In our society, lobbies and pressure groups constitute an essential part of the governmental process. They derive their authority from the Constitution, that is, the explicit right of citizens to petition their government (Ward, 1972). The AMA has been quite effective in maintaining the principle of fee-for-service solo practice and in fighting against third-party interference, although it has compromised little by little (Price, 1978).

Industrialism and Government Control. While some (Freidson, 1975b) see professional dominance as the major analytical key to the present state of health services, others (Carlson, 1975; Illich, 1976; Mechanic, 1974; Somers & Somers, 1977) address the broader perspectives of the medical-industrial complex.

For example, Illich (1976) traces the source of medical dominance to the ideology of industrialism. Industrialism in his view assumes technological determinism, which suggests that technology defines social structure, including the organization of medicine. Other components of the ideological construct of industrialism include productivity, efficiency, progress, and modernization.

Further, the theory of industrialism postulates that the process of industrialization is accompanied by the evolution of social stratification. As industrialization progresses, power is transferred first from owners of property and capital to the managers of that capital; and then is further shifted to the technocrats who have the skill and knowledge required to operate the social edifice of industrialism, that is, bureaucracy. Because of this evolution, Illich states that a new social order based on bureaucracy has transcended the capitalist order. At the top of this bureaucratic hierarchy are the technological experts and at the bottom are the recipients or consumers of goods and services. It is the medical technocrats who shape our medical practice.

But the expansionist force inherent in modern technology has gone beyond the private sector and has enlisted the support of the government. The advances in medical technology were accompanied by an increase in the overall costs of health care. Even if technology cuts some expenses, it will encourage a wider utilization of the service, incurring a higher expense. The soaring cost of health care eventually falls upon the government because it is the only social group that has the necessary financial resources.

Somers and Somers (1977) call it "the honeymoon of technology and government." The early results of this government funding and administrative control of medical technology are likely to be positive. The direct benefits are seen in the form of more services for a greater number of people.

However, there are a series of negative results derived from the expansion of technology facilitated by government involvement.

The growth of medical technology and advances in medical science have caused a growing emphasis on medical specialization and resulting fragmentation. At a highly advanced and complex level of medical technology, it is more efficient for physicians to pursue specialized areas rather than to attempt mastery of everything. This specialization in turn has resulted in a growing fragmentation of care in which no person or agency has responsibility for a patient as a whole individual. Since governments tend to be larger than private enterprises, the danger of fragmentation in government-sponsored medical enterprises is increased (Somers & Somers, 1977). Thus, the industrialization of medicine leads to the creation of engineers—the medical technocrats—who view the human body as a piece of equipment.

Medical technocracy operates under the assumption that if technology is available, all that is possible must be done to aid the individual patient regardless of the cost, the sentiment of the patient, or the needs of other people (Fuchs, 1974). The medical establishment advocates biomedical developments (e.g., antibiotics, polio immunization, kidney transplants, etc.), convincing the public that the money is well spent. However, a huge expenditure for secondary and tertiary medical care and research benefiting a small number of people almost insures that the larger segment of the population will receive less than a minimal standard of primary care.

There are some negative effects directly derived from sophisticated medical technology such as the side effects of potent drugs and unnecessary or experimental surgery. Indirectly, the medical establishment succeeds in keeping the public addicted to medicine, thereby extending its sphere of influence far beyond what was traditionally considered the medical domain. The discussion of medicalization of society and its ill effects (iatrogenesis) will be elaborated upon in Chapter 12 (Fuchs, 1974; Illich, 1976).

Finally, government assistance in the advancement of medical technology has helped to exacerbate inflation. Along with the rise in the government share of costs has come a phenomenal increase in the total cost itself. Since the money was available, there has been little restraint exercised on the part of providers and recipients of health services.

Capitalist Dominance. In analyzing the process of industrialization, some writers (Krause, 1977; Navarro, 1975, 1976, 197[illegible]a,b) assert the importance of capitalism as an underlying factor. According to these Marxian theorists, medical bureaucracy is merely the servant to a higher category of power: the dominant class that owns and manages capital. The medical profession is simply a stratum of trustworthy representatives to whom the bourgeoisie has delegated some of its power. Those who have the first and final voice in the most important decision-making in the health sector are not the physicians but rather the corporate groups composed of the upper, corporate, or capitalist class that owns and manages financial capital. For example, the famous Flexner Report was sponsored by the Carnegie foundation and represented the views of the corporate class of that period.

From the capitalist frame of reference, specialization and bureaucratization of medical practice are not the results of technological advances. Instead, they are the mechanisms by which employers can regulate the work process. Increased specialization, division of labor, and hierarchicalization of the health sector labor force help the owners and managers of production to optimize their control over workers. These health workers are so compartmentalized and alienated from one another that they lack the broader perspective needed to influence the design of the production process and to maintain autonomy.

Marxian theorists argue further that the concept of health and the type of health services have been defined according to the needs of the capitalist mode and relations of production, not by the medical profession. Capitalism needs for its survival the creation of consumption. The owners and controllers of the system must stimulate and maintain the consumers' dependency upon medical services through such expansion as that of the drug industry.

Even government intervention in the medical delivery system is interpreted as a class struggle, since the capitalist class has a dominant influence over the organs of the state. From the Marxist perspective, the nature of the law-making process is related to the patterns of ownership and wealth in a society. Those who have access to the wealth-producing process are the law makers because they can use their wealth and position to influence the political machinery.

The primary role of the state is viewed as establishing the conditions for the survival of the capitalistic economic system. The state may control some of the activities of specific capitalist groups, but it is because of the state's concern for promoting the interests of the capitalist economy as a whole.

In short, the politics of health care are geared by the capitalists, not by the medical profession.

The limitation of the above theories—professionalism, industrialism, and capitalism—in explaining the mechanisms of health politics is their determinism, unmindful of the importance of other factors. To illustrate, the medical profession is assumed to have had no status when it was not equipped with technology. However, technology along without the help of capital, even in the case of the AMA, could not have been so effective in suppressing legislation. On the other hand, by viewing everything from the angle of economic class struggles, one can overlook the importance of feedback relations among various factors, such as the interaction between economy and technology. These theoretical orientations provide us with useful instruments to analyze the politics of health care, but our task is to measure the magnitude of power exerted by each component pressure group and to study the group interaction rather than to postulate a deterministic explanation.

SUMMARY

The escalation in medical costs in the last two decades appears to be the main impetus for the development of national health insurance. However, the concept of social insurance did not emerge suddenly from the medical economic crisis.

American society prior to the depression of the 1930s was dominated by the value orientations of individualism, equalitarianism, and work ethic, derived from the Puritan and Revolutionary War traditions. These values were realized in liberal and decentralized political machinery, open-market economic practice, and open-class stratification among whites.

From the colonial years until 1935, health and welfare were almost entirely left to the responsibility of individual localities and states; the federal government only played a minimal role. Starting around 1900, large industries initiated medical programs for their employees, and organized medicine supported the drive for social health insurance. However, by 1920 the AMA came to denounce any health insurance, voluntary or compulsory, and also group practice.

During the depression years, American society underwent major structural changes. In order to cope with the national crisis, the power of the federal government was legitimated to regulate economic activities and to establish social welfare programs. The Social Security Act endorsed the value of equalitarianism by providing public assistance to the helpless and the aged. As the depression deepened, public interest in health insurance grew steadily. Finally, the AMA came to accept voluntary health insurance as the "American way."

The period between the Social Security Act (1935) and the passage of Medicare and Medicaid (1965) witnessed further concentration of power in the federal government, due to World War II, postwar prosperity, urbanization, bureaucratization, and increased unionization. The inclination toward collectivization also manifested itself in the cult of conformity, as noted by many social scientists in the 1950s. However, conformity did not mean passivity but rather was counterbalanced by efforts to realize equality through collective activities.

In the areas of health care, equalitarianism took the form of Medicare and Medicaid. The aged and the indigent were to be given special public assistance so that they could protect their rights to health on an equal basis with anyone else.

The ascendancy of federalism and collectivism came to be viewed with alarm by the 1970s. Proposals are being made to reach a new equilibrium between individualism and collectivism and between freedom and equality. Nevertheless, the quest for a national system of health care is stronger now than ever before as a direct result of medical inflation. The laissez-faire medical market operation has proven deficient in rendering medical care accessible to everyone, and governmental coordination and regulation are called for.

Having reviewed the history of social insurance in this country, can we say that we have come a long way in a relatively short time? Only 50 years ago any form of health insurance, public or private, was highly controversial. Everyone recognizes that a substantial change has taken place in the financing of health care services, but interpretations of the nature of the transformation vary depending upon the perspective taken.

From the functionalist perspective, the entire process can be viewed as an evolution of the medical delivery system. In the earlier undifferentiated stage, solo practitioners on a fee-for-service basis performed functions such as providing medical care, handling financial arrangements, and planning and distributing health care resources. The system was well integrated with a consensus on the values of voluntarism and laissez faire. The physicians' role was considered to be so important that their power was accepted as legitimate.

In the meanwhile, the health care system had to cope with both external and internal pressures. External forces included wars, depression, unionization, and federalism. Internally the system was faced with the emergence of specialization, hospital-based treatment, and private insurance. All of these currents threatened the autonomy of private physicians and thereby placed the system in disequilibrium.

However, the system did not fall apart but rather regained equilibrium after some repercussions within the system. Thus, the AMA came to accept private insurance as a lesser evil than compulsory insurance. Later, Medicare was tolerated by the AMA because its coverage was partial. By then, the AMA seemed to recognize that government financing does not necessarily entail undersirable restrictions on professional autonomy.

In the eyes of a functionalist, the American medical system has slowly evolved to its present state, all the while adhering to the central values of freedom. Even the bitter and protracted struggle over Medicare is now regarded as the system's adjustment to minor disturbances (Somers & Somers, 1972).

Conflict theorists, on the other hand, view the whole history as a process of dialectic conflict. To begin with, the basic values upon which the American nation was built consisted of mutually contradictory elements: freedom and equality. Whenever one is emphasized, the other must suffer.

American medicine began in the open market by competing against quacks and charlatans. In order to win this battle, the early AMA joined hands with scientific academia and progressive social philosophy, and it supported the idea of social welfare. By the time the AMA established its autonomy and power, it severed its affiliation with welfare promoters and switched its alliance to the private insurance industry to fight against their common enemy—socialized medicine.

However, society as a whole has been moving toward the value of equalitarianism rather than voluntarism. In recent years, organized medicine has done battle against such powerful opponents as organized labor, the civil rights movement, and consumerism, all of which advocate equalitarianism. The target of the war is national health insurance. Opposing teams are flooding Congress with proposals and counterproposals. Eventually a compromise or a synthesis will be reached. Yet national health insurance is not a panacea, and it contains the seed of its own destruction when viewed from a dialectic conflict perspective. If a comprehensive national health insurance proposal is adopted, it will challenge the whole social system, thus generating more conflict.

The aforementioned process of conflict generation and resolution has been interpreted by Marxian theorists as the manifestation of a class struggle. According to this view, the power that the medical profession commands is nothing but a delegated one from the bourgeois class. Even state intervention in medical practice in the form of national health insurance is seen as a mechanism to protect the capitalistic economy of the nation as a whole.

From the interactionist perspective, labels such as "voluntarism" and "American way" disguise any changes that have taken place, whether evolutionary or revolutionary. The "American way" represents democracy and freedom, juxtaposed against "alien" communism, socialism, and dictatorship. Both opponents and proponents of national health insurance have used these labels. In introducing the centrally controlled New Deal policy and the compulsory Social Security Act, Roosevelt appealed to the freedom from want and fear. When the AMA was pressured into accepting private health insurance, it declared that the voluntary way of private insurance was the only "American way."

The trouble with adherence to an old label is that substantial change can go unnoticed or is viewed as nonsignificant. Furthermore, in accordance with the labeling theory, the labeler is generally in a position of power and can compel the public to accept the label. Any proposal calling for a structural change of society will be stigmatized as "un-American" and therefore dangerous.

Despite varying political and sociological interpretations, a growing and converging socialization of the medical care system has been noted in modern nations. This convergence may be the result of the advances of medical technology and the rising expectations of populations for accessible and comprehensive care, or it may be interpreted in Marxian terms as an attempted solution to the crisis of contemporary capitalism (Navarro, 1978a,b). At any rate, many industrialized societies are faced with the dilemma of improving the quality of care with limited resources. In the next chapter we will examine whether or not socialized medicine in capitalist as well as communist social settings fares better than our system.

CHAPTER 11

International Health Care

Up to this point American health care services have been examined in historical as well as contemporary contexts. The analysis has revealed many problems which may make it appear that this country has less effective and more expensive health care than other developed countries. Criticism is usually expressed in terms of high medical costs, the absence of a coordinated medical system, a physician shortage, and the complexity of the medical bureaucracy. Remedies for these problems have been sought in measures such as the development of neighborhood health centers, health maintenance organizations, national health insurance, and paramedical professionals.

Faced with the quandary of how to improve the situation, Americans may look for possible alternatives in other countries. For instance, is it efficient to introduce the Chinese concept of the barefoot doctor (physician's assistant) into American rural areas to cope with the scarce medical work force?

In this chapter, the health care services in three countries, the USSR, the People's Republic of China, and the United Kingdom, are selected for comparison and analysis since socialized medicine is practiced in these countries, a medical approach that Americans have resisted throughout their history. Can a centrally controlled medical delivery system be the answer to the health problems in this country? What lessons can we learn from these countries?

Before an answer can be formulated, we must first recognize that the adoption of, say, the barefoot doctor, cannot be done in isolation from the historical and social milieu. A particular health care operation must be examined in the main contours of the political, economic, social, and ideological structures. Thus, in this chapter, the functionalist assumption is made that health services are a subsystem of the larger social system. The usual Parsonian functional prerequisites for a medical care system will be analyzed, and the alternative conflict and interactionist perspectives will be considered simultaneously.

Remember that the latency function refers to value orientations concerning health conduct as an integral part of the overall societal values. Health priorities and their rationale are influenced by different political and economic ideologies such as democracy, communism, laissez faire, and collectivism.

The task of integration in the medical care system will be explored in terms of the organization and administration of health services. In all three countries, the health administrations are centralized and medical networks are nationally coordinated.

The goal attainment function of health care systems will be analyzed through the ways in which physicians in the three countries practice medicine: the degree of professional autonomy in socialized medicine, the differentiation between specialists and general practitioners, and modern versus traditional medical practices.

Finally, the adaptive function will involve the financing and the supply of medical personnel resources. In all three countries, finance is centrally controlled, permitting the central control of medicine. The shortage in the medical work force in the USSR and the People's Republic of China is dealt with by developing paramedical personnel.

THE USSR

Social Background

The Union of Soviet Socialist Republics (USSR) occupies the largest territory of any country in the world. The vast lands of the Soviet Union are relatively sparsely populated, and slightly less than one-half of its population is said still to be rural (Lisitsin, 1972).

What is now called the USSR is a collection of old nations with a history of more than 1,000 years, but its new social and political system only dates back to the 1917 Revolution. Its transformation from an inefficient, autocratic serfdom to that of a technologically advanced nation that plays a leading role in the world was drastic. This transformation took place under extremely difficult conditions—economic chaos and famine caused by World War I. There was armed foreign intervention. The socialists fostered an internal revolution and the counterrevolution by the Bolsheviks took advantage of the resultant disorder and confusion (Walsh, 1958).

In order to achieve parity with the rest of the world in a little over half a century, the USSR adopted totalitarianism as a model for their political organization. As a result, Soviet society is one in which all of the political and most of the economic power has been gathered into the hands of a minority of the population, the Communist Party, which is a tightly knit hierarchic organization.

This totalitarianism operates by defining an attractive vision of the future that requires the consolidated efforts of the present society in order to realize it. The vision, conceived by Marx and Lenin, is that of a utopian, classless society. In order to implement this vision, the totalitarian society controls and mobilizes all human and material resources according to the program elaborated by the Communist Party leadership. Total political and economic power in the hands of the leaders permits the state to impose its scale of values and its order of priorities upon the entire society. Consumer goods and comforts are subjugated to scientific, technological, agricultural, industrial, and medical requirements (Shaffer, 1965). However, the development of limited autonomy in cultural institutions and independent public expressions can and do take place in Communist societies (Goldfarb, 1978). The intelligentsia actually constitutes a fairly large part of the population alongside the two major proletariat classes, the workers and the collective farmers.

The Polity versus the Medical Profession. When the Bolsheviks wrested power from the weak and disorganized Provisional Government, they were also faced with the plagues of the previous government: political corruption, economic bankruptcy, military collapse, and above all, a medical work force shortage and resultant epidemics.

The Bolsheviks needed the expertise and services of physicians to save the working and fighting capacity of the population from the tide of epidemics. There was, however, a conflict between the Bolsheviks and the medical profession. The former viewed the latter as enemies of the people and as an exploiting bourgeoisie, while the latter did not support the Communist revolution.

Physicians under the Tsardom were free agents who had united themselves into a medical corporation. With a sense of dedication and devotion to their calling, the prerevolutionary intelligentsia including physicians acquired definite political views. Without limiting their activities to medical subjects, the doctors entered the political field to attack the Tsarist government. During the period of democratic ferment that followed the 1917 Revolution, the medical profession attempted to reform the medical system along the lines of centralized planning required for government financing, but they also tried to maintain professional supervision and control of medical practices (Field, 1957).

The Bolsheviks, on the other hand, wanted the type of physicians who would do what they were bid. In order to alter the medical profession from being a self-governing, politically oriented, vocal corporate group into a docile body of state employees, state power was used to suppress physicians both individually and collectively. For instance, the state coerced individual physicians by taxing, confiscating property, or withholding food rations and living quarters. On an organizational level, the state replaced counterrevolutionary physicians with politically loyal individuals in the highest medical posts. Faced with the resistence by the leadership of the physicians' union, the state succeeded in undermining the union by approaching and winning the support of semiprofessional and nonprofessional medical personnel who had been exploited by the physicians (Field, 1957).

Despite opposition to and sabotage (Navarro, 1977) of the implementation of the Communist's program, by 1924 the physicians were recruited into the medical workers' union established by the state. The medical profession was captured, neutralized, and transformed into a group of expert officials trained and employed by the state.

In short, while the United States has enjoyed 200 years of relative political stability and technological proficiency in a land of wealth and resources, the

USSR undertook a drastic transformation from an inefficient, agrarian serfdom to a technologically advanced nation less than a century ago. This radical change was made possible by the political revolution championed by the Communists' whose totalitarian ideology altered the whole medical delivery system in a very short time.

Value Orientation

The development of Soviet medicine must be examined from the viewpoint of the Communist Party's interest in the welfare of the total population. Since Marxism-Lenninism is defined as a world view, it not only discusses the nature of reality and the unfolding of history but also provides an interpretation of medicine.

Within the framework of dialectic materialism (see Chapter 2 for a brief discussion of Marxism), the owners of capital are viewed as being interested only in monetary gain and are considered indifferent to the health of the workers. Just as in religious, political, and legal institutions, the medical system, according to Marxist theory, also serves only the interests of the ruling class. The elimination of private ownership of the means of production is believed to lead to the eradication of antagonistic classes and to the growth of a health system that serves the needs of the entire population (Field, 1967; Shaffer, 1965; Sigerist, 1937).

The position of Soviet health service within the national order of value priorities is determined by the Communist government and is imposed upon individuals. The aim of the health care delivery system is spelled out as "the minimum allocation necessary to maintain that state of health in the population that will most facilitate the realization of the regime's objective"—that is, the creation of a technically advanced classless society without jeopardizing other needs of equal or higher significance (Field, 1967, p. 11). Thus, the development of public health and medical capabilities must fit into the overall goals of the Communist state. The direction and supervision of all health activities is concentrated in a central governmental planning organization.

In reality, however, this central planning does not put medicine in a favorable position. The first priorities are given to military and industrial needs (Navarro, 1977), and the medical field is accorded only secondary importance. As a result, in many instances there is failure on the part of industrial ministries and the local soviets (legislative assemblies) to set aside sufficient resources for medical services. Physicians feel slighted by the authorities, who assume that their own activities are more important than the doctors' work (Field, 1957).

In order to carry out the goals of the state, the socialization of physicians is crucial. The Bolsheviks were not satisfied with simply neutralizing the psychological attitudes of physicians by making of them simple state employees. They tried to create a new intelligentsia of undoubted loyalty and commitment to the state, one with its feet solidly anchored in the working class. They considered that only the higher education of proletarian children would make this possible.

The state tried many strategies to recruit proletarian children. For instance, admission to the universities was made available to anyone 16 years of age or older. It also gave unconditional preference in admission to proletarian students by means of special stipends and by setting discriminatory fees for bourgeois children. The government went even further by providing remedial education for working class students.

In spite of all these efforts, the number of proletarian students did not increase substantially, and the quality of medical students declined. The Soviet Union could not afford to lower the standards of medical education and had to abandon the effort to proletarianize higher education. It is interesting to note that one of the reasons for this failure was that proletarian students who belonged to the Party were too absorbed in Party activities to devote themselves to academic work (Field, 1967).

Despite the failure to recruit proletarian students, or rather, because of that failure, it became all the more important to indoctrinate bourgeois students into Communist ideology at school. As a result, classes in Marxist-Leninist principles constituted an important part of the curriculum in the USSR medical schools. The completion of formal training was made contingent upon passing courses in political subjects. However, the extent of success of this indoctrination is suspect. Many students learned political textbooks by rote for fear of failing the examinations. Both physicians and students admitted in private interviews their distaste for political education because it takes so much time away from learning medicine (Field, 1957). There is evidence that after the mid-1930s the ideological slant in medical education was de-emphasized.

The implication is that if a well-planned comprehensive health care requires totalitarianism, it will not be feasible in the United States. From the beginning of this nation, Americans have cherished value orientations that are entirely different from those in the USSR. The dominant themes of American philosophy have been individual freedom, liberty, free enterprise, and the distrust of governmental intervention.

Organization and Administration of Health Services

Organization of Health Administration

The value orientations examined above give fundamental support to the machinery of Soviet medicine. The translation of ideals into action in medicine and public health is primarily the responsibility of the state and is carried out by a centralized administrative apparatus. The organization of health services corresponds to the general structure of the central and local governments (Anderson, 1973; Field, 1967; Navarro, 1977).

In formal terms, the executive and administrative power is vested in a Council of Ministers, of which the Health Minister is a member. At the highest national level, the Health Ministry of the USSR is entrusted with the responsibility for the health of the Soviet nation. As such, it possesses certain legislative power, and health legislation issued at this level supersedes policies adopted by the individual republics (which are administratively similar states in the United States).

More specifically, the Health Ministry is charged with (1) making overall plans for the future development of the national health service; (2) setting up standards for the allocation of health resources to the population; (3) providing technical assistance to the republican health ministries; (4) coordinating medical research; (5) maintaining international relations in the field of health, and (6) with administering other miscellaneous tasks.

The USSR is divided into republics, each of which has its own Ministry of Health. Each is headed by a minister who is appointed by the Central Soviet of the Republic and who is subject to the approval of the Ministry of Health of the USSR. Below the republican level, such as in a province, region, district, or city, the top executive health organ is the health department of that soviet (soviets are elected legislative councils at the local, regional, and national levels, culminating in the Supreme Soviet; see Figure 11.1).

The degree of centralization has fluctuated in the past. For instance, until Stalin's death, the Soviet administrative structure featured extreme centralization. The Khrushchev government decentralized the system somewhat by giving local administrations a limited autonomy, thereby decreasing the importance of the executive function performed by the Health Ministry of the USSR.

Merits of this centralized medical bureaucracy reside in its efficiency in making overall plans and coordinating activities. Medical needs are locally and nationally assessed; budgets are allocated in proportion to other needs in society; and available resources are rationally distributed throughout the country. In principle, this medical system can eliminate the problems of maldistribution of physicians by specialty and locality and of overlap of facilities, which plague the American medicine system based on free enterprise.

While American medicine can learn some lessons from the Soviet model, the latter suffers from its own shortcomings. Uniformity and standardization of this monolithic structure cause it to lack resilience because it does not allow self-evaluation and criticism nor does it accept new ideas and methods. Bureaucracy also has a tendency to be accompanied by individual members' lack of initiative, avoidance of personal responsibility, and indifference to their work (Fry, 1969). Finally, centralization of medical service has resulted in serving the interests of the Communist Party rather than the masses of the population (Navarro, 1977).

Networks of Health Services

In order to realize one of the major values of the Communist state—the availability and accessibility of medical care to everyone, their medical networks, as reported by Fry (1969), are closely integrated into a system of first-contact care, specialist care for the ambulatory, and inpatient services at hospitals (Field, 1967; Hyde, 1974).

Soviet cities, towns, and rural areas are divided into districts, which, in turn, are subdivided into microdistricts. Typically, as conceived in Soviet planning, a district has a population of 40,000, and it is divided into ten microdistricts of 4,000 adults and children each (Field, 1967, p. 89*f.*). Under the microdistrict

Figure 11.1: Health Service Organization–USSR

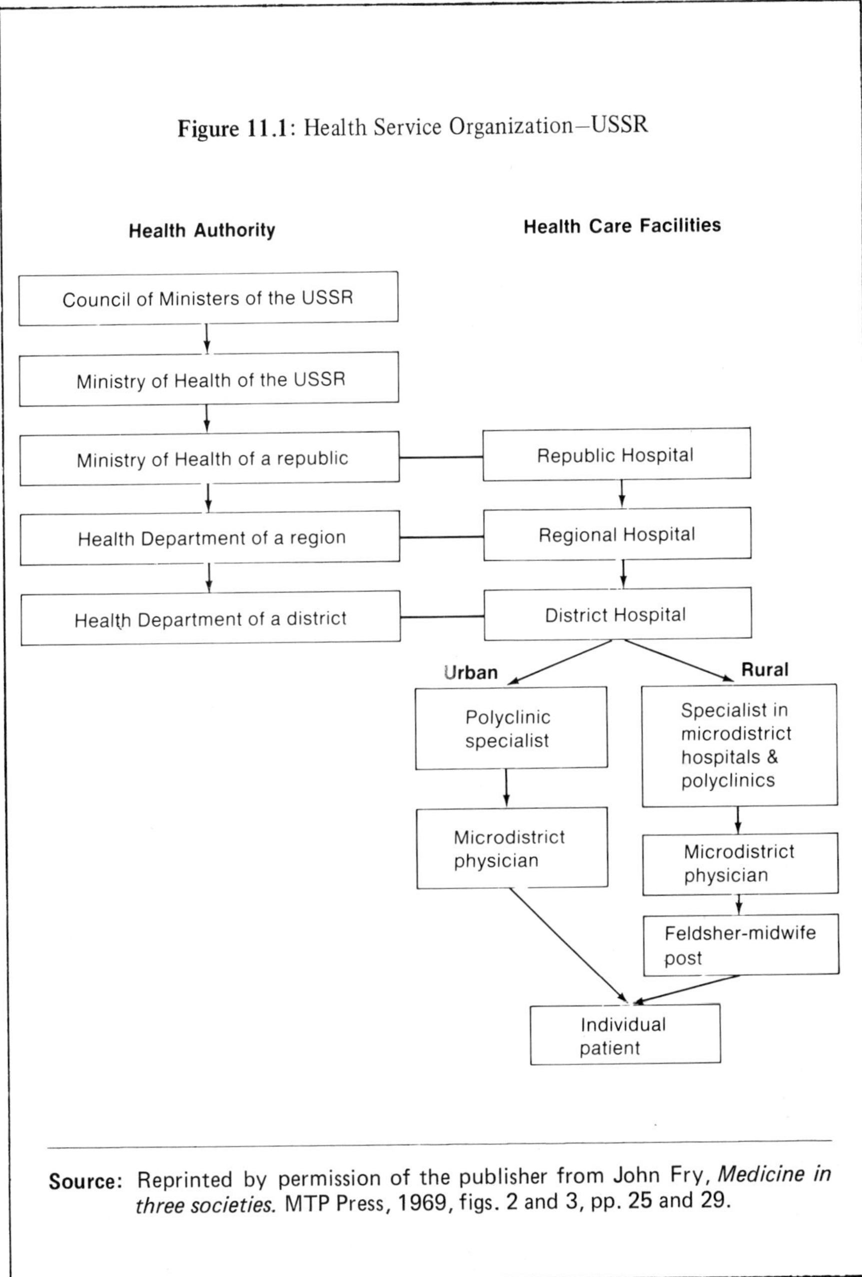

Source: Reprinted by permission of the publisher from John Fry, *Medicine in three societies.* MTP Press, 1969, figs. 2 and 3, pp. 25 and 29.

system, a person is assigned to a health territorial unit on the basis of residence.

First-contact care is based on the microdistrict principle. An urban microdistrict is served by its own physicians: a therapist (internist or general physician), a pediatrician, and an occupational physician. People living in a particular microdistrict are assigned to the care of the physician appointed for that area. Specificially, the occupational physician works in a large industrial unit in the area and provides first-contact care for 1,000 to 2,000 workers.

In the urban areas with a high population density, the microdistricts have no medical facilities of their own. There, the district is the smallest unit to have its own facilities, usually a polyclinic. Physicians in an urban microdistrict work from local polyclinics where they have special rooms, equipment, and nurses.

In larger cities, the polyclinics specialize according to the category of their patients—children, adults, and industrial workers, and according to different types of problems—psychiatric disorders, skin and venereal diseases, obstetric and gynecological conditions, tuberculosis, neoplasms, and the like. Thus, even in first-contact care, there is a considerable degree of division of labor. No arrangements are made for general practitioners to provide family care. Furthermore, polyclinics also provide the specialists, such as surgeons, opthalmologists, and psychiatrists, to whom patients may be referred. This combination of first-care and specialist care at the district polyclinics offers comprehensive health services in the community, with the exception of hospitalization, which will be discussed later.

In rural areas, a widely scattered population, difficulty with transportation, and above all, the physician shortage make it impossible for patients to receive regular first-contact care from a physician. As a substitute for physician services, a system of paramedical auxiliary care has been established. There are *feldsher*-midwife posts which are staffed by middle-grade health care personnel with nursing and medical training. The *feldsher* is what we would call the physician's assistant who works in close communication with and under the supervision of microdistrict physicians.

Some rural microdistricts have their own small hospitals, and the inhabitants do not have to travel long distances for health care. Such hospitals are combined with polyclinic (outpatient) services and are linked to the *feldsher*-midwife posts.

Americans can learn a great deal from the Soviet approach to first-contact care. In order to ensure ready and direct accessibility to medical services, it is practical to assign appropriate-sized populations to local physicians whether on a geographical basis or by some other criteria. In the United States there is no strong tradition whereby the physician feels bound to make himself or herself available and accessible to patients at all times. The nature and pattern of primary care vary according to the locale, social class, income, and other extraneous factors. Consequently, barriers have been created for some people, for example, the poor, in obtaining primary care services. The neighborhood health center and health maintenance organizations are examples of American efforts to remedy the situation, but as discussed in previous chapters, their impact has so far been limited.

In general, the hospitals in the USSR are primarily concerned with inpatient care and are graded according to the type of facilities provided. The first-level large hospitals in all areas are district hospitals. These are general hospitals, which deal with common acute and chronic medical, surgical, gynecological, and obstetric conditions. More specialized hospital units, such as cardiology, neurology, and neurosurgery, are situated in regional hospitals. Patients are normally referred to them through the district hospitals. The republic hospitals, which perform teaching functions, are at the top of the hospital hierarchy.

In addition to the territorial medical network described above, and through which the majority of the population receives its initial care, there are other, closed networks that cater exclusively to special categories of people. First there are the extensive facilities for the top political elite, including the Kremlin clinics. Second, the Academy of Sciences, a prestigious organization of the top cultural elite, has superior services reserved for its members. Third, members of the armed forces have their own health care system (Navarro, 1977).

On the other hand, the greatest number of users of closed health networks are found among industrial workers. In these cases, the health facilities are built and maintained by industrial plants and other organizations with their own budgetary resources. Health personnel, however, are appointed and paid by the local health department.

Medical Practice

The Soviet strategies for attaining the goal of national health are legitimized by the Marxist view that interprets illness as the result of defective social conditions. The state's efforts are directed toward changing the social structure, a goal which they believe will eliminate disease. Specifically, emphasis is placed on preventive medicine, public participation in health care services, health team practice, and the proletarianization of physicians.

Preventive Medicine. The importance assigned to preventive medicine is directly derived from the Marxian premise that a change in unhealthy environment—such as crowded substandard slums, unsanitary factories resulting from exploitation by the capitalists—will lead to the prevention of disease (Field, 1967, p. 159). As a result, much of the work in the polyclinics is for preventive purposes. It is reported that out of an average of ten annual polyclinic visits per person, one-half are for preventive examination (Fry, 1969, p. 61). In addition to regular clinical work, local physicians are actively engaged in health education and preventive measure (Lisitsin, 1972). The principle of prevention and health maintenance, such as in the form of the regular annual checkup, have been developed in the United States over the years. However, it has been confined to those who are either able to pay or to those who are covered by prepaid medical plans.

Public Participation. The ideology of a classless society inspires a mass participation in health administration. Although the medical profession is directly involved in administration, the base of the health delivery system is open to active trade union members, factory committees, collective farm associations, and to health committees of local soviets. There are also street committees, such as associations of local residents, that provide sociomedical assistance. Furthermore, by a decision of the Party General Committee and the Council of Ministers, public committees are formed at all medical establishments to attract more volunteers and to raise all-round medical standards (Hyde, 1974). However, Navarro (1977) says that public participation is limited to active and loyal members of the Party, and does not involve the grassroots.

Health Team. The health care team developed from pragmatic necessity as well as ideological commitment. The shortage of physicians compelled the transfer of some of the health care responsibilities from physicians to ancillary health workers. Physicians, *feldshers,* nurses, and others were made to cooperate in order to maximize scarce personnel resources. Ideologically, the notion of team work coincides with the proletarianization of physicians. With the physician as a manager, the middle-grade medical workers have no hierarchical relation to one another as team members.

Forgotson and Forgotson (1970) praised this equalitarian teamwork as a lesson to be learned by American medicine, which has only recently begun to nourish the idea. With the tradition of private fee-for-service practice, American medicine has provided few opportunities and incentives for bringing middle-grade workers into a health team. Also, patients who have paid for physicians are reluctant to be cared for by paramedical workers.

However, health teams in the USSR are not free from conflicts. Stresses have been reported when a young and relatively inexperienced physician on rural duty encounters a *feldsher* with many years of local experience. Viewing the physician as a threat to his or her antonomy and prestige, such a *feldsher* is not very cooperative. Another source of strain has been found between a physician who is not a Communist Party member and an ancillary personnel who is a Party member. The physician's medical authority is likely to be undermined by medically subordinate members who have political power (Field, 1957).

In short, the Soviet health team is not free from built-in conflicts. Nevertheless, it has a longer history than the American health team concept and its experience may be able to offer valuable lessons to Americans.

The Physicians. As already discussed, the efforts of the state to proletarianize medical students were not effective. However, the elitist status of the prerevolutionary physician was reduced to that of public employee.

The Soviet government broke up the traditional training system by closing the university medical schools and by placing the facilities at the disposition of separate institutions. This resulted in shortening the courses, speeding up the process toward specialization, and thereby attracting more students to a medcial education (Kaser, 1976).

Professional training of physicians consists of six years at a medical institute upon completion of a secondary school, usually at the age of 17 or 18. There is no formal internship parallel to the American system except that the sixth year constitutes a clinical experience. Physicians are trained in one of the three basic specialities—general medicine, pediatrics, or public health—but students usually postpone further specialization until they fulfill the mandatory obligation to work in the countryside for three years after graduation from a medical institute (Field, 1967, p. 120).

As salaried employees, physicians are expected to work a set number of hours. They generally have a five-day week schedule of six and a half to seven hours a day. A "day" refers to one three-hour consulting session plus a three-hour visiting session. At the polyclinic, the local pediatrician or therapist is supposed to see 15 patients during the three hour session, which allows each patient about 12 minutes. Visiting sessions consist of making six house calls, and each visit should average half an hour, including the travel time. In addition, 30 minutes to an hour of the physician's day is devoted to health education (Fry, 1969, p. 62).

Pressed for time, the Soviet physician might have a tendency to process patients as fast as possible. However, this is not unique to Soviet medicine; it is also common in a prepaid program that is conducted on a capitation basis. As a matter of fact, Soviet physicians, as state employees and public officials, are under stricter control with respect to the quality of their practice than physicians in other countries (Field, 1957, p. 967).

Physicians are hired either by the health departments at the different administrative levels or by the industrial organizations, and they are paid according to a scale of wages. Their salaries are lower than corresponding salaries for the technical intelligentsia, such as engineers or architects (Field, 1957), although higher than school teachers (Ryan, 1970).

This lower status of physicians as compared to that of American counterparts (Navarro, 1977) is primarily due to the high priority given to the productive sector of the economy rather than the service sector. In the light of the overall work force shortage and the priority commitment to industrialization, an expansion of the medical sector has been made possible by the large-scale recruitment of women into medicine. The great majority, 80 percent, of local or microdistrict physicians are women, although the top positions tend to be held by men (Swafford, 1978).

It is true that all top hospital administrators, from the Minister of Health on down, are practicing physicians. But this does not give power to the physicians as a group. Frequently, administrative posts are occupied by Communist Party physicians, who tend to exert some pressure over the non-Party practitioners. Physicians who join the Party, either from ideological belief or for opportunistic gain, represent a threat to the medical profession since their primary allegiance is to the Party rather than to their occupation (Field, 1967, p. 127).

Not only have Soviet physicians lost their professional autonomy, but their title and rights in the Medical Workers' Union are the same as those of their health union members, such as nurses, orderlies, and hospital gatekeepers. In addition, the union is not in a position to bargain with or to strike against the employer because the employer, whose position is unassailable, is the state itself. In fact, the trade union has become an instrument of the state to control the workers.

It should be noted, however, that in addition to the regular physicians described above, there are two higher-grade physicians: the academician and the professor. The professors must have obtained one or two advanced academic degrees with rigorous requirements after having completed the regular medical education. The academicians are elected from the group of professors. Ascending the medical hierarchy, the number of physicians decreases, while status and income increases dramatically (Field, 1967). The high-status physicians hold responsible positions in health service administration, in research, and in clinical work. The task of treating the sick falls upon regular physicians who consitute the bulk of the physicians. Thus, the medical profession in the USSR is highly stratified (Navarro, 1977), and the two top ranks of physicians appear to occupy a status rank corresponding to that of American physicians.

The Quality of Care. The quality of medical care can be evaluated by such measures as availability and accessibility of medical services, the level of medical technology (science of medicine), the therapist–patient relationship (art of medicine), and the outcome of medical practice. However, comparison of the quality of medical care in the USSR and the United States is rendered difficult by the inadequacy of published statistics and research data (Kaser, 1976).

In the USSR, availability and accessibility to medical care is high since everyone is assigned to a physician who is required to make himself or herself available at all times and to make frequent house calls. Further, there is little shortage of doctors or paramedical personnel. Between 1910 and 1970 the number of physicians in the United States increased 2.5 times, while in the Soviet Union the increase was almost 25 times. The number of physicians per unit of population remains fairly stable in the United States, as compared with an increase of 16 to 18 times in the Soviet Union, which now has about a 50 percent higher proportion than in the United States (Field, 1975, U.S. DHEW, 1975; U.S. National Center for Health Statistics, 1974).

Medical utilization rates are higher in the USSR than in the United States. While the United States has a per capita utilization rate of 4 to 6 visits per year, the USSR has a rate of 9 to 12 visits to physicians per year. However, health care-seeking behavior is not simply a function of the availability of facilities but is affected by sociocultural values and other factors (see Chapter 5).

The level of technical proficiency in Soviet medicine is difficult to assess. Many foreign visitors are impressed by the emergency care system, which is made possible by the abundance of personnel and financial resources. On the other hand, the bulk of the patients are attended by regular doctors who have received a shorter period of education than their American counterparts. In the rural areas the sick are frequently cared for by *feldshers,* who have had even less training (Navarro, 1977).

As for the art of medicine, the absence of freedom of choice of physicians, the bureaucratization of salaried physicians, and the pressure of the work norm may be considered as obstacles to physician–patient rapport. However, many patients seem to appreciate the structural pressures upon physicians and also note a large individual variation in physicians' attitudes toward patients (Field,

1957). Yet, the erosion of the physician's authority is noted as in other societies, which is partially attributable to increasing sophistication of clients in medical matters (Haug, 1976).

As for the outcome of this health care, there are still no systematic comprehensive survey series on mortality or morbidity in the USSR, although total secrecy has been broken in recent years. By the mid-1970s the death rate in the two countries was comparable: 8.9 per 1,000 population in the United States in 1976 and 9.3 in the USSR in 1975. However, the infant mortality rate is still considerably higher in the USSR (17.7 per 1,000 live births) than in the United States (15.1).

Finance and Personnel Resources

In the USSR, the individual patient does not have to pay the doctor, hospital, or clinic directly for medical services, but drugs prescribed for outpatient use are exceptions.

Financing of Health Care

In order to make the national health care service work efficiently, careful planning and budgeting of health expenditures are made. The planning starts with estimates of future requirements based on the projected general population (Popov, 1971).

In each district, a health inventory is carried out, which regularly measures the standards of equipment, staffing, and various social facilities. At the same time, analyses are made concerning the age, sex, and occupational composition of the population; the morbidity rates; and the nature of the local climate, geography, and economy. Deficiencies are estimated, and an arrangement for the forthcoming period is made that will attempt to meet national standards and norms. Similar analyses are performed at the higher regional, republic, and eventually at the national level.

Indirect financing of health care can be separated into government resources, social insurance, and other sources.

The government finances are obtained largely by the turnover tax, essentially a sales or excise tax applied to all consumer goods. Another source for the state treasury consists of payments based on a percentage of profits by industrial organizations (Field, 1967, p. 190).

These taxes are balanced at various territorial levels in that shortfalls from or excesses above planned expenditures are corrected against the territorially accrued revenue (Kaser, 1976, p. 62). These taxes are channelled into the state treasury and are reallocated to the health sector according to the approved state plan.

The extensive system of social insurance operated through the trade unions and the collective farmers' groups provide for partial or full salary compensation to workers who have been officially declared sick or injured. In addition, the social insurance covers the costs for resort cures, dietetic needs, and prosthetics.

An example of the category of other types of financing is the contributions made by businesses both to the capital and current costs of health posts, polyclinics, and hospitals on their premises (Kaser, 1976).

Despite this well-planned socialization of medicine, legal private practices do exist, although not extensively. They are limited because the consulting room must be authorized as properly equipped and the practitioner's income is subject to a very high rate of tax (Kaser, 1976).

Work Force Supply

Despite the ideology of equal accessibility by everyone to health care services, the uneven distribution of medical personnel and the physician shortage in rural areas have been problems in the USSR. This was partly due to the state's initial heavy emphasis on industrialization, improvement of the status of the proletariat, and neglect of rural conditions (Field, 1975).

One solution has been found in the assignment of a three-year rural duty to graduating medical students. This is considered to be a means for them to repay the government and the "people" for financing their education.

Another compromise has been achieved whereby paramedical workers, such as nurses, midwives, and *feldshers,* provide some of the initial care to the rural inhabitants. The *feldsher* (Field, 1967; Forgotson & Forgotson, 1970; Sidel, 1968) is a semiprofessional health worker, officially known as a physician's assistant. The *feldsher* was originally introduced into Russian armies in the seventeenth century. In the nineteenth century, civilian *feldshers,* mostly retired military *feldshers,* began to practice in rural areas. Though the Soviet Union once intended to eliminate this second-class medical practice, that proved impractical because of the shortage of medical workers in the villages. In theory, the *feldshers* are only physician's assistants, but in practice they fulfil many medical functions in the absence of physicians.

There are both positive and negative appraisals of *feldshers* in Soviet writings. For instance, in a study of 30 *feldsher* stations in 1967 (Sidel, 1968), the *feldshers* are given credit for the fall of 10 percent in the morbidity rate for children in the first year of life, a fall of 14 percent among children up to age 15, and an overall reduction of 73 percent in childhood mortality over a five-year period.

On the other hand, the rural *feldshers* are also criticized:

> Of the 180,000 inhabitants of the villages in the Berezin, . . . 75.4% live in areas served by feldsher-midwife stations.
>
> In one year over 96,000 calls were made to medical institutions: 52.5% to doctors and 41.9% to feldshers. . . . Unfortunately, the inexpertness of rural medium-trained medical workers has been demonstrated many times.
>
> Feldshers have most difficulty in diagnosing diphtheria, dysentery, and tuberculosis. Very often they are slow to recognize symptoms of ulcer disease of the stomach or of the duodenum, and they make not a few mistakes in diagnosing diseases of the cardio-vascular system and of the upper respiratory tract (Sidel, 1968, p. 938).

In summary, the USSR medical delivery system is an example of a centralized system, the opposite of the American laissez-faire voluntary practice. It has attained the goal of providing free comprehensive medical service to everyone through third-party control of medical practice.

However, the basic nature of Soviet medicine is not significantly different from that in the United States. In an attempt to overtake Western technology and industrialization, the USSR has adopted the kind of scientific medicine advocated by the 1910 Flexner Report, led by hospital-based specialists in urban areas, rather than a decentralized model with the massive participation of the population in preventive medicine, paramedical work, and health administration. Even the institution of *feldshers* has not helped much because, as physician's assistants, they are likely to accompany physicians into urban areas.

In other words, as Navarro (1977) points out, nationalization of Soviet medicine is not the same as socialization. In the USSR the take-over of the state by a minority group representing the working class has not been accompanied by the extension of power to the majority. Power is concentrated in the Communist Party, which delegates some authority to medical professionals. Nationalization of medicine becomes socialization only when it is used as a political vehicle toward the democratization and self-government of the people. In this sense, the experience of the People's Republic of China may provide a better model of socialized medicine, in that citizen control over the medical delivery system, deprofessionalization, and rustification are emphasized.

THE PEOPLE'S REPUBLIC OF CHINA

Social Background

The historical background of the People's Republic of China resembles that of the USSR in that both countries have long histories of ancient civilizations occupying vast land areas, each experienced drastic revolutionary changes during this century, each entered into radically different sociopolitical systems. At first, China adopted the Leninist type of Party dictatorship. However, similarities end there. Some 700 million people, more than the combined populations of the United States, the USSR, and the United Kingdom, live in an area about the size of the continental United States. The Chinese population is concentrated in agricultural areas—approximately 80 percent of the people work on farms.

In the history of the rapidly changing society of the People's Republic of China, two dates are significant: the Liberation of 1949 that resulted from the victory of the Communist forces headed by Mau Zedong (Mao Tse-tung), and the Cultural Revolution that began in 1965.

Pre-Liberation. For over three hundred years, China was a self sufficient empire that saw itself as the center of civilization. Prior to the Communist Liberation, however, the country was desolated by years of war (Fairbank, 1971), which disrupted agricultural and industrial production and caused extensive food shortage and consequent malnutrition and disease. The populace's medical resources were meager, health facilities were scarce, and physicians were ill-trained traditonal practitioners of herb medicine (Sidel & Sidel, 1973).

After the Liberation. During the 1950s the Communists attempted to develop an agricultural surplus as an investment in the future while they simultaneously encouraged industrialization. The policy of the Great Leap Forward (1958–1962) called for the people to work longer hours. Then, to mobilize labor more efficiently, the leaders changed the already collectivized agricultural cooperatives into communes of about 5,000 households. Unlike the cooperatives, which were purely economic organizations, the communes became units of both political and economic organizations. Assemblies of representative commune members now function as the congress of the townships and the people (Sidel & Sidel, 1973). This labor allocation on a massive scale through the communes accomplished remarkable economic productivity, but it also drove the people to exhaustion. The leaders were finally forced to relax the process and to decentralize the communes (Welty, 1973).

Their pragmatic revolutionary leader, Mau Zedong, placed a high priority on health care. He set the direction for the future health system and specified that it would serve the working people—workers, peasants, and soldiers; place priority upon preventive over curative medicine; unite traditional and Western medicine; and integrate the masses into public health activities (Liang et al., 1973). Implementation of these principles was facilitated by an influx of consultants, technology, and organizational methodology from the Soviet Union.

The Cultural Revolution. Agricultural productivity and economic development were curtailed somewhat when, in 1965, Chairman Mau summoned millions of Red Guards to spearhead the Great Proletarian Cultural Revolution. Mau tried to ferret out all the counterrevolutionaries in the Party, government, communes, unions, factories, and elsewhere.

The Ministry of Health and the Chinese Medical Association were particular targets of that criticism. Despite the fact that the Ministry of Health carried out its assigned job reasonably well from 1950 to 1965, especially considering the paucity of its resources, the Ministry was blamed by Mau for the persistence of inferior service in rural areas, continued emphasis on curative rather than preventive medicine, and the neglect of traditional medicine. Mau's corrective prescription consisted of shortening medical education, emphasizing practical training, stressing research in preventive medicine, and improving medical practice in rural areas.

Post-Cultural Revolution. Following the death of Mau and the dethronement of the Gang of Four (a small ingroup headed by Mau's wife) in late 1976, drastic shifts in policy occurred. The new ideological line emphasized the four areas of modernization—agriculture, defense, science, and technology. Correspondingly, the official attitude toward education and research changed. The Gang of Four was blamed for the severe disruptions of education and research that occurred during the Cultural Revolution. Thus, full university curricula were restored, graduate training was resumed, and above all, intellectual ability was recredited (Abelson, 1979).

In the following sections the consequences of the Cultural Revolution in the health field will be examined in some detail.

Value Orientation

Mau Zedong inherited Marx's perception of class conflict and Lenin's technique for revolution. However, Mau tailored his precursors' principles to fit Chinese tradition and his own observations of Chinese social reality.

While Lenin acknowledged the need for intensive industrialization, Mau focused his attention on the transformation of the Chinese "soul" as a prerequisite to modernization. He aligned himself less with Marx than with the romantic utopians who had interpreted history as determined by the spiritual rather than by material forces (An, 1972; Chen, 1975; Karnow, 1972; North, 1963).

Mau's ideology, with its stress on human perfectibility, is largely moralistic. Deprecating those who strive only for personal fame, profit, and power, Mau called for the cultivation of humanity dedicated to his new morality: Communists who are wholeheartedly devoted to the people. Mau proclaimed that this spiritual approach elevated Marxist-Leninism to a higher and completely new stage.

Despite his disavowal of Confucius, whose doctrine of social harmony was opposed to his preoccupation with revolution, Mau was never free from Chinese tradition. Like the ancient dynastic founders, he relied upon military strength to gain power, all the while nurturing a personality cult designed to portray himself as a charismatic leader. Moreover, he subscribed to the Confucian tenet of virtue as a key principle in public conduct.

Mau's authoritarianism was also tempered by Western influences such as Biblical axioms, homiles by Benjamin Franklin, and the romantic utopianism of Rousseau. Mau accused Stalin of neglecting to transform the Russian soul in his single-minded pursuit of industrialization.

It should be added that Mau's ideas were not accepted by many circles, including some Chinese Communists, and this necessitated the Cultural Revolution to purge his opponents.

Health Values. The Chinese Communists quickly recognized the need to protect China's largest resources—its population, and so health problems became the concern of economic and political strategies (Rifkin, 1973). Thus, Mau's moral-political messages included the implementation of correct health conduct. An ideological attachment to Mau was used as a basis to motivate patients and health workers to achieve and maintain good health. The most serious functional disability of an illness was interpreted as the inability to perform acts appropriate for Mau. In short, individual or collective acts of health conduct were raised to the highest moral and political plane (Chin, 1973).

More specifically, Mau's idea of human perfectibility is translated in the health field as the elimination of the feudal mentality anchored in the ancient belief that natural calamities are fixed by heaven. Preventive medicine and the mobilization of the general public in health activities are emphasized in the fight against one's own diseases (Sidel & Sidel, 1973).

The Chinese claim that their health care system is superior to that of the Soviet Union because the USSR lacks concern for the peasants. In contrast, not only are medical students but also urban doctors, teachers, and researchers of China assigned to rural duties in order to be re-educated in the needs of peasants (Gibson, 1972).

The efforts to remove traditional elitism are also apparent in medical training. Pre-Liberation attitudes, that of the superiority of intellectual endeavor as compared to manual labor, persisted to some extent in the 1950s and 1960s. During the Cultural Revolution, however, the "massification" of medical education was enforced. Students usually left school at the age of 15 or 16 after completing a junior middle school. Then they went to work in a commune or factory for two or three years. After that, fellow workers chose those who were to be proposed for admission to medical schools. The criteria for selection was not based on academic ability but on attitudes and political ideology (Sidel & Sidel, 1973). Then, while at medical school, students were required to attend lectures on history and the doctrines of the Communist Party in order to internalize the value that health conduct is a higher-order political act.

Since the denunciation of the Gang of Four, however, there has been a complete ideological twist. In order to train technically competent scientists and engineers, educational standards observed prior to 1966 were restored. In particular, educational attainment as measured by examination rather than by peer review, was re-emphasized (Abelson, 1979).

Organization and Administration of Health Service

Organization of Health Administration

The politicization of health care services was attempted from various angles (Chen, 1976): placing politically reliable nonprofessionals in key positions of health administration and bringing medical professionals into the Party in order to transform their ideology. Yet, the power of the medical profession was strong enough to work through the Ministry of Public Health to oppose Party politics, at least, from time to time. The health care system posed a potential threat to the polity since the latter was ill equipped to evaluate the technical expertise of health workers.

The relationship between the Chinese government and the medical profession has been viewed by some from the functionalist perspective of system integration. For example, Gibson (1972) claimed that even during the Cultural Revolution, the latent malintegration between the medical profession and Party politics was resolved by the use of ideology. Communist ideology penetrated all spheres of the social system: it defined societal goals and resolved tensions among conflicting groups. Gibson reached this conclusion by analyzing the *Peking Review,* an official theoretical journal of social and political ideas. He did not claim, however, that the *Peking Review* reflected the reality of the Chinese health system but only that it portrayed the official dogma presented to the outside world.

In contrast to Gibson's functional assumption of social integration, Lampton (1974) viewed the developmental process of health administration in China as a sequential conflict resolution among competing interest groups with different leadership and different mixtures of social values. Within this framework, Lampton examined the succession of health policy-making patterns as a cyclic rise and fall of a bureaucratic model.

1949–1955: Bureaucratic System. When Chairman Mau came to power in 1949, the Chinese Communist Party was inadequately prepared to handle health administration. Most Party cadre had too little formal education or training to be placed in core positions. The new leadership had to use all available personnel resources at the cost of ideological purity (Karnow, 1972). As a result, the Ministry of Public Health was established and staffed largely by Western-style medical doctors. Being entrusted with relatively comprehensive policy-making authority, this ministry attempted to resist the complete political absorption of its professional work.

This type of system was called "bureaucratic" by Lampton (1974) because it combined elements of central control with relative independence of various ministries (see Figure 11.2). The central Party and the state assumed the role of referee to resolve interministry disputes according to broad programmatic objectives.

Nevertheless, the power of the Ministry of Public Health was limited since it was obliged to cooperate and negotiate with other ministries and agencies that also dealt with health issues. For example, the health ministry encountered difficulties in persuading the Commercial and Chemical ministries to lower the price of drugs (Lampton, 1974). Another constraint was placed upon the ministry by specific directives coming from the higher Party organs and Mau himself, who believed that "it is a general rule for the layman to lead the expert . . . only the layman is capable of leading an expert" (Chen, 1976, p. 5).

1955–1960: Divided System. Because of fear of the perceived independence of the Ministry of Public Health, the central Party undertook a transformation in health administration during 1955–1960. Important policy responsibilities were removed progressively from the health ministry to the newly created Nine-Man Subcommittee headed by nonmedical personnel. While the ministry dealt with educational, research, and administrative programs, the subcommittee devoted itself to rural health needs, particularly to the establishment of communal health centers and antiparasitic work.

The central Party accused the ministry of not fulfilling the goals set by Mau, especially in rural areas. The ministry defended itself by saying that it was hesitant to assume responsibility for communal health clinics when the budget was so scanty. Health centers were built by the subcommittee as basic parts of communes and were administered by nonmedical cadre who viewed the program as an inducement to peasants to participate in the commune movement.

Figure 11.2: Health Policy-Making Systems—People's Republic of China

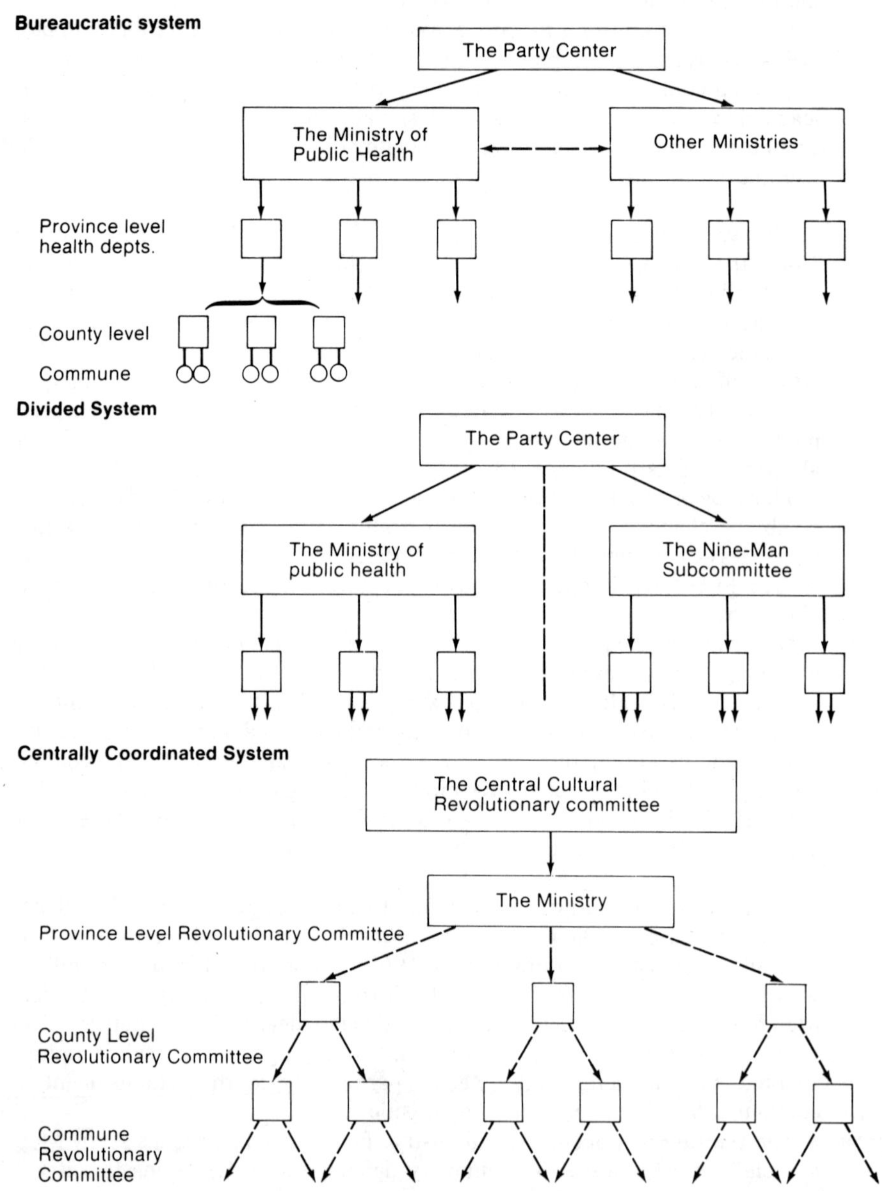

Source: Reprinted from *Health, Conflict, and the Chinese Political System* by David M. Lampton by permission of the University of Michigan Center for Chinese Studies, © 1974, charts 1, 2, & 3 on pp. 96, 98, and 99.

A program to eliminate parasitic diseases was established by the subcommittee, which had no regular channels for consulting with medical and scientific organizations. As a consequence, there were some negative effects such as adverse reactions to highly toxic drugs administered by untrained personnel (Lampton, 1974, p. 101).

The divided health policy system suffered from a lack of coordination. For example, the rapidly rising need for health personnel caused by the creation of communal health centers and antiparasitic projects was not accompanied by an increased supply of physicians. Curricula in some prestigious medical schools were lengthened in response to the health ministry's appeal for quality education (Cheng, 1973). In general, though Mau believed that the rural–urban gap in health care services was being reduced, doctors, researchers, and educators lamented a decline in professional standards.

However, the divided system had definite advantages as well. It made health policy more responsive to a broader range of social inputs. Prior to 1955 rural health needs were largely neglected (Almond & Powell, 1966). It was the antiparasitic policy and the communal curative facilities that enlisted provincial, local, and communal opinions, energies, and activities.

1960–1965: Return to the Bureaucratic System. The divided health policy system was replaced by the bureaucratic system from 1960 to 1965. The subcommittee became inactive during this period.

1966–1970: Centrally Coordinated System. During the Cultural Revolution, the health ministry became a nominal administrative body. Major directives were issued from the Revolutionary Committee. This centralization in policy making was accompanied by decentralization in policy implementation. Local units were encouraged to take an active role in carrying out the centrally determined policies (An, 1972; Chen, 1975; Risse, 1973). However, there was no middle-level bureaucracy that could serve an intermediary function between the Revolutionary Committee and local units.

The advantage of this system was the central coordination of policies; these included a shortening of medical education, autonomous financing in rural areas, and universalizing of commune clinics.

Aside from these three major areas, however, the range of policy was limited because of the concentration of power in the elite, who resisted input from other sources. Therefore, the Revolutionary Committee was prone to ignore such important fields as medical research, professional life and association, and mass campaigns.

Another shortcoming of a centralized system with no middle-level bureaucracy was the lack of clarity in policy interpretation at the local level, hence slow policy implementation. For example, the directive for shortening medical education to three years was issued in 1968, but it was not put into practice until 1970–1971 (Berger, 1973). Further, the concentration of power in a few people means that any change in the composition of the elite can result in a large difference in policy making, hence, policy instability.

The Bureaucratic System Again. Because of these difficulties, the system again reverted to the bureaucratic model in 1970.

The bureaucratic model is not an ideal arrangement but it appears to have the strength of both the divided and centralized systems. The bureaucratic system is more coordinated than the divided apparatus and is more receptive to a wide range of social input than the centralized system. Yet, the bureaucracy suffers from its unique weakness—structural rigidity, which generates the seed for its own destruction.

Networks of Health Services

Urban Areas. The health services of the cities are coordinated by the local bureau of public health, which deals not only with health care services and personnel but also with educational programs for allied health care workers (Sidel & Sidel, 1973).

The next lower level of urban organization is the district (covering an area with a population of 250,000–500,000), which is subdivided into streets (with a population of 50,000–100,000), and neighborhoods (2,500–12,000). This is the lowest level of the formal governmental organization in the cities (New & New, 1975).

The people are grouped into resident committees, which encompass about 2,000 people. These committees usually provide health stations and other social functions.

In addition, factories in urban areas offer highly organized medical services. There is a central clinic as well as health stations in individual workshops; sometimes there may even be a factory hospital.

The backup institution for the neighborhood resident committees and factory health stations is the neighborhood hospital. The public health department serving a neighborhood is located in the hospital. Hospitals in the cities range from small neighborhood facilities for ambulatory patients to large hospitals for technologically sophisticated research and teaching.

Rural Areas. The commune is the lowest level of formal state power in the rural areas, analogous to the neighborhood in the cities, and it is responsible for the overall planning, education, and provision of health and social services. The commune is divided into production brigades (with a population of 2,000–5,000) that in turn, are subdivided into production teams (200–800) ("China . . . ," 1974; New & New, 1975; Rifkin, 1973; Sidel & Sidel, 1973).

A production brigade has its own health station from which patients are referred to the commune hospital. County hospitals are generally located in the towns, and they serve the people in that area as well as those referred from the commune hospitals. The size and availability of facilities at brigade health stations and commune hospitals vary widely from commune to commune (Sidel & Sidel, 1973).

Medical Practice

Every revolutionary regime, no matter how radical, must work with what it has inherited from the past. The Chinese Communist Party found itself ruling a predominantly peasant population with very few Western-trained physicians available (Croizier, 1968). The limited production of physicians that resulted from following Western educational models seemed inappropriate and inadequate to meet China's massive needs for medical care. Thus, Mau undertook the task of restructuring medical training programs and of promoting Chinese traditional medical practice along with Western medicine.

Medical Training. One of the first actions taken in the post-Liberation period was to increase the number of medical personnel being trained. Following the Soviet model, many medical schools were split into adult therapeutic medicine, pediatrics, public health, and stomatology. The length of formal medical education was reduced to three years.

The curriculum emphasized practical clinical experience rather than classroom lectures on theories of medical matters (Heller, 1973). For example, the faculty and students were organized into mobile medical teams that visited rural areas in order to see and participate in the entire spectrum of medicine (Dimond, 1971).

Postgraduate residency training in clinical specialties still exists in China, but the number of specialty trainees appears to be far fewer than that of primary care students. Candidates for specialty education are chosen by their fellow workers, and their salaries are continued during the training period. They are expected to return to their work units such as factories or communes upon completion of their residency at teaching universities. The requirements for completion of the training are not standardized through national boards. Department members, including physicians, nurses, technicians, and others, determine whether or not a resident is ready, after about one year of training, to become a full-fledged physician (Sidel & Sidel, 1973, p. 124).

Traditional Medicine. The inclusion of traditional Chinese medicine into the mainstream health care system was necessitated by the difficulty of increasing the number of Western-style physicians in a short period of time. Traditional practitioners constituted the only work force available in many rural areas. Also, some rural residents would refuse to accept Western-style treatment if it were available.

Ideologically, traditional medicine was interpreted as an expression of the wisdom of the masses and a symbol of antielitism. It also represented cultural nationalism. During the time of the Chinese reaction against Soviet dominance in the 1950s, traditional medicine was given special support as a source of Chinese cultural heritage (Vogel, 1973). This support was reinforced by the belief that some traditional medical techniques are efficacious. Thus, traditional Chinese medicine became politically legitimate.

The main features and techniques of traditional medicine are based on a unique therapeutic concept and philosophy: there are assumed to be two elements, yin (negative, dark, and feminine) and yang (positive, bright, and masculine), whose interaction influences the destinies of creatures and things (Croizier, 1968; Sidel & Sidel, 1973).

The Chinese have used medicinal herbs from earliest times. Their effectiveness has been established only by trial-and-error empiricism. Chinese physicians use herbs to restore internal harmony of patients; thus they prescribe something to make up a deficiency of yang, or to aid the fire element against an excess of water, or to remove an impediment to the free circulation of the vital life force. Among the herbs which have been widely used are: *ma huang* (ephedra) for the treatment of hay fever, asthma, and nasal congestion; *securinega suffruticos* for chronic paralysis; and *thevetja peruviana* for cardiac problems.

Since disease is considered to rise out of a disequilibrium of yin and yang in the human organism, the basic cure is to restore harmony. Acupuncture is another technique for doing this; it is used on a wide variety of maladies, including mental illness. The basic theory of acupuncture is that channels which run throughout the internal organs of the body are connected to sites on the skin. Stimulation of these sites by inserting needles or by applying electric shock equalizes the balance between the opposite forces in the body.

Chinese manipulative arts—massage, reduction of dislocations, and bone setting—again go beyond relieving sore muscles or realigning bones to setting the patient's entire mind and body at rest. They accomplish the task by relying heavily upon the natural healing power of the human body. For example, the Chinese treat fractures by a gradual realignment, often using a splint, leaving the neighboring joints free to exercise. This is quite different from the American method of bringing two ends of broken bones into realignment in a single forcible thrust under anesthesia.

Traditional medicine is no longer passed on through apprenticeship but is taught in medical schools modeled after modern Western schools. A traditional physician in a clinic is considered to be equal to the specialists and is placed on the same salary scale as a Western-style physician (Sidel & Sidel, 1973).

According to the study by Lee (1975), physicians trained in Western-style medicine are likely to consider Western medicine to be superior, while traditional practitioners are inclined to perceive no significant difference in competence between the two styles of medicine. Patients, however, tend to believe in the effectiveness of Western medicine for the treatment of infectious diseases; to consider Chinese herbs as more effectual than Western drugs in promoting and maintaining good health (Lee, 1975); and to initially seek care from Western physicians (Gale, 1975).

Physicians' Status. In Communist societies, the health care system is not allowed much flexibility to decide its own goals nor the autonomy to exercise professional judgment. Since political ideology rather than professional stature is the criteria for clinical success, status distinction among physicians, other health workers, patients, manual laborers, and others cannot be maintained on the basis of professional expertise (Gibson, 1972).

Physicians are paid salaries determined by their labor classification because the self-employment system has almost completely disappeared (Wen & Hays, 1976). Manual workers frequently earn more than physicians, which does not seem to bother the latter greatly. Willox (1966) explains that physicians need less food than heavy manual workers and that money is of small value in a Communist society where there is so little to spend it on.

However, unlike the pattern in the Soviet Union, where separate professional medical associations were abolished, the Chinese Medical Association has remained exclusively a physician's organization. Since it is closely intertwined with the Ministry of Public Health, the Chinese Medical Association can occasionally exert pressure on the government (Lampton, 1974; Sidel & Sidel, 1973).

Finance and Personnel Resources

Financing of medical care is not nationalized in Communist China. The scarcity of funds, medical facilities, and personnel still renders free and universally available health care a distant vision (Vogel, 1973).

Financing of Health Care

The strategy of the Chinese government in financing health care is to transfer the burden to those whom it benefits directly: the rural communes, production brigades, and production teams (Heller, 1973). Although the central government subsidizes elements of health programs, it requires the local units to demonstrate their ability to mobilize their own resources.

Rural Areas. A typical budget allocation for a production team consists of the fund for maintenance, a public accumulation fund (including reserves for reinvestment, education, health, and welfare), and a remainder, which constitutes between 40 to 60 percent of the total. This last category of money is redistributed to the members according to their labor output, once the individual is assured of an adequate food ration (Lampton, 1974; Wen & Hays, 1976).

Each brigade owns and manages a Coop Medical Care Plan, which provides prepaid insurance coverage. A variable amount of matching funds are added from the brigade (or commune) to the premiums paid by the members. Subscribers to the plan are entitled to receive diagnostic and therapeutic treatments and drugs free of charge.

Most of the charges at hospitals are reimbursable through this plan except for the registration fees, the hospital meal expenses, and the amount that exceeds the coverage ceiling. For an emergency, a Public Accumulation Fund and/or low interest loans are available in most communes.

Urban Areas. Factory workers, office employees, and schoolteachers are fully covered under a governmental health plan. They have unlimited access to inpatient and outpatient services at the affiliated clinics and hospitals, and no payment is required.

Their families enjoy a 50 percent cost reduction for all health services. For those that may not be completely covered, there is an employer-initiated and locally administered Collective Group Care Plan that provides supplementary medical coverage (Wen & Hays, 1976).

Each street and lane in the urban areas has a Mass Prevention–Mass Treatment Clinic that provides primary care for the residents in its jurisdiction. A fee is collected for each curative service. The policy of financial self-sufficiency applies to both hospitals and clinics.

In short, a modification of fee-for-service along with prepayment plans is the method of payment for curative services. The government assumes major responsibility for the provision of free preventive services such as immunization, cancer screening, and flouridation (Jonas et al., 1975).

Work Force Supply

The shortage of physicians in China is alleviated by the creation of paramedical personnel for primary and preventive medical services (Cheng, 1973).

Barefoot Doctors. In the late 1950s efforts were begun to train indigeneous personnel who participated in agricultural production to also deliver health care (New & New, 1975; Sidel & Sidel, 1973).

Despite the fact that they spend much of their time doing medical work, these paramedics, called barefoot doctors, receive the usual wages of agricultural workers, and they perceive themselves primarily as peasants rather than as health workers. The term "barefoot" is used to emphasize a peasant orientation, not a lack of footwear.

Their formal training may be accomplished during three to four months on the job supervised by physicians, which usually spread over successive years. It may also be completed in three to six months of training followed by a period of practical experience.

Their duties vary from area to area, commune to commune, and even from brigade to brigade within the same commune. In general, however, barefoot doctors have responsibility for environmental sanitation (e.g., proper collection, treatment, storage, and use of human feces as fertilizer; and pest control), health education (e.g., teaching hygiene and birth control to commune members and training auxiliary health workers), immunization, first aid, aspects of personal primary care and postillness follow-up, planting and collecting herbs, and so on. More complicated medical problems are referred to the commune health station. However, many communes are moving in the direction of upgrading training so that the barefoot doctors may advance from the position of an aide giving first aid to that of an allied health worker who can deliver curative services (Wang, 1975).

The efficacy of the barefoot doctors is frequently measured by the amount of work productivity they save. If the barefoot doctors were not in the brigade, the population would be compelled to go to the communes for treatment, which could take a whole day for the round trip and require the accompaniment of a healthy adult. Thus, the reduction in working days lost to sickness and the amount of traveling and waiting time saved by the availability of barefoot doctors are important indexes of effectiveness of medical care. Also, the cost for training the barefoot doctors is lower than that required for Western-style doctors. Apart from the cost efficiency, the barefoot doctors are credited with practicing preventative medicine, thereby reducing the probability of their patients incurring serious illness. Further, the sense of patients' psychological security and a comfortable point of entry into the health care system are by no means minor benefits (Hu, 1976).

From the therapeutic viewpoint, the quality of care delivered by the barefoot doctors seems to be appropriate to the level of the problems presented, since consultation and referral for more specialized clinical care is available. However, the increase of barefoot doctors has resulted in a greater number of referrals from rural areas, burdening unprepared urban hospitals (Lampton, 1974; Sidel & Sidel, 1973).

Unlike Soviet health officials, who are attempting to phase out the *feldsher,* the Chinese feel that the barefoot doctors are playing an indispensable role, and so they are likely to survive for many years to come.

Red Medical Workers. Within each residential committee, encompassing about 2,000 people in the urban areas, there are organized groups of 50 to 150 people that conduct social and welfare work (Sidel & Sidel, 1973; Wen & Hays, 1976).

The health workers at the resident committee level are local housewives called red medical workers. Their basic medical training (four to six weeks) is acquired at the street-and-lane clinics. Their tasks include primary curative services as well as preventive measures.

Worker-Doctors. The worker-doctor in the factory is the analogue of the red medical worker and barefoot doctor. Just as a peasant is chosen by his or her peers to become a barefoot doctor, a factory employee is chosen by fellow workers to become a doctor.

As a poor country committed to economic development, Communist China has maximized its available human resources to increase efficiency. Although medical service is not yet free, Chairman Mau introduced, for the first time in Chinese history, the idea that access to health care is a right, not a privilege.

Overview

The People's Republic of China shares with the USSR the advantages and disadvantages of centralized medicine in a totalitarian society. Aside from this common feature, China departs from the USSR significantly in her emphasis on the rustification of medicine and reliance on traditional medicine.

What are the implications of the Chinese experience for other countries? Can we learn lessons from it, or is Chinese medicine peculiar to China? At one extreme is the position that the Chinese health care model is not applicable to the United States because of political, social, demographic, ideological, and developmental differences (Geiger, 1975).

In the first place, China is a developing nation that is predominantly rural, poor, and short of trained medical personnel, and has high mortality and morbidity rates due to communicable and parasitic diseases. China thus needs different types of medical service than does the highly industralized and affluent

United States, which is plagued with heart disease, cancer, stroke, and degenerative diseases.

There is also a difference in the tasks of changing the medical systems. The People's Republic of China needed to change medical practice from a near-zero basis to an advanced stage. This may cause less disturbance than a change of the highly developed and sophisticated system in the United States, which is maintained in equilibrium by the vested interests of many groups. It is simpler to establish a new medical care system on an empty lot than in a land already crowded with multiple complexes.

More generally, there are basic differences between the United States and the People's Republic of China in value orientations and sociopolitical systems. As compared with the state control of medicine and promotion of health in the People's Republic of China, Americans adhere to individualism, viewing health as a personal matter and cherishing the notion of medical free enterprise. In this regard, it may cost the United States a revolution to adopt the Chinese medical care model.

A good example of the nontransferability of Chinese medicine to other countries is shown in the failure of barefoot doctors in rural Iran (Ronaghy & Solter, 1974). The Chinese solution to the shortage of physicians by the creation of barefoot doctors, half of whom were females, appeared to provide an interesting model to other countries. In China, the barefoot doctors serve as a carrier of tradition in a rapidly changing society. There is free acceptance of these subprofessionals because they are familiar neighbors to their patients rather than strange professionals.

In Iran the project failed because that society did not possess the sociopsychological setting necessary to cultivate the concept of the barefoot doctor. The Iranians resisted the selection of barefoot doctors from the masses, particularly from the female population; they were unaccustomed to training methods on the job; and community members were unwilling to utilize the services of barefoot doctors once they began to practice.

There is an opposite, nonpessimistic view that the Chinese experience offers many good ideas to the United States in improving health delivery methods (Sidel & Sidel, 1973). While American medicine is suffering from massive bureaucratization, rising cost, duplication of facilities, shortage and maldistribution of physicians, deterioration of the doctor–patient relationship, and so on, the People's Republic of China is praised for such accomplishments as the elimination of poverty, the equalization of access to comprehensive medical care, widespread health education and preventive medicine, the public participation in health care delivery and decision-making, and the like (Karefa-Smart, 1975).

However, an exact comparison of the quality of medical care between the People's Republic of China and other countries is difficult because of the lack of systematic and reliable Chinese data and also because of biases of political propanganda.

A limited but an interesting application of the Chinese experience to the United States has been suggested by Geiger (1975). Geiger observes that the health care approaches of China as a developing nation are relevant to those areas and specific populations in the United States which, because of impoverishment and discrimination, possess developing-nation characteristics-—hazardous and unsanitary environment; high birth and death rates; high rates of communicable disease; malnutrition; and low levels of income, education, and employment. Populations such as the rural blacks in the south, Chicanos in the southwest, rural whites in Appalachia, and inner-city urban-ghetto racial minorities may be useful strategic targets for selective implementation of the Chinese model without undergoing a national revolution.

So far, we have concerned ourselves with societies in which the health delivery system is an integral part of the politically centralized system. Health values and health conduct are prescribed by the government according to political ideologies. We will now shift our attention from such politicized medicine in the USSR and the People's Republic of China to the United Kingdom, where socialized medicine is practiced within liberal-democractic and capitalistic frameworks.

THE UNITED KINGDOM

Historical Background

In contrast to the USSR, with the largest land area in the world, and the People's Republic of China, with the greatest number of inhabitants, the United Kingdom is a small nation that is one-ninth the size of the USSR. Its population density, however, is almost three-fold that of China.

Unlike the USSR and the People's Republic of China, which have gone through major revolutions, the United Kingdom has evolved gradually over many centuries to reach its present stage of modernization. It is a nation with established traditions and customs, and it is also a birthplace of parliamentary democracy and laissez-faire economy.

The emergence of the National Health Service (NHS) in 1948 was a phase of the evolutionary process rather than a revolutionary transformation into a socialistic state. The origin of the NHS and of its predecessor, National Health Insurance (1911), are traced by many writers to the noblesse oblige tradition in the United Kingdom (Abel-Smith, 1964; Abel-Smith & Gales, 1964; Anderson, 1972; Eckstein, 1970; Hodgkinson, 1967).

Noblesse oblige (i.e., the moral obligation of the rich or nobility to act honorably or charitably) is the underpinning for the functionalist assumption that the British aristocracy held well-motivated altruistic values of carrying the burden of society toward the realization of societal integration. For example, even in the famous Poor Law of 1601, which was promulgated to make the local parish responsible for its destitute, the noblesse oblige pattern persisted. Hospitals were supported by private charity, and state intervention was kept to a minimum.

In contrast, others (Navarro, 1978a,b) take a conflict perspective by viewing historical processes as geared to class struggle. Thus, National Health Insurance (NHI) emerged in response not to noblesse oblige but to economic and political forces that were generated by class conflict during and after the Industrial Revolution.

As industrialization and urbanization progressed in the nineteenth century, the concentration of the poor in cities induced some welfare service beyond what was then made available through voluntary hospitals. The Metropolitan Poor Act of 1867 acknowledged the obligation of the state to provide hospitals for the poor (Abel-Smith, 1964; Abel-Smith & Gales, 1964). The medical profession supported free medical care for the destitute because it felt that its income would be better secured if the indigent were taken care of by the state and if the affluent continued to pay for their treatment.

By the turn of the century, dissatisfaction with the Poor Law was mounting. To begin with, destitution was not decreasing despite the Poor Law. In the meanwhile, the concept of social insurance was gaining popularity throughout Europe (Stevens, 1966). To make matters worse, the first Soviet revolution and other uprisings on the continent alarmed the British upper and middle classes over lurking revolutionary socialism. Also, the growing power of the working class and trade unions made health insurance a worthwhile political response to gain the working class vote, to mitigate social unrest, and to stop the spread of socialism (Navarro, 1978a,b). It was under these circumstances that NHI was enacted in 1911.

The National Health Insurance (1911). National Health Insurance (NHI) was basically a working class program to provide wage earners, but not their families, with the services of a general practitioner. Based on the concept of insurance, that is, accumulation of reserves for future risk, NHI was financed mainly by insurance premiums along with small contributions from the general fund.

Professional autonomy was maintained by such stipulations as (1) free choice of a physician; (2) administration of medical benefits by the local health committee consisting of physicians; (3) professional autonomy in medical quality control; (4) capitation rather than fixed salary as a method of remuneration; and (5) an adequate representation of the medical profession in the NHI administration. These were essentially the conditions set by the British Medical Association for its giving approval to NHI.

The NHI system placed general practitioners in a relatively advantageous position over the specialists. For example, NHI furnished a general practitioner with a secure source of income through capitation fees from a panel of patients. In comparison, consultants were attached to voluntary hospitals as honorary unpaid staff members, and they were entirely dependent on their private practices. Furthermore, general practitioners were politically organized within the NHI scheme, while specialists remained isolated from one another.

With all of its shortcomings, NHI served at least as a first minimum line of defense against the financial hazards of diseases. Why then did the British decide to discard it completely instead of modifying it?

For one thing, it was becoming apparent that the plight of medical practice was such that it could not be solved within the boundaries of the existing apparatus. The health care system was plagued with shortages and maldistributions of physicians and hospital facilities, disorganization in administration of services, and even financial insolvency. All of these weaknesses of the old health delivery system were uncovered through the emergency needs of World War II. The war experience drew public attention to the importance of health as a tool of the work force.

Another important development during the 1920s through the 1940s was the increasing public sentiment in favor of the socialization of medical services as compared to insurance principles. While insurance is embedded in self-help contractual relations, socialization refers to a completely state-owned, state-financed, and state-controlled service.

The Socialist Medical Association within the Labor Party advocated (1) free comprehensive medical care to everyone; (2) renumeration of physician service by salary; (3) group practice by general practitioners; and (4) coordination of medical facilities by local authorities (Murray et al., 1971). The British Medical Association was against a salary system, but it did not object to free medical care for everyone.

The National Health Service (1948). Although the general climate of opinion was in support of the principles of socialized medicine, there was disagreement among various interest groups on the specific content of the program. Compromise led to the National Health Service Act in 1948. As an outcome of the evolutionary process, the NHS inherited structural irrationalities and problems of the past.

Value Orientation

An emphasis on individual freedom has dominated the British value orientation. The main contours of the liberal-democratic political system and laissez-faire economic structures appeared during the late nineteenth and early twentieth centuries (Anderson, 1972; McNeill, 1963). Through the Industrial Revolution and the establishment of a nation state, British society in the nineteenth century witnessed the emergence of the middle class, their full participation in the political process, and their dominance over private enterprise.

It was assumed that rationality would be promoted by free competiton in the development and allocation of economic resources. Individual pursuit of economic interests was believed to lead to the economic welfare of society as a whole. Parlimentary democracy through open debate and voting was also considered to be an assurance of rationality in the distribution and management of political power (Lindblom, 1965).

Within any liberal democratic framework, the government is, of course, the ultimate recourse for law and order. It plays the role of the umpire for private actors and groups during their contests in the political and economic arenas (Dahl & Lindblom, 1953). However, the British model is now a pluralist one of mutual checks and balances where power is distributed more or less equally among the different constituents of society, such as the private versus public sectors. Their government can now be viewed as another interest group that cooperates, competes, or negotiates with private individuals or groups.

This basic principle of pluralism evolved in Britain in the twentieth century, and it is evident in the socialization of medicine. The shift, according to

Anderson (1972), resulted from the gradual change in the proportion of private versus public functions and responsibilities. To illustrate, during the early stages of the evolution of the liberal-democratic capitalistic states, the role of the public sector was limited. Since World War II, the increased productivity of modern economy permits the redistribution of social surplus, which in turn increases the governmental function as the central coordinator of redistributive activities.

Health Values. In the NHS system, the Minister of Health is entrusted with the responsibility for providing all necessary medical and related services to all patients, free of charge. Why was medicine singled out to be the object of such an extraordinary equalitarianism and centralization in a society that adheres to democracy and laissez faire?

Several interpretations have been proposed. First of all, there is the British tradition of noblesse oblige and Christian socialism (Eckstein, 1970). Benevolence and paternalism characterized charitable health care activities in the seventeen century.

Any conflict between philanthrophic medicine and laissez-faire economy was resolved by economic reasoning. That is, disease is one of the primary causes of destitution, which, in turn, causes a heavy burden upon taxes, specificially, the purses of the well-to-do. This is an irresistible argument in favor of welfare collectivism. Thus, medical matters were excluded from laissez-faire policies prior to 1948 (Hodgkinson, 1967).

Another way of rationalizing the coexistence of socialized medicine and capitalistic economy is to view the treatment of illness as incidental and tangent to the redistribution of societal resources. It is assumed that collective effort to mitigate the effects of so accidental a matter as physical incapacity will not affect the fundamentals of an individualistic society (Eckstein, 1970).

In other words, even the Labor government, which put the NHS program forward, was cautious and conservative. It had no intention of breaking or even modifying the class-structured society. The strategy of the Labor government was to rely on class alliance. By granting privileges and decision-making power to the medical profession, it tried to weaken opposition from the upper classes, and at the same time curtail a movement toward socialism (Navarro, 1978a,b).

Organization and Administration of Health Service

The original NHS had a tripartite administration structure coordinated under a national Department of Health and Social Security (DHSS). The administrator of the DHSS is a member of parliament. Theoretically and legally, the health minister has enormous potential power. The health minister possesses the authority to approve financial allocations; to appoint administrative personnel; to review proposals and decisions of subsidiary authorities; and to scrutinize and rearrange activities of subsidiary agencies. However, unlike the USSR or the People's Republic of China, the British political tradition inhibits the minister from issuing arbitrary directives. The formal structure is built upon a matrix of informal understandings, agreements, consultations, and negotiations.

The minister is not likely to sabotage the system by deviating from this tradition (Anderson, 1972; Eckstein, 1970; Stevens, 1966).

The first of the three parallel parts consisted of the hospitals (see Figure 11.3), which drew from regions with a population base ranging from two to five million. Almost all hospitals, public or voluntary, were taken over by the health ministry. The chief reason for this nationalization of voluntary hospitals was to ameliorate maldistribution and to exercise national control over quality.

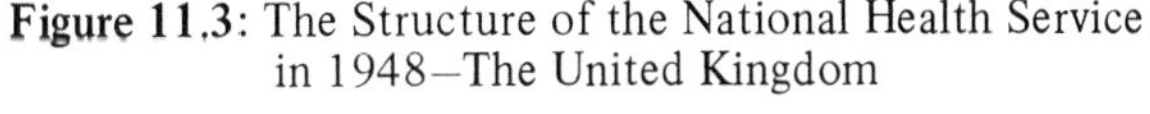
Figure 11.3: The Structure of the National Health Service in 1948—The United Kingdom

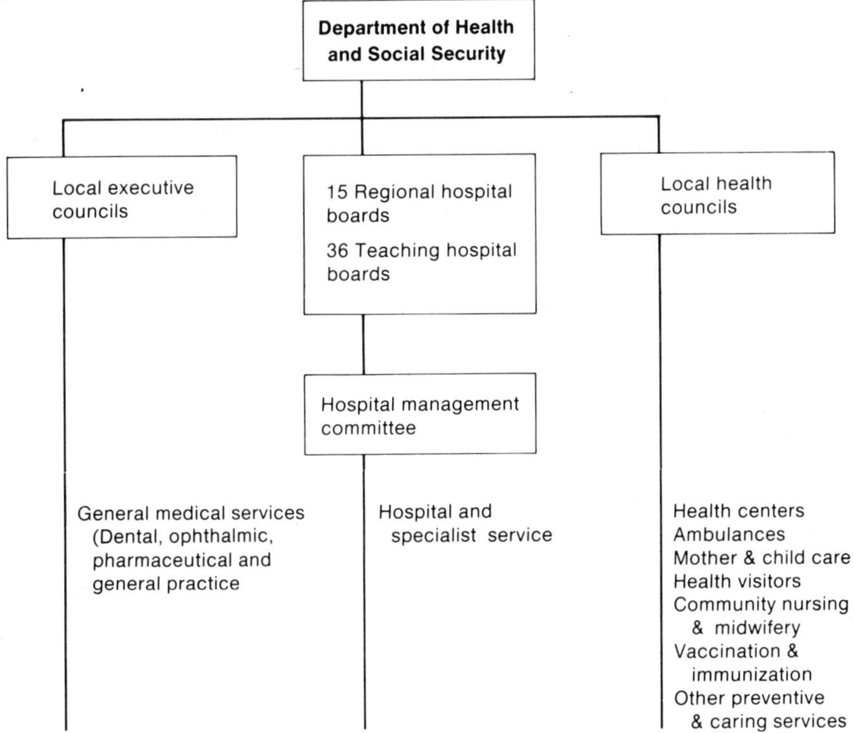

Source: Reprinted by permission of the publisher from *The NHS reorganization*. London: Office of Health Economics, 1974, fig. 1, p. 3.

The top governing body in each hospital region was the Regional Hospital Board, whose members, serving free of charge, were representatives of groups concerned with hospital affairs. The members of the board were appointed by the minister after consultation with universities, medical organizations, and other interested parties.

Each board reviewed the distribution, delivery, and costs of hospital-based services, and the maintenance, improvements, and construction of hospital facilities. The board hired all medical personnel and had a paid administrative staff. Despite this enormous responsibility, the board did not have taxing power, which placed it in an amorphous position.

Each region had at least one teaching hospital that was not part of the regional hospital body. Teaching hospitals were separate fiscal and administrative entities and were directly accountable to the minister.

The second division was made up of local executive councils, which dealt with the general practitioner and dental and pharmaceutical services. Each council made up contracts with the foregoing providers and paid them. The lists of patients and general practitioners were kept by this administrative unit, which made payment to the general practitioners on a capitation basis.

The third division consisted of the local health councils, which were the original local public health agencies. Financially, they depended mainly upon local taxes, and they discharged the traditional public health functions that are part of the NHS.

Thus, the traditional partition of medical services into hospital, general practice, and public health sectors was reinforced in the NHS. Since these three parallel divisions had their own budgets and their own boards accountable directly to the minister, there was no administrative necessity for interaction among them.

Reorganization. The need for interservice coordination in the tripartite system became manifest as the services expanded and proliferated. The growth of the NHS underscored the need for unification to ensure more efficient management of limited resources.

Reorganization of the NHS administration was undertaken in 1974 (see Figure 11.4). All the former functions of the tripartite NHS were incorporated into the new, unified structure, although parts of the environmental health services remained under local control (OHE, 1974).

An important element of the new system is the concept of a natural district for health care that encompasses an average of a quarter of a million residents. The district boundaries are defined "naturally," that is, in accordance with the prevailing pattern of the population's use of community and hospital services. Districts are seen as the basic units for which evaluation and management of the full range of health services are carried out.

The lowest-level statutory authority within the new NHS rests with the Area Health Authorities (AHA). One of the major functions of the AHA is to coordinate its own services and those of the new local authorities. The AHA are corporately responsible for health care in their geographical areas, while those grouped together under the Regional Health Authorities are themselves accountable to the DHSS (Wolman, 1976).

The restructuring of the health services was intended to improve the evaluative and rational planning capabilities by integrated management. However, from the functional perspective, one major criticism of the reorganization is its overemphasis on managerial efficiency. A centralized and strongly hierarchical organization tends to discourage communication and consultation between consumers and providers of health care services. Also, the sense of autonomy and general morale of the professional staff can be detrimentally affected by the rigidity of organizational structure (Jonas et al., 1975; Pain, 1976).

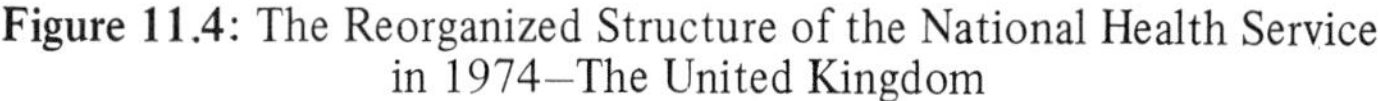

Figure 11.4: The Reorganized Structure of the National Health Service in 1974—The United Kingdom

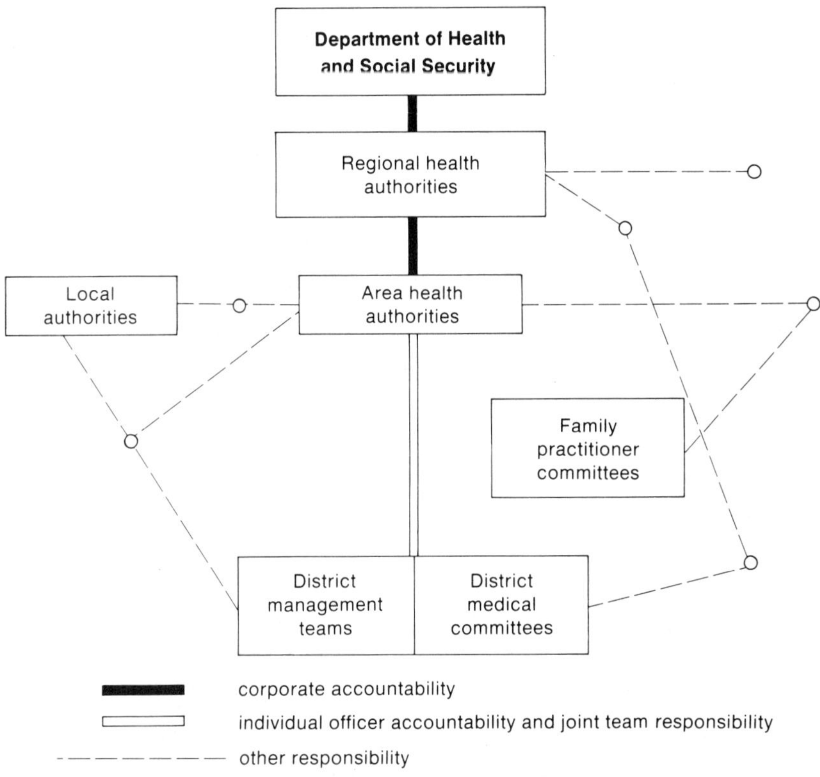

Source: Reprinted by permission of the publisher from *The NHS reorganization.* London: Office of Health Economics, 1974, fig. 2, p. 9.

Viewing the reorganization from the conflict perspective, an enterprise as large and complex as the NHS that is built upon many compromises among various groups is bound to have built-in strains. This implies that no single group is totally satisfied with the operation, or else the balance of the system will be disturbed (OHE, 1974).

Going a step further, a Marxian analysis of class conflict is adopted by some (Navarro, 1978a,b). According to this view, the reorganization of the NHS is a triumph for the upper classes because it has not changed the basic class structure of the medical delivery system, which is dominated by hospital-based specialists and deprives local health authorities of power.

Medical Practice

Since it does deliver health care services, the NHS is not merely a state insurance system. As a service organization, it defines its goals in terms of medical practices, and as an outcome of the evolutionary process, the NHS aims to preserve the old sytem of private practice as much as possible (Eckstein, 1970). It also retains the traditional demarcation between general practice and specialty care (Mechanic, 1968a,b). In other words, the NHS has emerged from a mixture of the NHI and private medical service; it is a new type of service embedded in an old structure (Eckstein, 1970; Farndale, 1964; Fry, 1969; McLachlan, 1971).

General Practitioners. Under the NHS, general practitioners are paid on a capitation basis. This is a compromise between a salary and the fee-for-service payment method. The capitation approach at least rewards practitioners in proportion to the number of their patients, thereby reserving the element of competition for patients in the open marketplace. However, some restrictions are set by the government to avoid malpractice. For example, physicians are not allowed to take on more than a fixed maximum number of patients, i.e., an annual limit of 3,500.

The NHS physicians can still engage in private practice, but this is restricted by limited consumer demand. The high cost of physician services and drugs discourage patients from seeking private care (Lindsey, 1962).

There is free choice of physicians by patients and vice versa since the majority of the population uses the NHS. Technically, it is easy for patients to change a physician by simply going through the necessary administrative procedure of registering with another physician. However, such changes are reported to be infrequent (Fry, 1969; Lindsey, 1962).

The general practitioner, or the family doctor, is the single portal of entry under the NHS. In principle, the general practitioner is expected to be concerned with the sociopsychological as well as medical problems of patients (Gillie, 1963). This presumably close understanding between patients and general practitioner has been cherished as a unique characteristic of British medical practice (Teeling-Smith, 1975).

One of the charges made against the National Health Service is that the doctor–patient relationship has deteriorated because of the abuse of the free service by patients and because of the demoralizing effects of a capitation system upon general practitioners.

Eckstein (1970) reports that there is little evidence to suggest that patients have abused the services by making inordinate demands on practitioners. For comparison, in 1946, while low-income Americans earning less than $1,000 made 2.2 calls to physicians per year and high-income Americans with over $10,000 made 5.5 calls, the United Kingdom indicated an average of 5 calls per patient under the National Health Insurance. It was thus noted that most people use a free health service about as frequently as private services are used by those who can afford them. However, there does seem to be an increase of health service utilization by the lower-income population when the medical care is free of charge.

Against the allegation that doctors serve private patients better than public patients, Eckstein (1970) found a relative absence of misconduct under the NHS—only 22 practitioners out of over 40,000 were expelled and no more than 322 disciplinary actions were taken during the first five years of the NHS. Further, there is a report indicating that the amount of time spent on a patient by a dentist is mainly affected by the clinical severity of the dental problem rather than whether the patient belongs to the NHS or not. Lindsey (1962) also claims that the NHS increased little, if any, the amount of work per patient on the doctor's list. A prewar survey disclosed an annual average of 4.81 to 5.39 consultations and visits per individual, while in 1950 the rate was 4.8 items of service per person.

Nevertheless, there exists the image of an overworked British general practitioner hurriedly taking care of patients who are crowding the waiting room. Comparing the workload of primary care doctors, Fry (1969) points out that British general practitioners see almost twice as many patients as do their colleagues in the United States and the USSR, and that they spend much less time (an average of 6 to 7 minutes per patient) on each office consultation.

Some (Lindsey, 1962) have observed that the excess workload of general practitioners in the United Kingdom existed prior to the enactment of the NHS. In the years before 1948, many practitioners, although overworked, were grossly underpaid. The NHS improved the lot of most doctors by redistributing them more evenly, thereby generating a better overall doctor–patient ratio than before.

Yet, there is still variation in the size of practice. According to Mechanic's (1968a,b) studies, general practitioners with a smaller practice are more likely to be satisfied with their practice, show more sociopsychological concern for their patients, and complain less about remuneration despite their lower income than physicians who have larger numbers of patients. Since the number of work hours per week does not vary significantly by size of practice, physicians who have a large number of patients cope with the problem not by extending their work hours but by decreasing the amount of consultation time per patient's visit (Abel-Smith & Gales, 1964). Whether this lowers the quality of care is subject to debate. Lindsey (1962) cites surveys which reveal that competent physicians with heavy workloads do give first-class clinical services, albeit without any frills. The trend is nevertheless toward smaller and more evenly distributed assignment of patients.

Given the decision to minimize the deviation from traditional operation, the NHS needed to move slowly in its attempt to develop corporate practice among general practitioners. Partnerships were encouraged by giving the partners certain advantages such as permission to carry larger lists of patients.

The concept of a health center was also advocated, one in which general practitioners practice in partnership not only with one another, but also with other health care personnel such as dentists, ophthalmologists, home nurses, environmental health officers, and maternity and child welfare workers. The health center was intended to efficiently integrate institutional and noninstitutional services (SMA, 1973). However, the health center is far from a state of fruition partly because of the cost of developing such facilities and also because of the lack of general practitioners' interest in this form of organization (Ryan, 1968).

Specialists. Within the NHS system, specialists became salaried employees of the nationalized hospitals. The basic salary scale is identical for all specialties in all hospitals. Salary level is determined by the number of half-day (3.5 hour) sessions per week that the specialist agrees to work in one or more hospitals. Full-time employment is the equivalent of 11 sessions or 5.5 days per week, and the full-time consultants are not allowed to undertake private practice (Stevens, 1966).

It appears that while general practitioners have retained their independence, specialists have been subjugated to bureaucracy. Be that as it may, the specialists do have considerable freedom to organize their professional activities and to maintain their autonomy.

Specialist–General Practitioner Separation. Traditionally, there has been a clear demarcation between specialists and general practitioners in the United Kingdom. Physicians practicing in the community as general practitioners serve as doctors of first contact and are expected to deal with not only physical but also emotional, family, and social problems of the patient. General practitioners provide services only on an outpatient basis and do not have access to hospital facilities. After the patients are referred to the hospital, they are treated exclusively by hospital-based specialists This is in a sharp contrast to the American practice in which the doctor of first contact is usually the one who sends the patient to the hospital where he or she continues to look after the patient.

The advantage of the specialist–general practitioner separation is that both groups can concentrate on limited areas and therefore reach a higher technical competence than otherwise. There is less likely to be a situation where a nonspecialist performs surgery, as is frequently seen in American practice (Nickerson et al., 1976). However, there are shortcomings in this separation, such as the lack of continuity in medical care for the patient who is transferred from a general practitioner to specialists, and the status discrimination between the two types of doctors. Due to the progress in medical science and increasing specialization, specialists enjoy prestige because of their high level of technical expertise as compared to that required of general practitioners. This status differentiation, which has been the source of dissatisfaction among general practitioners, did not change significantly under the NHS before or after the reorganization (Jonas et al., 1975).

Professional Autonomy. It is interesting to note the difference between the Communist Party in the USSR and the Labor Party in the United Kingdom in their dealings with the medical profession during the creation of socialized medicine. In the USSR the medical profession represented class interests, and the Communist strategy toward it was a political one of deprofessionalization and democratization of the health sector. In contrast, the Labor Party in the United Kingdom viewed the whole process as one of management (i.e., the integration of the medical profession and its co-optation within the NHS) rather than that of class conflict (Navarro, 1978a,b).

Although the NHS produced an employment monopoly, it has not interfered with professional independence and freedom, and many and various professional bodies and colleagues are free to engage in activities without state intervention. Negotiations on medico-political matters, such as rates of remuneration and terms of service, are largely in the hands of the British Medical Association. Maintenance of quality care is still largely a professional responsibility; there is no general system of built-in quality checks (Fry, 1969).

Administratively, the NHS allows for professional advice and opinion to be expressed to the health service management. For instance, each area has a local advisory committee elected by the professional groups. In short, within the new structure of the NHS, the medical profession retains much of its status and power.

Finance and Personnel Resources

Financing of Health Care

In state-owned economic systems such as those in the USSR and the People's Republic of China, it is the state authority that determines the hierarchy of priorities in allocating the budget. In the United Kingdom, on the other hand, as a liberal-democratic country, constant political debate is used to reach an appropriate working relationship between the private and public sectors or to produce a consensus regarding the amount to be assigned to the health care budget.

Approximately 80 percent of the NHS funds are financed by the central government, mainly through the general tax revenue and to some extent from employer and employee deductions. A remnant of the historical responsibility of the local government for public health services is seen in a small proportion (5 percent) of the funds obtained from local governments (Anderson, 1972; Fry, 1969).

The remaining 15 percent of the total NHS budget comes directly from the patients. Most of this arises from payment for private medical care such as private consultation and private hospital beds, and for charges for prescriptions and dental care.

Less than one percent of the fund is derived from voluntary health insurance. Within the British context, the benefits from private health insurance are formulated as an extremely minor rather than a major supplement to the NHS (Anderson, 1972).

Thus, the British system depends primarily upon a single source—the public fund, as compared with an American mixed financial type of funding based on large-scale private and public investments. Some experts argue that mixed investment has the advantage of stimulating improvement and experimentation while single-source financing tends to perpetuate the status quo as prescribed by the financial agency in control (Anderson, 1963).

Over the years the NHS has suffered from a failure to invest sufficient funds to realize its stated goals. The United Kingdom has spent consistently 1.5 to 2 percent less of her gross national product on health care than has the United States (Cooper & Worthington, 1973; "Medical care . . . ," 1973). However, it is difficult to determine whether this is due to the single-source financial mechanism or because of the general economic difficulties of the country. The NHS must develop within the context of many pressing problems resulting from World War II and overall economic scarcity (Mechanic, 1968a,b).

Work Force Supply

There are very few problems concerning the access to or the accessibility of first-contact care in the United Kingdom since it is a small territory with a well-established general practice system. Nevertheless, the attainment of a uniform geographical distribution of physicians was one of the major goals of the NHS.

In order to bring about a gradual change, the NHS did not undertake a radical redistribution of physicians. When the Service first went into operation, general practitioners were allowed to practice wherever they pleased. No one was forced to move to another territory.

After some time, however, a national agency, the Medical Practice Committee, began to control the physicians' entry into certain areas so as to achieve a gradual shift of practitioners from oversupplied to undersupplied locales. The committee now makes a continuous survey of the country to evaluate the adequacy of the physician supply in every local unit. Local areas are classified into (1) open areas where physicians are critically needed; (2) more or less restricted areas; and (3) closed areas where physicians are overabundant. If a physician applies to a closed area, he or she is likely to be rejected unless that person can offer a compelling reason (Eckstein, 1970).

In general, the redistribution of general practitioners has been fairly successful. The number of persons living in areas officially designated as underdoctored has been reduced from 50 percent in 1948 to less than 20 percent in 1963 (Jonas et al., 1975). Outlying rural areas are reported to suffer less from a deficiency of medical services than the less attractive industrial areas (Fry, 1969). Specialists, however, are not as evenly distributed as general practitioners, and nonteaching hospitals are still worse off in staffing than teaching hospitals.

Due to the unequal geographical distribution of physicians and differential ability in communication, there are social class distinctions in health service utilization. Middle class people make more use of preventive service and receive better quality care than members of the working class (Cartwright & O'Brien, 1976). Thus, one of the fundamental principles of the NHS—equity in health care delivery—has not yet been met satisfactorily.

Overview

The health service models of the Communist countries tend to be rejected by Americans, who perceive an unbridgeable gap between democratic and Communistic value orientations and social structures. In contrast, the socialized medicine of the United Kingdom has been closely examined as a possible model. The British NHS reveals both the potentialities and limitations of central medico-economic planning within a capitalist and democratic context. These have serious implications to Americans who are currently debating the pros and cons of various national health insurance proposals.

One of the crucial purposes of the NHS was to impose rational planning upon the chaotic patterns of medical service that existed before. Rationality here refers to achieving a desired end with the least expenditure of effort and least compromise of other valued ends. The experience of the NHS indicates difficulties in carrying out rational planning because of several factors, which American society shares.

While rational action requires internal consistency of ends, the NHS aims at a large number of objectives, some of which are related but not consistent with one another. For example, it attempts to provide a greater number of medical personnel and facilities, while trying to reduce expenditures. Another incongruence is that the NHS has developed a centralized bureaucratic structure, although it wishes to maintain a democratic administration. Unlike in the USSR and the People's Republic of China, priorities of value and actions in the United Kingdom are not monolithically determined by the state. Therefore, a decision between an improvement in, say, mental health versus the tuberculosis service, involves emotional sensitivity and political power of planners as well as rational calculation of means and ends.

One of the effects of these barriers to rationality is the tendency toward routinization, rigidity, inertia, and centralization of power in place of innovative experimentation. Thus, rather than going through an objective appraisal of individual cases and reaching an agreement among a multitude of decision-makers, there is a propensity to develop standardized routing procedures. Also, decisions are likely to become a product of influence and persuasion rather than rational calculation (Eckstein, 1970).

Rather critically, Watkin (1978) has asked an overall question: Are the British people healthier today because of the NHS? He suggests that major improvements in the health status in the United Kingdom since 1948 are attributable to developments (e.g., better nutrition, housing, living standards, and technological advances) that would have taken place whatever system had been chosen to administer and finance health services. For example, the NHS did not create any new hospitals or new doctors. It did not even make available to the poor what had been enjoyed by the rich, although it made it simpler for the poor to gain access to health services.

One of the fundamental difficulties in implementing socialized medicine in the British capitalist society was that while the administrative structure was centralized for rational management, the NHS left intact the more basic ideological, professional, and historical structures. With the commitment to bringing about a change gradually by adhering as closely as possible to the traditional medical delivery patterns, the NHS did not attempt to deal with basic health problems that result from the continuation of private physician entrepreneurship, private part-time practice by specialists, the specialist–general practitioner separation, and physician dominance over paraprofessionals and patients (Jonas et al., 1975; Wolman, 1976). After all, the first and foremost goals of the Labor government was to restore capitalist economy, not to implement socialism in the form of self-government of the masses (Navarro, 1978a,b).

These are some of the issues Americans must face in developing a full-scale national health program. However, a distinction must be made between limitations inherent in any public planning and control, and hurdles imposed by specific socioeconomic conditions such as national financial problems (McCurdy et al., 1977).

SUMMARY

Behind varied medical care patterns in different countries exists the common denominator that Fry (1969) calls the insolvable equation of medical care. It is a precarious balance between consumer needs, professional needs, and available resources. Therefore, a compromise between maximum health and minimum cost becomes the common goal. Major international differences in attaining this goal seem to be (1) the extent to which payment for services comes from individuals rather than from the third party, and (2) the degree to which medicine and other sectors of society are centrally controlled.

This chapter has examined three kinds of socialized medicine in an attempt to derive implications for improving American health care services. Before any conclusion is reached, however, care must be taken in recognizing the difficulties in cross-national comparison and the relative lack of cross-cultural transferability.

To begin with, the quality of care is a multi-dimensional concept that has many operational facets, such as superb technology for organ transplantation, accessibility to primary care doctors with sociopsychological concern for patients, development of preventive medicine, and so on. It is extremely difficult to standardize and measure such a concept, particularly in the cross-cultural context. To make it worse, international studies involve political ideologies and propanganda that bias whatever few materials each country is able or willing to disclose.

Even if a certain method of medical service is proven best, it is not always possible to transfer it from one society to another because it is deeply embedded in the cultural tradition of the society. Among the three countries studied in this chapter, the USSR and the People's Republic of China are so vastly different from the United States in sociopolitical backgrounds and value orientations that a direct transfer of any aspect of medical practice is likely to encounter resistence. Even the socialized medicine in the United Kingdom within a democratic-capitalistic social system cannot easily be imported to the United States because this country lacks the British tradition of social welfare.

With these limitations in mind, we can summarize briefly the relevance of socialized medicine in these three countries.

Value Orientation. Both in the USSR and the People's Republic of China, the hierarchy of values is imposed upon individuals by the Communist governments. Health is considered important not so much for the sake of an individual's happiness but as a necessity to carry out societal goals, that is, the realization of a classless society. In both countries, prerevolutionary physicians are viewed as exploitative bourgeoisie, and efforts are made to proletarianize them. Obviously, the American heritage of liberal democracy is not amenable to these ideas.

While Americans are struggling to resolve the dilemma of contradictory values, that is, individualism versus equalitarianism, the United Kingdom went through that stage years ago and enacted the NHI in 1911, and then the NHS in 1948. Under the NHS, health service is a national monopoly. However, within its liberal-democratic context, the priority to be placed upon health against other issues such as education, employment, and defense is not a decision dictated by the government but rather is a subject for regular debate and a source of constant conflict among interest groups.

Organization and Administration of Health Services. While American health services are criticized for having no system and for being fragmented into private insurance, social insurance, and no insurance schemes, the three countries reviewed in this chapter present officially integrated medical systems, although in practice they suffer from built-in conflict.

All three countries illustrate some of the potentialities and limitations of a centralized medical system. On the positive side, central planning coordinates all segments of health care activities. It helps to decrease unnecessary duplication of personnel, equipment, and other resources, problems that exist in the free enterprise system of American medicine. On the other hand, to the extent that centralized medical administration manages to suppress opposition and internal conflict, it is likely to become rigid and resistent to innovative ideas and practices.

Another advantage of central planning is its ability to enforce an even distribution of medical facilities among the people. The U.S. quest for providing care to the medically deprived population through neighborhood health centers seems to be well realized in other countries. Local clinics for preventive and first-contact curative medicine have been established for each local population unit in the USSR and China. In the United Kingdom, local health centers are not in full operation, but general practitioners serve as the portal of entry for patients.

Medical Practice. Without reliable and comparable data, it is difficult to determine which system—free enterprise or nationalized medicine—produces a better quality of medical care.

In the United States the capitalistic medical market has been scapegoated in recent years as the cause for defective medical service. Slowly but steadily the United States has been approaching the notion of social insurance by means of prepaid medical plans such as HMOs, social welfare such as Medicare and Medicaid, and finally the idea of national health insurance.

Since the proletarianization of physicians as realized in the Communist countries will not appeal to the AMA, which has enjoyed high status and income, and great power, the United Kingdom is a more likely candidate to provide some guidelines to the United States in developing national health insurance. In the United Kingdom, fee-for-service payment has been replaced by a capitation payment for general practitioners and by a salary for hospital physicians. The capitation method retains the element of free competition for patients, although there is a maximum limit of patients to be seen by a general practitioner. Despite the fact that the NHS produced an employment monopoly, both general practitioners and specialists maintain their professional autonomy.

Frequently, the NHS has been charged with overloading the physicians and thus causing a deterioration in the doctor–patient relationship. However, a distinction must be made as to how much of the physician's heavy workload is due to the mechanisms of the NHS itself, and how much is caused by other socioeconomic conditions of the country.

Although the loss of professional autonomy of physicians in the Communist countries will not provide an acceptable framework for American physicians, other practices such as the development of the health team and paramedical workers in the USSR and the People's Republic of China may prove to be useful in coping with the physician shortage. Naturally, barefoot doctors and *feldshers* cannot be directly transplanted into American urban ghettoes, but their experience may furnish some lessons to American paramedics. Also, the emphasis on preventive medicine practiced by ancillary health workers in the USSR and the People's Republic of China should be adopted by American medicine, which has leaned toward curative medicine.

Finance and Work Force Supply. In the United States, payment for medical services has traditionally been on a fee-for-service basis. Individuals are given the ultimate responsibility, unless they are poor. This tradition has been under severe attack in recent years because accessibility to health care is now considered a human right rather than a privilege.

In the United Kingdom and the USSR, the major portion of the health funds are financed by the central government through general taxes. The difference lies in the manner in which a decision is reached concerning the allocations of the health budget. While budgetary priorities are determined by the central government in the USSR, they are subject to open debate and democratic procedures in the United Kingdom.

The strategy of the Chinese government for financing health care is to transfer the burden to the organizations that benefit directly: the rural communes, production brigades, and production teams. A subsidy from the central government is contingent upon the ability of the local units to mobilize their own resources.

The strength and weakness of single-source financing has been debated in the United States in conjunction with various national health insurance proposals. A conclusive answer to this question is not easy to reach because it is intertwined with other factors such as the national financial situation; priorities given to health as against the priorities of defense, industry, housing, and education; and general value orientation. There is one advantage, however, in single-source central budgeting: that is the fair distribution of medical resources according to central planning.

The ultimate goal for a comparative study is to identify the most effective and efficient way of arranging health care resources. However, there are few studies that deal with the outcome (e.g., consumer utilization and satisfaction, quality of care, and efficiency) of different health delivery systems.

Among the few is the WHO/International Collaboration study of medical care utilization in seven industralized societies (the United States, the United Kingdom, Canada, Yugoslavia, Poland, Finland, and the Argentine) (Kohn & White, 1976). The results of this study support the postulate that consumer utilization of health care services is modified by differences in health services organization and resource allocation. For example, countries with scarce resources show greater concern with health as a societal value and with the manner in which services are distributed, organized, and financed. A greater degree of structuring in health care services, in turn, is associated with lower levels of health care expenditures. More specifically, the way in which health care personnel are organized, balanced, or work together (e.g., balance between primary and specialist care, and the relationship between the use of physicians and nurses) are more important than the sheer volume of work force resources in raising accessibility to medical care.

In sum, the problems faced by American medicine—consumer discontent, high medical costs, impersonality of medical bureaucracy, and the maldistribution of facilities—can be dealt with differently. The three countries discussed in this chapter possess more structured health service systems than does the United States. This does not mean, however, that systems in other societies are free from difficulties. In the United Kingdom, dissatisfaction is expressed within the medical profession regarding the availability of facilities. In the USSR and Communist China, discontent may be muted (Fry, 1969). The United States may be able to learn from these other countries. Yet, as mentioned earlier, medical services constitute a subsystem of a larger society. As such, any change in American medical service will be accompanied by evolutionary or revolutionary changes in society.

CHAPTER 12

Medical Ethics

In Chapter 1 we traced the history of medicine and sociology through three stages: (1) in the first stage theology, philosophy, medicine, and social thought were undifferentiated; (2) in the second stage philosophy, natural science, and social science diverged from one another; and (3) in the third stage facets of medicine and sociology converged into medical sociology.

In the beginning, the concept of health and illness, medical treatments, ideas about social relationships, and actual interpersonal and intergroup transactions were all submerged under theology and supernatural power was believed to govern everything.

However, the development of the germ theory during the second historical stage and the ensuing triumphs of medical biology and technology altered the morbidity patterns of society, bringing contagious disease well under control. Because of this technological advance as well as industrialization and modernization, the organization of medical care underwent significant changes, raising the status of physicians. At the same time, ideologies and research concerning social relationships grew into a distinct academic discipline, social science.

After a period of divergence of the natural and social sciences, the merging process began. This stage of convergence of medicine and sociology was in part a response to medicine's inability to control chronic and mental illnesses. The etiology of these illnesses must be sought not only in physical environments but also in sociological environments. Unlike acute diseases, which interfere with one's social role only temporarily, chronic and mental illnesses have lasting impacts upon the patient's social life and identity (Strauss, 1975). Recognition of the importance of social factors in health and illness resulted in the corroboration of medical and sociological disciplines.

Within the past twenty years, a further convergence has been observed: the integration of the scientific-technological and religious-philosophical spheres (Fox, 1974a,b). Medical issues were treated as an objective science during the 1950s, and they were rigorously separated from the so-called subjective, nonscientific orientations of philosophy and ethics. In contrast, during the

1960s and 1970s, ethical and moral questions became necessary ingredients of medical practices. This injection of existential and metaphysical themes into medicine is viewed by Fox (1974a,b) as part of the evolutionary process of social and cultural change in American society toward a "new stage of modernity."

The convergence of ethics and medicine was brought about partly because of medical progress. Medical science has enhanced the human capacity to preserve life through artificial means, to intervene and manipulate human bodies and minds, and to genetically design the human being itself. These developments have led to profound and troublesome questions: What is life? When does it begin and end? Who decides the length and quality of life and on what bases? These are ethical and existential questions that must be dealt with in contemporary medicine.

In this chapter we will examine both specific medical areas that involve ethical considerations and broader ethical problems in the organization of modern medicine.

THE RENAISSANCE OF MEDICAL ETHICS

That medicine involves ethical and moral dimensions has been evident since the Oath of Hippocrates. Throughout the history of medicine, ethics has been taught in some form to physicians (Etziony, 1973). Traditionally, it took two forms: Catholic moral theology taught in Catholic medical schools and medical etiquette courses in many secular schools.

For the last decade a new type of teaching has proliferated. What seems distinct about the current renaissance in modern ethics is that for the first time that topic is being recognized as a formal intellectual discipline integral to clinical medicine. In medical schools in the 1970s one sees significant activities such as seminars, experimental programs, internships, and national conferences on medical ethics (Fox, 1974a,b).

> Surveys in 1972 and 1974 revealed a dramatic growth and institutionalization of medical ethics teaching in medical schools. In 1972 there were thirty-seven elective courses and seventeen schools offering special lecture series or conferences out of ninety-five schools surveyed. They had nineteen faculty members teaching medical ethics at least half-time. Two years later there were forty-seven elective courses, fifty-six special lecture series or conferences, and thirty-one teachers devoting half their time to medical school medical ethics in 107 schools (Veatch, 1977, p. 2).

Several schools have established departments of medical ethics or medical humanities. Other humanistic disciplines have also been included, such as history, literature, and related fields. It is reported by Veatch (1977) that there are 42 medical humanities departments in American medical schools and more in the offing.

Furthermore, academic graduate programs in medical or biological ethics are becoming increasingly significant areas for teaching and research for trained professionals. Masters or doctoral degrees in medical ethics exist at several schools. As for the professional qualification of teachers of medical ethics, a consensus is emerging that teachers should have not only full professional qualifications in either ethics or the medical science, but also "competent amateur" status in the other field. Ideally, at least a year of "cross fertilization" is being promoted (Veatch, 1977).

There is also a growing network of new organizations that deal with medical ethics, for example, the Institute of Society, Ethics, and Life Sciences, founded in 1969 in Hastings-On-Hudson, New York; and the Society for Health and Human Values, founded in 1969 in Philadelphia. The wide mass media coverage of ethical subjects in professional as well as in popular journals and daily newspapers indicates public concern with these problems. Medical ethics has entered the political domain as well, and the result is a series of legislation affecting the principles of medical research and the legal rights of individuals in matters of life and death.

Where did the movement come from? Perhaps the most urgent impetus for ethical concern arose from publicized episodes of hazards in human experimentation and dilemmas caused by the utilization of advanced medical techniques. For instance, the New York City example of human experimentation in 1964, (cancer cells were injected into elderly and chronically ill individuals who were not sufficiently informed about the nature of the research) alerted the public to the necessity of protecting their interests against the negative consequences of science (Langer, 1966). Then, the prolongation of the life of Karen Ann Quinlan in a vegetative state on an artificial life-sustaining system made people ponder about the quality of life and the wisdom of human intervention in what had been considered the natural process of biological organisms. Documentation of these and other instances (Beecher, 1966; Pappworth, 1967) sensitized the public to consider ethical issues in medical practice.

Next, the rise of medical ethics is a response to what Ogburn (1964) called a cultural lag. According to this concept, changes in material culture (e.g., a change in technology) are not immediately followed by appropriate modifications of the social structure and public attitudes. Consequently, a new medical technology can solve physical problems, but it may create unanticipated adjustment difficulties in society. The pursuit of scientific knowledge without corresponding attention to human needs may lead to impersonal scientific abuses.

In addition, the growth of ethical concern in medicine can be viewed as part of the contemporary civil rights movement. The ideology of quality, dignity, and equity of life, particularly for the underprivileged, has been expressed since the mid-1960s through racial equality, antipoverty, peace, ecology, and pollution control movements. Our age, as Barber (1973) put it, is the age of civil rights.

Those protests against authority have also challenged the medical establishment. Our social climate has turned against the dominance by expert professionals whose decision-making powers involve life and death. This increasing public reaction against professional encroachment is partly due to the rising education and sophistication of the masses. It is also due to the specialization and bureaucratization of medicine (Simmons & Simmons, 1971). Patients who hardly know their physicians personally in bureaucratic hospitals now are suspicious of their doctors' intentions. Thus, patients, as consumers of health care, are demanding the power to influence the specifications of medical ethics lest their human rights should be sacrificed for scientific or medical needs.

While health has come to be claimed as a basic human right, the "right to death" also has become a current ethical concern. In recent years, as a result of several social forces, a great deal of attention and open discussion have been devoted to death and dying. The advances in medical science have changed mortality statistics, producing a larger proportion of older people who will be facing death. Medical technology has also made it possible to sustain a person on a life-support device even if he or she can never function autonomously again. These technological changes as well as secularization have challenged the traditional ethical position with respect to the sanctity of life: viewing life as sacred and nonmanipulable by humans.

THREE AREAS OF ETHICAL CONCERN

The term *medical ethics* is currently used in a variety of ways. In one of its tradition-honored definitions, *medical ethics* refers to a "body of thinking and conduct developed by the medical profession" (Reiser, Dyck, & Curran, 1977, p. 1). It assumes professional autonomy in that physicians' self-conscious reflection on standards of conduct will be the guidelines for the patients and the general public to follow in medical matters.

That the public can no longer leave medical ethics to professional self-regulation has been discussed in previous chapters. Consumer participation and third-party intervention in some areas of medical ethics—the physician–patient relations, allocation and financing of medical facilities, and the concept of health as a right—have already been dealt with.

Our attention in this chapter is focused upon the types of ethical concerns that in recent years have become crucial because of scientific advances: metaphysical questions concerning the desirability of human control over humanity and nature. The specific topics chosen for discussion are human experimentation, death and dying, and genetic engineering.

Human Experimentation

Human experimentation is defined as "deliberately inducing or altering body or mental functions, directly or indirectly, in individuals or in groups primarily for the advancement of health, science, and human welfare" (Ladimer, 1955).

Some of the most important preventive and therapeutic treatments in contemporary medicine could not have been developed without the use of human experimentation. Actually, all medical acts are more or less experimental. Human experimentation is endorsed by our societal values: the search for truth, faith in progress, survival of individual species, and above all, advancement of social and political goals (Katz, 1972). Science is viewed as a tool for national progress, defense, and security.

However, the issue is not so simple. While national progress is important,

Americans also cherish the welfare of individual citizens. In human experimentation, the individual risks and social benefits must be balanced. The physician-scientists must weigh the professional norm of advancing medical knowledge against the ethical norm of protecting patients from experimental risks.

Historical Examples of Mass Experimentation

A familiar historical example of human experimentation took place in Brookline, Massachusetts, in 1721. When an epidemic of smallpox swept over the colonists in Boston and eastern New England in the early eighteenth century, the Reverend Cotton Mather and Zabdiel Boylston undertook the type of smallpox inoculation they had learned from Turkish and African practices. It consisted of the intentional infection of a normal person with virulent smallpox virus obtained from a patient.

In the midst of riotous opposition by medical practitioners as well as the public, Boylston inoculated 247 persons, including his own 13-year-old son; six of them died. The experiment was successful in the sense that those who were inoculated rarely contracted the epidemic disease.

Could this experiment be conducted today? The answer is an emphatic no. It was a lethal experiment with a prohibitive mortality rate of over two percent. Also, Boylston had little idea of the nature of the disease. There was no scientific basis or preliminary laboratory work.

Other examples of initial therapeutic trials—the first use of ether as an anesthesia, insulin, liver extract, and a host of new drugs—all involved the same type of ethical problems of human experimentation. At present, women are engaged in the largest single mass experiment, the widespread use of oral contraceptives whose long-term side effects, if any, are still unknown (Moore, 1970).

Organ Transplantation and Hemodialysis

New surgical operations raise ethical problems similar to those in therapeutic innovations. In earlier days, surgeons could depend on the natural healing power of the patient because the operation was relatively simple. In contemporary medicine, however, surgery is affected by complicated physiological and pharmacological interactions.

Organ transplantation and chronic hemodialysis are among the most recent and important experimental developments in clinical medicine (Fox, 1970). At the present stage of development, both hemodialysis and transplantation are surrounded by a number of major, unsolved scientific and technical problems.

The First Artificial Heart Transplant. In 1969 Denton A. Cooley implanted the first totally mechanical heart into the chest of Mr. Karp, a 46-year-old patient, who had a 10-year history of cardiac problems. The mechanic device sustained him for about 65 hours until a donor for a heart could be obtained. The patient died 26 hours after the heart transplantation (Curran, 1974; Fox & Swazey, 1974).

Mrs. Karp brought legal action against Cooley, alleging gross negligence, a lack of informed consent, and improper experimentation. She alleged that Mr. Karp was abused for human experimentation because the mechanical heart had not been tested adequately even on animals and never on a human being. And it was the artificial heart that caused Mr. Karp to enter a process of irreversible deterioration from which he could not be saved.

It was also averred that the consent to the operation was fraudulently obtained. Mrs. Karp accused Cooley of initially informing herself and her husband that there was a donor for a human heart available at a nearby hospital, which was false. Only after the open-heart surgery started was Mrs. Karp told that no human heart was available and that a nationwide search for a donor must be made while the artificial heart sustained his life. Also, Cooley led Mr. Karp to believe, falsely, that unless the experimental operation was performed immediately, he would die. Cooley failed to inform Karp that the experimental mechanical heart had not been adequately tested.

Cooley testified that he told the patient about the heart pump in detail and said that it could be used to sustain him for a time while a donor was being sought. Cooley firmly asserted that he told the patient about the experimental nature of the operation and gave no guarantee of success. On the day before the surgery, a detailed consent form was signed by the patient.

The case was tried in the federal district court, but was withdrawn from the jury's consideration on the grounds that the allegations were not legally established because they were not legally attested to by medical doctors. Mrs. Karp appealed to the federal court of appeals, which dismissed the case. Having examined the patient's own involvement and his consent, the court ruled that the wife's understanding and consent were not legally necessary.

The case of *Cooley* v. *Karp* raised several crucial issues in medical ethics. First of all, there is a question of whether or not the mechanical heart had been sufficiently tested. Cooley was convinced that enough laboratory work had been done to warrant its use on humans. He therefore maintained that Karp's death from pneumonia and renal complications was not directly attributable to the mechanical heart. Technically speaking, the artificial heart did perform its pumping function during the 65 hours it was in Karp's chest. But immediately after the implant, physiological and biochemical negative signs appeared. In contrast to Cooley's optimism, DeBakey, a prominent cardiac surgeon who is in professional competition with Cooley, asserted that a human trial with the device was premature. Laboratory experiments on animals are a technical and ethical prerequisite to clinical trials of a new therapy on human beings. However, there are no absolute criteria for determining when it is proper to move from the laboratory to the clinic.

The second ethical question is whether death was imminent. Cooley avowed that his primary reason for implanting the artificial heart was to deal with an emergency situation by doing everything technically possible to save the life of a dying patient. However, the chronology of Cooley's activities shows that the use of the artificial heart was premediated. Months of preparation had gone into making the device ready for human use. The circumstantial evidence suggests that Cooley had a vested interest in human experimentation as a scientist-investigator as well as motivation as a doctor to save a specific patient.

Admitting that Cooley was anxious to experiment with his new apparatus on humans, the third ethical dilemma pertains to the criterion of societal risk versus benefit. According to the guidelines established by the National Institute of Health, the risk to an individual is outweighed by the potential benefit to him or her or by the importance of scientific knowledge to be gained. Cooley deliberately eschewed these guidelines and peer review procedures, and declared his right to professional individualism and autonomy without interference from a government agency or his colleagues. Cooley believes in the important of pioneering works for the advancement of science and criticizes physicians and patients who cowardly retreat from therapeutic innovations.

Related to this schism in professional orientations toward scientific research is the fourth ethical problem, that of competitiveness and rivalry among the professionals. The reason why the court decided not to use DeBakey's testimony in public hearing was because the alleged friction between DeBakey and Cooley might prejudice the jury unfairly. It had been well publicized that these two cardiac surgeons were rivals and that Cooley wanted to beat out DeBakey by being the first to implant an artificial heart into a human body.

It should be noted that the *Cooley* v. *Karp* case also involved questions about the ethical responsibility of the media. The media hailed the use of the artificial heart in man as a great new scientific accomplishment. It proclaimed that cardiac transplantation was a miraculously effective procedure for saving a dying patient.

This publicity particularly affected the donor of the heart. Moved by Mrs. Karp's piteous entreaty for a heart donation and the optimistic prediction of the success of the transplant, the donor's daughter decided to grant permission to donate the heart of her mother, who had been in a coma, suffering from irreversible brain damage. The donor was flown from Massachusetts to Texas, which created moral doubts about an encroachment upon the dignity of her death. It also deprived local candidate-recipients who had better chances of successful scarce organ transplants than Mr. Karp did. Moreover, the donor was technically and morally alive until the physicians declared her dead after her cross-country flight.

In sum, the case of the first artificial heart transplant has raised scores of ethical questions regarding human experimentation and organ transplantation.

Organ Transplantation. Since heart transplantation is so symbolic in promising human power to prolong life, the public became optimistic and ambitious about the future of human life. However, a lack of basic knowledge of the body's immunological defense against a transplanted organ makes the surgery highly risky. Due to the low success rate, heart transplantation has been discouraged in recent years (Fox & Swazey, 1974).

Vital organs for transplantation such as the heart, the liver, and the lungs can be obtained only from cadavers. Any attempt to take them from living sources runs afoul of state and federal suicide and homicide laws. The removal of nonvital parts—one kidney, small pieces of skin, and bone marrow—can be made from a living source but even this raises questions of coerced consent

("The sale . . . ," 1974). Although the Uniform Anatomical Gift Act has made it legal for adults to will their organs to medical science, there are still some states in which individuals do not have the legal right to donate parts of their bodies. In those states, and in cases where the person has not previously expressed an opinion about donation, consent for donation is given by the next of kin. This poses a problem because the decision has to be during a period of grief and therefore has psychological ramifications.

Another major ethical concern in organ transplantation is the protection of a donor against the pressure to save another human being. Since tissues should be matched, organs donated by close relatives have a far better chance for survival after transplantation than those from strangers. Therefore, there is likely to be pressure in the family for healthy siblings and cousins to contribute organs for ailing relatives. However, giving up of one kidney may affect the donor's future ability to recover from kidney disease. Also, there is the risk of the operation itself. The law imposes greater restrictions on the donation of nonvital organs when the source is a minor or an incompetent.

In case of a cadaver donation, the problem of determining the exact time of a potential donor's death becomes extremely serious because the organ must be alive to be of value. To avoid a conflict of interest, it has been generally agreed that the medical practitioners who take care of and declare the death of prospective donors shall be separate from the transplant surgeons (Simmons & Simmons, 1971).

Hemodialysis. While waiting for a donor of a kidney, a patient can be sustained by hemodialysis. Hemodialysis is the process of purification of the blood by means of an artificial kidney machine to which a patient is attached for several hours a day, two or three times a week.

> The machine . . . looks something like an old-fashioned washing machine. I fill its stainless steel tub with twenty-five gallons of water to which I add a large bottle of concentrated dialsate, a sort of brine with many of the chemical properties of blood. To a hollow rod in the tub I attach a coil that consists of a cellophane-like membrane wound round and round inside a plastic holder. . . .
>
> After I have filled the tub and tested the coil by pumping air into it to make sure the membrane won't leak or rupture under pressure, I rig the machine. This procedure involves stringing and connecting yards of complex plastic tubing and priming the tubing by pumping saline solution through it . . . inserts two thick hollow needles into a vein in my arm and connects them by means of slender saline-filled tubes to the tubing already attached to the machine. . . .
>
> After the machine is switched on, my blood flows from one of the needles through a tube to the coil that contains the membrane. The blood is on one side of the membrane, the dialsate bath on the other. Since the salt, urea, creatinine, potassium, uric acid, and other substances are in higher concentration in my blood than in the bath, they filter from the blood through the membrane into the bath by a process of osmosis. Thus my blood is cleansed as it passes by the membrane (Foster, 1976, pp. 5-6). 5–6).

Scarce and expensive therapy such as hemodialysis raises a serious problem in selecting the patients to whom the therapy should be applied. This is the decision of "who shall live when not all can" (Childress, 1970; Kulge, 1975).

The measure of social worth has frequently been adopted. Social worth is evaluated by the magnitude of past and future potential contribution to society in terms of social roles, relations, and functions. Important dimensions of social worth consist of the patient's motivation and intelligence, that is, "the need to prevail," the ability to adhere to therapeutic premises and restrictions, and the capacity to recognize any deviations from normal functioning (Fox & Swazey, 1974).

Functionalists would argue that these are exactly the attributes that make people occupationally and socially successful, and therefore important to society. Hence, the over-representation of middle class patients in the therapeutic pool for hemodialysis does not reflect prejudice against the socially disadvantaged. Value judgments exist at all levels and by common consent. The adoption of social worth based on the commonly shared value of material success therefore is not unethical, it is functional (Westervelt, 1970).

However, this perspective is valid only on the condition that everyone ought to do all of those things that contribute to the productive efforts of society. In addition, the difficulty of this premise is that societal standards of worth are reduced to one common denominator, material success, to the exclusion of all other values (Katz, 1976).

Unethical Experiment

Since World War II the increase in research funds and the importance attached to scientific investigation, when juxtaposed to the growing awareness of human rights, has heightened public sensitivity to moral issues in human experimentation. Beecher's (1966) documentation of unethical experiments is recognized as a significant contemporary effort to warn the medical profession and the public about errors of judgment and the overstepping of ethical boundaries. Beecher and others have illustrated various types of ethical errors, such as the withdrawal of known effective treatments and the administration of placebos. It was evident in most of these cases that the subjects would not have volunteered if they had been informed of the risks involved.

A frequently quoted example is the injection of live cancer cells into subjects who were not informed of the nature of the cells. The subjects for this experiment were 22 seriously ailing and debilitated patients at a relatively obscure chronic disease hospital in New York City. The researchers wanted to test the hypothesis that healthy persons would reject the cancer tissue culture much faster than individuals already suffering from advanced cancer. In order to make sure that the slower rate of rejection in the cancer patients was really due to their cancer and not to the general debility of chronically ill patients, a chronic disease hospital was chosen as an ideal place to select research subjects.

The researchers explained to the subjects that this study was to discover their resistence to disease. However, the subjects were not informed that the substance to be injected consisted of live cancer cells. The investigators were convinced that the procedure involved no risk of transplanting cancer to the experimental subjects, and they did not think it imperative to frighten the subjects unnecessarily by the word "cancer," which would hinder their study.

The charge brought against the researchers was that the patients used for research were in such a debilitated physical and mental state that they were incapable of giving informed consent. Further, if they had been told and had understood that live cancer cells were to be transplanted, they would have not volunteered to participate. The researchers were found guilty and their licenses were suspended for one year, although execution of the sentence was stayed. They were placed on probation but allowed to continue practicing (Langer, 1966).

The development of the Salk vaccine against polio was also based on several unethical experiments in the 1950s. Having successfully immunized monkeys in the laboratory, Jonas Salk was confident that he had found the key to immunization in a killed virus vaccine. Salk proceeded to test his discovery on humans. The first test was conducted on children from the Home for Crippled Children. Risk was reduced by vaccinating the children who already had polio and were thus immune to the injection. These children showed no adverse reactions (Brandt, 1978).

Then, he inoculated children who were mentally defective and had no history of polio. Fortunately, there were no negative reactions in these children. However, had the experiment gone wrong at this point, there might have been a tremendous outcry. It seems that if an experiment is successful, it is accepted as ethical; if a failure, it is condemned as unethical.

Later the large-scale field trial for polio vaccine was conducted with volunteers who were divided into two groups: half received the vaccine and the other half received placebos. The ethical dilemma is that if researchers are aware of the fact that the presence of the antibody is effective in preventing the disease, then there is no moral justification for intentionally injecting subjects with placebos. But the effectiveness of the vaccine could be proven only by a contraction of polio in those children who received placebos.

Informed Consent

From the functionalist perspective, contemporary American society subscribes to the common values of scientific research and progress, and those functions demand human subjects for experimentation. For example, society cannot afford to discard the organs of a hopelessly unconscious patient when they could be used to restore other individuals (Kulge, 1975). However, individuals are presumably protected by another set of values that require that no person will be used for experimentation without his or her informed consent. Functionalists further postulate the internalization of societal values into individuals. Thus, volunteers for human experimentation are expected to be highly motivated and dedicated persons who are intellectually capable of grasping the purposes and procedures of the experiment (Jonas, 1970).

The concern, however, is the extent to which experimental subjects have full knowledge of the potential risks before they participate. Under the best of circumstances, informed consent is problematic because of the uncertainty of the risk–benefit ratio even in the minds of the investigators. Furthermore, informed consent is not attainable from those who cannot make rational decisions, such as a fetus, children, the mentally ill, or the senile.

Fetus research involves at least three parties: an unseen patient (the fetus), the mother, and the father. The central issue of informed consent lies in who might be permitted to give it. One problem is to decide whether the fetus is considered to be a fully developed human. Another issue involves the interest of the mother, particularly her health (Academy Forum, 1975). Even if the fetus is given a right to life, it is not guaranteed the right to the continued use of another person's body. That privilege may infringe upon women's right or society's right to control the size of the population.

For functionalists, societal survival is the ultimate goal, but their concept of society is ambiguously defined. Society may refer to a particular political community or an interest group rather than the human race or a nation as a whole (Katz, 1976). The worst abuse of "society" was seen in the Nazi government. While functionalists assume that informed consent guarantees the balance of interests between individuals and society, conflict theorists point to the inequality of the way in which experimental advantages and risks are distributed among different individuals and groups. Those who are most exposed to experiments appear to belong to specific subservient categories such as fetus, children, patients, military, prisoners, and the poor, all of whom are powerless or are viewed as expendable (Lasagna, 1970).

Those poor who have the least education and sophistication are also the least able to understand the ways in which physicians communicate. Thus, they are not able to give an "informed" consent. In addition, the life situations of the poor that make them feel helpless place them in a position inherently vulnerable to external coercion.

Another reason for the disproportionately frequent use of the poor for experiments is that they are administratively more accessible than others. As recipients of welfare, health, and other public assistance, the destitute can be more effectively standardized, classified, treated, and observed than can the middle class patients of private physicians.

As mentioned earlier, when it comes to receiving the benefits of scientific advances such as hemodialysis or kidney transplants, the indigent are likely to be left out because they do not measure up to the criteria of social worth as defined by the dominant middle class (Beecher, 1970; Shatin, 1967).

A population that is better for certain kinds of controlled studies than the poor consists of prisoners, mental hospital patients, or nursing home residents, because their diets and lifestyles are easily observed and controlled. They are also under strict conditions of isolation and prolonged observation. There are positive aspects to experimentation with such groups, such as the enhancement of self-determination and self-esteem through contribution to worthy causes (Wells et al., 1974).

On the other hand, conflict theorists would claim that no person can be a free agent in institutions such as mental hospitals, nursing homes, or prisons, and that consent without coercion is impossible. They are not so much concerned with the actual, occasional abuse of captive human subjects as with subtle types of coercion or seduction—temporary escape from boredom and unpleasant surroundings, financial reward for participation, or a possibility for an earlier release (Academy Forum, 1975).

Another concern about experimentation on prisoners and mental patients is derived from the fact that inmates are state controlled. The state, which has possession and command of inmates, delivers their bodies to the scientists. Under these circumstances, the meaning of voluntary consent is suspect.

Whether we accept the functionalist assumption of value consensus regarding the importance of scientific progress or not, we cannot ignore the role of the mass media in generating symbolic halo effects over medical research and in labeling scientists celebrities.

Breakthroughs in medical technology make front-page news in our contemporary society. The press makes national heroes of research physicians and patient-subjects, and extolls them as courageous, daring, enduring, idealistic, and altruistic (Fox, 1970). The coverage of cardiac transplantation has been especially spectacular. However, the results have been both positive and negative. The mass media publicized the need for live and cadaver donors, but it also facilitated the competitive and commercialized behavior of physician-investigators who seek out and identify potential donors.

Informed, voluntary consent as defined by the functionalists is perceived by the interactionists as subtle coercion exercised by the physician-investigators upon their patients (Academy Forum, 1975). Through reading of reports and by interviewing physicians and patients, Fletcher (1976) found that many investigators and administrators worked from the assumption that a sick person would do almost anything a physician suggested. Patients often felt dependent and committed to their physicians and were reluctant to challenge them or to disagree with their decisions. Gray (1975) reported that some patients participated in a medical experiment against their wishes because they were afraid of weakening their physicians' sense of obligation to them. Whether this is true or not, the fact remains that the patients interpreted the situation as such.

The willingness to consent is also associated with the symbols used and the manner in which the physician advocates a project. Communication can be subtle in the phrasing of requests and the imposition of authority. For example, there is a great difference in people's willingness to try a "new" drug against an "experimental" drug (Gray, 1975). Modification of the vocabulary or even the tone of voice can constrain or expand the patient's readiness to consent (Fletcher, 1976).

Sometimes the guilt a patient feels for being ill and the accompanying need for self-sacrifice may be exploited by the investigator. The ultimate coercion is the manipulation of the patient's emotions and forcing him or her to "will" that which the physician wants.

In short, from interactionist perspectives, medical ethics refers to the strategic manipulation of symbols and of face-to-face interactions by physician-scientists in an attempt to justify their medical research and progress.

Death and Dying

Definition of Death

The difficulty in determining the appropriate time to remove a prospective donor's organs for transplantation, that is, the time of death, has been complicated by the development of artificial life-supporting mechanisms such as supportive therapy, resuscitation, and assisted circulation.

Because of their physicial interdependence, the three major life-sustaining body systems—respiratory, circulatory, and nervous—fail almost simultaneously if left to themselves. Thus, in the past, the cessation of the heartbeat marked the onset of death not only because the heart was considered to be the central organ of the body but also because the failure of the heart was accompanied by the breakdown of the other physiological systems.

Now, various medical techniques can retain life functions mechanically and chemically so that the heart may continue to beat even after the nervous system has ceased to operate. This presents grave social, legal, and technical problems. Financially, the expense of these life-supporting systems may be devastating to the patient's family or the national revenue. From a societal perspective, the use of rare techniques and the prolonged occupation of hospital space for a dying patient may interfere with the chance of saving another patient who is more likely to recover. Psychologically, the family of a patient on a life-support system must endure the pain of an extended death. The patient, if conscious, might have experienced a loss of dignity in being sustained in a vegetative state.

All of these questions point to the need for a redefinition of death. One new definition is brain death, that is, irreversible coma. Brain death refers to the permanent cessation of brain functioning. It is determined by the absence of responsivity to externally applied stimuli and to inner needs: the lack of spontaneous muscular movement and spontaneous respiration. A flat or isoelectric electroencephalogram is held to be of great confirmation value. These tests must be performed twice in 24 hours (Fox, 1974a,b).

The introduction of the concept of brain death has not solved all the questions but rather has created new uncertainties. Now the debate is between the destruction of the whole brain against that of a particular part of the brain—the seat of the highest mental functions. Another dimension of the controversy is concerned with whether death is a process (Morison, 1971) or a discrete event (Kass, 1971). Further, one of the criteria for death is that the patient cannot survive without the life-support systems.

Karen Ann Quinlan

The case of Karen Ann Quinlan (Quinlan & Quinlan, 1977; Reiser, Dyck, & Curran, 1977) was an unprecedented and agonizing attempt to determine what is legally required of health professionals and family members in case a comatose person does not meet the criteria of brain death.

On April 15, 1975, 21-year-old Karen Ann Quinlan went into a deep coma from undetermined causes. When it became clear after a few weeks that she would be extremely unlikely to regain consciousness, her parents decided to remove her artificial life supports. Her body was also deteriorating: over a period of time her body, which was reduced to 60 pounds, was described as shriveled, scarcely human, grotesque, and curled up in a fetal position.

Their Catholic church took the position that people's first obligation is to use all "ordinary means" to sustain life because life is sacred, but that if the life has to be maintained by "extraordinary means," such as a respirator, a human being may be allowed to die.

However, legal complications arose because Karen was declared legally and medically alive, even using the definition of brain death. Also, since Karen was of age, her father could not act as her legal guardian. To permit Karen to die would make the doctors, the hospital, or her father vulnerable to charges of malpractice or homicide.

After months of trials at a county court and the state Supreme Court, Karen's father was finally decreed on March 21, 1976 to be a legal guardian of his daughter. The Supreme Court eliminated any criminal or civil liability for removing the life-support system. The legal issue was finally settled, but the hospital showed reluctance to remove the life support on medical and moral grounds. Karen was subsequently weaned from the respirator and moved to a nursing home on June 9, 1976, and is still there at the time of this writing.

While legal issues were resolved, ethical issues just began to come to the surface. Quinlan's case may be generalized to other life-and-death situations, and therefore it stirred up all kinds of views and contentions (Kastenbaum, 1977; Ramsey, 1978).

On the technological side, there is the problem of inability to determine when life ends and death begins. Due to a rapid change in science, the definition of death must change with science. Also the decision to discontinue a life-support system requires a judgment concerning the prospect of recovery. A person in a coma now may recover later if he or she is sustained until a new scientific therapy is discovered.

On the part of a dying person, there is a dilemma in "death with dignity" (Cantor, 1973). If Karen Ann has already died as a person, death with dignity is meaningless because she has no consciousness. On the other hand, if she actually has some functions operating, the withdrawal of a respirator is considered as homicide. Another issue involves the quality of life: How important is survival regardless of the quality of life? How much impairment is acceptable to Karen Ann? Which would she choose, a quick death or a prolonged useless existence?

From the perspectives of survivors, continued use of life-supporting services may mean a prolongation of grief. The family members cannot place the death behind them and their daily life continues to be influenced by a hope that becomes psychological agony.

Finally, Quinlan's case raises the same controversies for society as does euthanesia: Who determines whose life should be sustained regardless of the expense? What should be the criteria for deciding to continue or discontinue life support?

The Right to Death

There are thousands of Karen Ann Quinlans every year who are terminally ill, sustained by respirators, and who are fed intravenously. The primary difficulty in finding a definition of death that is acceptable to the medical, legal, and religious sectors, and to the general public, is that there are many traditional concepts of death (Issacs, 1978). The questions may be phrased: What is it that has died when we speak of death? What is it that is so essential to human life? Does death mean the biological cessation of the artificial respirator, the loss of consciousness, the soul, or the capacity of social interaction? (Kastenbaum, 1977) Determination of the death of the biological organism and the death of the "person" involves medical, ethical, and social considerations.

Despite the difficulties, or because of the difficulties in defining death, there has been a growing tendency in recent years toward advocating the right to death. The public's concern to retrieve control of their bodily integrity from technological and impersonal forces has resulted in their claim for elective death.

There are a variety of "elective deaths" involving a number of legal and medical issues. Fletcher (1968) distinguished four types based on two dimensions: direct versus indirect, and voluntary versus involuntary. The direct method refers to executing some measure directly to end a life, while the indirect method means refraining from providing medical care so that death will come.

Fletcher's first type is the *direct voluntary death* wherein a patient consciously and deliberately chooses to end his or her life with or without medical intervention. In this case a patient may secretly take an overdose of drugs or pull out a tube. The second type is called *indirect voluntary death.* Here, a patient, before reaching an unconscious or comatose state, gives permission to physicians to use their discretion about letting death come. The third kind of elective death is *indirect involuntary,* which is caused by the decision of a doctor and/or family and friends to let the patient stop fighting off death, while the patient's wishes are unknown. This takes place when a patient's pain, subhuman condition, irreversibility of the condition, cost, and/or injustice to others outweigh the benefits of keeping the patient alive. The fourth type refers to *direct involuntary death.* This occurs when a patient's wishes are not known, yet physicians, family, or friends think it better to end a patient's life by a "mercy killing" than to keep alive a patient whose cerebral cortex has been shattered in an auto accident and who is unable to move a muscle.

Some people accept only types 2 and 3 (indirect death) and reject types 1 and 4 (direct method). Catholics, for example, differentiate ordinary and extraordinary means to sustain life. To them the withdrawal of extraordinary methods for sustaining life is acceptable since it is an indirect method. Others claim that the important thing is the end (the right to death) rather than the means (the direct or indirect method) (Fletcher, 1968).

A good example of indirect voluntary death is seen in the Natural Death Act. In 1977 California became the first state in the nation to allow terminally ill persons to authorize, by prior directive (sometimes called a "living will"), the withdrawal of life-sustaining procedures when death is believed imminent (Raible, 1977; Ramsey, 1978).

According to this Natural Death Act, a directive means a written document voluntarily executed by the declarant in the presence of two witnesses other than the attending physician, an employee of the physician or health facility, or anyone who has a claim against the declarant's estate. The directive will be kept in a patient's medical record and is effective for five years. Thus, the patient is protected from various people who might possibly gain from his or her death in the form of obtaining live organs for transplantation, inheritance, or release from the burden of caring for the patient.

However, there still remain ambiguities in this law. It is sometimes not easy to determine whether or not the patient is treatable: Can the patient somehow recover, and if so, what will the quality of life be? Another question concerns the state of mind, or rationality, in which a person makes the decision to die.

Apart from religious, moral, or metaphysical arguments over death, in actual practice passive euthanasia (indirect involuntary death) is not a rare occurrence. For example, Crane (1975) found that physicians make distinctions between physiological and sociological aspects of illness and treat patients accordingly. Based on extensive interviews of over 3,000 physicians in several medical specialties and studies of hospital patients, Crane showed that many physicians use social criteria (the extent to which a person is capable of interacting with others and performing social roles) in deciding upon the withdrawal of treatment from critically ill patients. Thus, the physically damaged but salvageable patient whose life can be maintained for a relatively long time and who shows the potentiality to participate in social life is more likely to be actively treated than the severely brain-damaged patient or the patient who is in the last stage of terminal illness.

In short, while active euthanasia is relatively rare, passive euthanasia with respect to certain types of cases (e.g., prescription of narcotics to terminal patients in pain, or the termination of the respirator for a patient with irreversible brain death) is widespread. Duff and Campbell (1973) also reported that of 299 consecutive deaths occurring in a special-care nursery, 43 (14 percent) were related to withholding treatment because of the prognosis that meaningful life was extremely poor.

Thus, in actual fact the practice of death control is increasing, depending, of course, upon circumstances. Fletcher (1968) and others advocate that since society is accepting the morality of abortion (the termination of lives at the beginning) for therapeutic reasons of mental, emotional, and social well-being, so the termination of lives at the end should be accepted as therapeutic euthanasia.

Debates on abortion and euthanasia share some common dilemmas, such as (1) difficulty in defining when human life begins and ends, and (2) conflicting interests of the parties involved—the fetus versus the mother in case of abortion, and the dying patient versus the healthy population in case of euthanasia. However, overall liberalization of attitudes toward abortion and euthanasia seems to indicate a growing sense of the right of individual human beings to resist religious as well as medico-technical encroachment upon the human body.

Genetic Engineering

Recent advances in biology and medicine have created the feasibility of various forms of genetic engineering, which in turn creates new ethical problems (Humber & Almeder, 1976; Reilly, 1977; Wertz, 1973). Certain methods are already in use, others need only minor adjustments, while still others are in the offing and are awaiting further basic research. Biologists and physicians disagree as to how much is possible how soon, and they view these developments both with enthusiasm and with alarm. Genetic engineering presents different problems from those arising from other medical treatments. While medicine affects existing individuals—their health, illness, and death—genetic manipulation can make changes that can be transmitted to succeeding generations. Hence, it has more serious consequences to humanity.

Intrauterine Testing

A genetic technology that has a high level of accuracy is the detection of certain abnormal genes and chromosonal conditions in the intrauterine fetus. The increasing ability to identify and diagnose genetic characteristics of a developing baby generates ethical issues concerning abortion. Since treatment of the intrauterine fetus is largely unavailable at present, diagnosis has to be followed by a decision on abortion, which entails the rights of the fetus to life and the consequences of the birth of an abnormal child to itself, to its family, and to society.

A genetic technology with more direct means for influencing eugenic ends is the artificial insemination of a woman with sperm from a donor other than her husband. This eugenic proposal (Muller, 1962) has been possible for some time because of the perfection of methods for long-term storage of human spermatozoa.

Test Tube Baby

Concern over genetic engineering was triggered recently by the birth of the world's first "test tube" baby in England on July 25, 1978. Patrick Steptoe surgically removed a cluster of eggs from a woman who could not have children because of a blockage of her fallopian tubes. The eggs were fertilized in a laboratory with her husband's sperm and their growth was examined through a microscope. The one that was doing the best was implanted in the mother's uterus, and subsequently a baby girl was born.

Prior to the birth of England's test tube baby attracting worldwide press attention, the Del Zio trial started in the United States. The Del Zios sued for $1.5 million for emotional distress caused by the destruction of their test tube embryo in 1973. The Del Zios alleged that Raymond V. Wiele "maliciously and wantonly" destroyed an in-vitro culture of Del Zio's eggs and her husband's sperm and thereby caused her emotional pain and suffering. Wiele claimed that by blocking the implantation of the culture into her uterus, an untried procedure in 1973, he prevented the performance of "an unauthorized human experiment" and perhaps saved Del Zio's life. In 1978 a four woman-two man jury in Manhattan federal court awarded $50,000 to Del Zio ("$50,000 award . . . ," 1978).

The above two incidents reveal scientific, legal, social, moral, and emotional difficulties involved in human experimentation. In 1973 opinions were divided among physicians as to the success of a test tube conception. Though some doctors believed that they had achieved a history-making operation, Wiele considered it immoral to carry out such procedures until there was more knowledge of the possible consequences.

The success of the British test tube baby in 1978 means a scientific breakthrough and a great joy to thousands of women with fallopian tube problems. Seeing in the mass media pictures of this happy couple with a new-born baby, one readily shares the view that outwitting nature to create a happy family environment is a positive step.

However, the test tube baby raises legal and moral questions. Some criticize the event as "tinkering with nature" and circumventing the natural way. Even if a baby created in a test tube does not turn out to be a monster, this procedure disrupts the relationship between the procreation (life-giving) and the integrative (love-giving) aspects of human sexual intercourse, and may have an adverse effect upon the child as well as upon parents. Also it is a human experimentation without the consent of the child. The question is raised as to whether or not we have a right to experiment with the life of a human being ("Test-tube baby . . . ," 1978).

From a legal aspect there are many problems, such as, embryo selling and suits by children born with defects as a result of test tube fertilization. Above all, the issue of who will regulate test tube fertilization stirs memories of Nazi experiments by which about 2,800 children were born at a Nazi maternity home. That experiment did not involve laboratory conception as in the British case but rather a strict and sometimes forced selection of prospective parents with the aim of expanding the Aryan race. There is always a possibility of someone's abusing test tube procreation (Minthorn, 1978).

Cloning

A development with a far more suitable technique for eugenic purposes, but one which is in the stage of experimentation with nonhumans, is cloning, or asexual genetic replication (Lederberg, 1966). In this process the nucleus of a mature but unfertilized egg is removed and replaced with a nucleus obtained from a specialized cell of the same or any other individual. Since almost all the hereditary material of a cell is contained within its nucleus, the individual who develops from the renucleated egg is genetically identical to the donor of the nucleus.

Currently there is controversy over the validity of the alleged successful cloning of a human being. A widely advertized and heavily promoted book recounts incidents surrounding the claim of successful cloning (Rorvik, 1978). The author narrates the efforts undertaken to satisfy the desire of a 67-year-old millionnaire bachelor to have an heir who would be his exact, genetic replica.

The identities of all the people in his book are concealed. The millionnaire is presented only as Max; the physician who performed the experiment is called Darwin; and the surrogate mother is known as Sparrow. To give the right touch of authenticity, Darwin is alleged to have boasted that his procedure, or timing, for implantation of an embryo is superior to that of Steptoe's.

Many people find this book of interest without questioning its authenticity. Some condemn the report as fraudulent because of Darwin's refusal to present the results in a medical or scientific journal with documentation that can be subjected to peer evaluation (Holman, 1978). Presented as it is, the validity of the report is open to question: Could Darwin really produce a clone? Even if he did, was it accidental? Whether the book tells a true story or not, it does raise ethical and moral issues about the procedure and consequences of human cloning.

On the positive side is the therapeutic use of genetic copying. The hope is that normal copies of appropriate genes, obtained biologically or otherwise, can be implanted into defective individuals to cure genetic disease. However, the possibility of abuse is even more devastating than in the case of test tube babies.

The fundamental issue in genetic engineering centers around the pros and cons of eugenics. If a superior individual is identified, why not copy it directly instead of letting nature take its course for the recombination of various genotypes? The problem then is to establish who will decide what constitutes a superior individual worthy of replication? Who will decide which individuals may or must not reproduce? The example of Nazi Germany's genocide makes people apprehensive about what can happen under the pretext of eugenics.

Another issue is whether or not the laboratory reproduction of a human being dehumanizes social interaction. Social bonds such as marriage, family, and the socialization of children may be undermined by asexual reproduction and test tube babies.

MEDICAL ETHICS, MEDICAL BUREAUCRACY, AND SOCIETY

Ethics

There are some who claim that the quetion of ethics, or what "ought to be," must not be confused with science, or what "is" (Lundberg, 1963). However, the examples in preceding sections clearly indicate that ethical issues enter into the domain of science. There are others who assert that science per se is a value, and that the problem in ethics is to determine the relationship between one kind of value (science) and other kinds of value (Ladd, 1976).

Ethics is defined by Parsons (1970, p. 1140) as a "system of control of human behavior in the interest of maintaining and implementing values." Hence ethical theories must be justified in terms of the welfare of both individuals and society. And thus for medical ethics (Jonas, 1970), the problem is to resolve the conflicts between the long-range interests of society and the immediate rights of individuals. Systematic intellectual reflection on what is right and wrong in the practice of medicine has traditionally occurred within both the religious and philosophical spheres.

Religion has had profound direct and indirect impact upon human behavior as well as on legal rules. Christianity defines the meaning of life and death, and it presupposes the belief in a personal God, the immortality of the human soul, and the existence of moral laws binding all human beings. Since supreme dominance over life is believed to belong to God alone, the state or an individual has no right to kill an innocent citizen for societal or individual utility (Kohl, 1975).

Various philosophical theories, such as utilitarianism and ethical naturalism, have been adopted by some as justification for medical ethics. Utilitarianism appears to solve the conflict between the interests of the individual and the welfare of society. According to this theory, an act is morally right only when it promotes the greatest amount of good for the greatest number of people (Albee, 1962; Kulge, 1975; Mill, 1871). Since the happiness of the greatest number takes precedence over that of the few, the individual who is a burden to society can justifiably be abandoned.

However, the calculus of the greatest number is not based on the assumption that members of the biological species, Homo Sapiens, are counted as equals. The greatest happiness principle is not concerned simply with numbers but with the power and the other social attributes of the members.

A different approach to medical ethics is found in ethical naturalism (Hart, 1965; Ulrich, 1976). This theory postulates that there are certain intrinsic principles of human conduct that can be discovered by human reason. Laws made by people, including the Constitution, must conform to natural human rights if they are to be valid. The Nuremberg trials of those Nazis who were accused of war crimes exemplify a situation in which human rights took precedence over legal rights.

The theory of ethical naturalism raises the important issue of whether human rights are indeed inalienable and non-negotiable. For one thing, what we call natural rights are likely to reflect the claimant's cultural heritage and social power. Human rights can be defined as nothing more than claims that are made with regard to the performance or prohibition of certain actions and are so acknowledged by other members of society. Social acknowledgment is a crucial factor in authorizing claims as human rights (Ulrich, 1976). For example, our contemporaries may view health as a natural right, but it would not have occurred to the eighteenth-century poor to claim such a right. Natural rights, when recognized as claims, seem to be associated with the social environment, the state of individual awareness (i.e., the claimant's definition of the situation), and above all, the power of the individual to make others accept his or her claims.

In sum, what appears to be an absolute ethical theory is likely to be affected by social factors. In fact, *ethics* can be used to refer to the *ethos* of a given society and to connote the customary practices in that society. Ethics as ethos reflects the structure and process of society. Therefore, the specific medical issues discussed in preceding sections are an integral part of the broader ethical problems in the structure and practice of modern medicine, which in turn are affected by the social, economic, political, and other forces of society. The broader ethical problems in the practice of modern medicine appear to be currently labeled by the public as the "medical crisis."

Medical Crisis

We are today spending several times as much of the nation's resources for health and medical care as we did twenty years ago. Health expenditures for individuals have risen faster than other costs. Yet, despite the soaring medical costs, problems seem to multiply—inaccessibility of physicians and persistently poor and even deteriorating health conditions. Clearly something must be wrong in the organization of medicine: there is a medical crisis.

In Chapter 10 and 11 our discussion focused on financial reorganization—in effect, socialized medicine—as a way to cope with the medical crisis. In contrast to such an economic approach to the problems we are facing today, some recent critics (Carlson, 1975; Fuchs, 1974; Illich, 1976) have attacked the cultural and structural aspects of the existing medical system in this country.

Fuchs and Carlson claim that medicine has been oriented toward acute illness and curative treatment rather than chronic illness and preventive treatment. However, those kinds of illness (the infectious diseases) that can be cured with this type of after-the-fact therapy have declined in prevalence relative to chronic and mental illnesses. Thus, the medical delivery system is unable to cure most of the major illnesses (e.g., cancer, arthritis, and heart disease) and has probably reached the point of diminishing returns in effectiveness to promote health. The new drugs and techniques discovered during the 1930s and the 1950s have reduced mortality rates from contagious diseases as much as they can be expected to.

At this point, factors other than medical care are more important in determining the status of one's health. They include heredity (genetic and physiological variations, etc.), environment (sanitation, pollution, housing, etc.), life (diet, exercise, smoking, stress, etc.), and attitudes (self-reliance, psychological well-being, etc.).

According to Fuchs and Carlson, costly yet ineffective medical care is partly due to the high utilization rate of medical services by the public, which has grown too dependent upon medicine. This dependency has been generated by the physician, the captain of the team, who controls not only the quality, type, and cost of services, but also the attitudes and behavior of consumer-patients. Physicians assume that they must do everything technically possible to promote medical scientific advances, while neglecting the question of patients' rights and wishes. They fail to see that there are other important goals in life.

Fuchs therefore proposes that individuals make value choices without being influenced by the medical profession. Value alternatives may include saving lives by organ transplantation versus reducing accidental traffic deaths by building better roads; or spending money on prescribed drugs versus improving diet. In other words, changes in cultural beliefs about health and illness are being proposed. Carlson suggests further a drastic reorganization of the structure of the health maintenance system by means of health education of the population, research on health behavior, deprofessionalization of the medical profession, and emphasis on preventive and environmental health.

While Fuchs maintains that medical care is no longer as effective in promoting health as it once was, Illich (1976) and Carlson (1975) go a step further and say that medicine is not only not useful but in fact is harmful.

Medical Nemesis

Crisis in medicine, according to Illich, is the unwarranted byproduct of the overexpansion of medical care and the concomitant medicalization of society. Illich calls this process "medical nemesis"—retribution for the pursuit of inhuman goals. Instead of being satisfied with what is humanly possible, physicians have aspired to control nature, humans, and society. Negative side effects of this ambition are analyzed by Illich as three phases of iatrogenesis (damages caused by physicians): clinical, social, and structural.

Clinical Iatrogenesis. Clinical iatrogenesis deals with "the undersirable side effects of approved, mistaken, callous, or contraindicated technical contacts with the medical system" (Illich, 1976, p. 32). Illich maintains that clinical iatrogenesis is caused primarily by the physicians' engineering approach to medicine, which views the individual as a machine. Therapeutic intervention here implies putting an aggregate of different pieces of human body together so that the human machinery functions properly. With this attitude, injury, sickness, or even death occurring as a result of medical treatment can be dismissed as a simple technical failure without much concern with the rights and sentiments of the patients as human beings (Coombs, 1978).

Another source of clinical iatrogenesis is attributed by Illich to the physician's arrogance in convincing the patients of the effectiveness of medical care. The doctors do not explicitly acknowledge that every treatment is nothing more than an experiment with only a certain probability of success and with a great chance of negative side effects. Illich provides historical evidence that the doctor's effectiveness has been an illusion:

> The combined death rate from scarlet fever, diphtheria, whooping cough, and measles among children up to fifteen shows that nearly 90 percent of the total decline in mortality between 1860 and 1965 had occurred before the introduction of antibiotics and widespread immunization (Illich, 1976, p. 16).

Social Iatrogenesis. If clinical iatrogenesis is the reality, how can there be anyone who would volunteer to participate in human experimentation? Illich interprets this as a result of social iatrogenesis: the addictive dependency of the populace on the medical care institutions.

In Illich's view, the cause for this addiction is the manipulative power of the medical bureaucracy in perpetuating and encouraging the passive and blind faith of the public in medicine. The medical bureaucracy monopolizes the power to define what health is and what methods of care should be utilized and therefore publicly funded. Physicians can decide who needs what kind of expensive and exotic medical devices and can appeal for public support. Conspicuous therapies such as heart transplantation serve as powerful means to persuade people to pay more taxes for medical research.

Medicine can justify its power as unbiased of any specific values because it is based on scientific foundations. As an unprejudiced umpire, medicine has extended its territory into various aspects of social deviation—labeling drug addicts, overactive children, and overaggressive social rebels as ill rather than as delinquent or criminal. The medical profession serves as an agency of social control over individuals who are deprived of the opportunities to make their own decisions.

Structural Iatrogenesis. When the medical bureaucracy succeeds in not only creating addiction to medicine but in stealing the autonomy of the patient, Illich calls this damage structural iatrogenesis. It sets in when the medical enterprise drains the will of people to face their reality, to express their own values, and to cope with human vulnerability such as pain, impairment, and death.

Illich elaborates upon the effect of medical technology on the experience of pain, which in his eyes is identical to the experience of life itself. Individuals learn from culture how to cope with pain. For example, traditional Japanese culture taught Japanese women that "real" love for children was derived from the pain of childbirth without anesthesia. Myriad virtues associated with persevering while in pain—duty, love, courage forebearance, compassion—traditionally enabled people to recognize painful sensation as a challenge and an integral part of "living."

Modern medicine, however, turned pain into a technical matter: a demand for drugs, hospitals, and medical services. Pain is no longer the experience of the soul, but is a symptom of dysfunction of the body machinery to be controlled by drugs and doctors. The appearance of pain-killers transformed doctors and patients into unfeeling spectators of the human apparatus. This is the context that makes human experimentation easy because both doctors and patients have been made insensitive to pain as well as other types of human feelings.

Traditional culture was also able to help people meet their death with dignity as individuals. The corpse had been treated almost like a person. For example, its dissection was considered a sacrilegious profanation. Now the physician whose scalpel has access to the corpse, has the power to determine the rules that designate how people ought to die (e.g., under intensive care) and that forbid them to choose any other fashion of departing from life. Thus, people do not die when their hearts stop beating but may be sustained on machines so long as they serve as evidence of technological advancement. According to Illich, people have lost the autonomy to choose the way to live and to experience pleasure and pain, and the manner in which to die.

Illich's solution to this medical nemesis lies within the individualistic orientation, similar to those proposed by Fuchs and Carlson. Illich advocates self-care and self-reliance, stating that health is primarily a personal task of autonomous adaptation of self to others and to the environment. Collective responsibility for care should be reduced so that individuals regain confidence and ability to cope with stress without depending on medicine. For this purpose he also proposes the breakdown of the centralization and bureaucratization of medical industrialization. The self-reliance approach by Illich and Fuchs stems from their concern with the separation of body and soul of humans as seen in the practice of modern medicine. They attempt to reintegrate body and soul so that individuals have control over their life again.

The limitations of "doing one's own thing" have been pointed out by many who assume that the basic cause of sickness is the social system, not the individual. For example, Navarro (1978a,b) asserts that emphasis on self-responsibility detracts us from the real cause of the medical crisis, namely, the political and economic structure of society. The critical factor in solving the medical crisis is to identify who controls the economy and the process of industrialization. Thus, according to Navarro, the only effective measure for solving the medical crisis is the change of the social structure to decentralize economic and political power and take it away from the dominant oligarchies.

Specific issues of medical ethics—human experimentation, genetic engineering, attitudes toward life and death, life-prolonging devices, and the like—are reflections of the medical crisis. Thus, the resolution of these ethical dilemmas must be accompanied by a solution to the medical crisis, which may require the joint effort of individuals and society. In other words, medical ethical issues must be dealt with on several levels: individual psychology, medical technology, cultural values, and social structure.

SUMMARY

Until the end of the Dark Ages, science, medicine, and social thought were largely submerged in the domain of theology. It was their inability to control nature that caused people to fear supernatural power and to seek answers in divinity.

Along with advances in science, however, medicine parted from both religious and philosophical ethics. The overwhelming emphasis on technological phenomena resulted in the isolation of medicine from a philosophical or religious orientation toward health and illness, life and death.

Within the past decade or two, medicine and ethics have begun to turn back toward each other. This came about through the dread of ungoverned human power to control nature, and it has led people to seek guidance in ethics. Our contemporary system of medicine has reached a stage of development characterized by "diffuse ethical and existential self-consciousness" (Fox, 1974a,b). This state of awareness involves searching out new interpretations of life and death, and questioning the desirability of human engineering of humanity and nature.

Answers to contemporary ethical questions are not found in the Hippocratic Oath, which prohibited active euthanasia but did not directly deal with, say, the termination of life-maintaining techniques, sometimes called passive euthanasia. The 1968 version of the Hippocratic Oath (Butler, 1968) declares that the rational ethical principles of minimizing suffering and of adhering to the humanitarian approach to medicine are basic to the medical profession. Among various ethical issues that are being raised and examined at present are the rights of every individual to some modicum of integrity, dignity, autonomy, and fulfillment.

More specifically, there is, first of all, the need to protect the interests of human subjects in experimentation. In 1966 the National Institute of Health (NIH) and the Public Health Service (PHS) mandated that all medical research supported by the NIH and PHS that involved human subjects must be reviewed concerning the rights and welfare of the parties concerned. By 1971, these requirements were extended to all research projects supported by any agency of the Department of Health, Education, and Welfare (which is the parent organization of both the NIH and PHS). In 1974 the National Research Act established a temporary two-year National Commission for the protection of human subjects of biomedical and behavioral research.

Moratoriums now being considered or that have been accepted in various states include the halting of medical experimentation on captives of the states such as prisoners and mental patients; the prohibition of fetus research; and the suspension of the use of procedures on medical or surgical patients that are still experimental (Fox & Swazey, 1974).

The second group of ethical issues centers around the rights of life and death. The individual's right to death with dignity can be protected by the appearance of a definition of brain death and by the legal right to terminate life-sustaining mechanisms, as is granted by the Natural Death Act enacted in 1977 in California. As for the right to life by means of scarce and expensive medical instruments, using social worth as the criterion for choosing the patients has been seriously questioned. Instead of a concept of social worth biased toward the middle class, randomization has been proposed. Also, the abortion debate partly involves the right-to-life issue.

Finally, genetic engineering is viewed by many people with alarm because of its impact on future generations. Biologists, physicians, theologists, and philosophers as well as members of the antiabortion movement have actively worked to deter genetic control.

All of these assertions of human rights indicate that there is apprehension about the consequences of unlimited biomedical scientific research: dehumanization, dependency upon medicine, rising medical expenses, and the like. Thus, specific issues of medical ethics must be examined with reference to the problems of the broader organization and practice of modern medicine.

Ineffectiveness of medical care coupled with soaring medical costs have engendered the medical crisis. Underlying causes for the medical crisis have been attributed by some to medical technocracy, in which medicine has turned into the engineering of the human body machinery. Others go further, saying that medical practice is managed but is not controlled by medical bureaucrats and technocrats because these people are subordinate to a greater power: the corporate class who owns and manages financial capital.

Two distinct kinds of solutions have been suggested: (1) liberation from medical domination and encouragement of a self-care approach to health; and (2) the change of social structure to decentralize political and economic power. To be effective, both approaches will probably have to be combined.

At any rate, neither medicine nor ethics stands in a sociological vacuum. Not only is there a convergence of medicine and ethics today, but also a growing interdependence of the various sectors of society, such as politics, law, economy, science, medicine, ethics, and religion.

For Aristotle, ethics was a branch of politics (Callahan, 1976). Whatever the merits of that view, recent events in the United States illustrate the enormous extent to which ethical problems have been transformed into political, legal, social, and medical controversies. These new developments have prompted medical professionals to join with experts in other disciplines as well as with lay people to work toward resolving their moral dilemmas.

EPILOGUE
The Changing Structure of American Medicine

In an attempt to provide an integrative framework for medical sociology, three major sociological theories—functionalism, conflict theory, and interactionism—have been used to interpret available sociomedical data.

Functionalism as a system approach is used as the point of departure (Davis, 1959) for identifying a unit of analysis as a social system; then the interdependence within the system and among systems is examined. Thus, within a society a subsystem of medicine exists, interlocked with other sectors such as the polity and the economy.

The functionalist premise of value consensus and integration is tested against the conflict theory assumption that society is an ongoing process of conflict generation and resolution.

As opposed to the above two theoretical perspectives, interactionism is concerned with the study of social behavior on a micro level. Here, the unit of analysis is the small-group, face-to-face interaction that is carried out both in an integrative and conflictive manner.

Using these theoretical perspectives, this book discusses (1) the development of the medical profession as a cohesive and dominant social system and (2) the current move toward the restructuring of that medical delivery system.

Development of the Medical Profession

In the ancient world medicine was undifferentiated from politics, social thought, economy, and other social institutions, all of which were subsumed under the domain of religion. Healing practitioners did not even possess an occupational identity and were socially powerless.

The turning point toward a successful consolidation of the medical profession is seen in the emergence of the germ theory and the ensuing advances in medical technology in the late eighteenth and early nineteenth centuries. From the functionalist perspective, it is argued that physicians attained a position of eminence because of their technical ability to perform indispensable functions for society. In order to be able to perform these functions, medicine "cleaned its own house." Since the Flexner Report, physicians have endeavored to maintain high educational standards and to socialize physicians-to-be with professional values.

Marxian conflict theorists, on the other hand, view modern medicine as "a child of capitalistic societies sired by the emergence of modern science" (Twaddle & Hessler, 1977, p. 313). Medicine was one of many divergent groups—homeopathy, thomsonianism, osteopathy, and chiropractic—competing in a laissez-faire marketplace. With the aid of the state in establishing licensure as well as with the weapon of technology, medicine won the power contest over other healing practitioners. Through continuous political lobbying and other tactics to fight against various third-party interference, medicine has succeeded in developing a closed system in which the physician enjoys autonomy and power.

The strategy for winning the battle was not limited to open confrontation. In fact, most of the transactions were carried out by bargaining, negotiating, and exchanging intangible resources with other interest groups. Throughout the alliance and re-alliance with various groups, organized medicine used the shibboleth "American way" to its advantage. For example, for fear of the enactment of compulsory health insurance, the AMA supported private health insurance as the "only American way." The symbolic power of medicine as the labeler is seen in the phenomenon called the medicalization of society, whereby social behavior is defined in terms of a medical perspective.

Restructuring of the Medical Care System

Now that the medical profession has established a dominant status, it is under attack both from within and without. Within the medical care system (the first party), there are dissenters who are against the physicians' autonomy and authority. The consumers (the second party) are no longer compliant clients to professionals but are critical of the way medical services are delivered. The government (the third party) is increasingly gaining control over medical care through governmental funding.

From the functionalist perspective, these attacks on the medical profession generate minor disturbances, and through repercussions among various components of the system a re-equilibrium will be reached. The assumption is that even after some rearrangement, the health service system will be maintained with the same basic value orientations of democracy, liberalism, and capitalism.

In contrast, conflict theorists reject the utility of such a premise when they see clashes of perspectives among competing interest groups such as the government, consumers, allied health workers, alternative health practitioners, the capitalist class, unions, and the like. Some believe that the driving force of the conflictive process lies in the hands of medical technocrats who are expanding the medical-industrial complex. Marxian theorists, on the other hand, claim that medical technologists are simply entrusted with power by the capitalist class, which is in command of the historical process.

Whether we label the emerging structure a "functional re-equilibrium" (i.e., the American way) or a "dialectic synthesis" (i.e., welfare state, socialism), we cannot deny that the American health service system is undergoing structural changes, and some alternatives are being predicted or proposed. Possible structural changes are summarized below in terms of the four Parsonian functional prerequisites: latency, integration, adaptation, and goal attainment.

Technology versus Humanitarianism (Latency)

Against the Disease Model. Since the germ theory and the reorganization of medical education following the Flexner Report, modern medicine has adhered to the disease model. This value orientation emphasizes (1) curing disease rather than caring about a patient; (2) treating acute rather than chronic illness; (3) training a specialist rather than a general practitioner; and (4) doing everything technically possible to save a patient's life regardless of the patient's sentiment, social utility, cost, and other factors. Physicians have been inculcated with these values through medical education, collegial reinforcement, and public expectation. Curing disease and saving life at any cost have been considered noble and progressive.

Within the past decade or two this disease orientation has been seriously questioned by the public as well as by medical practitioners. There is an increasing skepticism about the capacity of science and technology to improve life. Medicine, oriented toward acute care, is unable to cure chronic illnesses, which are the major causes of death in contemporary America (Carlson, 1975; Fuchs, 1974). Some people (Illich, 1976) deny any credit to medicine even in controlling contagious disease, claiming that improved living standards rather than medicine were responsible for the decline of infectious diseases. Further, medical research has created ethical dilemmas concerning human experimentation, genetic engineering, and human control over nature. Moratoria have been declared on many medical procedures.

From the cost efficiency viewpoint, the public has been alerted to the danger of expanding expensive specialization—specialized physicians, equipment, and research—at the cost of an adequate supply of primary care services. Carlson (1975) pointed out that saving one patient in a coronary care unit costs $70,000, which was then the yearly salary for two physicians delivering care to a medically underserved area. The disease model of medicine has been accused of causing inequity in health care delivery among different social strata.

The disease bias is also criticized by patients who are dissatisfied with impersonal doctor–patient relationships. The sudden upsurge of malpractice suits reflects patients' protests against doctors' lack of personal concern rather than the latter's technical incompetence, since patients are usually not able to evaluate the technical aspect of medical care.

Proposed or Projected Alternatives. There are two opposing views about the future of medical technology: (1) a deceleration of technological progress, and

(2) an acceleration of automation of medical care.

Those who are concerned with iatrogenesis argue that important determinants of health status are the lifestyle and environment instead of medicine. They therefore propose a new health care system (Carlson, 1975) based on (1) a "harmonious socio-environment"—better housing, improved nutrition, safe freeways, and clean air; (2) "readily obtainable resources to aid in becoming and staying healthy"—increase of primary care and preventive medicine and deprofessionalization of physicians; and (3) self-reliant health maintenance—public health education and improvement of lifestyle. The "end of medicine," as projected by Carlson, may not come in full force, but there is in recent years a greater interest shown by the public in preventive medicine (physicial fitness programs, health foods, etc.) and in a holistic approach (chiropractic, etc.).

In the iatrogenesis model, disease-oriented physicians are to be replaced by the public's self-reliant health maintenance system. Others predict the obsolescence of doctors caused by computarization of medicine.

Maxmen (1973) contends that within thirty years the United States will enter a "postphysician era" in which the physician's tasks—taking a history, performing a physicial examination, ordering ancillary tests, formulating a prognosis on the basis of past experience, and choosing the proper drug—will be usurped by medical technology and allied health workers. A computer can collect and synthesize a far greater amount of data than any physician can.

The emergence of a cybernated health care system, Maxmen argues, need not result in the submergence of medicine's humanistic orientation. The new automated medical order should reorient medical education to emphasize philosophical and social factors and develop schools of humanistic medicine. Maxmen asserts that a moratorium on medical research is unethical since it thwarts the humanistic desire for a healthier life.

Integration of the Health Care Delivery System

Against Professional Domination. The American health care delivery system has been integrated hierarchically with physicians at the top followed by ancillary health workers. Recently this physician dominance has been challenged by a series of events, promoting the power of allied health practitioners.

To begin with, new paramedical roles have been created to meet the needs of the physician shortage. The scarcity of physicians has been pronounced because of the increased utilization of health services due to (1) the public perception of health as a right rather than a privilege, and (2) government subsidies for medical care given to the poor and the aged, whose medical needs are great. The new allied health workers, such as physician's assistants and community health workers, are expected to play an important role in primary care by filling the communication gap between the medical bureaucracy and patients.

Successful development of allied health workers is well illustrated by the *feldshers* in the USSR and the barefoot doctors in the People's Republic of China. These workers were trained so that health standards could rise rapidly when the revolutionary governments decided to catch up with Western industrialized nations. In rural areas barefoot doctors and *feldshers* perform indispensable tasks not only as physician extenders but as the entry point to a complex medical care system. Farmers feel closer to these grassroot community workers than to physicians. However, a concept such as the Chinese barefoot doctors is not directly transferable to the United States because of different cultural patterns. Even the community health workers at the OEO-sponsored neighborhood health centers did not integrate well with the mainstream medical professionals.

Another factor that facilitated the awakening of consciousness of subordinate allied health workers was the civil rights movement of the 1960s, which subscribed to the ideals of equalitarianism and anti-elitism. The efforts of nurses, pharmacists, and other paramedics to professionalize themselves were slowly but steadily acknowledged. They began to extend their traditionally subordinate roles to more autonomous ones as nurse practitioners, clinical pharmacists, and the like.

Along with the growth of power among the lower- and middle-level health workers, the new concept of integration in the medical care system was introduced in the form of a health care team. The teamwork requires the performance of equalitarian and interdependent roles by physicians and ancillary health workers.

In order to implement this concept, it may be necessary not only to raise the status of allied health workers but also to lower the elitist position of physicians. In the USSR and the People's Republic of China physicians are state employees, receiving salaries from the state. Government effort to deprofessionalize physicians has been successful to the extent that physicians enjoy no higher status than other technicians and engineers. In the USSR physicians belong to the same labor union as other health workers. In a capitalistic society such as ours, deprofessionalization of this kind is unlikely. However, the professional authority of physicians has been eroded by various forces such as bureaucratization and centralization of medical financing as well as professionalization and unionization of lower-level health workers.

Government Control (Adaptation)

Over the years the medical profession has managed to cope with external threats. Physicians have established and maintained autonomy over the way in which they practice medicine without third-party intervention. They were also able, to a large extent, to adhere to the laissez-faire, fee-for-service manner of practice until recently.

Since 1965, however, the medical profession has been losing its financial autonomy to the government, which has become the major buyer of medical services. There are several causes that may be identified. First, the inequity of health services available to different social classes was attacked through the civil rights movements of the 1960s, which advocated the federal subsidy of health care for the indigent. Second, health care came to be regarded as a right rather than a privilege, which led the government to be responsible for providing health care to everyone. Third, technological advances and wider utilization of health services in conjunction with other factors have resulted in rising medical costs. The burden of financing medical care fell upon the government, which is the only social institution with the necessary resources.

Now that the government is financing the major portion of medical costs, it has the power to control the manner in which the money is spent. So far, government regulation has been limited to monitoring cost efficiency. However, such a practice is likely to touch upon other aspects of medical practice, such as quality control. Professional autonomy appears to be no longer unassailable.

Another aspect of government control is seen in administrative coordination. The increasing complexity and specialization in medical technology and the individualistic tradition of American society have generated a multiplicity of health services. Duplication of personnel and services, leading to medical inflation, calls for central coordination. The current interest in national health insurance reflects the public desire for government leadership in planning and allocating health resources instead of leaving them to the medical profession. Nevertheless, most of the national health insurance proposals are extensions of the existing insurance schemes with a minimum third-party control over medical practice.

The question is whether or not an American national insurance scheme will follow the pattern of the United Kingdom's and result in a national health service. Twaddle and Hessler (1977) described the present state of affairs as a "toxic combination of capitalism and socialism." Medicine, government, and industry are working together to patch up holes in the existing medical system without doing an overhaul.

From the labeling theory perspective, it is argued (Skidmore, 1970) that the American rhetoric of individualism could reduce the effectiveness of a radical idea such as national health insurance to no more than government-sponsored free enterprise. Dialectic theorists would argue that, after exchange, negotiation, and compromise among interest groups, the final version of a national health insurance bill will not satisfy any single group; hence, it contains the seed of its own destruction. From the Marxian viewpoint, the national health insurance proposals reflect the power of the capitalist class over the government. Functionalists, on the other hand, predict that a re-equilibrium will be attained after some redistribution of power and modification of functions among subsystems such as the government and the medical institution.

Consumer Power (Goal Attainment)

The ultimate goal of the medical profession is patient care. Physicians were applauded for their successful goal attainment when they brought contagious diseases under control. Also, each time the public hears about heart transplantation, the test-tube baby, and other spectacular events, confidence in physicians and medicine is reinforced.

However, contemporary American patients are no longer compliant and unquestioningly deferential to physicians. The doctor–patient relationship has changed from a client–professional one to a consumer–provider one. As consumers, patients are highly critical of the health services they receive. The most pronounced manifestation of patient rebellion is the upsurge of malpractice suits. Ironically, this is in part due to the patients' rising expectation of miraculous cures, which in turn is the product of technological progress. Frequently however, malpractice suits arise from deteriorated doctor–patient relationships aggravated by growing bureaucratization.

Another indication of consumer power over medical practice is the participation of community members in the decision-making process regarding medical administrative policies. Mass participation was encouraged in the neighborhood health center movement in the 1960s, although its impact upon the general public was not pervasive.

The massification of medical service was well exemplified in the People's Republic of China during the Cultural Revolution. The Communist government tried to develop health care services closely linked to the people. Thus, candidates for medical education were chosen from among the commune or factory workers by other workers. Upon completion of medical training, the new doctors were expected to return home. Note, however, that after the death of Mau and the denunciation of the Gang of Four, the massification of education was accused of lowering the educational standards.

Being an urban industrialized country with individualistic traditions, the United States is not likely to adopt the Chinese model. Rather, the American citizen's power may be exercised through various interest groups such as labor unions or consumers' advocate groups, which lobby for health legislation at local, state, and federal government levels.

Finally, consumer power over the medical delivery system can be expressed in a consumer's boycott of medical care. Increasing numbers of people are choosing to die rather than being sustained on a life-maintenance system. Self-care and self-reliance by means of changing lifestyles and diet, instead of medication, is an open announcement of the public's distrust of the efficacy of medical treatment and suspicions about iatrogenesis (Levin, Katz, & Holst, 1976; Pratt, 1973; Sehnert, 1975). Rebellion against medicalization of society is seen in the popularization of holistic and naturalistic medicine. People are seeking alternatives to medical treatment.

A possible model for a combination of modern and folk medicine is found in the People's Republic of China. The Chinese have consciously disfavored highly technological medicine and concentrated on the development of broad public health measures and individual responsibility.

Overview

Since the late nineteenth century, science and technology have been developed to control nature—regulate the natural environment, eliminate contagious disease, and extend life expectancy. Like sorcerers, human beings have learned to manipulate their apprentice, technology, to conquor the universe.

However, the spectacular development of technology and the medical-industrial complex during the past 40 years seems to have resulted in a situation in which human beings are no longer in command. As Somers and Somers (1977) describe it, Western people are dealing with a "Sorcerer's Apprentice" gone amuck, a theme which has haunted the imagination of Western poets and philosophers for centuries.

Western people created medical technology to serve humanity. Now, however, medical technology is enslaving humanity to technology. Technology has become an end in itself, less concerned with human health and happiness than with elegant theories and challenging procedures. People are committing themselves to health care policies that are no longer central to health and may even be threatening to life (Somers & Somers, 1977).

Current efforts to restructure the medical care system can be viewed as human attempts to regain control over technology and the medical-industrial complex.

REFERENCES

Abbott, Wilbur Cortez. 1918. *The expansion of Europe: A social and political history of the modern world, 1415–1789.* New York: Henry Holt & Co.

Abelson, Philip H. 1979. China in transition. *Science* 203:505–509.

Abel-Smith, Brian. 1964. *The hospitals in England and Wales: 1800–1948.* London: Heinemann.

Abel-Smith, Brian, and Gales, K. 1964. *British doctors at home and abroad* (Occasional papers on social administration, No. 8). Hertfordshire: Codicote Press.

Abrams, Richard, and Taylor, Michael Alan. 1976. Mania and schizo-affective disorder, manic type: A comparison. *American Journal of Psychiatry* 133:1445–1447.

Academy Forum. 1975. *Experiments and research with humans: Values in conflict.* Washington, D.C.: National Academy of Sciences.

Ackerknecht, Erwin H. 1942. Primitive medicine and culture pattern. *Bulletin of the History of Medicine* 12:545–574.

Adams, Bert H. 1966. Coercion and consensus theories: Some unresolved issues. *American Journal of Sociology* 71:714–717.

Adams, Jane. 1910. *Twenty years at Hull House.* New York: Macmillan.

Adams, Ruth, ed. 1966. *Contemporary China.* New York: Random House, Pantheon Books.

Aday, Lu Ann, and Anderson, Ronald. 1974. A framework for the study of access to medical care. *Health Services Research* 9:208–220.

———. 1975. *Development of indices of access to medical care.* Ann Arbor: Health Administration Press.

Aday, Lu Ann, and Eichhorn, R. 1972. *The utilization of health services: Indices and correlates.* Rockville, Md.: National Center for Health Services Research and Development.

Adler, Israel, and Shuval, Judith. 1978. Cross pressures during socialization for medicine. *American Sociological Review* 43:693–704.

Adler, Leta M. 1953. The relationship of marital status to incidence of recovery from mental illness. *Social Forces* 32:185–194.

Adler, Leta M., et al. 1952. *Mental illness in Washington County, Arkansas* (Institute of Science and Technology Research Series No. 23). Fayetteville: University of Arkansas.

AFT will organize health professionals. 1979. *American Teacher* 63:1, 20.

Again, a slowdown. 1976. *Time,* 19 January, p. 42.

Akers, Ronald L. 1968. The professional association and the legal regulation of practice. *Law and Society* 2:463–482.

Akers, Ronald L., and Quinney, Richard. 1968. Differential organization of health professions: A comparative analysis. *American Sociological Review* 33:104–121.

Albee, Edward. 1962. *A history of English utilitarianism.* New York: Collier.

Albrecht, Gary L. 1977. The negotiated diagnosis and treatment of occlusal problems. *Social Science and Medicine* 11:277–283.

Alexander, F., and French, T. 1948. *Studies in psychosomatic medicine.* New York: Ronald Press.

Alford, Robert. 1975. *Health care politics: Ideological and interest group barriers to reform.* Chicago: University of Chicago Press.

Allied health education. 1977. *Journal of the American Medical Association* 238: 2809–2814.

Allport, Floyd. 1934. The J-curve hypothesis of conformity behavior. *Journal of Social Psychology* 5:141–183.

Almond, Gabriel, and Powell, Bingham. 1966. *Comparative politics: A developmental approach*. Boston: Little, Brown & Co.

Altman, I. 1975. *The environment and social behavior*. Monterey, Calif.: Brooks-Cole.

The AMA antitrust suit: Viewpoint from a plaintiff. 1978. *International Review of Chiropractic* 32:14-16.

American Dental Association. 1969. *Annual report on dental education, 1968-1969*. Chicago.

_____. 1975. *The American dental association: Its structure and function*. Chicago.

_____. 1976. *Current policies adopted, 1954-1975*. Chicago.

_____. 1977. *The 1975 survey of dental practice*. Chicago.

American Hospital Association. 1968. *Classification of health care institutions*. Chicago.

_____. 1977. *Hospital statistics*. Chicago.

American Medical Association. 1959. *Digest of official actions, 1846-1958*. Chicago.

_____. 1976. *State by state report on the professional liability issue*. Chicago.

_____. 1978. *Profile of medical practice*. Chicago.

American Nurses Association. 1974. *Facts about nursing*. Kansas City.

American Psychiatric Association. 1968. *Diagnostic and statistical manual, mental disorders*. Washington, D.C.

American Sociological Association. 1965, 1974, 1975, 1977, 1978. *Guide to graduate departments of sociology*. Washington, D.C.

Amundsen, D. W. 1977. The liability of the physician in classical Greek legal theory and practice. *Journal of the History of Medicine and Allied Sciences* 32:172-203.

An, Tai Sung. 1972. *Mao Tse-tung's cultural revolution*. New York: Bobbs-Merrill, Pegasus.

Anderson, C. L. 1973. *Community health*. St. Louis: The C. V. Mosby Co.

Anderson, Elizabeth, et al. 1976. *The neighborhood health center program: Its growth and problems*. Washington, D.C.: National Association of Neighborhood Health Centers.

Anderson, Odin W. 1952. The sociologist and medicine. *Social Forces* 31:38-42.

_____. 1963. Health services systems in the United States and other countries–Critical comparisons. *New England Journal of Medicine* 269:839-843, 896-900.

_____. 1972. *Health care: Can there be equity? The United States, Sweden, and England*. New York: Wiley.

_____. 1973. *Health services in the USSR* (Selected papers, No. 42). Chicago: University of Chicago, Graduate School of Business.

_____. 1976. PSROs, the medical profession and public interest. *Milbank Memorial Fund Quarterly* 54:379-388.

Anderson, Odin W., and Sheatsley, P. B. 1967. Hospital use–A survey of patients' and physicians' decisions (Research Series No. 24). Chicago: University of Chicago, Center for Health Administration Studies.

Anderson, Robert E., and Morgan, S. 1973. *Comprehensive health care: A southern view*. Atlanta: Southern Regional Council.

Anderson, R. Bruce W. 1975. Choosing a medical specialty: A critique of literature in the light of 'curious findings'. *Journal of Health and Social Behavior* 16:152-162.

Anderson, Ronald M.; Kravits, Joanna; and Anderson, Odin W., eds. 1975. *Equity in health services: Empirical analysis in social policy*. Cambridge, Mass.: Ballinger Publishing Co.

Anderson, Ronald M., and Newman, John F. 1973. Societal and individual determinants of medical care utilization in the United States. *Milbank Memorial Fund Quarterly* 51:95-124.

Anderson, Ronald M., and Anderson, Odin W. 1979. Trends in the use of health services. *Handbook of medical sociology*, 3rd ed., ed. Howard E. Freeman, Sol Levine, and Leo G. Reeder. Englewood Cliffs, N.J.: Prentice-Hall.

Anderson, Ronald M., et al. 1972. *Health service use: National trends and variations–1953-1971* (DHEW Publications No. (HSM) 73-3004). Washington, D.C.: U.S. Government Printing Office.

Anderson, Theodore, and Warkov, S. 1961. Organizational size and functional complexity. *American Sociological Review* 26:23–27.

Andrew, G. 1968. Racial differences in time of identification and institutionalization of retarded children. *Mental Retardation* 6:9–12.

Antonovosky, Aaron. 1967a. Social class and illness: A reconsideration. *Sociological Inquiry* 37:311–322.

______. 1967b. Social class, life expectancy, and overall mortality. *Milbank Memorial Fund Quarterly* 45:31–73.

Apple, D. 1960. How laymen define illness. *Journal of Health and Human Behavior* 1:219–225.

Apple, William. 1970. Problems facing pharmacists under Medicare and Medicaid. *Journal of American Pharmaceutical Association* NS10:494–500.

Appleby, Lawrence, et al. 1967. Institution-centered and patient-centered mental hospitals. In *The sociology of mental disorder,* ed. S. Kirson Weinberg. Chicago: Aldine.

Arnstein, Sherry R. 1969. A ladder of citizen participation. *Journal of American Institute of Planners* 35:216–224.

Arthur, R. J. 1974. Extreme stress in adult life and its psychic and psychophysiological consequences. *Life stress and illness,* ed. E. K. Gunderson, and R. H. Rache. Springfield, Ill.: Charles Thomas.

Association of Physician Assistant Programs. 1976. *National new health practitioner program profile.* 2nd ed. Washington, D.C.

Atchley, Robert C. 1972. *The social forces in later life.* Belmont, Calif.: Wadsworth.

Atkinson, Donald T. 1956. *Magic, myth, and medicine.* New York: Books for Libraries Press.

Bachrach, Leona L. 1975. *Marital status and mental disorder: An analytical review* (DHEW Publication No. (ADM) 75-217). Washington, D.C.: U.S. Government Printing Office.

Badgley, Robin, and Bloom, S. 1973. Behavioral science and medical education: The case of sociology. *Social Science and Medicine* 7:927–941.

Baird, Leonard. 1975. The characteristics of medical students and their views of the first year. *Journal of Medical Education* 50:1092–1099.

Baker, Donald G. 1975. *Politics of race.* London: Butler & Tanner.

Baker, J. Jay, et al. 1976. Against legalization of laetrile. *New England Journal of Medicine* 295:679.

Bakke case views mixed. 1978. *Sacramento Union,* 29 June, p. A1, A7.

Bakke, E. W. 1940. *Citizens without work.* New Haven: Yale University Press.

Baldwin, Beverly Ann; Floyd, H. Hugh; and McSeveney, D. R. 1975. Status inconsistency and psychiatric diagnosis: A structural approach to labeling theory. *Journal of Health and Social Behavior* 3:257–267.

Balfe, B. E., and McNamara, M. E. 1968. *Security of medical groups in the United States: 1963.* Chicago: American Medical Association.

Balint, M. 1957. *The doctor, his patient, and the illness.* New York: International University Press.

Banta, H., and Fox, R. David. 1972. Role strains of a health care team in a poverty community. *Social Science and Medicine* 6:697–722.

Barbee, Robert A., and Dinham, Sarah M. 1977. Student decision-making and performance in a flexible-time curriculum. *Journal of Medical Education* 52:882–887.

Barber, Bernard. 1959. The sociology of science. In *Sociology today,* ed. Robert K.

Merton and Leonard S. Cottrell. New York: Basic Books.

———. 1973. Experimentation with human beings: Another problem of civil rights. *Minerva* 2:415–419.

Barenthin, I. 1977. Dental health status and dental satisfaction. *International Journal of Epidemiology* 6:73–79.

Barkin, Roger. 1974. Directions for statutory change: The physician extender. *American Journal of Public Health* 64:1132–1137.

Barrabee, R., and Mehring, O. V. 1953. Ethnic variations in mental stress in families with psychotic children. *Social Problems* 2:48–53.

Barrows, C. H., et al. 1978. The effect of various dietary restricted regimes on biochemical variables in the mouse. *Growth* 42:71-85.

Bartel, Mark, and Weisser, Lawrence. 1971. The street people and the straight society. In *The free clinic: Community approach to health care and drug abuse,* ed. D. E. Smith et al. Beloit, Wis.: Stash Press.

Baseheart, J. R. 1975. Nonverbal communication in the dentist–patient relationship. *Journal of Prosthetic Dentistry* 34:4–10.

Bashshur, Rashid, et al. 1967. Consumer satisfaction with group practice, the CHA case. *American Journal of Public Health* 57:1991–1999.

Basowitz, H., et al. 1955. *Anxiety and stress.* New York: McGraw-Hill.

Bates, Frederick L., and Whites, R. F. 1961. Differential perceptions of authority in hospitals. *Journal of Health and Human Behavior* 2:262–267.

Bateson, G., et al. 1956. Toward a theory of schizophrenia. *Behavioral Science* 1: 251–256.

Bauman, Patricia. 1976. The formulation and evolution of the health maintenance organization policy, 1970–1973. *Social Science and Medicine* 10:129–142.

Beale, L. V., and Kriesberg, L. 1959. Career relevant values of medical students–A research note. *Journal of the American Medical Association* 171:1447–1448.

Bean, Judy L. 1977. Pills, pantyhose, or patients? A sociological exploration of pharmacy. Unpublished master's thesis, California State University at Sacramento.

Becker, Howard S. 1963. *Outsiders: Students in the sociology of deviance.* New York: Free Press.

Becker, Howard S., and Barnes, Harry Elmer. 1961. *Social thought from lore to science,* 3 vols. New York: Dover Publications.

Becker, Howard S.; Geer, Blanche; Hughes, E. C.; and Strauss, A. L. eds. 1961. *Boys in white.* Chicago: University of Chicago Press.

Becker, Howard S.; Geer, Blanche; and Miller, Stephen J. 1972. Medical education. In *Handbook of medical sociology,* 2nd ed., ed. Howard E. Freeman, Sol Levine, and Leo G. Reeder. Englewood Cliffs, N.J.: Prentice-Hall.

Becker, M. H. 1974. The health belief model and sick role behavior. *Health Education Monographs* 2:409–419.

———. 1979. Psychosocial aspects of health-related behavior. *Handbook of medical sociology,* 3rd ed., ed. Howard E. Freeman, Sol Levine, and Leo G. Reeder. Englewood Cliffs, N.J.: Prentice-Hall.

Becker, M. H., and Maiman, Lois A. 1975. Sociobehavioral determinants of compliance with health and medical care recommendations. *Medical Care* 13:10–24.

Becker, M. H., et al. 1977. The health belief model and prediction of dietary compliance. *Journal of Health and Social Behavior* 18:348–366.

Becker, S. W., and Gordon, G. 1966. An entrepreneurial theory of formal organizations. *Administrative Science Quarterly* 11:315–344.

Becker, S. W., and Neuhauser, D. 1975. *The efficient organization.* New York: Elsevier Scientific Publishing Co.

Beecher, Henry K. 1959. *Measurement of subjective responses.* New York: Oxford University Press.

_____. 1966. Ethics and clinical research. *New England Journal of Medicine* 274:1354-1360.

_____. 1970. Scarce resources and medical advancement. In *Experimentation with human subjects,* ed. Paul A. Freund. New York: George Braziller.

Belknap, I. 1956. *Human problems of a state mental hospital.* New York: McGraw-Hill.

Bell, D. 1967. The post-industrial society: A speculative view. In *Scientific progress and human values,* ed. E. Hutchings and E. Hutchings. New York: American Elsevier Publishing Co.

Bell, R. R. 1971. *Marriage and family interaction.* Homewood, Ill.: Dorsey Press.

Bellin, Lowell E. 1970. The new left and American public health–Attempted radicalization of the APHA through dialectic. *American Journal of Public Health* 60:973-981.

Bellin, Lowell E., and Kavaler, Florence. 1970. Policing publicly funded health care for poor quality, overutilization, and fraud–The New York City medical experience. *American Journal of Public Health* 60:811-820.

Bellin, Seymours, and Geiger, H. J. 1970. Actual public acceptance of the neighborhood health center by the urban poor. *Journal of the American Medical Association* 214:2147-2153.

_____. 1972. The impact of a neighborhood health center on patients' behavior and attitudes relating to health care: A study of low income housing project. *Medical Care* 10:224-239.

Ben-David, Joseph. 1958. The professional role of the physician in bureaucratized medicine. *Journal of Human Relations* 11:255-274.

Ben-Sira, Zeev. 1976. The function of the professional's affective behavior in client satisfaction: A revised approach to social interaction theory. *Journal of Health and Social Behavior* 17:3-11.

Bennet, Edward H., III. 1976. Medical group practice in the United States, 1975. In *Reference data on profile of medical practice,* ed. James R. Cantwell. Chicago: American Medical Association.

Berger, Roland. 1973. Medical training in China. *Far Eastern Horizon* 12:31-34.

Berkanovic, Emile, and Reeder, Leo G. 1974. Can money buy the appropriate use of services? Some notes on the meaning of utilization data. *Journal of Health and Social Behavior* 15:93-99.

Berki, Sylvester. 1972. National health insurance: An idea whose time has come? *Annals of the American Academy of Political and Social Science* 399:125-144.

Berki, Sylvester, and Kobashigawa, B. 1976. Socioeconomic and need determinants of ambulatory care use: Path analysis of the 1970 health interview survey data. *Medical Care* 14:405-421.

Berlant, J. L. 1975. *Profession and monopoly.* Berkeley: University of California Press.

Bernard, Viola W. 1965. Why people become the victims of medical quackery. *American Journal of Public Health* 55:1142-1147.

Bernzweig, Eli R. 1966. *Legal aspects of PHS medical care* (DHEW Publication No. 1486). Washington, D.C.: U.S. Government Printing Office.

Berry, R. E. 1973. On grouping hospitals for economic analysis. *Inquiry* 10:5-12.

Betten, Neil, and Austin, M. 1977. Organizing for neighborhood health care: An historical reflection. *Social Work in Health Care* 2:341-349.

Bice, Thomas W. 1969. Factors related to the use of health services. *Medical Care* 7: 124-133.

Bice, Thomas W.; Eichhorn, R. L.; and Fox, P. D. 1972. Socioeconomic status and use of physician services: A reconsideration. *Medical Care* 10:261-271.

Biddle, Bruce J., and Thomas, Edwin. 1966. *Role theory.* New York: Wiley.

Bierman, Pearl, et al. 1968. Certifying independent laboratories under Medicare: Medicare's effect on medical care. *Public Health Reports* 83:731-739.

Binstock, Robert H., and Ely, Katherine. 1971. *The politics of the powerless.* Cambridge, Mass.: Winthrop Publishers.

Binstock, Robert H., and Shanas, Ethel, eds. 1977. *Handbook of aging and the social sciences.* New York: Van Nostrand Reinhold Co.

Biro, P. S., et al. 1976. A survey of patient's attitudes to their dentist. *Australian Dental Journal* 21:388–394.

Birren, James E., and Schaie, K. Warner, eds. 1977. *Handbook of the psychology of aging.* New York: Van Nostrand Reinhold Co.

Black, Max. 1961. *The social theories of Talcott Parsons.* Englewood Cliffs, N.J.: Prentice-Hall.

Blackwell, Gordon W. 1953. Behavioral sciences and health. *Social Forces* 32:211–215.

Blankenship, L. V., and Elling, R. H. 1962. Organizational support and community power structure: The hospital. *Journal of Health and Human Behavior* 3:257–269.

Blau, Peter M. 1963. *The dynamics of bureaucracy.* Chicago: University of Chicago Press.

_____. 1964. *Exchange and power in social life.* New York: Wiley.

Blau, Peter M., and Scott, W. Richard. 1964. *Formal organization.* San Francisco: Chandler.

Blau, Peter M., et al. 1966. The structure of small bureaucracies. *American Sociological Review* 31:179–191.

Bliss, Ann, and Cohen, Eva D., eds. 1977. *The new health professionals.* Germantown, Md.: Aspen Systems Corp.

Bloom, Samuel M. 1963. *The doctor and his patient.* New York: Russell Sage Foundation.

_____. 1965. The sociology of medical education. *Milbank Memorial Fund Quarterly* 63:143–184.

_____. 1973. *Power and dissent in the medical school.* New York: Free Press.

Bloom, Samuel W., and Wilson, R. N. 1972. Patient-practitioner relationships. In *Handbook of medical sociology,* 2nd ed., ed. Howard E. Freeman, Sol Levine, and Leo G. Reeder. Englewood Cliffs, N.J.: Prentice-Hall.

Blum, R. H. 1957. *The psychology of malpractice suits.* San Francisco: California Medical Association.

_____. 1960. *The management of the doctor-patient relationship.* New York: McGraw-Hill.

Blumer, Herbert. 1969. *Symbolic interactionism: Perspective and method.* Englewood Cliffs, N.J.: Prentice-Hall.

Bockoven, J. Sanbourne. 1957. Some relationships between cultural attitudes toward individuality and care of the mentall ill: An historical study. In *The patient and the mental hospital,* ed. M. Greenblatt et al. Glencoe, Ill.: Free Press.

Bogardus, Emory S. 1929. *A history of social thought.* Los Angeles: Josse Ray Miller.

Bonner, Paul, and Decker, Barry. 1973. *PSRO: Organization for regional peer review.* Cambridge, Mass.: Ballinger Publishing Co.

Bonner, Thomas. 1957. *Medicine in Chicago, 1850–1950.* Madison, Wis.: The American History Research Center.

Booth, A. 1972. Sex and social participation. *American Sociological Review* 37:183–192.

Bottomore, T. B., ed. 1973. *Karl Marx.* Englewood Cliffs, N.J.: Prentice-Hall.

Bourdillon, J. 1973. *Spinal manipulation.* New York: Appleton-Century-Crofts.

Bourgeois, C. 1975. The situational perspectives of premedical students and their effect on academic goals. Unpublished doctoral dissertation, Brown University.

Bourne, Patricia G., and Wikler, Norma J. 1978. Commitment and the cultural mandate: Women in medicine. *Social Problems* 25:430–440.

Bowers, John Z., and Purcell, Elizabeth F., eds. 1974. *Medicine and society in China.* New York: Josiah Macy, Jr. Foundation.

Boyer, John M.; Westerhaus, Carl L.; and Coggeshall, John H. 1975. *Employee relations and collective bargaining in health care facilities.* St. Louis: The C. V. Mosby Co.

Boyle, E., et al. 1967. An epidemiological study of hypertension among racial groups of Charleston County, South Carolina. In *The epidemiology of hypertension,* ed. J. Stamler, R. Stamler, and T. N. Pullman. New York: Grune & Stratton.

Bradburn, Norman, and Caplovitz, D. 1965. *Reports on happiness.* Chicago: Aldine.

Braden, Charles. 1958. *Christian science today.* Dallas: Southern Methodist University Press.

Brandon, William. 1977. Politics, administration, and conflict in neighborhood centers. *Journal of Health Politics* 2:79–99.

Brandt, Allan M. 1978. Polio, politics, publicity, and duplicity: Ethical aspects in the development of the Salk vaccine. *International Journal of Health Services* 8: 257–270.

Braucher, Charles I., and Evanson, R. V. 1963. Academic factors related to success in community pharmacy management. *American Journal of Pharmacy Management,* Winter, pp. 56–66.

Breslau, Naomi; Wolf, Gerrit; and Novack, Alvin H. 1978. Correlates of physician's task delegation in primary care. *Journal of Health and Social Behavior* 19:374–384.

Bremner, M. D. K. 1959. *The story of dentistry.* London: Dental Items of Interest Publishing Co.

Brenner, M. Harvey. 1973. *Mental illness and the economy.* Cambridge, Mass.: Harvard University Press.

Breyer, Peter. 1977. Neighborhood health centers: An assessment. *American Journal of Public Health* 67:179–182.

Breytspraak, Linda M., and Pondy, Louis R. 1969. Sociological evaluation of the physician's assistants' role relations. *Group Practice,* March, pp. 32–33, 37–41.

Britt, David W. 1975. Social class and the sick role: Examining the issue of mutual influence. *Journal of Health and Social Behavior* 16:178–182.

Brod, Jan. 1971. The influence of higher nervous processes induced by psychosocial environment on the development of essential hypertension. In *Society, stress, and disease,* ed. Lennart Levi. London: Oxford University Press.

Brody, Stanley. 1973. Comprehensive health care for the elderly: An analysis. *Gerontologist* 11:412–418.

Brook, R. H. 1974. *Quality of care: Methodologies of assessment.* Rockville, Md.: National Center for Health Services and Development.

Broverman, I. K., et al. 1970. Sex role stereotypes and clinical judgments of mental health. *Journal of Consulting Clinical Psychology* 34:1–10.

Brown, Esther Lucile. 1970. *Nursing reconsidered: A study of change.* Philadelphia: J. B. Lippincott.

Brown, G. W., and Birley, J. 1968. Crisis and life changes and the onset of schizophrenia. *Journal of Health and Social Behavior* 9:203–214.

Brown, G. W., et al. 1973. Life events and psychiatric disorders: Some methodological issues. *Psychological Medicine* 3:74–87.

Brown, Julia; Swift, Y. B.; and Oberman, M. L. 1974. Baccalaureate students' images of nursing: A replication. *Nursing Research* 23:53–59.

Bucher, Rue. 1972. Pathology: A study of social movements within a profession. In *Medical men and their work,* ed. Eliot Freidson and J. Lorker. Chicago: Aldine-Atherton.

Bucher, Rue, and Stelling, J. 1969. Characteristics of professional organization. *Journal of Health and Social Behavior* 10:3–15.

Bucher, Rue, and Strauss, Anselm. 1961. Professions in process. *American Journal of Sociology* 66:325–334.

Buckley, Walter. 1967. *Sociology and modern systems theory.* Englewood Cliffs, N.J.: Prentice-Hall.

Buerki, R. 1965. Pharmacist Smyth and druggist Smith: A study in the development of professionalism. Unpublished manuscript. Quoted in Disillusionment in pharmacy students, by Deanne E. Knapp and D. A. Knapp. *Social Science and Medicine* 1:445–447.

Bullough, Bonnie. 1972. Poverty, ethnic identity, and preventive health care. *Journal of Health and Social Behavior* 13:347–359.

——— 1976. The law and the expanding nursing role. *American Journal of Public Health* 66:249–254.

Bullough, Bonnie, and Bullough, Vern L. 1975. Sex discrimination in health care. *Nursing Outlook* 23:40–45.

Bullough, Vern L., and Bullough, Bonnie. 1969. *The emergence of modern nursing.* New York: Macmillan.

Burgess, Ernest W. 1939. The influence of Sigmund Freud on sociology in the United States. *American Journal of Sociology* 45:356–374.

Burke, Yvonne B. 1977. Minority admissions to medical schools: Problems and opportunities. *Journal of Medical Education* 52:731–738.

Burlage, R. K. 1968. The municipal hospital affiliation plan in New York City: A case study and critique. *Milbank Memorial Fund Quarterly* 46:171–203.

Burling, Temple, et al. 1956. *The give and take in hospitals.* New York: G. P. Putnam's Sons.

Burrow, James G. 1963. *AMA: Voice of American medicine.* Baltimore: Johns Hopkins University Press.

Burtt, E. A. 1954. *The metaphysical foundations of modern physical science.* Garden City, N.Y.: Doubleday.

Bury, J. B. 1932. *The idea of progress.* New York: Dover Publications.

Butler, A. M. 1968. Letter to the editor: Hippocratic oath, 1968. *New England Journal of Medicine* 278:48.

Butterfield, Herbert. 1960. *The origins of modern science.* New York: Macmillan.

Cain, Rosalyn M., and Kahn, Joel S. 1971. The pharmacist as a member of the health team. *American Journal of Public Health* 11:2220–2228.

Calahan, Don, et al. 1957. Career interest and expectations of U.S. medical students. *Journal of Medical Education* 32:557–563.

Callahan, Daniel. 1973. The WHO definition of health. *The Hastings Center Studies* 1:77–88.

Callahan, Daniel. 1976. The emergence of bioethics. In *Science, ethics, and medicine,* ed. H. Tristram Engelhardt and Daniel Callahan. New York: Institute of Society, Ethics, and the Life Sciences.

Calnek, M. 1970. Racial factors in the counter transference: The black therapist and the black client. *American Journal of Ortho-psychiatry* 40:39–46.

Campbell, Augus, et al. 1976. *The quality of American life: Perceptions, evaluations, and satisfactions.* New York: Russell Sage Foundation.

Campbell, John. 1971. Working relationships between providers and consumers in a neighborhood health center. *American Journal of Public Health* 60:97–103.

Campbell, Margaret A. 1973. *Why would a girl go into medicine?* New York: The Feminist Press.

Cannon, Mildred, and Locke, Ben Z. 1977. Being black is detrimental to one's mental health: Myth or reality? *Phylon* 38:408–428.

Cantor, Norman L. 1973. A patient's decision to decline lifesaving medical treatment: Bodily integrity versus the preservation of life. *Rutgers Law Review* 26:228–264.

Cantwell, James R., ed. 1976. *Reference data on profile of medical practice.* Chicago: American Medical Association.

Caplan, Robert. 1971. *Organizational stress and individual strain.* Unpublished doctoral dissertation, University of Michigan, Ann Arbor.

Caplow, Theodore. 1954. *The sociology of work.* Minneapolis: University of Minnesota Press.

Cardiac mortality and socioeconomic status. 1967. *Statistical Bulletin, Metropolitan Life Insurance Company* 48:9–11.

Carlson, Clifford L., and Athelstan, Gary T. 1970. The physician's assistant. *Journal of the American Medical Association* 214:1855–1861.

Carlson, Rick J. 1975. *The end of medicine.* New York: Wiley.

Carnegie Commission on Higher Education. 1970. *Higher education and the nation's health: Policies for medical and dental education.* New York: McGraw-Hill.

Carr, Leslie, and Krause, N. 1978. Social status, psychiatric symptomatology, and response bias. *Journal of Health and Social Behavior* 19:86–91.

Carr-Saunders, A. M., and Wilson, P. A. 1933. *The profession.* Oxford: Clarendon Press.

Carson, Joseph. 1869. *A history of the medical department of the University of Pennsylvania from its foundation in 1765.* Philadelphia: Lindsay & Blackiston.

Carter, H., and Glick, P. C. 1976. *Marriage and divorce: A social and economic study.* Cambridge: Harvard University Press.

Cartwright, Ann. 1967. *Patients and their doctors.* New York: Atherton Press.

Cartwright, Ann, and O'Brien, Maureen. 1976. Social class variations in the health care and in the nature of general practitioner consultations. In *The sociology of the National Health Service* (Sociological Review Monograph 22), ed. Margaret Stacy. Keele, Staffordshire: University of Keele.

Cartwright, Lilian K. 1971. Women in medical school. Unpublished doctoral dissertation, University of California, Berkeley.

———. 1972a. Conscious factors entering into decisions of women to study medicine. *The Journal of Social Issues* 28:201–215.

———. 1972b. Personality differences in male and female medical students. *Psychological Medicine* 3:212–218.

Casamassimo, P. S. 1977. Some perspectives on leadership in dentistry. *Journal of American College of Dentists* 44:219–226.

Cashing, James A., ed. 1970. *The impact of the advent of Medicare on hospital costs.* New York: Hofstra University.

Cashman, John W., and Myers, B. A. 1967. Medicare: Standards of service in a new program–Licensure, certification, accreditation. *American Journal of Public Health* 57:1107–1117.

Cassell, John. 1970. Physical illness in response to stress. In *Social stress,* ed. Sol Levine and Norman A. Scotch. Chicago: Aldine.

Cassell, John, and Tyroler, H. A. 1961. Epidemiological studies of culture change, I. *Archives of Environmental Health* 3:25–33.

Castiglioni, Arturo. 1958. *A history of medicine.* New York: Knopf.

Cater, Douglas, and Lee, P. R. 1972. *Politics of health.* New York: Medcom Press.

Caudill, William. 1953. Applied anthropology of medicine. In *Anthropology Today,* ed. A. L. Kroeber. Chicago: University of Chicago Press.

———. 1958. The psychiatric hospital as a small society. Cambridge: Harvard University Press.

———. 1961. Effects of social and cultural systems in reacting to stress. *New York Social Science Research Council* 26:51–58.

Celentano, David D. 1978. Critical policy issue concerning new health practitioners–Quality of care. *Sociological Symposium* 23:61–77.

Chabot, Marion Johnson; Garfinkel, J.; and Pratt, M. W. 1975. Urbanization and differentials in white and nonwhite infant mortality. *Pediatrics* 56:777–781.

Chambliss, Rollin. 1954. *Social thought.* New York: Henry Holt & Co.

Chandrasekhar, Sripati. 1959. *Infant mortality in India, 1901–1955.* London: George Allen & Unwin.

———. 1972. *Infant mortality, population growth, and family planning in India.* London: George Allen & Unwin.

The changing status of the relationships between medicine and nursing. 1978. *Connecticut Medicine* 42:247–251.

Channing, Edward. 1917. *A history of the United States.* New York: Macmillan.

Charlety, Sebastien. 1931. *Histoire du Saint-Simonisme (1825–1864).* Paris: Paul Hartmann.

Chen, Jack. 1975. *Inside the cultural revolution.* New York: Macmillan.

Chen, Pi-chao. 1976. *Population and health policy in the People's Republic of China.* Washington, D.C.: Interdisciplinary Communications Program, Smithonian Institution.

Cheney, H. Gordon. 1977. Effect of patient behavior and personality on treatment planning. *Dental Clinics of North America* 21:531–538.

Cheng, Chu-Yuan. 1973. Health manpower: Growth and distribution. In *Public health in the People's Republic of China,* ed. Myron E. Wegman et al. New York: Josiah Macy, Jr. Foundation.

Childress, James F. 1970. Who shall live, when not all can live? *Soundings* 53:339–362.

Chin, Robert. 1973. The changing health conduct of the "new man." In *Public health in the People's Republic of China,* ed. Myron E. Wegman et al. New York: Josiah Macy, Jr. Foundation.

China: Science walks on two legs (A report for Science for the People). 1974. New York: Avon Books.

Chiropractors: Healers or quacks? The eighty-year war with science. 1977. *Delaware Medical Journal* 49:277–300.

Christian Science and legislation. 1905. Boston: Christian Science Publishing Society.

Christie, Richard, and Merton, R. K. 1958. Procedure for the sociological study of the value climate of medical schools. *Journal of Medical Education* 33:125–153.

Chu, Franklin, D., and Trotter, Sharland. 1974. *The madness establishment.* New York: Grossman Publishers.

Clancy, Kevin, and Gove, Walter. 1974. Sex differences in mental illness. *American Journal of Sociology* 80:205–216.

Clark, Harry W. 1974. How relevant is the free clinic movement to black people? *Journal of Social Issues* 30:67–72.

Clark, M. 1959. *Health in the Mexican-American culture.* Berkeley: University of California Press.

———. 1971. Patterns of aging among the elderly poor of the inner city. *Gerontologist* 11:58–66.

Clark, Robert E. 1949. Psychoses, income, and occupational prestige. *American Journal of Sociology* 54:433–440.

Clausen, John A., and Huffine, Carol L. 1975. Sociocultural and social/psychological factors affecting social responses to mental disorder. *Journal of Health and Social Behavior* 16:405–420.

Clausen, John A., and Kohn, M. L. 1954. The ecological approach in social psychiatry. *American Journal of Sociology* 60:140–151.

———. 1959. Relation of schizophrenia to the social structure of a small city. In *Epidemiology of mental disorder,* ed. B. Pasamanick. Washington, D.C.: American Association for Advancement of Science.

———. 1960. Social relations and schizophrenia. In *The etiology of schizophrenia,* ed. Don D. Jackson. New York: Basic Books.

Clendening, Logan, ed. 1960. *Source book of medical history.* New York: Dover Publications.

Clevelend, E. J., and Longaker, W. D. 1957. Neurotic patterns in the family. In *Explorations in social psychiatry,* ed. Alexander H. Leighton et al. New York: Basic Books.

Clyne, M. G. 1961. *Night calls: A study in general practice.* London: Tavistock Publications.

Cobb, Beatrix. 1954. Why do people detour to quacks? *Psychiatric Bulletin* 3:66–69.

Coburn, D., and Pope, C. R. 1974. Socioeconomic status and preventive health behavior. *Journal of Health and Social Behavior* 15:67–78.

Coe, Rodney M. 1967. The impact of Medicare on the utilization of health care facilities: A sociological interpretation. *Inquiry* 4:42–47.

———. 1978. *Sociology of medicine.* 2nd ed. New York: McGraw-Hill.

Coe, Rodney M.; Pepper, Max; and Mattis, Mary. 1977. The "new" medical student: Another view. *Journal of Medical Education* 52:89–98.

Coe, Rodney M., and Sigler, Jack. 1970. Physicians' perceptions of the impact of Medicare. *Medical Care* 8:26–34.

Cohen, Albert, and Hodges, H. 1963. Characteristics of the lower blue-collar class. *Social Problems* 10:303–334.

Cohen, Carl; Skhel, Willemel; and Berger, Dirk. 1977. The use of a mid-Manhattan hotel as a support system. *Journal of Community Health* 13:76–83.

Cohen, E. D., et al. 1974. An evaluation of policy-related research on new and expanding roles of health workers. New Haven: Office of Regional Activities and Continuing Education, Yale University School of Medicine.

Cohen, Harry. 1965. *Demonics of bureaucracy.* Ames: Iowa State University Press.

Cohn, Werner. 1960. Social status and the ambivalence hypothesis. *American Sociological Review* 25:508–513.

Cole, Stephen, and Lejeure, R. 1972. Illness and the legitimation of failure. *American Sociological Review* 37:347–356.

Coleman, James. 1957. *Community conflict.* Glencoe, Ill.: Free Press.

Coleman, James, et al. 1966. *Medical innovation: A diffusion study.* Indianapolis: The Bobbs-Merrill Co.

Colombotos, John. 1969a. Physicians and Medicare: A before-after study of the effects of legislation on attitudes. *American Sociological Review* 34:318–334.

———. 1969b. Social origins and ideology of physicians: A study of the effects of early socialization. *Journal of Health and Social Behavior* 10:16–29.

Commager, Henry Steele. 1950. *The American mind.* New York: Yale University Press.

Commission on chronic illness. 1957. *Chronic illness in a large city.* Cambridge: Harvard University Press.

Compulsory medical treatment and a patient's free exercise of religion. 1975. *Medical Legal Bulletin* 24:1–30.

Comstock, Donald E. 1975. Technology and context: A study of hospital patient care units. Unpublished doctoral dissertation, Stanford University.

Congressional Quarterly. 1977. *National health issues.* Washington, D.C.

Conrad, Peter. 1975. The medicalization of deviance in American culture. *Social Problems* 23:12–21.

Cons, Natham C. 1973. The clinical evaluation of Medicaid's patients in the state of New York. *Journal of Public Health Dentistry* 33:186–193.

Controversy over national health insurance proposals: Pro and con. 1977. *Congressional Digest,* August-September.

Cooley, Charles H. 1902. *Human nature and the social order.* New York: Scribner.

Cooley, C. S. 1949. Science sidelights. *Journal of the National Chiropractic* 19:35–38.

Coombs, Robert H. 1978. *Mastering medicine: Professional socialization in medical school.* New York: Free Press.

Cooper, Barbara S., and McGee, Mary F. 1971. Medical care outlays for three age groups: Young, intermediate, and aged. *Social Security Bulletin* 34:3–14.

Cooper, Barbara S., and Worthington, N. L. 1973. National health expenditures, 1929–1972. *Social Security Bulletin* 36:3–19, 40.

Cooperstock, Ruth, and Parnell, Penny. 1976. Comments on Clancy and Gove. *American Journal of Sociology* 81:1455--1457.

Corey, L., et al., eds. 1972. *Medicine in a changing society.* St. Louis: The C. V. Mosby Co.

Corlett, W. T. 1935. *The medicine-man of the American Indian and his cultural background.* Springfield, Ill.: Charles C Thomas, Publishers.

Cornford, F. M. 1957. *From religion to philosophy.* New York: Harper & Row.

Corning, Peter A. 1969. *The evolution of Medicare: From idea to law* (DHEW Social Security Administration, Research Report No. 29). Washington, D.C.: U.S. Government Printing Office.

Corwin, Edward H. 1946. *The American hospital.* New York: Commonwealth Fund.

Corwin, R. G. 1961. Role conception and career aspirations: A study of identity in nursing. *Sociological Quarterly* 2:69–86.

Coser, Lewis A. 1956. *The functions of social conflict.* New York: Free Press.

———. 1966. Some social functions of violence. *Annals of the American Academy of Political and Social Science* 364:8–18.

Coser, Rose L. 1958. Authority and decision-making in a hospital. *American Sociological Review* 23:56–64.

———. 1963. Alienation and the social structure. In *The hospital in modern society,* ed. Eliot Freidson. Glencoe, Ill.: Free Press.

Costonis, Anthony F. 1966. The mental hospital unit system. *Journal of Health and Human Behavior* 7:75–82.

Cowie, James B., and Roebuck, J. 1975. *An ethnography of a chiropractic clinic.* New York: Free Press.

Cowie, Leonard W. 1960. *Seventeenth-century Europe.* New York: Frederick Ungar Publishing Co.

Coye, Robert D., and Hansen, Marc F. 1969. The doctor's assistant. *Journal of American Medical Association* 209:529–533.

Crane, Diana. 1975. *The sanctity of social life: Physicians' treatment of critically ill patients.* New York: Russell Sage Foundation.

Crawford, F. R., et al. 1960. Variations between negroes and whites in concepts of mental illness and its treatment. *Annals of the New York Academy of Science* 84:918-937.

Crile, George. 1976. Legalization of laetrile. *New England Journal of Medicine* 295:116.

Crippen, David W. 1976. Laetrile: Cancer cure or quack remedy? *Hastings Center Report* 6:18–19.

Croizier, Ralph C. 1968. *Traditional medicine in modern China.* Cambridge: Harvard University Press.

Croog, Sydney H. 1961. Ethnic origins, educational level, and responses to a health questionnaire. *Human Organization* 20:65–69.

———. 1970. The family as a source of stress. In *Social stress,* ed. Sol Levine and Norman A. Scotch. Chicago: Aldine.

Cumming, Elaine, and Henry, William E. 1961. *Growing old: The process of disengagement.* New York: Basic Books.

Curran, William J. 1974. The first mechanical transplant: Informed consent and experimentation. *New England Journal of Medicine* 291:1015–1016.

Current DSM-III outline. *Psychiatric News,* 17 November, pp. 14–19.

Curti, Merle. 1943. *The growth of American thought.* New York: Harper & Row.

Curtis, James L. 1971. *Blacks, medical schools, and society.* Ann Arbor: University of Michigan Press.

Cussler, Margaret, and Gordon, Evelyn W. 1968. *Dentists, patients, and auxiliaries.* Pittsburgh: University of Pittsburgh Press.

Cuvillier, Armand, P. J. V. 1948. *Bûchez et les origines du socialisme Chréstien.* Paris: Presses Universitaires de France.

Dahl, Robert A., and Lindblom, Charles E. 1953. *Politics, economics, and welfare.* New York: Harper.

Dahrendorf, Ralf. 1958a. Out of utopia: Toward a reorientation of sociological analysis. *American Journal of Sociology* 64:115–127.

———. 1958b. Toward a theory of social conflict. *Journal of Conflict Resolution* 2: 170–183.

———. 1959. *Class and class conflict in industrial society.* Palo Alto: Stanford University Press.

———. 1967. *Essays in the theory of society.* Palo Alto: Stanford University Press.

Dainton, Courtney. 1961. *The story of England's hospitals.* Sprinfield, Ill.: Charles C Thomas Publishers.

Davidson, Lynn R. 1977. Choice by constraint: A comment on the selection and function of specialists among women physician-in-training. Paper presented at the annual meeting of the American Sociological Association, Chicago.

Davies, D. V., ed. 1969. *Gray's anatomy,* 34th ed. London: Longman's Green. Originally published, 1858.

Davis, Allinson. 1946. The motivation of the underprivileged worker. In *Industry and society,* ed. William Foote Whyte. New York: McGraw-Hill.

Davis, Fred. 1963. *Passage through crisis.* Indianapolis: The Bobbs-Merrill Co.

———. 1966. *The nursing profession: Five sociological essays.* New York: Wiley.

Davis, Fred; Olesen, Virginia L.; and Whittaker, E. W. 1966. Problems and issues in collegiate nursing education. In *The nursing profession,* ed. Fred Davis, New York: Wiley.

Davis, Karen, 1975a. Equal treatment and unequal benefits: The Medicare program. *Milbank Memorial Fund Quarterly* 53:449–488.

———. 1975b. *National health insurance.* Washington, D.C.: The Brookings Institute.

Davis, Kingsley. 1959. The myth of functional analysis as a special method in sociology and anthropology. *American Sociological Review* 24:757–772.

Davis, Kingsley, and Moore, W. E. 1945. Some principles of stratification. *American Sociological Review* 10:242–249.

Davis, Michael M. 1921. *Immigrant health and the community.* New York: Harper & Bros.

———. 1955. *Medical care for tomorrow.* New York: Harper & Bros.

Davis, Milton. 1968. Variations in patients' compliance with doctors' advice. *American Journal of Public Health* 58:274–288.

Davis, Milton, and Tranqueda, R. E. 1969. A sociological evaluation of the Watts neighborhood health center. *Medical Care* 7:105–117.

Davis, Peter. 1976. Compliance structures and the delivery of health care: The case of dentistry. *Social Science and Medicine* 10:329–337.

Dawson, M. M. 1898. *Practical lessons in acturial science.* New York: The Spectator.

Dawber, T. R., et al. 1967. Environmental factors in hypertension. In *The epidemiology of hypertension,* ed. J. Stamler et al. New York: Grune & Stratton.

Dayton, Neil A. 1949. *New facts on mental disorder.* Springfield, Ill.: Charles C Thomas.

Decker, B., and Bonner, P. 1973. *Professional standards review organizations.* Cambridge, Mass.: Ballinger Publishing.

Demerath, N. J., and Peterson, R. A. 1967. *System, change, and conflict.* New York: Free Press.

Dennis, Ruth. 1977. Social stress and mortality among nonwhite males. *Phylon* 38: 315–328.

Denton, John A. 1976. Motives for entering nursing and attitudes toward alternative models of unions and professions. *Nursing Research* 25:178–180.

———. 1978. *Medical sociology.* Boston: Houghton Mifflin.

Denzin, Norman K. 1968. The self-fulfilling prophecy and patient-therapist interaction. In *The mental patient,* ed. Stephen P. Spitzer and Norman K. Denzin. New York: McGraw-Hill.

Denzin, Norman K., and Mettlin, Curtis J. 1968. Incomplete professionalization: The case of pharmacy. *Social Forces* 46:375–381.

Denzin, Norman K., and Spitzer, S. P. 1968. Path to the mental hospital and staff prediction of patient role behavior. In *The mental patient,* ed. Stephen P. Spitzer and Norman K. Denzin. New York: McGraw-Hill.

Derbyshire, Robert C. 1974. Medical ethics and discipline. *Journal of the American Medical Association* 228:59–62.

Deutch, A. 1948. *The shame of the states.* New York: Harcourt, Brace.

Deutch, Morton, and Krauss, Robert M. 1965. *Theories in social psychology.* New York: Basic Books.

DHSS (Department of Health and Social Security). 1976a. *Prevention and health: Everybody's business.* London: Her Majesty's Stationary Office.

———. 1976b. *Priorities for health and personal social services in England.* London: Her Majesty's Stationary Office.

Dick, Harry R. 1960. A method for ranking community influentials. *American Sociological Review* 25:395–404.

Dietz, Lena Dixon. 1963. *History and modern nursing.* Philadelphia: F. A. Davis Co.

Dimond, E. Grey. 1971. Medical education and care in the People's Republic of China. *Journal of American Medical Association* 218:1552–1557.

Dintenfass, Julius. 1970. *Chiropractic, A modern way to health.* New York: Pyramid Books.

Dipalma, Joseph R. 1977. Laetrile: When is a drug not a drug? *American Family Physician* 15:186–187.

Dock, Lavina L., and Stewart, Isabel M. 1938. *A short history of nursing.* New York: G. P. Putnam's Sons.

Doctors hit the streets with a new strike law. 1975. *Businessweek,* 31 March, pp. 19–20.

Doctors on strike. 1975. *Newsweek,* 31 March, pp. 71–72.

———. 1975. *Time,* 31 March, p. 81.

Doctors' revolt, The. 1975. *Newsweek,* 12 May, p. 71.

Dodge, David L., and Martin, Walter T. 1970. *Social stress and chronic illness.* Notre Dame: University of Notre Dame Press.

Dodge, John, and Rodgers, Charles. 1976. Is NIMH's dream coming true? *Community Mental Health Journal* 12:399–404.

Dodge, W. F., et al. 1970. Patterns of maternal desires for child health care. *American Journal of Public Health* 60:1421–1429.

Dohrenwend, Bruce P. 1961. The social psychological nature of stress: A framework for causal inquiry. *Journal of Abnormal and Social Psychology* 62:294–302.

Dohrenwend, Bruce P., and Dohrenwend, Barbara S. 1969. *Social status and psychological disorder.* New York: Wiley.

_____. 1970. Class and race as status-related sources of stress. In *Social stress,* ed. Sol Levine and Norman A Scotch. Chicago: Aldine.

_____. 1974a. Psychiatric disorders in urban settings. In *American handbook of psychiatry,* vol. 2, ed. S. Arieti and G. Caplan. New York: Basic Books.

_____. 1974b. Sex differences and psychiatric disorders. Paper presented at the 8th World Congress of Sociology, Toronto.

_____, eds. 1974c. *Stressful life events.* New York: Wiley.

_____. 1976. Sex differences and psychiatric disorders. *American Journal of Sociology* 81:1447–1454.

_____. 1977. Reply to Gove and Tudor's comment on "sex differences and psychiatric disorders." *American Journal of Sociology* 83:1336–1345.

Dolan, John P., and Adams-Smith, William N. 1978. *Health and society.* New York: The Seabury Press.

Dorn, Harold F. 1954. Cancer morbidity survey. Paper presented at the Epidemiology and Statistics Section, American Public Health Association, Buffalo.

Dougherty, J. D. 1967. Cardiovascular findings in air traffic controllers. *Aerospace Medicine* 38:26–30.

Draughon, Margaret. 1975. Relationship between economic decline and mental hospital admissions continues to be significant. *Psychological Reports* 36:882.

Dubbs, G. 1970. Tomorrow's chiropractic school. *The ACA Journal of Chiropractic* 7:7–24.

Dube, W. F., et al. 1971. Study of U.S. medical school applicants, 1970–1971. *Journal of Medical Education* 46:837.

Dubin, Robert. 1969. *Theory building.* New York: Free Press.

Dublin, Louis I.; Lotka, A. J.; and Spiegelman, M. 1949. *Length of Life: A study of the life table,* rev. ed. New York: The Ronald Press.

Dubos, René. 1959. *Mirage of health.* Garden City, N.Y.: Doubleday.

_____. 1965. *Man adapting.* New Haven: Yale University Press.

Dubos, René, and Dubos, Jean. 1952. *The white plague: Tuberculosis, man, and society.* Boston: Little, Brown.

Duff, Raymond S., and Campbell, M. B. 1973. Moral and ethical dilemmas in the special-care nursery. *New England Journal of Medicine* 289:890–894.

Duff, Raymond S., and Hollingshead, A. 1968. *Sickness and society.* New York: Harper & Row.

Duffy, John. 1968. *A history of public health in New York City, 1625-1866.* New York: Russell Sage Foundation.

_____. 1976. *The healers: The rise of the medical establishment.* New York: McGraw-Hill.

Dumbaugh, Karin, and Neuhauser, Duncan. 1976. The effect of pre-admission testing on length of stay. In *Organizational research in hospitals,* ed. Stephen M. Shortell and M. Brown. Chicago: An Inquiry Book, Blue Cross Association.

Dunbar, Flanders, ed. 1943. *Emotions and bodily changes.* New York: Columbia University Press.

Dunham, H. W. 1947. Current status of ecological research in mental disorder. *Social Forces* 25:321–326.

_____. 1965. *Community and schizophrenia.* Detroit: Wayne State University Press.

Dunham, H. W., and Weinberg, S. F. 1960. *The culture of the state mental hospital.* Detroit: Wayne State University Press.

Dunn, John E., and Buell, P. 1959. Association of cervical cancer with circumcision of sexual partner. *Journal of the National Cancer Institute* 22:749–769.

Dunn, J. P., et al. 1962. Frequency of peptic ulcer among executives, craftsmen and foremen. *Journal of Occupational Medicine* 4:343–348.

Dunning, James M. 1976. *Dental care for everyone: Problems and proposals.* Cambridge: Harvard University Press.

Durgin, Jane M., et al. 1972. *Manual for pharmacy technician.* St. Louis: The C. V. Mosby Co.

Durkheim, Emile. 1950. *[Suicide]*, ed. and trans. George Simpson. Glencoe, Ill.: Free Press. Originally published, 1897.

Duttera, M. J., and Harlan, N. R. 1975. Evaluation of physician's extenders in the rural southeast: Patterns of practice and patient care. Paper presented at the meeting of the American College of Physicians, San Francisco.

Dutton, Diana B. 1978. Low use of health services by the poor. *American Sociological Review* 43:348–367.

Eaton, Joseph, and Weil, R. J. 1954. *Culture and mental disorders.* Glencoe, Ill.: Free Press.

Eaton, William. 1974. Residence, social class, and schizophrenia. *Journal of Health and Social Behavior* 15:289–299.

Eckstein, Harry. 1970. *The English health service: Its origins, structure, and achievement.* Cambridge: Harvard University Press.

Edinson, Jack. 1977. Discussion of papers presented at the session, "Have we narrowed the gaps in health status between the poor and the nonpoor?" *Medical Care* 15: 675–677.

Editorial: The committee on the cost of medical care. 1932. *Journal of the American Medical Association* 99:1950–1952.

Eddy, Mary Baker. 1934. *Science and health with key to the scriptures.* Boston: Christian Science Publishing Society.

———. 1936. *Manual of the mother church.* Boston: Trustee under will of Mary Baker Eddy.

Ehrenreich, Barbara, and Ehrenreich, John. 1971. *The American health empire.* New York: Random House.

Ehrenreich, Barbara, and English, D. 1973. *Witches, midwives, and nurses: A history of women healers.* Old Westbury, N.Y.: The Feminist Press.

Eilers, Robert D., and Moyerman, Sue S., eds. 1971. *National health insurance.* Homewood, Ill.: Richard D. Irwin.

Eisdorfer, Carl, and Wilkie, Frances. 1977. Stress, disease, aging and behavior. In *Handbook of the psychology of aging,* ed. James E. Birren and Warner Schaie. New York: Van Nostrand Reinhold Co.

Elesh, D., and Schollert, P. T. 1972. Race and urban medicine: Factors affecting the distribution of physicians in Chicago. *Journal of Health and Social Behavior* 13:236–250.

Elinson, Jack, and Herr, C. E. A. 1970. A sociomedical view of neighborhood health centers. *Medical Care* 8:97–103.

Engel, Gloria. 1969. The effect of bureaucracy on the professional autonomy of the physician. *Journal of Health and Social Behavior* 10:30–41.

Enos, Darryl, and Sultan, Paul. 1977. *The sociology of health care.* New York: Praeger Publishers.

Entralgo, P. Lain. 1969. *Doctor and patient.* New York: McGraw-Hill.

Epstein, F. H. 1971. Coronary heart disease and epidemiology. In *Trends in epidemiology,* ed. G. T. Steward. Springfield, Ill.: Charles C Thomas.

Epstein, F. H., et al. 1957. The epidemiology of atherosclerosis among a random sample of clothing workers of different ethnic origin in New York City. *Journal of Chronic Diseases* 5:300–328.

Erhardt, Carl, and Berlin, J. E. 1974. *Mortality and morbidity in the United States.* Cambridge: Harvard University Press.

Erikson, Kai T. 1962. Notes on the sociology of deviance. *Social Problems* 9:307-314.

Eron, Leonard D. 1955. Effect of medical education on medical students' attitudes. *Journal of Medical Education* 30:559-566.

Estes, E. H. 1970. The training of physicians' assistants: A new challenge for medical education. *Modern Medicine* 38:90-93.

Estes, E. H., and Howard, D. R. 1970. Potential for newer classes of personnel: Experiences of the Duke physician's assistant program. *Journal of Medical Education* 45:149-155.

Etzioni, Amitai, ed. 1961. *Complex organizations.* New York: Holt, Rinehart & Winston.

_____. 1969a. *Readings on modern organization.* Englewood Cliffs, N.J.: Prentice-Hall.

_____. 1969b. *The semi-professions and their organization.* New York: Free Press.

Etziony, M. B. 1973. *The physicians' creed.* Springfield, Ill.: Charles C Thomas.

Evang, Kral. 1960. *Health service, society, and medicine.* London: Oxford University Press.

Evans, D. O. 1951. *Social romanticism in France, 1830-1848.* Oxford: Clarendon Press.

Evans, Lester J. 1952. The next twenty years in medicine. *Journal of Medical Education* 27:326-329.

Fabrega, Horacio. 1974. *Disease and social behavior.* Cambridge, Mass.: M.I.T. Press.

Fagin, C. 1976. Can we bring order out of the chaos of nursing education? *American Journal of Nursing* 76:98-105.

Fain, Tyrus G., ed. 1977. *National health insurance* (Public Document Series). New York: R. R. Bowker Co.

Fairbank, J. 1971. *The United States and China.* Boston: Harvard University Press.

Falk, I. S. 1973. Medical care in the U.S.A.–1932-1972–Problems, proposals, and programs. *Milbank Memorial Fund Quarterly* 51:1-39.

_____. 1977. Proposals for national health insurance in the U.S.A.: Origins and evolution, and some perceptions for the future. *Milbank Memorial Fund Quarterly* 55: 161-192.

Farina, Amerigo, et al. 1963. Relationship of marital status to incidence and prognosis of schizophrenia. *Journal of Abnormal and Social Psychology* 67:624-630.

Faris, Robert E. L., and Dunham, H. W. 1939. *Mental disorders in urban areas.* Chicago: University of Chicago Press.

Farndale, James, ed. 1964. *Trends in the national health service.* New York: Macmillan.

Fauchard, Pierre. 1728. *Le Chirugien Dentiste, ou Traite des Dents.* Paris: J. Mariette.

Faulkner, Harold U. 1952. *American political and social history.* New York: Appleton-Century-Crofts.

Fauman, Michael A. 1977. A diagnostic system for organic brain disorders: Critique and suggestion. *Psychiatric Quarterly* 49:173-186.

Feder, Judith M. 1977. *Medicare: The politics of federal hospital insurance.* Lexington, Mass.: D. C. Heath & Co.

Feingold, Eugene. 1966. *Medicare: Policy and politics.* San Francisco: Chandler Publishing Co.

_____. 1970. A political scientist's view of the neighborhood health center as a new social institution. *Medical Care* 8:108-115.

Fenwick, Mrs. Bedford. 1901. A plea for the higher education of trained nurses. *American Journal of Nursing* 2:4-8.

Field, Mark G. 1957. *Doctor and patient in Soviet Russia.* Cambridge: Harvard University Press.

_____. 1966. Health personnel in the Soviet Union: Achievements and problems. *American Journal of Public Health* 56:1904-1920.

_____. 1967. *Soviet socialized medicine.* New York: Free Press.

_____. 1975. American and Soviet medical manpower: Growth and evolution, 1910–1970. *International Journal of Health Services* 5:455–474.

$50,000 award in "test tube" suit. 1978. *American Medical News,* 1 September, p. 1.

Finch, Caleb E., and Hayflick, Leonard, eds. 1977. *Handbook of the biology of aging.* New York: Van Nostrand Reinhold.

Firestein, Stephen K. 1976. Patient anxiety and dental practice. *American Dental Association Journal* 93:1180–1187.

Firman, G. J., et al. 1975. The future of chiropractic: A psychosocial view. *New England Journal of Medicine* 293:639–642.

Fischer, J. 1969. Negroes and whites and rates of mental illness: Reconsideration of a myth. *Psychiatry* 32:428–446.

Fisher, Donald W., and Horowitz, Susan M. 1977. The physician's assistant: Profile of a new health profession. In *The new health professionals,* ed. Ann Bliss and Eva D. Cohen. Germantown, Md.: Aspen Systems Corp.

Fishman, D., and Zimel, C. 1972. Specialty choice and beliefs about specialties among freshman medical students. *Journal of Medical Education* 17:524–533.

Fishman, Sherwin R., and Ortiz, Eduardo, 1977. Effective case presentation. *Dental Clinics of North America* 21:539–548.

Fletcher, John. 1976. Relations of patient consent to medical research. In *Biomedical ethics and law,* ed. James Humber and Robert F. Almeder. New York: Plenum Press.

Fletcher, Joseph. 1968. Elective death. In *Ethical issues in medicine,* ed. E. Fuller Torrey. Boston: Little, Brown.

Fletcher, Ronald. 1971. *The making of sociology.* London: Michael Joseph.

Flexner, A. 1910. *Medical education in the United States and Canada* (Bulletin No. 4). New York: Carnegie Foundation for the Advancement of Teaching.

Flood, Ann Barry, and Scott, W. Richard. 1978. Professional power and professional effectiveness: The power of the surgical staff and the quality of surgical care in hospitals. *Journal of Health and Social Behavior* 19:240–254.

Fogg, Susan. 1979. Role of insurance firms only point of agreement. *Sacramento Union,* 10 June, p. C4.

Ford, Ann Suter. 1975. *The physician's assistant: A national and local analysis.* New York: Praeger Publishers.

Forgotson, E. H., and Cook, J. L. 1967. Innovations and experiments in uses of health manpower–The effect of licensure laws. *Law and Contemporary Problems* 32:731–750.

Forgotson, E. H., and Forgotson, Judith. 1970. Innovations and experiments of health manpower: A study of selected programs and problems in the United Kingdom and the Soviet Union. *Medical Care* 8:3–14.

Form, W. H., and Miller, D. C. 1960. *Industry, labor, and community.* New York: Harper.

Foster, Lee. 1976. Man and machine: Life without kidneys. *Hastings Center Report* 6:5–8.

Foucault, Michael. 1965. *Madness and civilization: A history of insanity in the age of reason.* New York: Pantheon Books.

Fox, Daniel M., and Crawford, Robert. 1979. Health politics in the United States. *Handbook of medical sociology,* 3rd ed., ed. Howard E. Freeman, Sol Levine, and Leo G. Reeder. Englewood Cliffs, N.J.: Prentice-Hall.

Fox, David, et al. 1961. *Career decisions and professional expectations of nursing students.* Ithaca, N.Y.: Cornell University, Bureau of Publications.

Fox, H. M., et al. 1957. Some methods of observing humans under stress. *Psychiatric Research Report* 7:14–26.

Fox, Renée C. 1957. Training for uncertainty. In *The student-physician,* ed. R. K. Merton et al. Cambridge: Harvard University Press.

——. 1970. A sociological perspective on organ transplantation and hemodialysis. *Annals of the New York Academy of Science* 169:406–428.

——. 1974a. Is there a new medical student? In *Ethics of health care,* ed. L. R. Tancredi. Washington, D.C.: National Academy of Sciences.

——. 1974b. Ethical and existential developments in contemporary American medicine: Their implications for culture and society. *Milbank Memorial Fund Quarterly,* Fall, 445–483.

Fox, Renée C., and Swazey, Judith P. 1974. *The courage to fail.* Chicago: The University of Chicago Press.

Frank, Jerome D. 1973. *Persuasion and healing: A comparative study of psychotherapy,* rev. ed. Baltimore: Johns Hopkins University Press.

Frank, J. P. 1941. [The people's misery: Mother of disease], (trans. and intr. E. Sigerist). *Bulletin of the History of Medicine* 9:81–100. Address originally delivered, 1790.

Fredericks, Marcel A.; Mundy, Paul; and Kosa, John. 1974. Willingness to serve: The medical profession and poverty problems. *Social Science and Medicine* 8:51–57.

Fredericks, Marcel A., and Mundy, Paul. 1976. *The making of a physician.* Chicago: Loyola University Press.

Freeborn, Donald K., and Darsky, Benjamin J. 1974. A study of the power structure of the medical community. *Medical Care* 12:1–12.

Freedman, A.; Kaplan, H.; and Sadock, B., eds. 1975. *Comprehensive textbook of psychiatry,* 2nd ed., 2 vols. Baltimore: Williams & Wilkins.

Freedman, Ronald. 1950. *Recent immigration to Chicago.* Chicago: University of Chicago Press.

Freeman, Howard E., and Kassebaum, G. C. 1960. Relations of education and knowledge to opinions about mental illness. *Mental Hygiene* 44:43–47.

Freeman, Howard E.; Levine, Sol; and Reeder, Leo G., eds. 1972. *Handbook of medical sociology,* 2nd ed. Englewood Cliffs, N.J.: Prentice-Hall.

——. 1979. *Handbook of medical sociology,* 3rd ed. Englewood Cliff, N.J.: Prentice-Hall.

Freidson, Eliot. 1960. Client control and medical practice. *American Journal of Sociology* 65:374–382.

——. 1970. *Professional dominance: The social structure of medical care.* New York: Atherton Press.

——. 1973. Prepaid group practice and the new 'demanding patient'. *Milbank Memorial Fund Quarterly* 51:473–488.

——. 1975a. *Doctoring together: A study of professional social control.* New York: Elsevier.

——. 1975b. *Profession of medicine.* New York: Dodd, Mead, & Co.

——. 1979. The organization of medical practice. *Handbook of medical sociology,* 3rd ed., ed. Howard E. Freeman, Sol Levine, and Leo G. Reeder. Englewood Cliffs, N.J.: Prentice-Hall.

Freidson, Eliot, ed. 1963. *The hospital in modern society.* New York: Free Press.

——. 1971. *The professions and their prospects.* Beverly Hills, Calif.: Sage.

Freidson, Eliot, and Rhea, Buford. 1963. Processes of control in a company of equals. *Social Problems* 2:119–131.

French, John P., et al. 1965. Workload of university professor (Cooperative Research Project No. 2171. U.S. Office of Education). Ann Arbor: University of Michigan.

Freund, Paul A., ed. 1970. *Experimentation with human subjects.* New York: George Braziller.

Freymann, John Gordon. 1964. Leadership in American medicine. *New England Journal of Medicine* 270:5–6.

Fried, M. 1969. Social differences in mental health. In *Poverty and health,* ed. J. Kosa, A. Antonovsky, and I. Zola. Cambridge: Commonwealth Fund.

Friedlander, D. 1945. Personality development of 27 children who later became psychotic. *Journal of Abnormal and Social Psychology* 40:330–335.

Friedman, Jay W. 1966. Dental care programs: Prospects and perspectives. *Journal of Health and Human Behavior* 7:255–264.

Friedman, M., and Roseman, R. H. 1959. Association of specific overt behavior pattern with blood and cardiovascular findings. *Journal of American Medical Association* 169:1286–1296.

Friedman, M., et al. 1958. Changes in the serum cholesterol and blood clotting time in men subjected to cyclic variation of occupational stress. *Circulation* 17:852–861.

Friedman, S. B., et al. 1963. Behavioral observations on parents anticipating the death of a child. *Pediatrics* 32:610–625.

Friedrichs, Robert W. 1970. *A sociology of sociology.* New York: Free Press.

Frumkin, Robert S. 1955. Occupation and major mental disorders. In *Mental health and mental disorder,* ed. Arnold M. Rose. New York: W. W. Norton.

Fry, John. 1969. *Medicine in three societies.* Aylesbury, England: Medical and Technical Publishing.

Fuchs, Victor R. 1974. *Who shall live? Health, economics, and social choice.* New York: Basic Books.

Fusillo, Alice E., and Metz, A. Stafford. 1971. Social science research on the dental student. *Social sciences and dentistry: A critical bibliography,* ed. N. D. Richards and L. K. Cohen. London: Federation Dentaire Internationale.

Galdston, Iago. 1949. *Social medicine.* New York: The Commonwealth Fund.

Gale, James L. 1975. Patient and practitioner attitudes toward traditional and western medicine in a contemporary Chinese setting. In *Studies of health care in Chinese and other societies* (DHEW Publication No. (NIH) 75-653), ed. Arthur Kleinman et al. Washington, D.C.: U.S. Government Printing Office.

Galvin, Michael L., and Fan, Margaret. 1975. The utilization of physician's services in Los Angeles county, 1973. *Journal of Health and Social Behavior* 16:75-94.

Garfield, S. L., and Sundland, D. M. 1966. Prognostic scales in schizophrenia. *Journal of Consulting Psychology* 30:18–24.

Gaudet, F. J., and Watson, R. I. 1935. The relationship between insanity and marital conditions. *Journal of Abnormal and Social Psychology* 30:366–370.

Geerken, Michael, and Gove, Walter R. 1974. Race, sex, and marital status: Their effect on mortality. *Social Problems* 21:567–580.

Geiger, H. Jack. 1967a. Of the poor, by the poor, or for the poor: The mental health implications of social control of poverty programs. *Psychiatric Research Report* 21:55--65.

———. 1967b. The neighborhood health center. *Archives of Environmental Health* 14: 912–916.

———. 1975. Health care in the People's Republic of China: Implications for the United States. In *Studies of health care in Chinese and other societies* (DHEW Publication No. (NIH) 75-653), ed. Arthur Kleinman et al. Washington, D.C.: U.S. Government Printing Office.

Gelfand, Donald E. 1975. The challenge of applied sociology. *American Sociologist* 10:13–18.

Genovese, Eugene D. 1967. *The political economy of slavery.* New York: Random House, Pantheon.

Georgopoulos, Basis S. 1972a. The hospital as an organization and problem-solving system. In *Organization research in health institutions,* ed. Basil S. Georgopoulos.

Ann Arbor: University of Michigan, Institute for Social Research.
——, ed. 1972b. *Organization research on health institutions.* Ann Arbor: University of Michigan, Institute for Social Research.
——. 1975. *Hospital organization research: Review and source book.* Philadelphia: W. B. Saunders Co.
Georgopoulos, Basil, and Mann, Floyd C. 1962. *The community general hospital.* New York: Macmillan.
Georgopoulos, Basil, and Matejko, A. 1967. The American general hospital as a complex social system. *Health Service Research* 2:76–112.
Gerald, D. L., and Siegel, J. 1950. The family background of schizophrenia. *Psychiatric Quarterly* 24:47–73.
Gerkin, Michael, and Gove, W. R. 1974. Race, sex, and marital status. *Social Problems* 21:567–580.
Gersten, Joanne C., et al. 1977. An evaluation of the etiologic role of stressful life-change events in psychological disorders. *Journal of Health and Social Behavior* 18:228–244.
Gerth, Hans H., and Mills, C. W., eds. and trans. 1958. *From Max Weber: Essays in sociology.* New York: Oxford University Press.
Gerver, I., and Bensman, J. 1954. Toward a sociology of expertness. *Social Forces* 32:226–235.
Geschwender, J. A. 1967. Continuities in theories of status consistency and cognitive dissonance. *Social Forces* 46:160–172.
Getzels, John W., and Guba, E. C. 1954. Role, role conflict, and effectiveness. *American Sociological Review* 19:164–175.
Gibbons, Russell. 1979. Chiropractic as both medical and social protest: Notes on the survival years and after. Paper presented at the International Scientific Conference on the Spine, Anaheim, California.
Gibbs, Jack, and Martin, Walter. 1964. *Status integration and suicide.* Eugene: University of Oregon Press.
Gibson, Geoffrey. 1972. Chinese medical practice and the thoughts of Chairman Mao. *Social Science and Medicine* 6:67–93.
Gibson, Geoffrey; Bugbee, George; and Anderson, Odin W. 1970. *Emergency medical services in the Chicago area.* Chicago: University of Chicago, Center for Health Administration.
Gibson, Robert M., and Fisher, Charles R. 1978. National health expenditures, fiscal year 1977. *Social Security Bulletin* 41:3–20.
Gibson, Robert M., and Mueller, M. S. 1977. National health expenditures, fiscal year 1976. *Social Security Bulletin* 40:3–22.
Gillie, A. 1963. *The field work of the family doctor* (Report of the Subcommittee of the Standing Medical Advisory Committee). London: Ministry of Health.
Ginzberg, Elli, et al. 1951. *Occupational choice.* New York: Columbia University Press.
Glaser, Barney G., and Strauss, Anselm L. 1965. *Awareness of dying.* Chicago: Aldine.
——. 1968. *Time for dying.* Chicago: Aldine.
Glaser, William A. 1959. Internship appointments of medical students. *Administrative Science Quarterly* 4:337–356.
——. 1966a. Nursing leadership and policy: Some cross-national comparisons. In *The nursing profession: Five sociological essays,* ed. Fred Davis. New York: Wiley.
——. 1966b. "Socialized medicine" in practice. *The Public Interest* Spring, 90–106.
——. 1970. *Social settings and medical organization: A cross-national study of the hospital.* New York: Atherton.
Glass, A. J. 1958. Observations upon the epidemiology of mental illness in troops during warfare. In *Symposium on preventive and social psychiatry,* Walter Reed Army

Institute of Research. Washington, D.C.: U.S. Government Printing Office.

Glasser, M. 1972. Consumer expectations of health services. In *Medicine in a changing society,* ed. L. Corey et al. St. Louis: The C. V. Mosby Co.

Glazer, David L. 1977. National commission on certification of physician's assistants: A precedent in collaboration. *The new health professionals,* ed. Ann Bliss and Eva D. Cohen. Germantown, Md.: Aspen Systems Corp.

Glazer, Nathan. 1954. Ethnic groups in America: From national culture to ideology. In *Freedom and control in modern society,* ed. Morrow Berger et al. New York: Octagon Books.

glimpse at some future physician's assistants, A. 1972. *Journal of American Medical Association* 221:1100–1104.

Godkins, T. R., et al. 1974. Current status of the physician's assistant in Oklahoma. *Oklahoma State Medical Association Journal* 67:102–107.

Goering, J., and Coe, R. M. 1970. Cultural versus situational explanations of the medical behavior of the poor. *Social Science Quarterly* 50:309–419.

Goffman, Erving. 1959. *The presentation of self in everyday life.* New York: Doubleday.

_____. 1961. *Asylums.* New York: Doubleday.

Gold, Margaret. 1977. A crisis of identity: The case of medical sociology. *Journal of Health and Social Behavior* 18:160–168.

Gold, M. R., and Rosenberg, R. G. 1974. Use of emergency room services by the population of a neighborhood health center. *Health Service Reports* 89:65–70.

Goldberg, E. M., and Morrison, S. L. 1963. Schizophrenia and social class. *British Journal of Psychiatry* 109:785–802.

Goldberg, Hyman, et al. 1976. Survey of dentists' opinions on issues facing the profession. *American Dental Association Journal* 93:348–354.

Goldfarb, Jeffrey. 1978. Social bases of independent public expression in communist societies. *American Journal of Sociology* 83:920–939.

Goldman, Lee. 1974. Factors related to physicians' medical and political attitudes: A documentation of intraprofessional variations. *Journal of Health and Social Behavior* 15:177–187.

Goldman, Lee, and Ebbert, Arthur. 1973. The fate of medical student liberalism: A prediction. *Journal of Medical Education* 48:1095–1103.

Goldscheider, Calvin. 1971. *Population, modernization, and social structure.* Boston: Little, Brown & Co.

Goode, William J. 1957. Community within a community: The profession. *American Sociological Review* 22:194–200.

_____. 1960a. Encroachment, charlatanism, and the emerging profession: Psychology, sociology, and medicine. *American Sociological Review* 25:902–914.

_____. 1960b. A theory of role strain. *American Sociological Review* 25:483–496.

_____. 1961. The librarian: From occupation to profession? *Library Quarterly* 31: 307–320.

_____. 1969. The theoretical limits of professionalization. In *The semi-professions and their organization,* ed. Amitai Etzioni. New York: Free Press.

Goodnow, Minnie. 1930. *Outlines of nursing history.* Philadelphia: W. B. Saunders.

Goran, Michael J., et al. 1975. The PSRO hospital review system. *Medical Care* 13:1–33.

Gordon, Gerald. 1966. *Role theory and illness.* New Haven, Conn.: College and University Press.

Gordon, Gerald, et al. 1968. *Disease, the individual, and society.* New Haven, Conn.: College and University Press.

Gordon, Gerald; Tanon, Christian P.; and Morse, Edward V. 1976. Decision-making criteria and organization performance. In *Organizational research in hospitals,* ed. Stephen M. Shortell and M. Brown. Chicago: An Inquiry Book, Blue Cross Association.

Gordon, Jeoffry. 1969. The politics of community medicine projects: A conflict analysis. *Medical Care* 7:419–428.

_____. 1976. Quality of care in free clinics. *American Journal of Public Health* 66: 955–956.

Gordon, Leon. 1973. Effectiveness of comprehensive care programs in preventing rheumatic fever. *New England Journal of Medicine* 289:331–335.

Gordon, Milton M. 1964. *Assimilation in American life.* New York: Oxford University Press.

Gordon, P. J. 1961–1962. The top management triangle in voluntary hospitals, I & II. *Journal of the Academy of Management* 4:205–215; 5:66–75.

Gordon, Tavia. 1957. Mortality experience among the Japanese in the United States, Hawaii, and Japan. *Public Health Reports* 72:543.

Gordon, Tavia, and Devine, Brian. 1966. *Hypertension and hypertensive heart disease in adults, United States, 1960–1962* (U.S. National Center for Health Statistics, Series 11, No. 13). Washington, D.C.: U.S. Government Printing Office.

Gordon, Travis L., and Dubé, W. F. 1976. Datagram: Medical student enrollment, 1971–1972 through 1975–1976. *Journal of Medical Education* 51:144–146.

Gordon, Travis L., and Johnson, Davis G. 1977. Study of U.S. medical school applicants, 1975–1976. *Journal of Medical Education* 52:707–730.

Gosfield, Alice. 1975. *PSROs: The law and health consumer.* Cambridge, Mass.: Ballinger Publishing.

Goss, M. E. W. 1962. Administration and physician. *American Journal of Public Health* 52:183–191.

_____. 1963. Patterns of bureaucracy among hospital staff physicians. In *The hospital in modern society,* ed. Eliot Freidson. New York: Free Press.

_____. 1970. Organizational goals and quality of medical care: Evidence from comparative research on hospitals. *Journal of Health and Social Behavior* 11:255-268.

Goss, M. E. W., and Reed, J. I. 1974. Evaluating the quality of hospital care through severity-adjusted death rates. *Medical Care* 12:202–213.

Goss, M. E. W., et al. 1977. Social organization and control in medical work: A call for research. *Medical Care* 15:1–10.

Gottschalk, Stephen. 1973. *The emergence of Christian Science in American Religious life.* Berkeley and Los Angeles: University of California Press.

Gough, Harrison G., and Hall, Wallace B. 1977. A comparison of medical students from medical and nonmedical families. *Journal of Medical Education* 52:541–547.

Gouldner, Alvin W. 1954. *Patterns of industrial bureaucracy.* New York: Free Press.

_____. 1956. Explorations in applied social science. *Social Problems* 3:169–181.

_____. 1957. Theoretical requirements of the applied social science. *American Sociological Review* 22:92–102.

_____. 1962. Anti-minotaur: The myth of a value-free sociology. *Social Problems* 9: 199–213.

Gove, Walter R. 1972a. The relationship between sex roles, marital status, and mental illness. *Social Forces* 51:34–44.

_____. 1972b. Sex, marital status and suicide. *Journal of Health and Social Behavior* 13:204–213.

_____. 1973. Sex, marital status and mortality. *American Journal of Sociology* 79: 45–67.

_____. 1975a. Labeling and mental illness: A critique. In *The labeling of deviance,* ed. Walter R. Gove. New York: Wiley.

_____, ed. 1975b. *The labeling of deviance.* New York: Wiley.

Gove, Walter R., and Fain, Terry. 1977. A comparison of voluntary and committed psychiatric patients. *Archives of General Psychiatry* 34:669–675.

Gove, Walter R., and Geerken, M. R. 1977. Response bias in surveys of mental health:

An empirical investigation. *American Journal of Sociology* 82:1289–1317.

Gove, Walter R., and Hughes, Michael. 1979. Possible causes of the apparent sex differences in physical health: An empirical investigation. *American Sociological Review* 44:126–146.

Gove, Walter R., and Tudor, J. F. 1973. Adult sex roles and mental illness. *American Journal of Sociology* 78:812–835.

——. 1977. Commentary and debate: Sex differences in mental illness: A comment on Dohrenwend and Dohrenwend. *American Journal of Sociology* 82:1327–1336.

Gowen, B. S. 1907. Some aspects of pestilences and other epidemics. *American Journal of Psychology* 18:1–60.

Graham, Saxon. 1963. Ethnic deviation as related to cancer at various sites. *Cancer* 6: 13–27.

——. 1972. Group versus solo practice: Arguments and evidence. *Inquiry* 9:49–60.

Graham, Saxon, and Lilienfeld, A. M. 1958. Genetic studies of gastric cancer in humans. *Cancer* 11:945–958.

Graham, Saxon, and Reeder, Leo G. 1979. Social epidemiology of chronic diseases. In *Handbook of medical sociology,* 3rd ed., ed. Howard E. Freeman, Sol Levine, and Leo G. Reeder. Englewood Cliffs, N.J.: Prentice-Hall.

Graham, Saxon, et al. 1960. The socio-economic distribution of cancer at various sites in Buffalo, New York, 1948–1952. *Cancer* 13:180–182.

Graham, Victoria. 1977. Helpless in a senseless world: Mentally disabled turned out to roam the streets. *The Sacramento Union,* 27 November, p. A6.

Gray, B. H. 1975. *Human subjects in medical experimentation.* New York: Wiley-Interscience.

Gray, Charlotte. 1977. Laetrile: Canada's legal position firm but pressure in the south grows. *Canadian Medical Association Journal* 117:1068–1074.

Gray, Lois. 1977. The geographic and functional distribution of black physicians. *American Journal of Public Health* 67:519–526.

Gray, Robert M., et al. 1965. An analysis of physicians' attitudes of cynicism and humanitarianism before and after entering medical practice. *Journal of Medical Education* 40:760–766.

Greenblatt, Milton. 1957. Implications for psychiatry and hospital practice: The movement from custodial hospital to therapeutic community. In *The patient and the mental hospital,* ed. Milton Greenblatt et al. Glencoe, Ill.: Free Press.

Greenblatt, Milton, et al., eds. 1957. *The patient and the mental hospital.* Glencoe, Ill.: Free Press.

Greene, Jack P. 1976. Values and society in revolutionary America. *Annals of the American Academy of Political and Social Science* 426:53–69.

Greenley, James. 1972. The psychiatric patients' family and length of hospitalization. *Journal of Health and Social Behavior* 13:25–37.

Greenley, James R., and Mechanic, David. 1976. Social selection in seeking help for psychological problems. *Journal of Health and Social Behavior* 17:249–262.

Greenlick, Merwyn. 1972. The impact of prepaid group practice on American medical care: A critical evaluation. *Annals of the American Academy of Political and Social Science* 399:100–113.

Griffin, Gerald J., and Griffin, J. K. 1973. *History and trends of professional nursing.* St. Louis: The C. V. Mosby Co.

Grinker, R. 1953. *Psychosomatic research.* New York: W. W. Norton & Co.

Grosicki, T. W. 1963. History of pharmacy in the 5-year program. *American Journal of Hospital Pharmacy* Spring, pp. 237–241.

Gross, B. M. 1967. The coming general systems. *Human Relations* 20:357–374.

Gross, Edward. 1970. Work, organization, and stress. In *Social stress,* ed. Sol Levine and Norman A. Scotch. Chicago: Aldine.

Grosser, Henry, et al., eds. 1969. *Nonprofessionals in the human services.* San Francisco: Jossey-Bass.

Grotjahn, Alfred. 1915. *Soziale Pathologie,* 2nd ed. Berlin: August Hirschwald Verlag.

Guérin, Jules. 1848. Médicine sociale: Un corps médicale de France. *Gazette Médicale de Paris,* 11 March, p. 203.

Gunderson, E. K., and Rahe, R. H. 1974. *Life stress and illness.* Springfield, Ill.: Charles C Thomas.

Guralnick, L. 1963a. Mortality by occupation level and cause of death among men, 20 to 64 years of age, United States, 1950. *Vital Statistics, Special Reports* 53: 448–451.

_____. 1963b. Socioeconomic differences in mortality by cause of death: United States, 1950, and England and Wales, 1949–1953. Prepared for the International Union for the Scientific Study of Population, Ottawa.

Gurin, Gerald; Veroff, Joseph; and Feld, Sheila. 1960. *Americans view mental health.* New York: Basic Books.

Gustafson, Elizabeth. 1972. Dying: The career of the nursing home patient. *Journal of Health and Social Behavior* 13:226–235.

Habenstein, R. W., and Christ, E. A. 1963. *Professionalizer, traditionalizer, and utilizer.* Columbia: University of Missouri Press.

Haenszel, William. 1961. Cancer mortality among foreign born in the United States. *Journal of the National Cancer Institute* 26:37–132.

Haenszel, William, et al. 1962. Lung-cancer mortality as related to residence and smoking histories. *Journal of National Cancer Institute* 28:947–1001.

Hage, J. 1965. An axiomatic theory of organizations. *Administrative Science Quarterly* 10:294–301.

Haggard, Howard W. 1934. *The doctor in history.* New Haven: Yale University Press.

Hall, H. G. 1977. Molière satirist of seventeenth-century French medicine: fact and fantasy. *Proceedings of the Royal Society of Medicine* 70:425–431.

Hall, Oswald. 1946. The informal organization of the medical profession. *Canadian Journal of Economics and Political Science* 12:30–41.

_____. 1948. The stages of the medical career. *American Journal of Sociology* 53: 327–336.

_____. 1949. Types of medical careers. *American Journal of Sociology* 55:243–253.

_____. 1954. Some problems in the provision of medical services. *Canadian Journal of Economic and Political Science* 20:456–466.

Hall, R. H.; Hass, J. E.; and Johnson, N. J. 1967. Organizational size complexity, and formalization. *American Sociological Review* 32:903–911.

Hallowell, A. Irving. 1935. Primitive concepts of disease. *American Anthropologist* 37: 365–368.

Hammond, Kenneth R., et al. 1959. *Teaching comprehensive medical care.* Cambridge: Harvard University Press.

Hamolsky, Milton W. 1972. An integrated program in the liberal arts and medical sciences. In *The changing medical curriculum,* 2nd ed., ed. Vernon Lippard and Elizabeth Purcell. New York: Josiah Macy, Jr. Foundation.

Harburg, Ernest; Erfurt, John C.; Chape, Catherine; Hauenstein, Louis S.; Schull, William J.; and Schork, M. A. 1973. Socioecological stressor areas and black-white blood pressure: Detroit. *Journal of Chronic Diseases* 26:595–611.

Harburg, Ernest; Schull, William J.; and Erfurt, John C. 1970. A family set method for estimating heredity and stress. *Journal of Chronic Diseases* 23:69–81.

Hare, E. H. 1956. Family setting and the urban distribution of schizophrenia. *Journal of Mental Science* 102:753–760.

Harkey, John, et al. 1976. The relation between social class and functional status: A new look at the drift hypothesis. *Journal of Health and Social Behavior* 17: 194–204.

Harrey, E. 1968. Technology and the structure of organizations. *American Sociological Review* 33:247–258.

Harris, Richard. 1966. *A sacred trust.* New York: The New American Library.

Hart, H. L. A. 1965. *The concept of law.* Fair Lawn, N.J.: Oxford University Press.

Hartz, Louis M. 1955. *The liberal tradition in America: An interpretation of American political thought since the revolution.* New York: Harcourt, Brace.

Harvey, Edward. 1966. Some implications of value differentiation in pharmacy. *Canadian Review of Anthropology and Sociology* 3:23–37.

Haug, Marie R. 1972. Deprofessionalization: Alternative hypothesis for the future. *Sociological Review Monograph* 20:195–211.

_____. 1975. The deprofessionalization of everyone? *Sociological Focus* 8:197–214.

_____. 1976. The erosion of professional authority: A cross-cultural inquiry in the case of the physician. *Milbank Memorial Fund Quarterly* 54:83–106.

Haug, Marie R., and Lavin, Bebe. 1978. Methods of payment for medical care and public attitudes toward physician authority. *Journal of Health and Social Behavior* 19:279–291.

Haug, Marie R., and Sussman, Marvin B. 1969. Professional autonomy and the revolt of the client. *Social Problems* 17:153–160.

Havighurst, Clark C. 1970. Health maintenance organization and the market for health services. *Law and Contemporary Problems* 35:716–795.

Havighurst, Robert A. 1963. Successful aging. In *Process of aging,* ed. R. Williams, C. Tibbitts, and W. Donahue. New York: Atherton.

Hawkins, Richard, and Tiedeman, Gary. 1975. *The creation of deviance.* Columbus, Ohio: Charles E. Merrill Publishing Co.

Hayes-Bautista, David E. 1976. Termination of the patient-practitioner relationship: Divorce, patient style. *Journal of Health and Social Behavior* 17:12–21.

Haynes, G. 1967. Chiropractic education and curriculum flexibility. *The ACA Journal of the Chiropractic* 8:13.

HDFP (Hypertension Detection and Follow-up Program Cooperative Group, National Heart, Lung, and Blood Institute, NIH). 1977. Race, education, and prevalence of hypertension. *American Journal of Epidemiology* 106:351–361.

Heer, Friedrich. 1961. *The medieval world.* London: Weidenfeld & Nicolson.

Heist, P. 1962. The student. In *Education for the profession,* ed. Nelson B. Henry. Chicago: University of Chicago Press.

Heller, Peter. 1973. *The strategy of health-sector planning.* In *Public health in the People's Republic of China,* ed. Myron Wegman et al. New York: Josiah Macy, Jr. Foundation.

Hellman, L. M., et al. 1970. The use of health manpower in obstetric-gynecologic care in the United States. *Internist Journal of Obstetric Gynecology* 8:732–738.

Henderson, Lawrence J. 1935. Physician and patient as a social system. *New England Journal of Medicine* 212:819–823.

Hengst, Acco, and Roghmann, Klaus. 1978. The two dimensions in satisfaction with dental care. *Medical Care* 16:202–213.

Hennes, James D. 1972. The measurement of health. *Medical Care Review* 29:1268–1288.

Henry, Jules. 1954. The formal structure of a psychiatric hospital. *Psychiatry* 17: 139–151.

Henry, J. P., and Cassel, J. C. 1969. Psychosocial factors in essential hypertension. *American Journal of Epidemiology* 90:171–200.

Hepple, Lawrence. 1946. Selective service rejectees in Missouri. Unpublished doctoral dissertation, University of Missouri.

Herrington, B. S. 1978. Carter NHI ideas revealed: MH benefits uncertain. *Psychiatric News* 16:1 & 16.

Hershey, N. 1969. The inhibiting effect upon innovation of the prevailing licensure system. *Annals of New York Academy of Science* 166:951-956.

———. 1972. The defensive practice of medicine: Myth or reality? *Milbank Memorial Fund Quarterly* 50:69-98.

Hessler, R. M., and Griffard, C. D. 1976. Community health professional. *Inquiry* 13:90-96.

Hetherington, Robert W.; Hopkins, Carl E.; and Roemer, Milton I. 1975. *Health insurance plans: Promise and performance.* New York: Wiley.

Heydebrand, Wolf V. 1973. *Hospital bureaucracy.* New York: Dunellen.

Hill, R. 1958. Genetic features of families under stress. *Social Casework* 39:139-150.

Hillman, Bruce, and Charney, Evan. 1972. A neighborhood health center: What the patients know and think of its operation. *Medical Care* 10:336-344.

Himes, Joseph H. 1974. *Racial and ethnic relations.* Boston: W. C. Brown.

Hinkle, Lawrence E., and Wolff, H. G. 1957. Health and the social environment. In *Explorations in social psychiatry,* ed. Alexander H. Leighton, J. A. Clausen, and R. N. Wilson. New York: Basic Books.

Hinkle, Lawrence E., et al. 1952. A summary of experimental evidence relating life stress in diabetes mellitus. *Journal of Sinai Hospital* 19:537-570.

Hiscock, I. V. 1935. The development of neighborhood services in the United States. *Milbank Memorial Fund Quarterly* 13:30-51.

Hixson, H. H. 1965. Hospital governing boards and lay advisory boards: The challenge of the future. *Hospital Forum* 8:20-26.

Hochbaum, G. M. 1969. Consumer participation in health planning: Toward conceptual clarification. *American Journal of Public Health* 59:1698-1705.

Hodge, Robert W., et al. 1964. Occupational prestige in the United States, 1925-1963. *American Journal of Sociology* 70:286-302.

Hodgkinson, Ruth G. 1967. *The origin of the national health service.* Berkeley and Los Angeles: University of California Press.

Hoffman, L. 1958. How do good doctors get that way? In *Patients, physicians and illness,* 1st ed., ed. D. Gartly Jaco. New York: Free Press.

Hogstel, Mildred. 1977. Associate degree and baccalaureate graduates: Do they function differently? *American Journal of Nursing* 77:1598-1600.

Holden, Constance. 1973. Mental health: Establishment balks at innovative psychiatrist. *Science* 181:638-640.

Hollingshead, A. B. 1973. Medical sociology: A brief review. *Milbank Memorial Fund Quarterly* 51:531-542.

Hollingshead, A. B., and Redlich, F. C. 1953. Social stratification and psychiatric disorders. *American Sociological Review* 18:163-169.

———. 1954. Social stratification and schizophrenia. *American Sociological Review* 19: 302-306.

———. 1958. *Social class and mental illness.* New York: Wiley.

Hollingshead, A. B.; Ellis, R.; and Kirby, E. 1954. Social mobility and mental illness. *American Sociological Review* 19:577-584.

Hollingsworth, Mary F., and Hollingsworth, T. H. 1971. Plague, mortality rates by age and sex in the parish of St. Botolph's without Bishopsgate, London, 1603. *Population Studies* 25:131-146.

Hollingsworth, T. H. 1965. A demographic study of the British ducal families. In *Population in history,* ed. D. V. Glass and D. E. Eversley. London: Edward Arnold.

Hollister, Robert M. 1974. Neighborhood health centers as demonstrations. In *Neigh-*

borhood health centers, ed. Robert M. Hollister et al. Lexington, Mass.: D. C. Heath & Co.

Hollister, Robert M., et al. 1974a. Neighborhood health centers as a social movement. In *Neighborhood health centers,* ed. Robert M. Hollister et al. Lexington, Mass.: D. C. Heath & Co.

_____, eds. 1974b. *Neighborhood health centers.* Lexington, Mass.: D. C. Heath & Co.

Holloway, Robert G., et al. 1963. The participation patterns of "economic influentials" and their control of a hospital board of trustees. *Journal of Health and Human Behavior* 4:88–89.

Holman, Edwin J. 1978. Cloning: The book, the validity is open to question. *American Medical News,* 5 May, pp. 14–15.

Holmes, Thomas H., and Masuda, Minoru, 1974. Life change and illness susceptibility. In *Stressful life events,* ed. Bruce P. Dohrenwend and Barbara S. Dohrenwend. New York: Wiley.

Holmes, Thomas H., and Rahe, R. H. 1967. The social readjustment rating scale. *Journal of Psychosomatic Research* 11:213–218.

Holt, R. R., and Luborsky, L. 1958. *Personality patterns of psychiatrists.* New York: Basic Books.

Holton, W., et al. 1972. Citizen participation and interagency relations. Research report to the National Institute of Mental Health, Wasington, D.C.

Homans, George. 1950. *The human group.* New York: Harcourt, Brace & World.

_____. 1961. *Social behavior: Its elementary forms.* New York: Harcourt, Brace & World.

Honigfeld, G. 1964. Nonspecific factors in treatment. *Disease of Nervous System* 25: 145–156, 225–239.

Horan, Patrich M., and Gray, B. H. 1974. Status inconsistency, mobility and coronary heart disease. *Journal of Health and Social Behavior* 15:300–310.

Horowitz, Irving L. 1977. *Ideology and utopia in the United States, 1956-1976.* New York: Oxford University Press.

Horton, John. 1967. Time and cool people. *Transaction* 4:5–12.

House, James S. 1974. Occupational stress and coronary heart disease. *Journal of Health and Social Behavior* 15:12–27.

How to protect yourself against needless surgery. 1977. *Good Housekeeping,* October, pp. 245–246.

Howard, Jan, and Holman, B. L. 1970. The effects of race and occupation on hypertension mortality. *Milbank Memorial Fund Quarterly* 48:263–296.

Howard, John H., et al. 1976. Stress in the job and career of a dentist. *American Dental Association Journal* 93:630–636.

Howells, John G., ed. 1975. *Modern perspectives in psychiatry.* New York: Brunner-Mazel.

Hu, Teh-wei. 1976. The financing and the economic efficiency of rural health services in the People's Republic of China. *International Journal of Health Services* 6:239–249.

Hughes, Everett C. 1956. The making of a physician. *Human Organization* 14:21–25.

_____. 1958. *Men and their work.* Glencoe, Ill.: Free Press.

Hughes, H. Stuart. 1958. *Consciousness and society.* New York: Knopf.

Hulka, B. S., et al. 1972. Determinants of physician utilization. *Medical Care* 10:300–309.

Hull, William H. 1955. *Public relations for the pharmacists.* Philadelphia: J.B. Lippincott.

Humber, James, and Almeder, Robert F., eds. 1976. *Biomedical ethics and the law.* New York: Plenum Press.

Huntington, Mary Jean. 1957. The development of a professional self-image. In *The student physician,* ed. Robert K. Merton, G. G. Reader, and P. L. Kendall. Cambridge: Harvard University Press.

Hurwitz, Elliot. 1972. An analysis of the effect of OEO neighborhood health centers on the distribution of physicians. Unpublished doctoral dissertation, Temple University.

Hutchings, E., and Hutchings, E., eds. 1967. *Scientific progress and human values.* New York: American Elsevier.

Hyde, David R., et al. 1954. The AMA: Power, purpose and politics in organized medicine. *Yale Law Journal* 63:943–955.

Hyde, Gordon. 1974. *The Soviet health service: A historical and comparative view.* London: Lawrence and Wishwart.

Hyde, R. W. 1955. *Experiencing the patient's day.* New York: G. P. Putnam.

Hyde, R. W., et al. 1944. Studies in medical sociology. *New England Journal of Medicine* 231:543–548.

Hyler, Steven E., and Spitzer, Robert L. 1978. Hysteria split asunder. *American Journal of Psychiatry* 135:1500–1504.

Iglehart, John K. 1978. The Carter administration's health budget: Charting new priorities with limited dollars. *Milbank Memorial Fund Quarterly* 56:51–77.

Illich, Ivan. 1976. *Medical nemesis: The expropriation of health.* London: Calder & Boyars.

Ingmire, Alice E. 1952. Attitudes of student nurses at the University of California. *Nursing Research* 1:36–39.

In wake of Bakke case, medical schools finding need for "new commitment." 1978. *American Medical News,* 4 August, p. 9.

Issacs, Leonard. 1978. Death, where is thy distinguishing? *The Hastings Center Report* 8:5–8.

Israel, Elaine. 1973. Certification of need for and volumetric appraisal of medical care. In *PSRO: Organization for regional peer review,* ed. Paul Bonner and Barry Decker. Cambridge, Mass.: Ballinger Publishing Co.

Jackson, E. F. 1962. Status consistency and symptoms of stress. *American Sociological Review* 27:469–480.

Jaco, E. Gartly. 1959. Mental health of the Spanish American in Texas. In *Culture and mental health,* ed. Marvin Opler. New York: Macmillan.

———. 1960. *The social epidemiology of mental disorder.* New York: Russell Sage Foundation.

———. 1970. Mental illness in response to stress. In *Social stress,* ed. Sol Levine and Normal A. Scotch. Chicago: Aldine.

———, ed. 1972. *Patients, physicians and illness,* 2nd ed. New York: Free Press.

Jacob, Theodore. 1975. Family interaction in disturbed and normal families. *Psychological Bulletin* 82:33–65.

Janis, I. L. 1958. *Psychological stress.* New York: Wiley.

Jenkins, C. David. 1971. Psychologic and social precursors of coronary disease. *New England Journal of Medicine* 284:244–255, 307–317.

———. 1976. Recent evidence supporting psychologic and social risk factors for coronary disease. *New England Journal of Medicine* 294:987–994, 1033–1038.

Jenkins, C. David, et al., 1971a. Association of coronary-prone behavior scores with recurrence of coronary disease. *Journal of Chronic Diseases* 24:601–612.

———. 1971b. Progress toward validation of a computer-scored test for the type A coronary-prone behavior pattern. *Psychosomatic Medicine* 33:193–202.

Johnson, Allan. 1977. Sex differentials in coronary heart disease: The explanatory role of primary risk factors. *Journal of Health and Social Behavior* 18:46–54.

Johnson, D. G., and Hutchings, Edwin B. 1966. Doctor or dropout? *Journal of Medical Education* 41:1239.

Johnson, Malcolm L. 1975. Medical sociology and sociological theory. *Social Science and Medicine* 9:227–232.

Jonas, Hans. 1970. Philosophical reflections on experimenting with human subjects. In *Experimentation with human subjects,* ed. Paul A. Freund. New York: George Braziller.

Jonas, S., et al. 1975. The 1974 reorganization of the British NHS: An analysis. *Journal of Community Health* 1:91–105.

Jones, Edward G., et al. 1958. A study of epidemiologic factors in carcinoma of the uterine cervix. *American Journal of Obstetrics and Gynecology* 76:1010–1015.

Jones, W. H. S., ed. & trans. 1943. *Hippocrates.* London: William Heinmann.

Jorgenson, Cynthia L. 1978. A study of chiropractic spinal manipulation as it relates to the many human illnesses. *International Review of Chiropractic* 32:30–37.

Jowett, Benjamin, trans. 1927. *The Republic of Plato,* 3rd ed. Oxford: Clarendon Press.

Juan, I. R., et al. 1974. High and low levels of dogmatism in relation to personality characteristics of medical students. *Psychological Report* 34:303–315.

Jury awards paralyzed girl $7.6 million. 1978. *Sacramento Union,* 22 November, p. 1.

Kadushin, Charles. 1964. Social class and the experience of ill health. *Sociological Inquiry* 24:67–80.

———. 1969. *Why people go to psychiatrists.* New York: Atherton.

Kahn, H. A., et al. 1969. Serum cholesterol. *Israel Journal of Medical Science* 5:1117.

Kahn, Manford. 1964. Major trends in symbolic interaction theory in the past 25 years. *Sociological Quarterly* 5:61–84.

Kahne, Merton J. 1959. Bureaucratic structure and impersonal experience in mental hospitals. *Psychiatry* 22:363–375.

Kandel, Denise. 1960. Career decisions of medical students: A study of occupational recruitment and occupational choice. Unpublished doctoral dissertation, Columbia University.

Kaplan, Abraham. 1964. *The conduct of inquiry.* San Francisco: Chandler Publishing Co.

Kaplan, Howard B. 1979. Social psychology of disease. *Handbook of medical sociology,* 3rd ed., ed. Howard E. Freeman, Sol Levine, and Leo G. Reeder. Englewood Cliffs, N.J.: Prentice-Hall.

Kaplan, Howard B., and Warheit, G. J. 1975. Introduction to "recent developments in the sociology of mental illness." *Journal of Health and Social Behavior* 16: 343–346.

Kardiner, Abram, and Ovesey, L. 1951. *The mark of oppression.* New York: Norton.

Karefa-Smart, John. 1975. The relevance for developing countries of the Chinese experience in the health field. In *Medicine in Chinese culture: Comparative studies of health care in Chinese and other societies* (DHEW Publication No. (NIH) 75–653), ed. Arthur Kleinman et al. Washington, D.C.: U.S. Government Printing Office.

Kark, Sidney L. 1974. *Epidemiology and community medicine.* New York: Appleton-Century-Crofts.

Karmel, Madeline. 1970. The internalization of social roles in institutionalized chronic mental patients. *Journal of Health and Social Behavior* 11:231–235.

Karnow, Stanley. 1972. *Mao and China.* New York: Viking Press.

Kaser, Michael. 1976. *Health care in the Soviet Union and eastern Europe.* Boulder, Colo.: Westview Press.

Kasl, Stanislav V., and French, J. R. P. 1962. The effects of occupational status on physical and mental health. *Journal of Social Issues* 18:67–89.

Kasl, Stanislav V., and Hamburg, Ernest. 1975. Mental health and the urban environment: Some doubts and second thought. *Journal of Health and Social Behavior* 16:268–282.

Kass, Leon R. 1971. Death as an event: A commentary on Robert Morison. *Science* 173:698–702.

Kassebaum, Gene G., and Baumann, Barbara O. 1972. Dimensions of the sick role in chronic illness. In *Patients, physicians and illness,* 2nd ed., ed. E. Gartly Jaco. New York: Free Press.

Kasteler, Josephine, et al. 1976. Issues underlying prevalence of "doctor-shopping" behavior. *Journal of Health and Social Behavior* 17:328–339.

Kastenbaum, Robert J. 1977. *Death, society, and human experience.* St. Louis: The C. V. Mosby Co.

Kastenbaum, Robert J., and Aisenberg, Ruth. 1972. *The psychology of death.* New York: Springer Publishing Co.

Kastenbaum, Robert J., and Candy, S. 1973. The four percent fallacy: A methodological and empirical critique of extended care facility program statistics. *Aging and Human Development* 4:15–21.

Katz, D., and Kahn, R. L. 1966. *The social psychology of organizations.* New York: Wiley.

Katz, E., et al. 1963. Doctor-patient exchanges: A diagnostic approach to organizations and professions. *Human Relations* 22:309–324.

Katz, Jay. 1972. *Experimentation with human beings.* New York: Russell Sage Foundation.

Katz, Jay, and Capron, Alexander M. 1975. *Catastrophic diseases: Who decides what?* New York: Russell Sage.

Katz, Leon. 1976. Implications of prenatal diagnosis for the human right to life. In *Biomedical ethics and the law,* ed. James Humber and Robert F. Almeder. New York: Plenum Press.

Kaufman, Herbert. 1969. Administrative decentralization and political power. *Public Administration Review* 29:3–15.

Kavet, Joel, and Luft, Harold S. 1974. The implications of the PSRO legislation for the teaching hospital sector. *Journal of Medical Education* 49:321–330.

Keegeles, S. S. 1961. Why people seek dental care. *American Journal of Public Health* 51:1306–1311.

Keil, Julian E., et al. 1977. Hypertension: Effects of social class and racial admixture. *American Journal of Public Health* 67:634–639.

Kelly, Alfred H., and Miles, Richard D. 1976. Maintenance of revolutionary values. *Annals of the American Academy of Political and Social Science* 426:25–52.

Kelly, Lucie Young. 1975. *Dimensions of professional nursing.* New York: Macmillan.

Kempe, Duncan B. 1968. Joint education of medical students and allied health personnel. *American Journal of Diseases of Children* 116:499–504.

Kendall, Patricia, and Selvin, H. C. 1957. Tendencies toward specialization in medical training. In *The student physician,* ed. Robert K. Merton, G. G. Reader, and P. L. Kendall. Cambridge: Harvard University Press.

Kennaway, E. L. 1948. Racial and social incidence of cancer of the uterus. *British Journal of Cancer* 2:177–179.

Kessel, Reuben. 1958. Price discrimination in medicine. *Journal of Law and Economics* 1:20–53.

Kessner, D. K., et al. 1974. *Assessment of medical care for children.* Washington, D.C.: Institute of Medicine, National Academy of Science.

Keys, A., ed. 1970. Coronary heart disease in seven countries. *Circulation* 41, suppl. 1.

Kimmel, E. 1964. A critical evaluation of the chiropractic as a profession. *The ACA Journal of the Chiropractic* 1:8.

King, B. 1971. People versus commissioner. *Health Rights News* 4:11.

Kinlun, M. Lucille. 1972. Independent nurse practitioner. *Nursing Outlook* 20:22–24.

Kinston, W., and Rosser, R. 1974. Disaster: Effects on mental and physical state. *Journal of Psychosomatic Research* 18:437–456.

Kisch, Arnold I., and Reeder, Leo G. 1969. Client evaluation of physician performance. *Journal of Health and Social Behavior* 10:51–58.

Kissam, Philip C. 1977. Physician's assistant and nurse practitioner laws for expanded medical delegation. In *The new health professionals,* ed. Ann Bliss and Eva D. Cohen. Germantown, Md.: Aspen Systems Corp.

Kitagawa, E. M., and Hauser, P. M. 1973. *Differential mortality in the United States: A study of socioeconomic epidemiology.* Cambridge: Harvard University Press.

Kitano, Harry H. L. 1969. Japanese-American mental illness. In *Changing perspectives in mental illness,* ed. Stanley C. Plog and R. B. Edgerton. New York: Holt, Rinehart & Winston.

Kitterie, Nicholas. 1971. *The right to be different.* Baltimore: Johns Hopkins University Press.

Klein, Alan J. 1978. Personal satisfaction for the dental practitioner. *Dental Clinics of North America* 22:187–196.

Kleiner, Robert J., and Parker, S. 1963. Goal-striving, social status, and mental disorder. *American Sociological Review* 28:169–203.

_____. 1966. *Mental illness in the urban negro community.* New York: Free Press.

_____. 1969. Social mobility, anomie, and mental disorder. In *Changing perspectives in mental illness,* ed. Stanley C. Plog and R. B. Edgerton. New York: Holt, Rinehart & Winston.

_____. 1971. Potential sources of error in epidemiological studies of mental illness. *International Journal of Social Psychiatry* 17:122–132.

Kleinman, Arthur, et al., eds. 1975. *Medicine in Chinese cultures: Comparative studies of health care in Chinese and other societies* (DHEW Publication No. (NIH) 75–653). Washington, D.C.: U.S. Government Printing Office.

Kluckhohn, Clyde. 1958. Have there been discernible shifts in American values during the past generation? In *The American style: Essays in values and performance,* ed. Eliting E. Morison. New York: Harper & Row.

Knapp, Deanne E., and Knapp, D. A. 1968. Disillusionment in pharmacy students. *Social Science and Medicine* 1:445–447.

Knopf, Lucille. 1972. *From student to RN: A report of the nurse career pattern study* (DHEW). Washington, D.C.: U.S. Government Printing Office.

Knowles, John H. 1970. U. S. health: Do we face a catastrophe? *Look Magazine,* June, pp. 74–78.

Kohl, Marvin, ed. 1975. *Beneficient euthanasia.* Buffalo, N.Y.: Prometheus Books.

Kohn, Melvin. 1968. Social class and schizophrenia. *Journal of Psychiatric Research* 6:155–173.

_____. 1972. Class, family, schizophrenia. *Social Forces* 50:295–304.

Kohn, Melvin, and Clausen, John A. 1956. Parental authority behavior and schizophrenia. *American Journal of Orthopsychiatry* 26:297–313.

Kohn, Robert, and White, Kerr L., eds. 1976. *Health care: An international study.* New York: Oxford University Press.

Kolko, Gabriel. 1963. *The triumph of conservatism: A reinterpretation of American history, 1900–1916.* Glencoe, Ill.: Free Press.

Komarovsky, M. 1964. *Blue collar marriage.* New York: Random House.

Koos, Earl L. 1954. *The health of Regionville.* New York: Columbia University Press.

Kosa, John, and Coker, R. E. 1965. The female physician in public health. *Sociology and Social Research* 49:294–305.

Kovar, Mary Grace. 1977. Mortality of black infants in the United States. *Phylon* 38: 370–397.

Koz, Gabriel, and Rosenblatt, Aaron. 1978. Psychiatric house staff on strike. *Journal of the American Medical Association* 239:1056–1060.

Krafchek, Steven. 1975. *The malpractice issue in Washington.* Seattle: University of Washington, Health Policy Analysis Program.

Kramer, M. 1967. Comparative study of characteristics, attitudes, and opinions of neophyte British and American nurses. *International Journal of Nursing Studies* 4:281.

_____. 1970. Role conception of baccalaureate nurses and success in hospital nursing. *Nursing Research* 19:428–439.

_____. 1974. *Reality shock: Why nurses leave nursing.* St. Louis: The C. V. Mosby Co.

Kramer, Ralph M. 1969. *Participation of the poor.* Englewood Cliffs, N.J.: Prentice-Hall.

Krause, Elliot A. 1977. *Power and illness: The political sociology of health and medical care.* New York: Elsevier.

Krehl, W. A. 1977. The nutritional epidemiology of cardiovascular disease. *Annals of the New York Academy of Science* 300:335–359.

Kremers, Edward, and Urdang, George. 1963. *History of pharmacy.* Philadelphia: J. B. Lippincott.

Kroeger, Gertrand. 1937. *The concept of social medicine and other writers in Germany, 1779--1932.* Chicago: Julius Rosenwald Fund.

Kroll, R. 1970. The free clinic complaints aired. *Berkeley Daily Gazette,* 9 June, pp. 1–2.

Kronous, Carol L. 1975. Occupational values, role, orientations, and work settings: The case of pharmacy. *Sociological Quarterly* 16:171–183.

Kruger, Helen. 1974. *Other healers, other cures.* Indianapolis: Bobbs-Merrill.

Küber-Ross, Elizabeth. 1969. *On death and dying.* New York: Macmillan.

Kuhn, J. W. 1960. Does collective bargaining usurp the manager's right to manage? *Modern Hospital* 95:70–73.

Kulge, Eike-Henner W. 1975. *The practice of death.* New Haven: Yale University Press.

Kurokawa, Minako. 1969. Cultural conflict and mental disorders. *Journal of Social Issues* 25:195–214.

_____, ed. 1970. *Minority responses: Comparative views of reactions to subordination.* New York: Random House.

Kurtz, R. A., et al. 1962. Hospital social systems and differential perceptions (Report No. 4). Lincoln: University of Nebraska, Hospital Research Project.

Ladd, John. 1976. Are science and ethics compatible? In *Science, ethics, and medicine,* ed. H. Tristram Engelhardt and Daniel Callahan. New York: Institute of Society, Ethics, and the Life Sciences.

Ladimer, I. 1955. Ethical and legal aspects of medical research on human beings, from law and medicine, a symposium. *Journal of Public Law* 3:467–511.

Lambert, Randall L., et al. 1977. The pharmacists' clinical role as seen by other health workers. *American Journal of Public Health* 67:252–253.

Lampton, David M. 1974. *Health, conflict, and the Chinese political system.* Ann Arbor: University of Michigan, Center for Chinese Studies.

Langer, E. 1966. Human experimentation: New York verdict affirms patients' rights. *Science* 151:663–666.

Langner, Thomas, and Michael, S. T. 1963. *Life stress and mental health.* New York: Free Press.

Langston, Joann H., et al. 1972. Study to evaluate the OEO neighborhood health center program at selected centers (vol. 1, PB-207-084). Springfield, Va.: National Technical Information Service.

Lapouse, Rema, et al. 1956. The drift hypothesis in socio-economic differentials in schizophrenia. *American Journal of Public Health* 46:978–986.

Larson, Donald E., and Rootman, Irving. 1976. Physician role performance and patient satisfaction. *Social Science and Medicine* 10:29–32.

Larson, W. R., and Palola, E. G. 1961. Exploration of job satisfaction among hospital personnel. Seattle: Washington State Health Department.

Lasagna, Louis. 1963. *The doctor's dilemma.* New York: Harper.

_____. 1970. Special subjects in human experimentation. In *Experimentation with human subjects,* ed. Paul A. Freund. New York: George Braziller.

Laue, James H. 1965. The changing character of the negro protest. *Annals of the American Academy of Political and Social Science* 357:119–126.

Lave, L. B., and Leinhardt, S. 1975. Medical manpower models: Need, demand and supply. *Inquiry* 12:97–125.

Lawrence, P. R., and Lorsch, J. W. 1967. *Organization and environment.* Boston: Harvard University Press.

Lawson, W. R. 1976. The choice of dentistry as a career. *New Zealand Dental Journal* 72:155–158.

Lazarus, J., et al. 1963. Migration differentials in mental disease. *Milbank Memorial Fund Quarterly* 41:25–42.

Lazarus, R. 1966. *Psychological stress and the coping process.* New York: McGraw-Hill.

Leacock, Eleanor. 1957. Three social variables and the occurrence of mental disorder. In *Explorations in social psychiatry,* ed. Alexander H. Leighton, J. A. Clausen, and R. N. Wilson. New York: Basic Books.

Leatherman, G. H. 1978. The challenges to the dental profession as an integral part of the health service. *Journal of American College of Dentists* 45:79–88.

Leavy, Stanley A., and Freedman, L. Z. 1956. Psychoneurosis and economic life. *Social Problems* 4:55–67.

Lederberg, J. 1966. Experimental genetics and human evolution. *American Naturalist* 100:519–526.

Lee, G. A. 1974. Marriage and anomie: A causal argument. *Journal of Marriage and the Family* 36:523–532.

Lee, M. L. 1971. A conspicuous production theory of hospital behavior. *The Southern Economic Journal* 38:48–58.

Lee, Rance P. L. 1975. Interaction between Chinese and Western medicine in Hong Kong: Modernization and professional inequality. In *Medicine in Chinese cultures: Comparative studies of health care in Chinese and other societies* (DHEW Publication No. (NIH) 75–653), ed. Arthur R. Kleinman et al. Washington, D.C.: U.S. Government Printing Office.

_____. 1976. The causal priority between socioeconomic status and psychiatric disorder. *International Journal of Social Psychiatry* 22:1–7.

Leerman, Jane. 1978. The professional values and expectations of medical students. *Journal of Medical Education* 53:330–336.

Lefton, Mark, and Rosengren, W. R. 1966. Organizations and clients: Lateral and longitudinal dimensions. *American Sociological Review* 31:802–810.

Leighton, Alexander H.; Clausen, John A.; and Wilson, R. N., eds. 1957. *Explorations in social psychiatry.* New York: Basic Books.

Leighton, Alexander H., and Leighton, Dorothea. 1945. *The Navaho door.* Cambridge: Harvard University Press.

Leininger, Madeleine. 1976. Doctoral programs for nurses: Trends, questions, and projected plans. *Nursing Research* 25:201–210.

Leis, Gordon Leroy. 1971. The professionalization of chiropractic. Unpublished doctoral dissertation, State University of New York at Buffalo.

Lemert, Edwin M. 1948. An exploratory study of mental disorders in a rural problem area. *Rural Sociology* 13:48–64.

_____. 1951. *Social pathology.* New York: McGraw-Hill.

_____. 1962. Paranoia and the dynamics of exclusion. *Sociometry* 25:14–19.

_____. 1967. *Human deviance, social problems and social control.* Englewood Cliffs, N.J.: Prentice-Hall.

Lena, Hugh Francis. 1975. The anatomy and functioning of the hospital. Unpublished doctoral dissertation, University of Connecticut.

Lennard, H. L., and Glock, C. Y. 1957. Studies in hypertension. *Journal of Chronic Diseases* 5:186–196.

Lenski, G. E. 1954. Status crystalization. *American Sociological Review* 19:405–413.

Lerner, Monroe, and Stutz, Richard N. 1977. Have we narrowed the gaps between the poor and the non-poor? Part II. Narrowing the gaps, 1959–1961 to 1969–1971: Mortality. *Medical Care* 15:620–635.

Levin, Lowell S.; Katz, Alfred; and Holst, Erik. 1976. *Self-care: Lay initiatives in health.* New York: Prodist.

Levin, Morton L., et al. 1962. Nursing, fertility, and other factors in the epidemiology of cancer of the breast. Paper presented at the meeting of the American Public Health Association, Miami.

Levine, D. N., ed. 1971. *Georg Simmel on individuality and social forms.* Chicago: University of Chicago Press.

Levine, Mortimer. 1973. Chiropractic analysis. In *Mental health and chiropractic,* ed. Herman S. Schwartz. New York: Sessions Publishers.

Levine, Sol, and Scotch, Norman A., eds. 1970. *Social stress.* Chicago: Aldine.

Levine, Sol; Scotch, Norman A.; and Vlasak, George J. 1969. Unravelling technology–culture in public health. *American Journal of Public Health* 59:237–244.

Levine, Sol, and White, Paul E. 1961. Exchange as a conceptual framework for the study of interorganizational relationships. *Administrative Science Quarterly* 5:583–601.

Levinson, Daniel J. 1967. Medical education and the theory of adult socialization. *Journal of Health and Social Behavior* 8:253–264.

Levinson, Daniel J., and Gallagher, E. B. 1961. *Patienthood in the mental hospital.* Boston: Houghton Mifflin.

Levinson, P., and Schiller, J. 1966. Role analysis of the indigenous nonprofessional. *Social Work* 11:95–101.

Levitan, Sar A. 1969. *The great society's poor law: A new approach to poverty.* Baltimore: Johns Hopkins University Press.

Levy, Leo, and Rowitz, Louis. 1975. The state mental hospital in transition. *International Journal of Social Psychiatry* 21:262–273.

Lewis, Aubrey. 1953. Health as a social concept. *British Journal of Sociology* 4:109–124.

Lewis, Charles E.; Fein, Rashi; and Mechanic, D. 1976. *A right to health: The problem of access to primary medical care.* New York: Wiley.

Lewis, Charles E., et al. 1969. Activities, events, and outcomes in ambulatory patient care. *New England Journal of Medicine* 12:645–649.

Lewis, Oscar. 1966. *La Vida.* New York: Random House.

Liang, Matthew H., et al. 1973. Chinese health care: Determinants of the system. *American Journal of Public Health* 63:102–109.

Liberman, R. 1962. An analysis of the placebo phenomenon. *Journal of Chronic Diseases* 15:761–783.

Lidz, R. W., and Lidz, T. 1949. The family environment of schizophrenia patients. *American Journal of Psychiatry* 106:343–344.

Lidz, T., et al. 1957. Schism and skew in the families of schizophrenics. *American Journal of Psychiatry* 64:241–248.

Lieberson, Stanley. 1958. Ethnic groups and the practice of medicine. *American Sociological Review* 23:542–549.

Liem, Ramsay, and Liem, Joan. 1978. Social class and mental illness reconsidered: The role of economic stress and social support. *American Sociological Review* 19: 139–156.

Lilienfeld, Abraham M. 1956. Variation in mortality from heart disease. *Public Health Reports* 71:545–552.

———. 1957. Epidemiological methods and inferences in studies of noninfectious diseases. *Public Health Reports* 72:51–60.

Lilienfeld, Abraham M., and Graham, S. 1958. Validity of determining circumcision status by questionnaire as related to epidemiological studies of cancer of the cervix. *Journal of the National Cancer Institute* 21:713–720.

Lin, P. 1972. The chiropractor, chiropractic, and process: A study of the sociology of an occupation. Unpublished doctoral dissertation, University of Missouri.

Lin, T. S. 1953. A study of the incidence of mental disorder in Chinese and other cultures. *Psychiatry* 16:313–336.

Lindblom, Charles E. 1965. *The intelligence of democracy: Decision making through mutual adjustment.* New York: Free Press.

Lindsey, Almond. 1962. *Socialized medicine in England and Wales.* Chapel Hill: University of North Carolina Press.

Linn, Erwin L. 1967. Role behaviors in two dental clinics: A trial of Nadel's criteria. *Human Organization* 26:141–148.

Linn, Lawrence A., and Davis, Milton S. 1973. Occupational orientation and overt behavior–The pharmacist as drug advisor to patients. *American Journal of Public Health* 63:502–508.

Linsky, Arnold S. 1970. Who shall be excluded: The influence of personal attributes in community reaction to the mentally ill. *Social Psychiatry* 5:166–171.

Lippard, Vernon W. 1972. Trends in the medical curriculum. In *The changing medical curriculum,* ed. Vernon Lippard and Elizabeth Purcell. New York: Josiah Macy, Jr. Foundation.

Lippard, Vernon W., and Purcell, Elizabeth, eds. 1972. *The changing medical curriculum,* 2nd ed. New York: Josiah Macy, Jr. Foundation.

Lipset, Seymour Martin. 1963. *The first new nation.* New York: Basic Books.

Lipton, E. 1932. England in the age of mercantilism. *Journal of Business History* 4: 697–707.

Lisitsin, Y. 1972. *Health protection in the USSR.* Moscow: Progress Publishers.

Litman, Theodor J. 1972. Public perception of the physicians' assistants–A survey of the attitudes and opinions of rural Iowa and Minnesota residents. *American Journal of Public Health* 62:343–346.

Litwak, Eugene. 1961. Models of bureaucracy which permit conflict. *American Journal of Sociology* 67:177–184.

Locke, B. Z., et al. 1960. Immigration and insanity. *Public Health Reports* 75:301–306.

Lockwood, David. 1956. Some remarks on "the social system." *British Journal of Sociology* 7:134–146.

Longest, B. 1974. Relationships between coordination, efficiency, and quality of care in general hospitals. *Hospital Administration* 19:65–86.

Lopate, Carol. 1968. *Women in medicine.* Baltimore: Johns Hopkins University Press.

Loupe, M. J., et al. 1976. Contrasting interest profiles of dental educators, practicing dentists, and graduate students. *Journal of Dental Education* 40:215–218.

Luft, Harold S. 1978. Why do HMOs seem to provide more health maintenance services? *Milbank Memorial Fund Quarterly* 56:140–168.

Lundberg, George. 1939. *Foundations of sociology.* New York: Macmillan.

———. 1963. The postulates of science and their implications for sociology. In *Philosophy of the social sciences,* ed. Maurice Natanson. New York: Random House.

Lynd, Robert S. 1939. *Knowledge for what? The place of social science in American culture.* Princeton: Princeton University Press.

Lynd, Robert S., and Lynd, Helen. 1929. *Middletown.* New York: Harcourt, Brace & Co.

_____. 1937. *Middletown in transition.* New York: Harcourt, Brace & Co.

Lyon, J. L., et al. 1976. Cancer incidence in Mormons and non-Mormons in Utah. *New England Journal of Medicine* 294:129–133.

MacMahon, Brian, and Pugh, Thomas F. 1970. *Epidemiology: Principles and methods.* Boston: Little, Brown.

Maddox, J. L. 1923. *The medicine man: A sociological study of the character and evolution of shamanism.* New York: Macmillan.

Madsen, William. 1973. *The Mexican-Americans of south Texas,* 2nd ed. New York: Holt, Rinehart, & Winston.

Magraw, Richard M. 1975. Medical specialization and medical coordination. In *Medical behavioral science,* ed. T. Millon. Philadelphia: W. B. Saunders.

Maiman, L. A., and Becker, M. H. 1974. The health belief model: Origins and correlates in psychological theory. *Health Education Monographs* 2:336–353.

Major, Ralph H. 1954. *A history of medicine,* 2 vols. Springfield, Ill.: Charles C Thomas.

Makofsky, David. 1977. Malpractice and medicine. *Society* 14:25–29.

Malina, Robert M. 1973. Biological substrata. In *Comparative studies of blacks and whites in The United States,* ed. Kent S. Miller and Ralph M. Dreger. New York: Seminar Press.

Malinowski, Bronislaw. 1944. *A scientific theory of culture.* Chapel Hill: University of North Carolina Press.

_____. 1948. *Magic, science, and religion and other essays.* Glencoe, Ill.: Free Press.

Maliphant, R. G. 1949. The incidence of cancer of the uterine-cervix. *British Medical Journal* 2:978–980.

Malpractice, MD's revolt. 1975. *Newsweek,* 9 June, pp. 58–61.

Malzberg, Benjamin. 1936a. Migration and mental disease among negroes in New York State. *American Journal of Physical Anthropology* 21:107–113.

_____. 1936b. Rates of mental disease among certain population groups in New York State. *Journal of American Statistical Association* 31:545–548.

_____. 1936c. Trends of mental disease in New York State. *Psychiatric Quarterly* 10: 667–707.

_____. 1940. *Social and biological aspects of mental disease.* Utica, N.Y.: State Hospitals Press.

_____. 1943. Increase of mental disease. *Psychiatric Quarterly* 17:488–507.

_____. 1959. Important statistical data about mental illness. In *American handbook of psychiatry,* ed. S. Arieti. New York: Basic Books.

_____. 1963. *The mental health of the negro.* Albany: Research Foundation for Mental Hygiene.

Malzberg, Benjamin, and Lee, E. S. 1956. *Migration and mental disease.* New York: Social Science Research Council.

Mangus, A. R. 1955. Medical sociology. *Sociology and Social Research* 39:158–164.

Mann, W. R., and Parkin, G. 1960. The dental school applicant. *Journal of Dental Education* 24:16–37.

Mannon, James Monroe. 1975. Time, work and decision-making in emergency medicine. Unpublished doctoral dissertation, Southern Illinois University.

March, J. G. 1965. *Handbook of organizations.* Chicago: Rand McNally.

March, J. G., and Simon, H. 1958. *Organization.* New York: Wiley.

Margolis, Richard J. 1977. National health insurance–The dream whose time has come? *New York Time Magazine,* 9 January.

Markovits, Andrew S. 1963. Let's kill autocracy in medicine. *Medical Economics* 40: 122–123.

Marks, Renee. 1967. Factors involving social and demographic characteristics. *Milbank Memorial Fund Quarterly* 45:51–108.

Markson, Elizabeth. 1973. A hiding place to die. In *Where medicine fails,* 2nd ed., ed. Anselm Strauss. New Brunswick, N.J.: Transactions Books.

Marmor, Theodore R. 1973. *The politics of Medicare.* Chicago: Aldine.

Marmot, M. G., and Syme, S. Leonard. 1976. Acculturation and coronary heart disease in Japanese-Americans. *American Journal of Epidemiology* 101:177–181.

Marti-Ibanez, Felix, ed. 1960. *Henry E. Sigerist on the history of medicine.* New York: M.D. Publications.

Martin, B. 1972. Physician manpower, 1972. In *'73 profile of medical practice,* ed. S. Vabovich. Chicago: American Medical Association.

Martin, Harry W., and Simpson, I. H. 1959. *Patterns of psychiatric nursing.* Chapel Hill, N.C.: American Nurses Foundation.

Martin, Walter T. 1976. Status integration, social stress, and mental illness. *Journal of Health and Social Behavior* 17:280–294.

Martin, William. 1957. Preference of types of patients. In *The student physician,* ed. Robert K. Merton, G. G. Reader, and P. L. Kendall. Cambridge: Harvard University Press.

Martindale, Don. 1960. *The nature and types of sociological theory.* Boston: Houghton Mifflin.

Marx, Karl. 1970. *[A contribution to the critique of political economy]*, Maurice Dobb. trans. New York: International Publishers. Originally published, 1859.

Mason, Aaron A., et al. 1960. Discharges from a mental hospital in relation to social class and other variables. *Archives of General Psychiatry* 2:1–6.

Matsumoto, Y. Scott. 1970. Social stress and coronary heart disease in Japan. *Milbank Memorial Fund Quarterly* 48:9–31.

Mauksch, Hans O. 1963. Becoming a nurse: A selective view. *Annals of the American Academy of Political and Social Science* 346:88–98.

———. 1965. The nurse. In *Social interaction and patient care,* ed. James K. Skipper, and R. C. Leonards. Philadelphia: J. B. Lippincott.

———. 1972. Nursing: Churning for change? In *Handbook of medical sociology,* 2nd ed., ed. Howard E. Freeman, Sol Levine, and Leo G. Reeder. Englewood Cliffs, N.J.: Prentice-Hall.

Maxcy, K. F., ed. 1941. *Papers of Wade Hampton Frost.* New York: Commonwealth Fund.

Maxmen, Jerrold S. 1972. Good-bye, Dr. Welby. *Social Policy* 3:97–106.

May, Jacques M. 1958. *The ecology of human disease.* New York: M.D. Publications.

Maykovich, Minako K. 1972. *Japanese American identity dilemma.* Tokyo: Waseda University Press.

McAdoo, Harriette. 1977. Family therapy in the black community. *American Journal of Orthopsychiatry* 47:75–79.

McCally, Michael, et al. 1977. Interprofessional education of the new health practitioner. *Journal of Medical Education* 52:177–182.

McCarthy, Eugene G., and Widmer, G. W. 1974. Effects of screening by consultants on surgical procedures. *New England Journal of Medicine* 291:1331–1335.

McCluggage, Robert W. 1959. *A history of the American Dental Association.* Chicago: American Dental Association.

McCormack, Thelma H. 1956. The druggists' dilemma: Problems of a marginal occupation. *American Journal of Sociology* 61:308–315.

McCorkle, Thomas. 1961. Chiropractic: A deviant theory of disease and treatment in contemporary western culture. *Human Organization* 20:20–22.

McCurdy, P. M., et al. 1977. The British experience: Thirty years of national health service. *Journal of Oklahoma State Medical Association* 70:497–505.

McDonald, Forrest. 1968. *The United States in the twentieth century.* Reading, Mass.: Addison-Wesley.

McDonough, J R.; Garrison, G. E.; and Hames, C. G. 1964. Blood pressure and hypertensive disease among negroes and whites. *Annals of Internal Medicine* 61:208–228.

McDonough, J. R., Hames, C. G.; Stulb, S. C.; and Garrison, G. E. 1965. Coronary heart disease among negroes and whites in Evans County, Georgia. *Journal of Chronic Diseases* 18:443–468.

McGrath, Ellen, and Zimet, Carl N. 1977. Female and male medical students: Differences in specialty choice selection and personality. *Journal of Medical Education* 52: 293–300.

MCHS (Maternal and child health service) 1971. *Promoting the health of mothers and children.* Washington, D.C.

McInnes, E. M. 1963. *St. Thomas's hospital.* London: Allen & Unwin.

McKinlay, John B. 1972. Some approaches and problems in the study of the use of services–An overview. *Journal of Health and Social Behavior* 13:115–152.

_____. 1975. Who is really ignorant–Physician or patient? *Journal of Health and Social Behavior* 16:3–11.

_____. 1977. The business of good doctoring or doctoring as good business: Reflection on Freidson's view of the medical game. *International Journal of Health Services* 7:459–483.

McKusick, Victor A. 1978. *Medical genetic studies of the Amish.* Baltimore: Johns Hopkins University Press.

McLachlan, Gordon, ed. 1971. *Challenge for change.* London: Oxford University Press.

McMahon, B., et al. 1960. *Epidemiological methods.* Boston: Little, Brown & Co.

McManners, J. 1967. *Lectures on European history, 1789-1914.* New York: Barnes & Noble.

McNeill, William H. 1963. *The rise of the west, a history of the human community.* Chicago: University of Chicago Press.

McPartland, Thomas S. 1957. *Formal education and the process of professionalization* (Publication 107). Kansas City: Community Study.

Mead, George H. 1934. *Mind, self, and society,* ed. Charles Morris. Chicago: University of Chicago Press.

_____. 1964. *Selected writings,* ed. Andrew J. Reck. Indianapolis: Bobbs-Merrill.

Mead, Margaret, ed. 1953. *Cultural patterns and technical change.* New York: World Federation for Mental Health, UNESCO.

Means, James H. 1953. *Doctors, people, and government.* Boston: Little, Brown.

_____. 1961. *The association of American physicians.* New York: McGraw-Hill.

Mebs, James E., and Brewer, John W. 1971. Pre-admission testing. *Hospitals* 45:48–51.

Mechanic, David. 1962a. The concept of illness behavior. *Journal of Chronic Diseases* 15:189–194.

_____. 1962b. Some factors in identifying and defining mental illness. *Mental Hygiene* 46:66–74.

_____. 1962c. Sources of power of lower participants in complex organizations. *Administration Science Quarterly* 7:349–364.

_____. 1964. The influence of mothers on their children's health attitudes and behavior. *Pediatrics* 33:444–453.

_____. 1968a. General medical practice in England and Wales. *New England Journal of Medicine* 279:680–689.

_____. 1968b. General practice in England and Wales. *Medical Care* 6:245–260.

_____. 1968c. *Medical sociology,* 1st ed. New York: Free Press. 2nd ed. published 1978.

_____. 1970. Correlates of frustration among British general practitioners. *Journal of Health and Social Behavior* 11:87–104.

———. 1972a. General medical practice: Some comparisons between the work of primary care physicians in the United States and England and Wales. *Medical Care* 5: 402–420.

———. 1972b. *Public expectations and health care.* New York: Wiley.

———. 1972c. Social class and schizophrenia. *Social Forces* 50:304–313.

———. 1974. *Politics, medicine, and social science.* New York: Wiley.

———. 1976. *The growth of bureaucratic medicine.* New York: Wiley.

———. 1978. *Medical Sociology,* 2nd ed. New York: Free Press.

———. 1979. Physicians. *Handbook of medical sociology,* 3rd ed., ed. Howard E. Freeman, Sol Levine, and Leo G. Reeder. Englewood Cliffs, N.J.: Prentice-Hall.

Mechanic, David, and Faich, Ronald G. 1970. Doctors in revolt: The crisis in the English national health service. *Medical Care* 8:442–445.

Mechanic, David, and Tessler, Richard. 1973. Comparisons of consumer response to prepaid group practice and alternative insurance plans in Milwaukee County (Research and analytic report series, no. 5–73). Madison: University of Wisconsin, Center for Medical Sociology and Health Services Research.

Mechanic, David, and Volkart, E. H. 1961. Stress, illness behavior and the sick role. *American Sociological Review* 26:51–58.

Medalie, J. H., et al. 1973. Five-year myocardinal infarction incidents–II. Association of single variables to age and birthplace. *Journal of Chronic Diseases* 26:329–350.

Medical care expenditures in seven countries. 1973. *Social Security Bulletin* 36:39–88.

Medical education in the United States. 1976, 1977, 1978. *Journal of American Medical Association* 236, No. 26; 238, No. 26; 240, No. 26.

Medical World News, 30 June 1975, pp. 5–60.

Meile, Richard L., and Haese, P. N. 1969. Social status, status incongruence and symptoms of stress. *Journal of Health and Social Behavior* 10:237–244.

Meile, Richard L., et al. 1976. Marital role, education, and mental disorder among women. *Journal of Health and Social Behavior* 17:295–301.

Melick, Mary Evans. 1978. Life changes and illness: Illness behavior of males in the recovery period of a national disaster. *Journal of Health and Social Behavior* 19: 335–342.

Meltzer, Bernard N. 1964. *The social psychology of George Herbert Mead.* Kalamazoo: Western Michigan University, Center for Sociological Research.

Memmler, Ruth, and Rada, R. B. 1970. *The human body in health and disease,* 3rd ed. Philadelphia: J. B. Lippincott.

Mendel, Ed. 1978. UCD admission program having little effect on local minority health care. *Sacramento Union,* 31 July, p. A3.

Mendelson, Mary A., and Hapgood, David. 1974. The political economy of nursing homes. *Annals of the American Academy of Political and Social Science* 401: 95–105.

Merrison, A. 1976. Dentists and doctors: The concept of the professional man. *British Dental Journal* 141:157–161.

Merton, Robert K. 1948. Division of Parson's "the position of sociological theory." *American Sociological Review* 13:164–168.

———. 1949. *Social structure and social theory.* New York: Free Press.

———. 1957. The role set. *British Journal of Sociology* 8:106–120.

———. 1973. *The sociology of science: Theoretical and empirical investigations.* Chicago: University of Chicago Press.

Merton, Robert K.; Bloom, Samuel; and Rogoff, Natalie. 1956. Studies in the sociology of medical education. *Journal of Medical Education* 31:552–564.

Merton, Robert K.; Broom, Leonard; and Cottrell, Leonard S., eds. 1959. *Sociology today.* New York: Basic Books.

Merton, Robert K. Reader, G. G.; and Kendall, P. L., eds. 1957. *The student physician.* Cambridge: Harvard University Press.

Metsch, Jonathan M., and Veney, James E. 1976. Consumer participation and social accountability. *Medical Care* 14:283–293.

Metzer, Helen L.; Harbury, E.; and Lamphier, D. 1977. Early life social incongruities, health risk factors and chronic disease. *Journal of Chronic Diseases* 30:225–245.

Metzger, Norman, and Pointer, D. D. 1972. *Labor-management relations in the health service industry: Theory and practice.* Washington, D.C.: Science and Health Publications.

Meyer, Genevieve R. 1960. Tendencies and technique: Nursing values in transition (Monograph Series No. 6). Los Angeles: University of California, Institute of Industrial Relations.

Meyer, H. J. 1969. Sociological comments. *Nonprofessionals in the human services,* ed. C. Henry Grosser et al. San Francisco: Jossey-Bass.

Meyers, R. M. 1970. *Medicare.* Bryn Mawr, Penn.: McCahan Foundation.

Michell, A. R. 1978. Salt appetite, salt intake, and hypertension: A deviation of perspective. *Perspectives in Biology and Medicine* 21:335–347.

Milgrom, Peter, et al. 1978a. Dental examinations for quality control: Peer review versus self-assessment. *American Journal of Public Health* 68:394–400.

_____. 1978b. Dentists' self-evaluations: Relationship to clinical performance. *Journal of Dental Education* 42:180–185.

Mill, John Stuart. 1871. *Utilitarianism.* London: Longmans, Green, Reader, and Dyer.

Miller, J. D., and Shortell, S. M. 1969. Hospital unionization: A study of the trends. *Hospitals* 43:67–73.

Miller, Kent S., and Dreger, Ralph Mason, eds. 1973. *Comparative studies of blacks and whites in the United States.* New York: Seminar Press.

Miller, Michael H. 1973. Who receives optimal medical care? *Journal of Health and Social Behavior* 14:176–182.

Miller, Stephen. 1970. *Prescription for leadership.* Chicago: Aldine.

Millis, John S. 1975. *Pharmacists for the future: The report of the study commission on pharmacy.* Ann Arbor: Health Administration Press.

Millman, Marcia. 1976. *The unkindest cut.* New York: William Morrow & Co.

Mills, C. Wright. 1959. *The sociological imagination.* New York: Oxford University Press.

Minthorn, David. 1978. "Test tube" baby stirs memories of Nazi experiments. *Sacramento Union,* 10 September, p. A4.

Minter, Richard E., and Kimball, C. P. 1978. Life events and illness onset: A review. *Psychosomatics* 19:334–339.

Miofsky witnesses' stories unveiled. 1979. *Sacramento Union,* 31 March, p. 2.

Mishler, E., and Scotch, N. 1963. Sociocultural factors in the epidemiology of schizophrenia. *Psychiatry* 26:315–351.

Mitchell, Wayne. 1975. Medical student career choice. *Social Science and Medicine* 9:641–653.

Moffet, Toby. 1971. *The participation put-on.* New York: Dell Publishing.

Montag, Mildred L. 1972. *Evaluation of graduates of associate degree nursing programs.* New York: Teachers College Press.

Monteiro, Lois. 1973. Expense is not object . . . : Income and physician visits reconsidered. *Journal of Health and Social Behavior* 14:99–115.

Montoye, H. J., et al. 1967. Serum uric acid concentration among business executives with observations on other coronary heart disease risk factors. *Annals of Internal Medicine* 66:838–850.

Moody, P. M., and Gray, R. M. 1972. Social class, social integration and the use of preventive health services. In *Patients, physicians and illness,* ed. E. G. Gartly Jaco. New York: Free Press.

Mooney, Anne. 1977. The great society and health: Policies for narrowing the gaps in health status between the poor and the non-poor. *Medical Care* 15:611-619.

Moore, Francis D. 1970. Therapeutic innovation: Ethical boundaries in the initial clinical trials of new drugs and surgical procedures. In *Experimentation with human subjects,* ed. Paul A. Freund. New York: George Braziller.

Moore, G. T., et al. 1972. Effect of a neighborhood health center on hospital emergency room use. *Medical Care* 10:240-247.

Mora, G. 1975. Historical and theoretical trends in psychiatry. In *Comprehensive textbook of psychiatry,* ed. A. Freedman et al. Baltimore: Williams & Wilkins.

More, D. M. 1959. Social origins of future dentists. *The Midwest Sociologist* 21:69-76.

———. 1960. A note on occupational origins of health service professions. *American Sociological Review* 25:403-404.

———. 1961a. Choice of a career in dentistry. *Journal of the American College of Dentists* 28:28-35.

———. 1961b. The dental student. *Journal of the American College of Dentists* 28:5-93.

More, D. M., and Kahn, N. 1960. Some motives for entering dentistry. *American Journal of Sociology* 66:48-53.

Morehead, M. A.; Donaldson, R. S.; and Burt, F. E. 1964. *A study of the quality of hospital care secured by a sample of teamster family members in N. Y. C.* New York: Columbia University, School of Public Health, Administration Medicine.

Morehead, M. A., et al. 1971. Comparison between OEO neighborhood health centers and other health care providers of ratings of the quality of health care. *American Journal of Public Health* 61:1294-1306.

Morgan, T., et al. 1978. Hypertension treated by salt restriction. *Lancet* 1:227-230.

Morison, E. E., ed. 1958. *The American style: Essays in values and performance.* New York: Harper & Row.

Morison, Robert S. 1971. Death: Process or event? *Science* 173:694-698.

Morison, Samuel E., and Commager, H. S. 1950. *The growth of the American republic.* New York: Oxford University Press.

Moriyama, I. M.; Krueger, D. E.; and Stamler, J. 1971. *Cardiovascular diseases in the United States.* Cambridge: Harvard University Press.

Morris, J. N. 1959. Health and social class. *Lancet* 2:303-305.

———. 1964. *Uses of epidemiology.* Edinburgh: E. & S. Livingstone.

Morris, Lynn M. C. 1976. Change or exchange? The transition of the public mental hospital. Unpublished doctoral dissertation, University of Michigan.

Morse, E. V.; Gordon, G., and Moch, M. 1974. Hospital costs and quality of care: An organizational perspective. *Milbank Memorial Fund Quarterly* 52:315-346.

Moss, Gordon E. 1973. *Illness, immunity, and social interaction: The dynamics of biosocial resonation.* New York: Wiley.

Mountin, Joseph W. 1940. Administration of public medical service by health department. *American Journal of Public Health* 30:138-144.

Moynihan, D. 1969. *Maximum feasible misunderstanding: Community action in the war on poverty.* New York: Free Press.

Mueller, Daniel P., et al. 1977. Stressful life events and psychiatric symptomatology: Change or undesirability? *Journal of Health and Social Behavior* 18:307-317.

Muller, Hermann J. 1962. *Studies in genetics: The selected papers of H. J. Muller.* Bloomington: Indiana University Press.

Murray, B. P., et al. 1975. A study of the professional role satisfaction of dentists. *Journal of American College of Dentists* 120:107-117.

Mustard, H. S. 1945. *Government in public health.* New York: The Commonwealth Fund.

Myers, J. K., and Roberts, R. H. 1959. *Family and class dynamics in mental illness.* New York: Wiley.

Myers, J. K., and Schaffer, L. 1954. Social stratification and psychiatric practice: A study of an outpatient clinic. *American Sociological Review* 19:307-310.

Myers, J. K., et al. 1974. Social class, life events, and psychiatric symptoms. In *Stressful life events,* ed. Bruce P. Dohrenwend and Barbara S. Dohrenwend. New York: Wiley.

Myers, Robert J. 1970. *Medicare.* Homewood, Ill.: McCahan Foundation.

NACHC (National Association of Community Health Centers, Inc.). 1978. *Policy and issues guidebook for community health centers and migrant health centers.* Washington, D.C.

NAIC (National Association of Insurance Commissioners). 1976. *Medical professional liability survey,* vol. 1, no. 2. Milwaukee.

Nagel, Ernest. 1953. Teleological explanations and teleological systems. In *Readings in the philosophy of science,* ed. H. Feigel and M. Broadbeck. New York: Harper & Bros.

Nathanson, Constance A. 1975. Illness and the feminine role: A theoretical review. *Social Science and Medicine* 9:57-62.

———. 1977. Sex, illness, and medical care: A review of data, theory, and method. *Social Science and Medicine* 11:13-25.

National health service reorganization: England. 1972. Presented to Parliament by the Secretary of State for Social Services by Command of Her Majesty. London: Her Majesty's Stationary Office.

Navarro, Vicente. 1973. National health insurance and the strategy for change. *Milbank Memorial Fund Quarterly* 51:223-252.

———. 1975. The industrialization of fetishism or the fetishism of industrialization: A critique of Ivan Illich. *International Journal of Health Services* 5:351-371.

———. 1976. Social class, political power and the state and their implications in medicine. *Social Science and Medicine* 10:437-457.

———. 1977. *Social security and medicine in the USSR.* Lexington, Mass.: D. C. Heath & Co.

———. 1978a. *Class struggle, the state and medicine.* New York: Neale Watson Academic Publications.

———. 1978b. The crisis of the western system of medicine in contemporary capitalism. *International Journal of Health Services* 8:179-212.

Neff, W. S. 1968. *Work and human behavior.* New York: Atherton.

Nelson, Eugene C., et al. 1974. Patients' acceptance of physician's assistants. *Journal of the American Medical Association* 228:63-67.

Nelson, Lowry, et al. 1960. *Community structure and change.* New York: Macmillan.

Nelson, R. J. 1977. The essence of professional worth. *Journal of the American College of Dentists* 44:17-25.

Neuhauser, Duncan. 1966. Hospital size and structure. In *Hospital size and efficiency: Proceedings of the Ninth Annual Symposium on Hospital Affairs.* Chicago: University of Chicago, Center for Health Administration Studies.

———. 1971. *The relationship between administrative activities and hospital performance* (Research Series 28). Chicago: University of Chicago, Center for Health Administration Studies.

Neuhauser, Duncan, and Anderson, Ronald. 1972. Structural studies of hospitals. In *Organizational research on health institutions,* ed. Basil S. Georgopoulos. Ann Arbor: University of Michigan, Institute for Social Research.

New, Peter Kong-ming, and Hessler, R. M. 1972. Neighborhood health centers: Traditional medical care at an outpost? *Inquiry* 9:45-58.

New, Peter Kong-ming, and New, Mary Louie. 1975. The links between health and political structure in New China. *Human Organizations* 34:237-251.

New, Peter Kong-ming, et al. 1973. Consumer control and public accountability. *Anthropological Quarterly* 46:196–213.

New York, State of, Special Advisory Panel on Medical Malpractice. 1976. *Report: New York.* New York.

Newcomb, Theodore M. 1950. *Social psychology.* New York: Dryden.

Newman, Howard N. 1972. Medicare and Medicaid. *Annals of the American Academy of Political and Social Science* 399:114–124.

Nichaman, M. Z., et al. 1962. Cardiovascular disease mortality by race, based on a statistical study in Charleston, South Carolina. *Geriatrics* 17:724–737.

Nickerson, Rita J., et al. 1976. Doctors who perform operations: A study of in-hospital surgery in four diverse geographic areas. *New England Journal of Medicine* 295: 921–926.

Nofz, Michael. 1978. Paradigm identification and organizational structure: An overview of the chiropractic health care profession. *Sociological Symposium* 22:18–32.

Normile, F. R. 1969. A formula for estimating bed needs. *Hospitals* 43:57–58.

Norris, George W. 1866. *The early history of medicine in Philadelphia.* Philadelphia: n.n.

North, Robert C. 1963. *Moscow and Chinese communists.* Stanford: Stanford University Press.

Norwood, William F. 1971. *Medical education in the United States before the civil war.* New York: Arno Press & the New York Times.

Notkin, J., and Notkin, M. S. 1970. Community participation in health services. *Medical Care Review* 27:537–543.

Notterman, J. M., and Trumbull, R. 1959. Note on self-regulating systems and stress. *Behavioral Sciences* 4:324–327.

Nudelman, Arthur E., and Nudelman, Barbara E. 1972. Health and illness behavior of Christian Scientists. *Social Science and Medicine* 6:253–262.

Nunnally, J. 1959. *Tests and instruments.* New York: McGraw-Hill.

Nutting, M. Adlaide, and Dock, Lavinia L. 1912. *A history of nursing,* 4 vols. New York: G. P. Putnams' Sons.

Oakes, T. W., et al. 1973. Social factors in newly discovered elevated blood pressure. *Journal of Health and Social Behavior* 14:198–204.

O'Brien, Davis J. 1975. *Neighborhood organization and interest-group processes.* Princeton: Princeton University Press.

Ødegaard, O. 1946. Marriage and mental disease. *Journal of Mental Science* 62:35–59.

———. 1956. The incidence of psychoses in various occupation. *International Journal of Social Psychiatry* 2:85–104.

O'Dell, M. L. 1974. Physician's perceptions of an extended role for the nurse. *Nursing Research* 23:348–351.

Odenheimer, K. J., et al. 1977. The importance of developing teamwork between dentists and physicians. *Journal of American Dental Association* 95:22–25.

OEO (Office of Economic Opportunity). 1969. Bulletin of the Office of Economic Opportunity: Neighborhood Health Center, Fact Sheet. Washington, D.C.: U.S. Government Printing Office.

Ogburn, William F. 1964. *Social change with respect to culture and original nature.* Gloucester, Mass.: P. Smith. Originally published, 1922.

O'Hara-Devereaux, Mary, et al. 1977. Economic effectiveness of family nurse practitioner practice in primary care in California. In *The new health professionals,* ed. Ann A. Bliss and Eva D. Cohen. Germantown, Md.: Aspen Systems Corp.

OHE (Office of Health Economics). 1974. *The NHS reorganization.* London.

Okada, L. M., and Sparer, G. 1976. Access to usual source of care by race in ten urban areas. *Journal of Community Health* 1.163–174.

Olmstead, A., and Pacet, M. 1969. Some theoretical issues: Professional socialization.

Journal of Medical Education 44: 663–671.
O'Malley, C. D. 1970. *The history of medical education*. Berkeley: University of California.
Omran, Abdel R. 1974. *Community medicine in developing countries*. New York: Springer Publishing Co.
O'Neil, M. F. 1973. A study of baccalaureate nursing student values. *Nursing Research* 22:437–441.
Opler, Marvin K. 1967. *Culture and social psychiatry*. New York: Atherton.
Opler, Marvin K., ed. 1959. *Culture and mental health*. New York: Macmillan.
Oppenheimer, Martin. 1972. The proletarianization of the professional. *Sociological Review Monograph* 20:213–227.
Osofsky, J. H. 1968. The walls are within: An examination of barriers between middle-class physicians and poor patients. In *Among the people*, ed. I. Deutscher and E. J. Thompson. New York Basic Books.
Ostrea, Enrique, and Schumar, Harriet. 1976. The role of the pediatric nurse practitioner in a neonatal unit. *Nursing Digest* 4:8–10.
Otis, G. N., et al. 1975. *Medical specialty selection, A review* (DHEW Publication No. (HRA) 75-8). Washington, D.C.: U.S. Government Printing Office.
Overall, Betty, and Aronson, H. 1963. Expectations of psychotherapy in patients of lower socioeconomic class. *American Journal of Orthopsychiatry* 33:421–430.
Owens, Arthur. 1976. How much have malpractice premiums gone up? *Medical Economics*, 27 September, pp. 102–108.

Packard, Francis R. 1963. *History of medicine in the United States*, 2 vols. New York: Hafner Publishing Co.
Page, Charles H. 1946. Bureaucracy's other face. *Social Forces* 25:88–94.
Pain, L. H. 1976. The reorganized national health service: Theory and reality. *CIBA Foundation Symposium* 43:21–30.
Palmore, Erdman. 1971. Attitudes toward aging as shown by humor. *Gerontologist* 2:181–186.
Palmore, Erdman, and Luikart, C. 1972. Health and social factors related to life satisfaction. *Journal of Health and Social Behavior* 13:68–80.
Palola, E. G., and Larson, W. R. 1965. Some dimensions of job satisfaction among hospital personnel. *Sociology and Social Research* 49:201–213.
Pappworth, M. H. 1967. *Human guinea pigs: Experimentation on man*. London: Routledge & Kegan Paul.
Parker, G., et al. 1976. The chiropractic patient: Psychosocial aspect. *Medical Journal of Australia* 2:373–378.
Parker, Seymour, and Kleiner, Robert J. 1966. *Mental illness in the urban negro community*. New York: Free Press.
Parker, Seymour, et al. 1962. Social status and psychopathology. Paper presented at the annual meeting of the Society of Physical Anthropology, Philadelphia.
Parsons, Talcott. 1949. *Essays in sociological theory*. Glencoe, Ill.: Free Press.
_____. 1951. *The social system*. Glencoe, Ill.: Free Press.
_____. 1957. The mental hospital as a type of organization. In *The patient and the mental hospital*, ed. Milton Greenblatt et al. Glencoe, Ill.: Free Press.
_____. 1960. *Structure and process in modern societies*. Glencoe, Ill.: Free Press.
_____. 1966. *Societies*. Englewood Cliffs, N.J.: Prentice-Hall.
_____. 1970. Research with human subjects and the professional complex. In *Experimentation with human subjects*, ed. Paul A. Freund. New York: George Braziller.
_____. 1972. Definitions of health and illness in the light of American values and social structure. In *Patients, physicians and illness*, 2nd ed., ed. E. Gartly Jaco. New York: Free Press.

———. 1975. The sick role and the role of physician reconsidered. *Milbank Memorial Fund Quarterly* 53:257–278.

Parsons, Talcott, and Fox, Renée. 1952. Therapy, and the modern urban family. *Journal of Social Issues* 8:31–44.

Parsons, Talcott, and Smelser, N. J. 1956. *Economy and society.* New York: Free Press.

Parsons, Talcott, et al., eds. 1961. *Theories of society,* 2 vols. New York: Free Press.

Paterson, T. T. 1964. The theory of the social threshold. In *Accident research: Methods and approaches,* ed. William Haddon, Edward A. Suchman, and David Klein. New York: Harper.

Paul, B., ed. 1955. *Health, culture and community.* New York: Russell Sage Foundation.

Pavalko, Ronald M. 1972. *Sociological perspectives on occupation.* Itasca, Ill.: F. E. Peacock Publishers.

Payne, Beverly C., and Lyons, Thomas F. 1972. *The episode of illness: Methods of evaluating and improving personal medical care quality.* Ann Arbor: University of Michigan School of Medicine.

Pearlin, L. I. 1962. Alienation from work: A study of nursing personnel. *American Sociological Review* 27:314–326.

Pearlin, L. I., and Johnson, J. S. 1977. Marital status, life strains and depression. *American Sociological Review* 42:704–715.

Peel, Robert. 1971. *Mary Baker Eddy,* 3 vols. New York: Holt, Rinehart & Winston.

Peller, S. 1944. Studies on mortality since the Renaissance. *Bulletin of the History of Medicine* 16:362–381.

Perlstadt, Harry. 1972. Goal implementation and outcome in medical schools. *American Sociological Review* 37:73–81.

Perrott, G.; Tibbitts, C.; and Britten, R. 1939. The national health surveys. *Public Health Reports* 54:1663–1687.

Perrow, C. B. 1960. *Authority, goals, and prestige in a general hospital.* Berkeley: University of California Press.

———. 1961. Organizational prestige: Some functions and dysfunctions. *American Journal of Sociology* 66:335–341.

———. 1963. Goals and power structure. In *The hospital in modern society,* ed. Eliot Freidson. New York: Free Press.

———. 1965. Hospitals: Technology, structure, and goals. In *Handbook of organizations,* ed. J. G. March. Chicago: Rand McNally.

———. 1967. A framework for the comparative analysis of organization. *American Sociological Review* 32:194–208.

———. 1969. The analysis of goals in complex organizations. In *Readings on modern organization,* ed. Amitai Etzioni. Englewood Cliffs, N.J.: Prentice-Hall.

Petersdorf, R. G. 1975. Health manpower: Numbers, distribution, quality. *Annals of Internal Medicine* 82:694–701.

Petersen, William. 1969. The classification of subnations in Hawaii: An essay in the sociology of knowledge. *American Sociological Review* 34:863–877.

Peterson, Osler L.; Andrews, L. P.; Spain, R. S.; and Greenberg, B. G. 1956. An analytical study of North Carolina general practice, 1953–1954. *Journal of Medical Education* 31:part 2.

Peterson, Ted. 1974. Operating a free clinic from day to day. *Journal of Social Issues* 30:27–51.

Pfeffer, Jeffrey. 1973. Size, composition, and function of hospital boards of directors: A study of organization-environment linkage. *Administrative Science Quarterly* 18:349–363.

Pflanz, Manfred. 1975. Relations between social scientists, physicians and medical organizations in health research. *Social Science and Medicine* 9:7–13.

Philips, Wilbur C. 1940. *Adventuring for democracy.* New York: Social Unit Press.

Phillips, Derek L. 1963. Rejection: A possible consequence of seeking help for mental disorders. *American Sociological Review* 28:963–972.

_____. 1964. Rejection of the mentally ill. *American Sociological Review* 29:679–687.

Phillips, Derek L., and Segal, Bernard E. 1969. Sexual status and psychiatric symptoms. *American Sociological Review* 34:58–72.

Phillips, J. J. 1977. The interrelationship between the American college of dentists and the American Dental Association. *Journal of American College of Dentists* 44: 17–25.

Pilati, Joe. 1969. The hospitals don't belong to the people. *The Village Voice,* 6 February, p. 21.

Piven, F. F., and Cloward, R. A. 1971. *Regulating the poor: The functions of public welfare.* New York: Random House.

Plog, Stanley C., and Edgerton, R. B., eds. 1969. *Changing perspectives in mental illness.* New York: Holt, Rinehart & Winston.

Plotnick, Robert, and Skidmore, F. 1975. *Progress against poverty.* New York: Academic Press.

Policy and issues guidebook for community health centers and migrant health centers. 1978. Washington, D.C.: National Association of Community Health Centers.

Pollack, J. 1969. *Aged people caught in the decay of the inner city.* New York: Central Bureau for the Jewish Aged.

Polsby, Nelson W., et al. 1963. *Politics and social life.* Boston: Houghton Mifflin.

Pomrinse, D. S. 1969. To what degree are hospitals publicly accountable? *Hospitals* 43:41–44.

Popov, G. A. 1971. *Principles of health planning in the USSR.* Geneva: World Health Organization.

Potter, David. 1954. *People of plenty.* Chicago: University of Chicago Press.

Powles, John. 1973. On the limitations of modern medicine. *Science, Medicine, and Man* 1:1–30.

Pratt, Henry. 1965. The doctor's view of the changing nurse–physician relationship. *Journal of Medical Education* 40.767–771.

Pratt, Lois. 1973. The significance of the family in medication. *Journal of Comparative Family Studies* 4:13–35.

Pratt, Lois, et al. 1957. Physician's views on the level of medical information among patients. *American Journal of Public Health* 47:1277–1283.

Price, Don K. 1978. Planning and administrative perspectives on adequate minimum personal health services. *Milbank Memorial Fund Quarterly* 56:22–50.

Proceedings of the special session. 1935. *Journal of the American Medical Association* 104:747–752.

Pugh, D. S. 1966. Modern organization theory: A psychological and sociological study. *Psychological Bulletin* 66:235–251.

Quadagno, Jill. 1976. Occupational sex-typing and internal labor market distribution: An assessment of medical specialties. *Social Problems* 23:442–453.

Quarantelli, Enrico L. 1961a. Career choice patterns of dental students. *Journal of Health and Human Behavior* 2:124–132.

_____. 1961b. The dental student image of the dentist–patient relationship. *American Journal of Public Health* 51:1312–1319.

Quarantelli, Enrico L., and Cooper, J. 1966. Self-conceptions and others: A further test of Meadian hypothesis. *The Sociological Quarterly* 7:281–297.

Queen, S. A. 1940. The ecological studies of mental disorders. *American Sociological Review* 5:201–209.

Quesada, Gustavo M., et al. 1978. Interracial depressive epidemiology in the Southwest. *Journal of Health and Social Behavior* 19:77–85.

Quinlan, Joseph, and Quinlan, Julia. 1977. *Karen Ann: The Quinlans tell their story.* New York: Doubleday.

Quinn, Joseph R., ed. 1973. *Medicine and public health in the People's Republic of China* (DHEW Publication No. (NIH) 73-67). Washington, D.C.: U.S. Government Printing Office.

Quinney, Earl R. 1963. Occupational structure and criminal behavior: Prescription violation by retail pharmacists. *Social Problems* 11:179-185.

_____. 1964. Adjustment to occupational role strain: The case of retail pharmacy. *The Southwestern Social Science Quarterly* 44:367-376.

Raba, Mariana. 1979. Mid-level health practitioners: A review and discussion of the state of the art. Unpublished master's thesis, California State University at Sacramento.

Radcliffe-Brown, A. R. 1935. On the concept of function in social science. *American Anthropologist* 37:394-402.

Radloff, Lenore. 1975. Sex differences in depression: The effects of occupation and marital status. *Sex Roles* 1:249-265.

Rahe, Richard H. 1974. The pathway between subjects' recent life changes and their near-future illness reports. In *Stressful life events,* ed. Bruce P. Dohrenwend and Barbara S. Dohrenwend. New York: Wiley.

Raible, Jane A. 1977. The right to refuse treatment and natural death legislation. *Medical News* 5:6-8.

Rainwater, Lee. 1969. *Fighting poverty: Perspectives from experience.* New York: Basic Books.

Ramsey, Paul. 1978. *Ethics at the edges of life.* New Haven: Yale University Press.

Rayack, Elton. 1967. *Professional power and American medicine.* Cleveland and New York: World Publishing Co.

Reader, George G., and Goss, Mary E. W. 1959. The sociology of medicine. In *Sociology today,* ed. Robert K. Merton, Leonard Broom, and Leonard S. Cottrell. New York: Basic Books.

Redick, R., and Johnson, C. 1974. Statistical Note 100. Marital status, living arrangements and family characteristics of admissions to state and county mental hospitals and outpatient psychiatric clinics, United States, 1970 (DHEW Public Health Service, Office of Program Planning Evaluation, Biometry Branch, Survey and Reports Section). Washington, D.C.: U.S. Government Printing Office.

Redlich, F. C., et al. 1953. Social structure and psychiatric disorders. *American Journal of Psychiatry* 109:729-734.

Reed, Louis. 1932. *The healing cults* (Publication No. 16 of the Committee on the Costs of Medical Care). Chicago: University of Chicago Press.

Reeder, Leo G. 1972. The patient-client as a consumer: Some observations on the changing professional-client relationship. *Journal of Health and Social Behavior* 13:406-412.

Reeder, Sharon J., and Mauksch, Hans. 1979. Nursing: Continuing change. *Handbook of medical sociology,* 3rd ed., ed. Howard E. Freeman, Sol Levine, and Leo G. Reeder. Englewood Cliffs, N.J.: Prentice-Hall.

Register General for England and Wales. 1951. *Decennial Supplement, England and Wales, 1951. Occupational Mortality, Part I.* London: Her Majesty's Stationary Office.

Reid, John D., and Lee, E. S. 1977. A review of the W. E. B. Dubois conference on black health. *Phylon* 38:341-351.

Reid, John D., et al. 1977. Trends in black health. *Phylon* 38:105-116.

Reilly, Philip. 1977. *Genetics, law, and social policy.* Cambridge: Harvard University Press.

Rein, Martin. 1970a. The demonstration as a strategy of change. In *Social policy,* ed. Martin Rein. New York: Random House.

——, ed. 1970b. *Social policy.* New York: Random House.

Reinhardt, A. M., and Gray, R. M. 1972. A social psychological study of attitude change in physicians. *Journal of Medical Education* 47:112–117.

Reinhardt, Uwe E. 1973. Proposed changes in the organization of health-care delivery: An overview and critique. *Milbank Memorial Fund Quarterly* 51:208–209.

Reiser, Stanley Joel; Dyck, Arthur J.; and Curran, William J., eds. 1977. *Ethics in medicine: Historical perspectives and contemporary concerns.* Cambridge: M.I.T. Press.

Reiss, Albert J. 1959. The sociological study of communities. *Rural Sociology* 24:118–130.

Reiss, David. 1976. The family and schizophrenia. *American Journal of Psychiatry* 133: 177–180.

Reitzes, Dietrich C. 1958. *Negroes and medicine.* Cambridge: Harvard University Press.

Renne, Karen S. 1971. Health and marital experience in an urban population. *Journal of Marriage and the Family* 33:338–350.

Reskin, Barbara, and Campbell, Frederick L. 1974. Physician distribution across metropolitan areas. *American Journal of Sociology* 79:981–998.

Retherford, R. 1975. *The changing sex differential in mortality.* Westport, Conn.: Greenwood Press.

Reuther, W. 1972. The need for comprehensive national health insurance and a national service corps. In *Medicine in a changing society,* ed. L. Corey et al. St. Louis: The C. V. Mosby Co.

Reynolds, Roger A. 1976. Improving access to health care among the poor—Neighborhood health center experience. *Milbank Memorial Fund Quarterly* 54:47–82.

Rezler, Agnes G. 1974. Attitude changes during medical school: A review of the literature. *Journal of Medical Education* 49:1023–1030.

Rhee, Sang-O. 1976. Factors determining the quality of physician performance in patient care. *Medical Care* 14:733–750.

——. 1977. Relative importance of physicians' personal and situational characteristics for the quality of patient care. *Journal of Health and Social Behavior* 18:10–15.

Rhoads, John M., et al. 1974. Motivation, medical school admissions, and student performance. *Journal of Medical Education* 49:1092–1099.

Rice, R. G. 1966. Analysis of the hospital as an economic organism. *Modern Hospital,* April, pp. 67–91.

Richard, S., and Tillman, G. 1950. Patterns of parent-child relationships in schizophrenia. *Psychiatry* 13:247–257.

Richardson, William C. 1972. Poverty, illness, and the use of health services in the United States. In *Patients, physicians and illness,* 2nd ed., ed. E. Gartly Jaco. New York: Free Press.

Riddick, F. A., et al. 1971. Use of allied health professionals in internists' offices. *Archives of Internal Medicine* 127:924–931.

Riesman, David. 1950. *The lonely crowd.* New Haven: Yale University Press.

Riessman, C. K. 1974. The use of health services by the poor. *Social Policy* 5:41–49.

Rifkin, Susan B. 1973. Health care for rural areas. In *Medicine and public health in the People's Republic of China* (DHEW Publication No. (NIH) 73–67), ed. Joseph R. Quinn. Washington, D.C.: U.S. Government Printing Office.

Riska, Elaine, and Taylor, James A. 1978. Consumer attitudes toward health policy and knowledge about health legislation. *Journal of Health Politics, Policy and Law* 3:112–123.

Risse, Guenter B., ed. 1973. *Modern China and traditional Chinese medicine.* Springfield, Ill.: Charles C Thomas.

Rivkin, M. O. 1972. Contextual effects on female responses to illness. Unpublished doctoral dissertation, Johns Hopkins University.

Roberts, Bertram H., and Myers, J. K. 1954. Religion, national origin, immigration, and mental health. *American Journal of Psychiatry* 110:754–764.

Robertson, L. S., et al. 1968. Anticipated acceptance of neighborhood health clinics by the urban poor. *Journal of the American Medical Association* 205:815–818.

Robin, Stanley S., and Wagenfeld, Morton O. 1977. The community mental health workers: Organizational and personal sources of role discrepancy. *Journal of Health and Social Behavior* 18:16–27.

Rodowskas, Christopher A. 1977. Pharmacy in the year 2000: The midpoint of your career. *Vital Speeches of the Day* 43:595–598.

Roebuck, Julian B., and Hunter, B. 1970. Medical quackery as deviant behavior. *Criminology* 8:46–62.

Roemer, Milton I., and Friedman, Jay W. 1971. *Doctors in hospitals: Medical staff organization and hospital performance.* Baltimore: Johns Hopkins University Press.

Roemer, Milton I., and Shonick, William 1973. HMO performance: The recent evidence. *Milbank Memorial Fund Quarterly* 51:271–371.

Roghmann, K. J., et al. 1971. Anticipated and actual effects of Medicaid on the medical care pattern of children. *New England Journal of Medicine* 285:1053–1057.

Rogoff, Natalie. 1957. The decision to study medicine. In *The student physician,* ed. Robert K. Merton, G. G. Reader, and P. L. Kendall. Cambridge: Harvard University Press.

Role of the nurse in primary health care. 1977. *Bulletin of Pan American Health Organization* 11:166–174.

Roman, Paul M., and Trice, Harrison M. 1967. *Schizophrenia and the poor.* Ithaca: New York State School of Industrial and Labor Relations.

Ronaghy, Hossain A., and Solter, Steven. 1974. Is the Chinese "barefoot doctor" exportable to rural Iran? *Lancet* 1:1331–1333.

Roos, Noralou P.; Shermerhorn, John R.; and Roos, Leslie L. 1974. Hospital performance: Analyzing power and goals. *Journal of Health and Social Behavior* 15: 78–92.

Rorvik, David M. 1978. *In his image: The cloning of a man.* Philadelphia: J. B. Lippincott.

Rose, Arnold M., ed. 1955. *Mental health and mental disorder.* New York: W. W. Norton.

_____. 1967. *The power structure.* New York: Oxford University Press.

Rose, Arnold M., and Stub, H. R. 1955. Summary of studies on the incidence of mental disorders. In *Mental health and mental disorder,* ed. Arnold M. Rose. New York: W. W. Norton.

Rosen, A. C., et al. 1977. Changes in role perceptions by first-year dental students. *Journal of Dental Education* 41:507–510.

Rosen, George. 1953. Cameralism and concept of medical policy. *Bulletin of the History of Medicine* 27:21–42.

_____. 1954. *The specialization of medicine.* New York: Free Press.

_____. 1955. Problems in the application of statistical analysis to questions of health: 1700–1880. *Bulletin of the History of Medicine* 29:27–45.

_____. 1958. *A history of public health.* New York: M. D. Publications.

_____. 1963. The hospital: Historical sociology of a community institution. In *The hospital in a modern society,* ed. Eliot Freidson. New York: Free Press.

_____. 1968. *Madness in society.* Chicago: University of Chicago Press.

_____. 1971. The first neighborhood health center movement—Its rise and fall. *American Journal of Public Health* 61:1620–1637.

_____. 1974. *From medical policy to social medicine: Essays on the history of health* care. New York: Science History Publications.

_____. 1976. Social science and health in the United States in the twentieth century. *Clio Medica* 11:245–268.

_____. 1979. The evolution of social medicine. *Handbook of medical sociology,* 3rd ed., ed. Howard E. Freeman, Sol Levine, and Leo G. Reeder. Englewood Cliffs, N.J.: Prentice-Hall.

Rosenblatt, D., and Suchman, E. A. 1964. Blue collar attitudes and information toward health and illness. In *Blue collar world,* ed. A. Shostak and E. Gomberg. Englewood Cliffs, N.J.: Prentice-Hall.

Rosenham, D. L. 1973. On being sane in insane places. *Science* 179:250–258.

Rosenkrantz, J. A. 1967. Should administrators serve on hospital boards? *Hospitals* 41:63–66.

Rosenstock, Irwin M. 1966. Why people use health services. *Milbank Memorial Fund Quarterly* 44:94–127.

_____. 1969. Prevention of illness and maintenance of health. In *Poverty and health: A sociological analysis,* ed. J. Kosa, A. Antonovsky, and I. K. Zola. Cambridge: Harvard University Press.

_____. 1974. Historical origins of health belief model. *Health Education Monographs* 2:328–335.

Rosow, Irving. 1967. *Social integration of the aged.* New York: Free Press.

_____. 1974. *Socialization into old age.* Berkeley: University of California Press.

Ross, Catherine E., and Duff, Raymond S. 1978. Quality of outpatient pediatric care. *Journal of Health and Social Behavior* 19:348–360.

Rossides, Daniel W. 1978. *The history and nature of sociological theory.* Boston: Houghton Mifflin.

Rostow, W. W. 1962. *The stages of economic growth.* Cambridge: At the University Press.

Roszak, T. 1969. *The making of a counter culture.* New York: Doubleday.

Roth, Julius. 1963. *Timetables: Structuring the passage of time in hospital treatment and other careers.* Indianapolis: Bobbs-Merrill.

_____. 1972. Some contingencies of the moral evaluation and control of clientele: The case of the hospital emergency service. *American Journal of Sociology* 77:839–856.

Rothstein, Robert J. 1970. *The dental health team.* Philadelphia: J. B. Lippincott.

Rothstein, William. 1972. *American physicians in the nineteenth century.* Baltimore: Johns Hopkins University Press.

Rowland, Howard S., ed. 1978. *The nurse's almanac.* Germantown, Md.: Aspen Systems Corp.

Rowntree, Leonard G., et al. 1945. Mental and personality disorders in selective service registrants. *Journal of the American Medical Association* 128:1084–1087.

Rubin, Irwin M., and Beckhard, R. 1972. Factors influencing the effectiveness of health teams. *Milbank Memorial Fund Quarterly* 50:317–335.

Rubinow, I. M 1915. Social insurance and the medical profession. *Journal of the American Medical Association* 64:381–386.

Ruch, Libby O. 1977. A multidimensional analysis of the concept of life change. *Journal of Health and Social Behavior* 18:71–83.

Rushing, William A. 1969. Two patterns in the relationship between social class and mental hospitalization. *American Sociological Review* 34:533–541.

_____. 1971. Individual resource, societal reaction and hospital commitment. *American Journal of Sociology* 77:511–526.

_____. 1978. Status resources, societal reactions, and type of mental hospital admission. *American Sociological Review* 43:521–533.

Rushing, William A., and Esco, Jack. 1969. The status resources hypothesis and length of hospitalization. In *Deviant behavior and social process,* ed. William A Rushing. Chicago: Rand McNally.

Rushmore, Stephen. 1922. The bill to register chiropractors. *New England Journal of Medicine* 206:614-615.

Russek, H. I. 1959. Role of heredity, diet, and emotional stress in coronary heart disease. *Journal of the American Medical Association* 171:503-508.

_____. 1962. Emotional stress and coronary heart disease in American physicians, dentists, and lawyers. *American Journal of Medical Science* 243:716-725.

Russell, J. C. 1948. *The British medieval population.* Albuquerque: University of New Mexico Press.

Ryan, Michael. 1968. Health center policy in England and Wales. *British Journal of Sociology* 19:34-46.

Ryan, T. M. 1970. Some current trends in the Soviet health services. *The Medical Officer,* 13 February, p. 83.

Sadler, Alfred M., et al. 1975. *The physician's assistant–Today and tomorrow.* Cambridge: Ballinger Publishing Co.

Salber, Eva J.; Feldman, Jacob J.; Johnson, Helen; and McKenna, Elizabeth. 1972. Health practices and attitudes of consumers at a neighborhood health center. *Inquiry* 9:55-61.

Salber, Eva J.; Feldman, Jacob J., Offenbacher, Hanna; and Williams, Shirley. 1970. Characteristics of patients registered for service at neighborhood health center. *American Journal of Public Health* 66:2273-2283.

sale of human body parts, The. 1974. *Michigan Law Review* 2:1182-1264.

Sales, S. M., and House, J. 1971. Job dissatisfaction as possible risk factor in coronary heart disease. *Journal of Chronic Diseases* 23:861-873.

Samora, J., et al. 1961. Medical vocabulary knowledge among hospital patients. *Journal of Health and Human Behavior* 2:83-92.

Sanders, Irwin T. and Brownlee, Ann. 1979. Health in the community. In *Handbook of medical sociology,* 3rd ed., ed Howard E. Freeman, Sol Levine, and Leo G. Reeder. Englewood Cliffs, N.J.: Prentice-Hall.

Sarason, Seymour B. 1977. *Work, aging, and social change.* New York: Free Press.

Saunders, Lyle. 1954. *Cultural differences and medical care.* New York: Russell Sage Foundation.

Savage, L. J. 1971. Call for peace among healing professions. *Journal of California Chiropractic Association,* April.

Schachter, Joseph; Lachin, John M.; and Wimberly, F. C. 1976. Newborn heart rate and blood pressure: Relation to race and to SES. *Psychosomatic Medicine* 38: 390-398.

Schachter, Joseph; Lachin, John M.; Kerr, Joyce L.; Wimberly, F. C.; and Ratey, John J. 1976. Heart rate and blood pressure in black newborns and in white newborns. *Pediatrics* 58:283-287.

Schachter, S., and Singer, J. 1962. Cognitive, social, and physiological determinants of emotional state. *Psychological Review* 69:379-399.

Schatz, Bernard E., and Ebraham, Fred. 1972. Free clinic patient characteristics. *American Journal of Public Health* 62:1354-1363.

Scheff, Thomas, 1966a. Users and non-users of a student psychiatric clinic. *Journal of Health and Human Behavior* 7:114-121.

_____. 1966b. *Being mentally ill.* Chicago: Aldine.

_____. 1974. The labelling theory of mental illness. *American Sociological Review* 39:444-452.

Schein, E. H. 1957. Reaction patterns to severe chronic stress in American army prisoners-of-war of the Chinese. *Journal of Social Issues* 13:21–30.

Schlenger, William E. 1976. A new framework for health. *Inquiry* 13:207–214.

Schmitt, Madeline H. 1978. The utilization of chiropractors. *Sociological Symposium* No. 22:55–74.

Schonfeld, H. K. 1969. Peer review of quality of dental care. *American Dental Association Journal* 79:1376–1382.

_____. 1970. Dentists, dental societies, and dental review committees. *Journal of Connecticut State Dental Association* 44:140–146.

Schonfeld, H. K.; Heston, J. F.; and Fals, I. S. 1972. Numbers of physicians required for primary medical care. *New England Journal of Medicine* 286:571–576.

Schroeder, Clarence W. 1942. Mental disorders in cities. *American Journal of Sociology* 48:40–47.

Schulman, Sam. 1972. Basic functional roles in nursing: Mother surrogate and healer. In *Patients, physicians and illness,* 2nd ed., ed. E. Gartly Jaco. New York: Free Press.

Schultz, R. 1972. Physicians on board: Survey examines level, extent of participation. *Hospitals* 46:51–54.

Schumaker, C. J. 1965. Hospital prestige and active participation of administrators in community affairs: A relationship study. *Hospital Management* 99:54–57.

Schumaker, Florence. 1977. The new pharmacology: More than pills and pantyhose. *Change* 9:16–17.

Schumpeter, Joseph. 1954. *History of economic analysis.* Fair Lawn, N.J.: Oxford University Press.

Schur, Edwin M. 1971. *Labeling deviant behavior.* New York: Harper & Row.

Schwartz, C. 1957. Perspectives on deviance: Wives' definitions of their husbands' mental illness. *Psychiatry* 20:275–291.

Schwartz, Daniel J. 1976. Societal responsibility for malpractice. *Milbank Memorial Fund Quarterly* 54:469–488.

Schwartz, Herman, ed. 1973. *Mental health and chiropractic.* New York: Sessions Publishers.

Schwartz, Howard D., and Kart, Carry S. 1978. *Dominant issues in medical sociology.* Reading, Mass.: Addison-Wesley.

Schwartz, Jerome L. 1968. *Medical plans and health care.* Springfield, Ill.: Charles C Thomas.

_____. 1971a. Sources of funding for free clinics and neighborhood medical programs. In *The free clinic: Community approach to health care and drug abuse,* ed. D. E. Smith et al. Beloit, Wis.: Stash Press.

_____. 1971b. Preliminary observations of free clinics. In *The free clinic: Community approach to health care and drug abuse,* ed. D. E. Smith et al. Beloit, Wis.: Stash Press.

Schwartz, M. S., and Shockley, E. L. 1956. *The nurse and the mental patient.* New York: Russell Sage Foundation.

Scotch, N. A., and Geiger, H. J. 1963. The epidemiology of essential hypertension. *Journal of Chronic Diseases* 16:1183–1213.

Scott, Robert, and Howard, Alan. 1970. Models of stress. In *Social Stress,* ed. Sol Levine and Norman A. Scotch. Chicago: Aldine.

Scott, W. Richard; Forrest, William H.; and Brown, Byron W. 1976. Hospital structure and postoperative mortality and morbidity. In *Organizational research in hospitals,* ed. Stephen M. Shortell and M. Brown. Chicago: An Inquiry Book, Blue Cross Association.

Scott, W. Richard, and Volkart, E. H., eds. 1966. *Medical care: Readings in the sociology of medical institutions.* New York: Wiley.

See, Joel, and Miller, Kent S. 1973. Mental health. In *Comparative studies of blacks and whites in the United States,* ed. Kent S. Miller and Ralph M. Dreger. New York: Seminar Press.

Seeman, K., et al. 1976. Psychopathology, feelings of confinement and helplessness in the dental chair, and relationship to the dentist in patients with disproportionate dental anxiety. *Acta Psychiatrica Scandinavia* 54:81–91.

Seeman, M., and Evans, J. W. 1961. Stratification and hospital care. *American Sociological Review* 26:67–80; 193–203.

Segal, B., et al. 1965. Emotional adjustment, social organization, and psychiatric treatment rates. *American Sociological Review* 30:548–556.

Segal, Steven P., and Aviram, Uri. 1977. *The mentally ill in community-based sheltered care: A study of community care and social integration.* New York: Wiley-Interscience.

Seguin, C. Alberto. 1950. *Introduction to psychosomatic medicine.* New York: International Universities Press.

Sehnert, Keith W. 1975. *How to be your own doctor (sometimes).* New York: Grossett & Dunlap.

Seigel, Barbara; Jensen, David A.; and Coffee, Earl M. 1977. Cost effectiveness of FNP versus MD-staffed rural practice. In *The new health professionals,* ed. Ann Bliss and Eva D. Cohen. Germantown, Md.: Aspen Systems Corp.

Seltzer, Carl C., et al. 1974. Differences in pulmonary function related to smoking habits and race. *American Review of Respiratory Disease* 110:598–608.

Selye, Hans. 1956. *The stress of life.* New York: McGraw-Hill.

Sewell, William H., and Haller, A. O. 1959. Factors in the relationship between social status and the personality adjustment of the child. *American Sociological Review* 24:511–520.

Shaffer, Harry G., ed. 1965. *The Soviet system in theory and practice.* New York: Appleton-Century-Crofts.

Shanas, Ethel, and Maddox, George. 1977. Aging, health, and the organization of health resources. In *Handbook of aging and the social sciences,* ed. Robert H. Binstock and Ethel Shanas. New York: Van Nostrand Reinhold Co.

Shapiro, A. K. 1959. The placebo effect in the history of medical treatment. *American Journal of Psychiatry* 116:298–304.

Sharaf, M. R., and Levinson, D. J. 1964. The quest of omnipotence. *Psychiatry* 27: 135–149.

Shatin, Deborah. 1977. Legalization and legitimation of a marginal profession: A socio-historical account of chiropractic. Paper presented at the Midwest Sociological Society meeting, Minneapolis.

Shatin, Leo. 1967. Medical care and the social worth of a man. *American Journal of Orthopsychiatry* 36:97–101.

Shaw, Marvin E., and Costanzo, Philip R. 1970. *Theories of social psychology.* New York: McGraw-Hill.

Sheehy, Elvin F., and Schaber, Gordon D. 1979. "Schaber report" (Report by special committee to investigate Miofsky affair on behalf of the board of trustees of Sutter Community Hospitals). Sacramento, California.

Shekelle, R. B. 1976. Status inconsistency, mobility, and coronary heart disease: A reply to Horan and Gray. *Journal of Health and Social Behavior* 17:83–87.

Sheps, Cecil G., and Seipp, C. 1972. The medical school, its products, and its problems. *Annals of the American Academy of Political and Social Science* 399:38–49.

Sheps, Cecil G., et al. 1965. Medical schools and hospitals. *Journal of Medical Education* 40:1–169.

Sherlock, Basil, and Morris, R. T. 1971. *Becoming a dentist.* Springfield, Ill.: Charles

C Thomas.

Shonick, William, and Price, Walter. 1977. Reorganizations of health agencies by local government in American urban centers: What do they portend for "public health"? *Milbank Memorial Fund Quarterly* 55:233–271.

Shortell, Stephen M. 1972. *A model of physician referral behavior: A test of exchange theory in medical practice* (Research Series 31). Chicago: University of Chicago, Center for Health Administration Studies.

_____. 1973. Patterns of referral among internists in private practice: A social exchange model. *Journal of Health and Social Behavior* 14:335–348.

_____. 1974a. Determinants of physician referral rates: An exchange theory approach. *Medical Care* 12:13–31.

_____. 1974b. Hospital staff organization: Structure, process and outcome. *Hospital Administration* 19:96–107.

_____. 1976. Organization theory and health services delivery. In *Organizational research in hospitals,* ed. Stephen M. Shortell and M. Brown. Chicago: An Inquiry Book, Blue Cross Association.

Shortell, Stephen M., and Anderson, Odin W. 1971. The physician referral process: A theoretical perspective. *Health Services Research* 5:39–48.

Shortell, Stephen M.; Becker, Selwyn; and Neuhauser, D. 1976. The effects of management practices on hospital efficiency and quality of care. In *Organizational research in hospitals,* ed. Stephen M. Shortell and M. Brown. Chicago: An Inquiry Book, Blue Cross Association.

Shortell, Stephen M., and Vahovich, Stephen G. 1975. Patient referral differences among specialists. *Health Services Research* 10:146–161.

Shortell, Stephen M., et al. 1977. The relationship among dimensions of health services in two provider systems: A causal model approach. *Journal of Health and Social Behavior* 18 139–159.

Shortell, Stephen M., and Brown, M., eds. 1976. *Organizational research in hospitals.* Chicago: An Inquiry Book, Blue Cross Association.

Shryock, Richard Harrison. 1947. *The development of modern medicine.* New York: Knopf.

_____. 1966. *Medicine in America.* Baltimore Johns Hopkins University Press.

Shulman, S. 1977. Labeling laetrile. *Hastings Center Report* 7:4.

Shuval, Judith J. 1970. *Social functions of medical practice: Doctor-patient relationships in Israel.* San Francisco: Jossey-Bass.

_____. 1975. From "boy" to "colleague": Processes of role transformation in professional socialization. *Social Science and Medicine* 9:413–420.

Sidel, Victor W. 1968. Feldshers and "feldsherism." *New England Journal of Medicine* 278:934–939.

Sidel, Victor W., and Sidel, Ruth. 1973. *Serve the people.* New York: Josiah Macy, Jr. Foundation.

Siegler, Miriam, and Osmond, H. 1974. *Models of madness: Models of medicine.* New York: Macmillan.

Sigerist, Henry E. 1937. *Socialized medicine.* New York. W. W. Norton.

_____. 1960. *On the sociology of medicine.* New York: M. D. Publications.

_____. 1961. *A history of medicine,* 2 vols. New York: Oxford University Press.

Silver, G. 1963. *Family medical care.* Cambridge: Harvard University Press.

Silverman, A. 1964. Religious background, participation and evaluation and the use of a psychiatric clinic. Unpublished master's thesis, University of Wisconsin.

Silverman, Milton, and Lee, P. R. 1976. *Pills, profits, and politics.* Berkeley and Los Angeles: University of California Press.

Silversin, Jacob, and Drolette, M. 1977. An analysis of admissions procedures in dental school. *Journal of Dental Education* 41:143–148.

Simmel, Georg. 1955. *[Conflict and the web of group affiliation]*, R. Bendix, trans. Glencoe, Ill.: Free Press. Originally published, 1922.

Simmons, Leo, and Wolff, Harold G. 1954. *Social science in medicine.* New York: Russell Sage Foundation.

Simmons, Roberta G.; Klein, Susan D., and Simmons, Richard L. 1977. *The social impact of transplantation.* New York: Wiley Interscience.

Simmons, Roberta G., and Simmons, Richard L. 1971. Organtransplantations: A societal problem. *Social Problems* 19:36–47.

1969 survey of dental practice, The. 1969. *Journal of American Dental Association* 78:342–346.

Skidmore, Max J. 1970. *Medicare and the American rhetoric of reconciliation.* Alabama: University of Alabama Press.

Skinner, J. S., et al. 1966. Social status, physicial activity and coronary proneness. *Journal of Chronic Diseases* 19:773–783.

Skipper, James K. 1978. Medical sociology and chiropractic. *Sociological Symposium* No. 22:1–5.

Skipper, James K., and Leonard, R. C., eds. 1965. *Social interaction and patient care.* Philadelphia: J. B. Lippincott.

SMA (Socialist Medical Association). 1973. *Health centers–The next step.* Birmingham, U.K.

Small, Albion W. 1909. *The cameralists: The pioneers of German social policy.* Chicago: University of Chicago Press.

Smith, Adam. 1976. *[An inquiry into the nature and causes of the wealth of nations]*, eds. R. H. Campbell and A. S. Skinner. Oxford: Clarendon Press. Originally published, 1776.

Smith, Clagett G. 1966. Some conditions and consequences of intra-organizational conflict. *Administrative Science Quarterly* 10:504–529.

Smith, David E. 1969. Runaways and their health problems in Haight-Ashbury during the summer of 1967. *American Journal of Public Health* 59:2046–2050.

Smith, David E., and Luce, John. 1970. *Love needs care.* Boston: Little, Brown.

Smith, David E., et al., eds. 1971. *The free clinic: Community approach to health care and drug abuse.* Beloit, Wis.: Stash Press.

Smith, Harvey L. 1955. Two lines of authority are one too many. *Modern Hospitals* 84:59–64.

——. 1957. Psychiatry in medicine. *American Journal of Sociology* 3:285–289.

——. 1958. Contingencies of professional differentiation. *American Journal of Sociology* 63:410–414.

Smith, Ralph Lee. 1969. *At your own risk: The case against chiropractic.* New York: Pocket Books.

Smith, Richard A. 1969. Medex–A demonstration program in primary medical care. *Northwest Medicine* 68:1023–1030.

Smith, Richard T. 1973. Health and rehabilitation manpower strategy: New career and the role of the indigenous paraprofessional. *Social Science and Medicine* 7: 281–290.

Smith, T. Lynn. 1948. *Population analysis.* New York: McGraw-Hill.

Snider, Arthur. 1973. Mental hospitals–Resorts for the poor? *Science Digest* 75:44–45.

Snow, Loudell F. 1974. Folk medical beliefs and their implications for care of patients. *Annals of Internal Medicine* 81:82–96.

Sodeman, William A., Jr., and Sodeman, William A. 1967. *Pathologic physiology: Mechanisms of disease,* 4th ed. Philadelphia and London: W. B. Saunders.

Somers, Ann R. 1971. *Health care in transition: Directions for the future.* Chicago: Hospital Research and Educational Trust.

———. 1972a. Medical education and the community: A consumer point of view. *The Pharos* 35:149–155.

———. 1972b. Who's in charge here? or Alice searches for a king in mediland. *New England Journal of Medicine* 287:849–855.

Somers, Ann R., and Somers, Herman M. 1977. *Health and health care.* Germantown, Md.: Aspen System Corp.

Somers, Herman M. 1977. The malpractice controversy and the quality of patient care. *Milbank Memorial Fund Quarterly* 55:193–232.

Somers, Herman M., and Somers, Ann R. 1961. *Doctors, patients, and health insurance.* Washington, D.C.: The Brookings Institute.

———. 1972. Major issues in national health insurance. *Milbank Memorial Fund Quarterly* 50:177–210.

Sorenson, James R. 1974. Biomedical innovation, uncertainty, and doctor-patient interaction. *Journal of Health and Social Behavior* 15:366–374.

Sparer, Gerald, and Anderson, A. 1972. Cost of services at neighborhood health centers–A comparative analysis. *New England Journal of Medicine* 286:1241–1245.

Sparer, Gerald, and Okada, Louise M. 1974. Chronic conditions and physician use patterns in ten urban poverty areas. *Medical Care* 12:549–560.

Sparer, Gerald, et al. 1970. Consumer participation in OEO-assisted neighborhood health centers. *American Journal of Public Health* 60:1091–1102.

Spiegel, Allen D., and Podair, Simon, eds. 1975. *Medicaid: Lessons for national health insurance.* Rockville, Md.: Aspen Systems Corp.

Spitzer, Robert L. 1979. Draft of the introduction to DSM–III. Unpublished draft prepared by the Task Force on Nomenclature and Statistics, American Psychiatric Association. New York.

Spitzer, Robert L.; Endicott, Jean; and Robins, Eli. 1975. Clinical criteria for psychiatric diagnosis and DSM–III. *American Journal of Psychiatry* 132:1187–1192.

Spitzer, Robert L., and Wilson, Paul T. 1975. Nosology and the official psychiatric nomenclature. In *Comprehensive textbook of psychiatry,* 2nd ed., ed. A. Freedman, H. Kaplan, and B. Sadock. Baltimore: Williams & Wilkins.

Spitzer, Stephen P., and Denzin, Norman K., eds. 1968. *The mental patient.* New York: McGraw-Hill.

Sprowbs, Joseph B., ed. 1970. *Prescription pharmacy.* Philadelphia: J. B. Lippincott.

Srole, Leo, et al. 1962. *Mental health in the metropolis.* New York: McGraw-Hill.

Stafford, Rita L. 1966. An analysis of consciously recalled motivating factors and subsequent professional involvement for American women in New York State. Unpublished doctoral dissertation, New York University.

Stallybrass, Clare O. 1931. *The principles of epidemiology and the process of infection.* New York: Macmillan.

Stamler, J., et al. 1960. Epidemiologic studies on cardiovascular-renal diseases. *Journal of Chronic Diseases* 12:448.

Stamler, J.; Stampler, R.; and Pullman, T. N., eds. 1967a. *The epidemiology of hypertension.* New York: Grune & Stratton.

———. 1967b. Socioeconomic factors in the epidemiology of hypertensive disease. In *The epidemiology of hypertension,* ed. J. Stamler, R. Stampler, and T. N. Pullman. New York: Grune & Stratton.

Stanford Research Institute. 1960. *Chiropractic in California.* Los Angeles: The Haynes Foundation.

Stanton, A. H., and Schwartz, M. S. 1954. *The mental hospital.* New York: Basic Books.

Starkweather, David B. 1970. Hospital size, complexity, and formalization. *Health Services Research* 5:330–341.

Stead, Eugene A. 1966. Conserving costly talents–Providing physicians' new assistants. *Journal of the American Medical Association* 198:182–183.

———. 1967. The Duke plan for physician's assistants. *Medical Times* 95:40–48.

Steeg, Donna, and Croog, Sydney H. 1979. Hospitals and related health care delivery settings. *Handbook of medical sociology,* 3rd ed., ed. Howard E. Freeman, Sol Levine, and Leo G. Reeder. Englewood Cliffs, N.J.: Prentice-Hall.

Stein, L. 1967. The doctor–nurse game. *Archives of General Psychiatry* 16:699–703.

Sternbach, R., and Tursky, B. 1965. Ethnic differences among housewives in psychophysical and skin potential responses to electric shock. *Psychophysiology* 1: 841–846.

Stevens, Robert. 1971. *American medicine and the public interest.* New Haven: Yale University Press.

Stevens, Robert, and Stevens, Rosemary. 1974. *Welfare medicine in America.* New York: Free Press.

Stevens, Rosemary. 1966. *Medical practice in modern England.* New Haven: Yale University Press.

Stoeckle, John D., and Candib, L. M. 1969. The neighborhood health center–Reform ideas of yesterday and today. *New England Journal of Medicine* 280:1385–1391.

Stoeckle, John D., et al. 1971. The free clinic movement: Present and future. In *The free clinic: Community approach to health care and drug abuse,* ed. D. E. Smith et al. Beloit, Wis.: Stash Press.

Stotsky, Bernard A. 1970. *The nursing home and the aged psychiatric patient.* New York: Appleton.

Strauss, Anselm L. 1969. Medical organization, medical care, and lower income groups. *Social Science and Medicine* 3:143–177.

———. 1973. *Where medicine fails.* New York: Transaction Books.

———. 1975. *Chronic illness and the quality of life.* St. Louis: The C. V. Mosby Co.

Strauss, Anselm L., and Glaser, B. G. 1970. *Anguish: A case history of dying in a hospital.* San Francisco: Sociology Press.

Strauss, Anselm L., et al. 1963. The hospital and its negotiated order. In *The hospital as a social system,* ed. E. Greidson. New York: Free Press.

Strauss, Anselm L., ed. 1964. *George Herbert Mead on social psychology.* Chicago: University of Chicago Press.

Strauss, Mark A., and Sparer, G. 1971. Basic utilization experience of OEO comprehensive health services projects. *Inquiry* 8:36–49.

Strauss, Robert. 1957. The nature and status of medical sociology. *American Sociological Review* 22:200–204.

Street, David P., and Weinstein, Eugene. 1975. Problems and perspectives of applied sociology. *American Sociologist* 10.65–72.

Streib, Gordon F. 1977. Social stratification and aging. In *Handbook of aging and the social sciences,* ed. Robert H. Binstock and Ethel Shanas. New York: Van Nostrand Reinhold Co.

Stroman, Duane. 1976. *The medical establishment and social responsibility.* Port Washington, N.Y.: Kennikat Press.

Suchman, Edward A. 1964. Sociomedical variations among ethnic groups. *American Journal of Sociology* 70:319–331.

———. 1965a. Social patterns of illness and medical care. *Journal of Health and Human Behavior* 6:2–16.

———. 1965b. Stages of illness and medical care. *Journal of Health and Human Behavior* 6:114–128.

Survey of operational "physician's assistant" programs: Numbers graduated and employed. 1971. Chicago: American Medical Association.

Suspended administrator speaks out. 1979. *Sacramento Union,* 10 April, p. 1.

Sutter nurses talk about Miofsky and doctors. 1979. *Sacramento Union,* 29 April, p. B1.

Sutter stripped of accreditation. 1979. *Sacramento Union,* 8 April, p. 1.

Sutton, Willis A., and Kolaja, J. 1960. The concept of community. *Rural Sociology* 25:197–203.

Swafford, Michael. 1978. Sex differences in Soviet earnings. *American Sociological Review* 43.657–673.

Swanson, Bert E. 1972. The politics of health. In *Handbook of medical sociology,* 2nd ed., ed. Howard E. Freeman, Sol Levine, and Leo G. Reeder. Englewood Cliffs, N.J.: Prentice-Hall.

Syme, S. Leonard, and Berkman, L. F. 1976. Social class, susceptibility and sickness. *American Journal of Epidemiology* 104:1–8.

Syme, S. Leonard, et al. 1974. Social class and racial differences in blood pressure. *American Journal of Public Health* 64:619–620.

Syndenstricker, Edgar. 1926. A study of illness in a general population group. *Public Health Reports* 41:2069–2088.

Szasz, Thomas. 1960. The myth of mental illness. *American Psychologist* 15:113–118.

———. 1963. *Law, liberty, and psychiatry: An inquiry into the social uses of mental health practices.* New York: Macmillan.

Tagliacozzo, Daisy L., and Mauksch, Hans O. 1972. The patients' view of the patients' role. In *Patients, physicians and illness,* 2nd ed., ed. E. Gartly Jaco. New York: Free Press.

Talbot, C. H. 1967. *Medicine in Medieval England.* London: Oldbourne.

Tawny, R. H. 1920. *The acquisitive society.* New York: Harcourt Brace.

Taylor, Carol. 1970. *Horizontal orbit: Hospitals and the cult of efficiency.* New York: Rinehart & Winston.

Taylor, H. L., et al. 1966. Railroad employees in the United States. *Acta Medical Scandinavica* 450:55–115.

Taylor, Lee. 1968. *Occupational sociology.* New York: Oxford University Press.

Taylor, Ronald L. 1976. Psychosocial development among children and youth: A reexamination. *American Journal of Orthopsychiatry* 46:4–19.

Teeling-Smith, George. 1975. *You and the national health service.* London: Arrow Books.

Terris, Milton, and Calmann, M. C. 1960. Carcinoma of the cervix. *Journal of the American Medical Association* 174 1487–1851.

Terris, Milton, ed. 1964. *Goldberger on pellagra.* Baton Rouge: Louisiana State University Press.

Tessler, Richard, and Mechanic, David. 1975. Consumer satisfaction with prepaid group practice: A comparative study. *Journal of Health and Social Behavior* 16:95–113.

———. 1978. Psychological distress and perceived health status. *Journal of Health and Social Behavior* 19:254–262.

Test-tube baby raises legal, moral questions. 1978. *Sacramento Union,* 23 August, p. B3.

Thibaut, John W., and Kelley, H. H. 1959. *The social psychology of groups.* New York: Wiley.

Thielens, W., Jr. 1957. Some comparisons of entrants to medical and law school. In *The student physician,* ed. Robert K. Merton, G. G. Reader, and P. L. Kendall. Cambridge: Harvard University Press.

Thomas, C. B., and Murphy, E. A. 1958. Further studies on cholesterol levels in the Johns Hopkins medical students. *Journal of Chronic Diseases* 8:661–668.

Thomlinson, Ralph. 1965. *Population dynamics.* New York: Random House.

Thompson, C. D. 1975. Teaching basic dental concepts to medical students. *Journal of Dental Education* 39:600–603.

Thompson, J. D. 1967. *Organization in action.* New York: McGraw-Hill.

Thompson, Theodis. 1974. The politics of pacification: The case of consumer participation in community health organization. Washington, D.C.: Howard University, Institute for Urban Affairs.

Thorner, Isidor. 1942. Pharmacy: The functional significance of an institutional pattern. *Social Forces* 20:321-328.

Thursz, Daniel. 1970. Consumer involvement in rehabilitation service (SRS-114 System of Documents). Washington, D.C.: U.S. Government Printing Office.

Tietze, Christopher, et al. 1942. Personality disorder and spatial mobility. *American Journal of Sociology* 48:29-39.

Tietze, Trude. 1949. A study of mothers of schizophrenic patients. *Psychiatry* 12: 55-65.

Tilson, H. H. 1973. Characteristics of physicians in OEO neighborhood health centers. *Inquiry* 10:27-38.

Tobin, Sheldon S., and Lieberman, Morton A. 1976. *Last home for the aged.* San Francisco: Jossey-Bass.

Todd, Malcolm C. 1972. National certification of physician's assistants by uniform examinations. *Journal of the American Medical Association* 222:563-566.

Todd, Malcolm C., and Foy, Donald F. 1972. Current status of the physician's assistant and related issues. *Journal of the American Medical Association* 200:1714-1720.

Toor, Mordecai, et al. 1960. Atherosclerosis and related factors in immigrants to Israel. *Circulation* 12:265-279.

Toren, Nina. 1975. Deprofessionalization and its sources: A preliminary analysis. *Sociology of work and Occupations* 2:323-337.

Townsend, J. Marshall. 1976. Self-concept and the institutionalization of mental patients: An overview and critique. *Journal of Health and Social Behavior* 17:263-271.

Trager, B. 1971. Home health services and health insurance. *Medical Care* 9:89-98.

Trustees to draft DSM-III criticisms. 1979. *Psychiatric News,* 18 May, pp. 1, 12-13.

Tuckman, Jacob, and Kleiner, R. H. 1962. Discrepancy between aspiration and achievement as a predictor of schizophrenia. *Behavioral Science* 7:443-447.

Tudor, William, et al. 1977. The effect of sex role differences on the social control of mental illness. *Journal of Health and Social Behavior* 18:98-112.

Tumin, Melvin. 1967. *Social stratification.* Englewood Cliffs, N.J.: Prentice-Hall.

Turk, H., and Simpson, R. L., eds. 1970. *The sociologies of Talcott Parsons and George Homans.* Indianapolis: Bobbs-Merrill.

Turner, C. 1931. *The rise of chiropractic.* Los Angeles: Powell Publishing.

Turner, Jonathan H. 1978. *The structure of sociological theory,* 2nd ed. Homewood, Ill.: Dorsey Press.

Turner, Ralph. 1968. Social roles: Sociological aspects. *International Encyclopedia of the Social Sciences.* New York: Macmillan.

Turner, Ralph H. 1947. The navy disbursing officer as a bureaucrat. *American Sociological Review* 12:342-348.

Turner, R. Jay. 1972. The epidemiological study of schizophrenia: A current appraisal. *Journal of Health and Social Behavior* 13:360-369.

Turner, R. Jay, and Gartrell, John W. 1978. Social factors in psychiatric outcome: Toward the resolution of interpretive controversies. *American Sociological Review* 43:368-382.

Turner, R. Ray, and Wagenfeld, M. O. 1967. Occupational mobility and schizophrenia. *American Sociological Review* 32:104-113.

Turner, R. Ray, et al. 1970. Marital status and schizophrenia. *Journal of Abnormal and Social Psychology* 76:110-116.

Twaddle, Andrew C., and Hessler, Richard M. 1977. *A sociology of health.* St. Louis: The C. V. Mosby Co.

Tyler, Varro E. 1968. Clinical pharmacy: The need and an evaluation of the professional concept. *American Journal of Pharmaceutical Education* 32:764-771.

Tyroler, H. A., and Cassel, J. 1964. Health consequences of culture change. *Journal of Chronic Diseases* 17:167-177.

U.S. Department of Commerce, Bureau of Census. 1960–1977. *Statistical abstract of the United States.* Washington, D.C.: U.S. Government Printing Office.

_____. 1970. *Current population reports: Projection of the United States by age and sex, 1970 to 2020.* Washington, D.C.: U.S. Government Printing Office.

_____. 1975. *Historical statistics of the United States,* 2 parts. Washington, D.C.: U.S. Government Printing Office.

U.S. DHEW (Department of Health, Education, and Welfare). 1962. *Medical care financing and utilization: Source book of data through 1961* (Health Economics Series 1, Publication 947). Washington, D.C.: U.S. Government Printing Office.

_____. 1966. *Characteristics of patients of selected types of medical specialists and practitioners, U. S. July 1963-June 1964.* Washington, D.C.: U.S. Government Printing Office.

_____. 1968. *Independent practitioners under Medicare, a report to Congress.* Washington, D.C.: U.S. Government Printing Office.

_____. 1970. *Recommendations of the task force on Medicaid and related programs–June 1970.* Washington, D.C.: U.S. Government Printing Office.

_____. 1971. *Facts and figures on older Americans: An overview, 1971.* Washington, D.C.: U.S. Government Printing Office.

_____. 1972. *Selected training programs for physician support personnel.* Washington, D.C.: U.S. Government Printing Office.

_____. 1973a. *Medical malpractice: Report of the U.S. secretary's commission on medical malpractice* (DHEW Publication No. (OS) 73–88). Washington, D.C.: U.S. Government Printing Office.

_____. 1973b. *Mortality trends: Age, color, and sex, United States–1950-1969* (DHEW Publication No. (HRA) 74–1852). Washington, D.C.: U.S. Government Printing Office.

_____. 1974. *Mortality trends for leading causes of death, United States–1950-1969* (DHEW Publication No. (HRA) 74–1853). Washington, D.C.: U.S. Government Printing Office.

_____. 1975. *Minorities and women in the health fields* (DHEW Publication No. (HRA) 76–22). Washington, D.C.: U.S. Government Printing Office.

_____. 1976. *Health, United States, 1975* (DHEW Publication No. (HRA) 76-1232). Washington, D.C.: U.S. Government Printing Office.

U.S. DHEW, Social Security Administration. 1968. *Medicare: A bibliography of selected references 1966-1967.* Washington, D.C.: U.S. Government Printing Office.

U.S. Department of Labor, Bureau of Labor Statistics. 1953–1977. *Consumer price index.* Washington, D.C.: U.S. Government Printing Office.

_____. 1976. *Occupational outlook for chiropractors* (Bulletin No. 1875–99). Washington, D.C.: U.S. Government Printing Office.

U.S. Department of Labor, Manpower Administration, Office of Manpower Policy, Evaluation, and Research. 1967. *Technology and manpower in the health service industry* (Manpower Research Bulletin No. 14). Washington, D.C.: U.S. Government Printing Office.

U.S. National Center for Health Statistics. 1974. Physician visits: Volume and interval since last visit, United States, 1971. *Vital and health statistics* (DHEW Publication No. (HRA) 75–1524). Washington, D.C.: U.S. Government Printing Office.

_____. 1976. *Monthly vital statistics report. Annual summary for the United States, 1975* (DHEW Publication No. (HRA) 76–1120). Washington, D.C.: U.S. Government Printing Office.

_____. 1976. *Vital statistics of the United States, 1900-1976.* Washington, D.C.: U.S. Government Printing Office.

_____. 1977a. *Characteristics, social contacts, and activities of nursing home residents* (DHEW Publication No. (HRA) 77–1778). Washington, D.C.: U.S. Government

Printing Office.

———. 1977b. *Charges for care and sources of payment for residents in nursing homes: U.S.: national nursing home survey, August 1973–April 1974* (DHEW Publication No. (PHS) 78-1783). Washington, D.C.: U.S. Government Printing Office.

———. 1977c. *Nursing homes in the United States: 1973-1974, National nursing home survey* (DHEW Publication No. (HRA) 78-1812). Washington, D.C.: U.S. Government Printing Office.

———. 1977d. *Profiles of chronic illness in nursing homes, United States: National nursing home survey* (DHEW Publication No. (PHS) 78-1780). Washington, D.C.: U.S. Government Printing Office.

———. 1977e. *Utilization of nursing homes: National nursing home survey* (DHEW Publication No. (HRA) 77-1779). Washington, D.C.: U.S. Government Printing Office.

U.S. Public Health Service. 1960. *Health statistics from the U.S. national health surveys: Dental care: Interval and frequency of visits: U.S.: July 1957–June 1959.* Washington, D.C.: U.S. Government Printing Office.

U.S. Senate Committee on Finance. 1970. *Medicare and Medicaid: Problems, issues, and alternatives* (Report of the Staff). Washington, D.C.: U.S. Government Printing Office.

Udry, J. R. 1974. *The social context of marriage,* 3rd ed. Philadelphia: J. B. Lippincott.

Ullman, L. P. 1967. *Institution and outcome.* New York: Oxford University Press.

Ulrich, Lawrence P. 1976. Reproductive rights and genetic disease. In *Biomedical ethics and the law,* ed. James Humber and Robert F. Almeder. New York: Plenum Press.

United Nations. 1948–1976. *Demographic yearbook.* New York.

Veatch, Robert M. 1977. Medicine, biology, and ethics. *Hastings Center Report* 6:2–3.

Venzmer, Gerhard. 1968. *Five thousand years of medicine.* New York: Taplinger Publishing Co.

Verbrugge, Lois M. 1979. Marital status and health. *Journal of Marriage and the Family* 41:267–285.

Veroff, J., and Feld, S. 1970. *Marriage and work in America.* New York: Van Nostrand Reinhold.

Vigners, R. T. 1961. Politics of power in a hospital. *Modern Hospital* 96:89–94.

Viseltear, A. J. 1973. Emergence of the medical care section of the American Public Health Association, 1926–1948. *American Journal of Public Health* 63:896–1007.

Vogel, Ezra. 1973. Organization of health services. In *Public health in the People's Republic of China,* ed. Myron E. Wegman et al. New York: Josiah Macy, Jr. Foundation.

Vollmer, Howard M., and Mills, Donald L., eds. 1966. *Professionalization.* Englewood Cliffs, N.J.: Prentice-Hall.

von Mering, O., and King, S. 1957. *Remotivating the mental patient.* New York: Russell Sage Foundation

Vorherr, H., et al. 1978. Breast cancer: Potentially predisposing and protecting factors. *American Journal of Obstetrics and Gynecology* 130:335–355.

Vuori, Hannu. 1968. Ideology versus interest: The case of Medicare. *Social Science and Medicine* 2:355–363.

Wagner, Helmut R. 1963. Types of sociological theory. *American Sociological Review* 28:735–742.

Waitzkin, Howard, and Waterman, Barbara. 1974. *The exploitation of illness in a capitalist society.* Indianapolis: Bobbs-Merrill.

Waldman, Bart. 1977. Economic and racial disadvantages as reflected in traditional medical school selection factors. *Journal of Medical Education* 52:961–970.

Waldman, H. Barry, and Schlissel, Edward. 1977. Honor codes and peer review. *Journal of Dental Education* 41:126–128.

Waldman, S. 1976. *National health insurance proposals: Provisions of bills introduced in the 94th Congress as of February 1976* (Office of Research and Scientific Statistics, DHEW Publication No. 76-11920). Washington, D.C.: U.S. Government Printing Office.

Walker, David B. 1974. How fare federalism in the mid-seventies? *Annals of the American Academy of Political and Social Science* 416:17–31.

Walker, Kenneth. 1955. *The story of medicine.* New York: Oxford University Press.

Wallace, Anthony F. C. 1959. Cultural determinants of response to hallucinatory experience. *Archives of General Psychiatry* 1:58–69.

Walsh, Warren B. 1958. *Russia and the Soviet Union.* Ann Arbor: University of Michigan Press.

Walters, Verle H., et al. 1972. Technical and professional nursing: An exploratory study. *Nursing Research* 21:124–131.

Wan, Thomas T. H., and Gray, Lois C. 1978. Differential access to preventive services for young children in low-income urban areas. *Journal of Health and Social Behavior* 19:312–324.

Wan, T., and Soifer, J. 1974. Determinants of physician utilization: A causal analysis. *Journal of Health and Social Behavior* 15:100–112.

Wang, Virginia Li. 1975. Training of the barefoot doctor in the People's Republic of China: From prevention to curative service. *International Journal of Health Services* 5:475–488.

Warbasse, James Peter. 1970. *The doctor and the public.* College Park, Md.: McGrath Publishing Co.

Ward, Paul D. 1972. Health lobbies: Vested interests and pressure politics. In *Politics of health,* ed. D. Carter and P. R. Lee. New York: Medcom.

Wardwell, Walter I. 1952. A marginal professional role: The chiropractor. *Social Forces* 30:339–348.

———. 1955. The reduction of strain in a marginal social role. *American Journal of Sociology* 61:16–25.

———. 1965. Christian Science healing. *Journal for the Scientific Study of Religion* 4:175–181.

———. 1978. Social factors in the survival of chiropractic: A comparative view. *Sociological Symposium* No. 22:6–17.

———. 1979. Limited, marginal, and quasi-practitioners. In *Handbook of medical sociology,* 3rd ed., ed. Howard E. Freeman, Sol Levine, and Leo G. Reeder. Englewood Cliffs, N.J.: Prentice-Hall.

Warheit, G.; Holzer, C., III; and Arey, Sandra A. 1975. Race and mental illness: An epidemiologic update. *Journal of Health and Social Behavior* 16:243–256.

Warheit, G.; Holzer, C., III; and Schwab, J. 1973. An analysis of social class and racial differences in depressive symptomatology: A community study. *Journal of Health and Social Behavior* 4:291–299.

Warheit, G., et al. 1976. Sex, marital status, and mental health: A reappraisal. *Social Forces* 55:459–470.

Watkin, Brian. 1978. *The national health services: The first phase, 1948–1974 and after.* Edison, N.J.: Allen and Unwin, Inc.

Weber, Max. 1958. *[The protestant ethic and the spirit of capitalism]*, T. Parsons, trans. New York: Charles Scribner's Sons. Originally published, 1904–1905.

Wegman, Myron E., et al., eds. 1973. *Public health in the People's Republic of China.* New York: Josiah Macy, Jr. Foundation.

Weiant, C. W. 1973. Chiropractic and mental health in the world of the future. In *Mental health and chiropractic,* ed. Herman Schwartz. New York: Sessions Publishers.

Weinberg, E., and Rodney, J. F. 1973. The academic performance of women students in medical school. *Journal of Medical Education* 48:240–247.

Weinberg, S. K. 1952. *Society and personality disorders.* Englewood Cliffs, N.J.: Prentice-Hall.

Weinberg, S. K., ed. 1967. *The sociology of mental disorder.* Chicago: Aldine.

Weiner, H. M., et al. 1957. Etiology of duodenal ulcer: I. Relation of specific psychological characteristics to rate of gastric secretion (serum pepsionogen). *Psychosomatic Medicine* 19:1–10.

Weingart, Peter. 1969. Beyond Parsons? A critique of Ralf Dahrendorf's conflict theory. *Social Forces* 48:151–165.

Weinlein, A. 1943. Pharmacy as a profession with special reference to the state of Wisconsin. Unpublished master's thesis, University of Chicago.

Weinstein, James. 1968. *The corporate ideal in the liberal state, 1900-1918.* Boston: Beacon Press.

Welch, Norman A. 1964. Medical care, its social and organizational aspects: The AMA. *New England Journal of Medicine* 270:178–182.

Wells, S. H., et al. 1974. *Pharmacological testing in a correctional institution.* Springfield, Ill.: Charles C Thomas.

Welty, Paul Thomas. 1973. *The Asians.* Philadelphia: J. B. Lippincott.

Wen, Chi-Pang, and Hays, Charles W. 1976. Health care financing in China. *Medical Care* 14:241–254.

Wenger, Dennis, and Fletcher, R. 1969. The effect of legal counsel on admissions to a state mental hospital. *Journal of Health and Social Behavior* 10:66–72.

Wershow, H. J., and Reinhart, G. 1974. Life change and hospitalization: A heretical view. *Journal of Psychosomatic Research* 18:393–401.

Wertz, Richard, ed. 1973. *Readings on ethical and social issues in biomedicine.* Englewood Cliffs, N.J.: Prentice-Hall.

Wessen, Albert F. 1972. Hospital ideology and communication between ward personnel. In *Patients, physicians and illness,* 2nd ed., ed. E. Gartly Jaco. New York: Free Press.

Westervelt, Frederic. 1970. A reply to Childress: The selection process as viewed from within. *Soundings* 53:339–362.

Wexler, Murray. 1976. The behavioral sciences in medical education. *American Psychologist* 3:275–283.

Wheaton, Blair. 1978. The sociogenesis of psychological disorder: Reexamining the causal issues with longitudinal data. *American Sociological Review* 43:383–403.

Wheeler, C. E. 1914. *The case for homeopathy.* London: The British Homeopathic Association.

When doctors went out on strike. 1975. *U.S. News and World Report,* 26 May, p. 34.

White, Jack E. 1977. Cancer differences in the black and caucasian population. *Phylon* 38 297–314.

White, Marjorie, and Skipper, James K. 1971. The chiropractic physician: A study of career contingencies. *Journal of Health and Social Behavior* 12:300–306.

Whyte, William H. 1956. *The organization man.* New York: Simon and Schuster.

Wilber, Joseph A. 1977. Hypertension: An editorial. *Phylon* 38:352–355.

Wild, Patricia. 1978. Social origin and ideology of chiropractors: An empirical study of the socialization of the chiropractic student. *Sociological Symposium* No. 22: 33–54.

Wilensky, H. L. 1962. Dynamics of professionalism: The case of hospital administration. *Hospital Administration* 7:6–24.

Wilk, Chester A. 1973. *Chiropractic speaks out: A reply to medical propaganda, bigotry, and ignorance.* Park Ridge, Ill.: Wilk Publishing Co.

Williams, K. J. 1978. "Williams report" (Report of study on the proposed position of the director of medical affairs and some related problems, prepared for the board of trustees of Sutter Community Hospitals). Napa, Calif.: K. J. Williams & Associates, Inc.

Williams, Robin M. 1960. *American Society.* New York: Knopf.

Williams, Roger. 1977. Are they closing the mental hospitals too soon? *Psychology Today* 10:124–129.

Willox, G. L. 1966. Contemporary Chinese health, medical practice, and philosophy. In *Contemporary China,* ed. Ruth Adams. New York: Random House, Pantheon Books.

Wilson, Bryan R. 1961. *Sects and society.* Berkeley and Los Angeles: University of California Press.

Wilson, Robert N. 1970. *The sociology of health.* New York: Random House.

Wilson, Ronald W., and White, Elijah L. 1977. Changes in morbidity, disability, and utilization differentials between the poor and the nonpoor: Data from the health interview survey: 1964 and 1974. *Medical Care* 15:636–646.

Wilson, William J. 1973. *Power, racism, and privilege.* New York: Macmillan.

Wing, J. K. 1967. The modern management of schizophrenia. In *New aspects of the mental health services,* ed. Hugh Freeman and James Frandale. New York: Pergamon.

Winick, C. 1961. Diffusion of innovation among physicians in a large city. *Sociometry* 24:384–396.

Winkelstein, W., et al. 1975. Epidemiologic studies of coronary heart disease and stroke in Japenese men living in Japan, Hawaii, and California: Blood pressure distributions. *American Journal of Epidemiology* 102:502–513.

Winokur, G., et al. 1960. Stress as an inhibitor of pathological processes. *Psychiatric Research Report* 12:73–80.

Winslow, Charles-Edward Amory. 1967. *The conquest of epidemic disease.* New York and London: Hafner Publishing Co.

Wise, Harold B., et al. 1968. The family health worker. *American Journal of Public Health* 58:1828–1838.

Wittemann, J. K., and Currier, G. Frans. 1976. Motives to enter the dental profession: Students, practitioners, faculty. *Journal of Dental Education* 40:265–268.

Wittemann, J. K., et al. 1975. Dentistry, medicine, pharmacy: Treatment interests, ability and socioeconomic index of three stable career groups. *Journal of Dental Research* 54:548–552.

Wolf, S. 1959. The pharmacy of placebos. *Pharmacology Review* 11:689–704.

Wolff, H. G. 1953. *Stress and disease.* Springfield, Ill.: Charles C Thomas.

Wolff, K. H., ed. 1950. *The sociology of Georg Simmel.* New York: Free Press.

Wolinsky, Frederick D. 1978. Assessing the effects of predisposing, enabling, and illness-morbidity characteristics on health service utilization. *Journal of Health and Social Behavior* 19:384–396.

Wolman, Dianne Miller. 1976. Quality control and the community physician in England: An American perspective. *International Journal of Health Service* 6:79–102.

Woodley, Rose F., and Kane, Robert L. 1977. *Approaches to the validation of manipulation therapy.* Springfield, Ill.: Charles C Thomas.

Woodward, J. 1965. *Industrial organization: Theory and practice.* London: Oxford University Press.

Wootton, A. C. 1971. *Chronicles of pharmacy.* Boston: Milford House.

World Health Organization. 1946. *Constitution of WHO, Preamble.* Geneva.

____. 1976, 1977, 1978. *World health statistics, Annual, 1973–1976.* Geneva.

Wren, G. R. 1971. Some characteristics of freshmen students in baccalaureate, diploma, and associate degree programs. *Nursing Research* 20:167–172.

Wrestler, Frank A. 1974. The development of professional identification among chiropractic students. Unpublished doctoral dissertation, University of Oregon.

Wright, Edith. 1976. Registered nurses' opinions on an extended role concept. *Nursing Research* 25:112–114.

Wrigley, E. A. 1969. *Population and history.* London: Weidenfeld & Nicolson.

Wylie, Charles M. 1970. The definition and measurement of health and disease. *Public Health Reports* 85:100–104.

Wynder, Ernest, et al. 1954. Study of environmental factors and carcinoma of the cervix. *American Journal of Obstetrics and Gynecology* 72:1016–1052.

Wynder, E. L., et al. 1977. Diet and cancer of the gastrointestinal tract. *Advances in Internal Medicine* 22:397–419.

Wynne, Lyman C., et al. 1958. Pseudo-mutuality in the family relations of schizophrenics. *Psychiatry* 21:205–220.

Yabura, Lloyd. 1977. Health care outcomes in the black community. *Phylon* 38:194–202.

Yallow, Marion, R., et al. 1955. The psychological meaning of mental illness in the family. *Journal of Social Issues* 11:12–24.

Yankauer, Alfred, et al. 1970. Pediatric practice in the United States. *Pediatrics* 45: 521–554.

Yette, Samuel. 1971. *The choice: The issue of black survival in America.* New York: G. P. Putnam's Sons.

Young, James H. 1961. *The toadstool millionnaires.* Princeton: Princeton University Press.

———. 1967. *The medical messiahs: A social history of health quackery in twentieth century America.* Princeton: Princeton University Press.

Young, Wesley O., and Cohen, Lois K. 1979. The nature and organization of dental practice. *Handbook of medical sociology,* 3rd ed., ed. Howard E. Freeman, Sol Levine, and Leo G. Reeder. Englewood Cliffs, N.J.: Prentice-Hall.

Young, Wesley O., and Smith, Lawrence. 1972. The nature and organization of dental practice. *Handbook of medical sociology,* 2nd ed., ed. Howard E. Freeman, Sol Levine, and Leo G. Reeder. Englewood Cliffs, N.J.: Prentice-Hall.

Zahn, Stella. 1968. Neighborhood medical care demonstration training program. *Milbank Memorial Fund Quarterly* 46:309–321.

Zald, M. N. 1969. The power and functions of boards of trustees: A theoretical synthesis. *American Journal of Sociology* 75:97–111.

Zalokar, J. 1960. Marital status and major causes of death in women. *Journal of Chronic Diseases* 11:50–60.

Zborowski, M. 1952. Cultural components in responses to pain. *Journal of Social Issues* 8:16–30.

Zelditch, M., and Hopkins, J. K. 1961. Laboratory experiments with organization. In *Complex organizations,* ed. Amitai Etzioni. New York: Holt, Rinehart & Winston.

Zola, Irving K. 1966. Culture and symptoms—An analysis of patients' presenting complaints. *American Sociological Review* 31:615–630.

———. 1975. In the name of health and illness: On some sociopolitical consequences of medical influences. *Social Science and Medicine* 9:83–87.

Zola, Irving K., and Miller, S. J. 1971. The erosion of medicine from within. In *The professions and their prospects,* ed. Eliot Freidson. Beverly Hills, Calif.: Sage.

Zwick, Daniel I. 1972. Some accomplishments and findings of neighborhood health centers. *Milbank Memorial Fund Quarterly* 50:387–420.

INDEXES

INDEX OF NAMES

INDEX OF SUBJECTS